ATHEROSCLEROSIS
Metabolic, Morphologic, and Clinical Aspects

ADVANCES IN EXPERIMENTAL MEDICINE AND BIOLOGY

Recent Volumes in this Series

Volume 82
ATHEROSCLEROSIS: Metabolic, Morphologic, and Clinical Aspects
Edited by George W. Manning and M. Daria Haust • 1977

Volume 83
FUNCTION AND BIOSYNTHESIS OF LIPIDS
Edited by Nicolás G. Bazán, Rodolfo R. Brenner, and Norma M. Giusto • 1977

Volume 84
MEMBRANE TOXICITY
Edited by Morton W. Miller and Adil E. Shamoo • 1977

Volume 85A
ALCOHOL INTOXICATION AND WITHDRAWAL – IIIa: Biological Aspects of Ethanol
Edited by Milton M. Gross • 1977

Volume 85B
ALCOHOL INTOXICATION AND WITHDRAWAL – IIIb: Studies in Alcohol Dependence
Edited by Milton M. Gross • 1977

Volume 86A
PROTEIN CROSSLINKING: Biochemical and Molecular Aspects
Edited by Mendel Friedman • 1977

Volume 86B
PROTEIN CROSSLINKING: Nutritional and Medical Consequences
Edited by Mendel Friedman • 1977

Volume 87
HYPOTHALAMIC PEPTIDE HORMONES AND PITUITARY REGULATION
Edited by John C. Porter • 1977

Volume 88
AVIAN IMMUNOLOGY
Edited by Albert A. Benedict • 1977

Volume 89
MUCUS IN HEALTH AND DISEASE
Edited by Max Elstein and Dennis V. Parke • 1977

Volume 90
PARKINSON'S DISEASE: Neurophysiological, Clinical, and Related Aspects
Edited by Fathy S. Messiha and Alexander D. Kenny • 1977

ATHEROSCLEROSIS

Metabolic, Morphologic, and Clinical Aspects

Edited by

George W. Manning
and M. Daria Haust

University of Western Ontario
London, Ontario, Canada

PLENUM PRESS • NEW YORK AND LONDON

Library of Congress Cataloging in Publication Data

International Workshop-Conference on Atherosclerosis, University of Western Ontario, 1975.
Atherosclerosis.

(Advances in experimental medicine and biology; v. 82)
Includes indexes.
1. Arteriosclerosis–Congresses. I. Manning, George William, 1911- II. Haust, Maria Daria. III. University of Western Ontario. IV. Series. [DNLM: 1. Atherosclerosis–Congresses. W1 Ad559 v. 82 / WG550 I623a 1975]
RC692.I56 1975 616.1'36 77-5066
ISBN 978-1-4613-4222-9 ISBN 978-1-4613-4220-5 (eBook)
DOI 10.1007/978-1-4613-4220-5

Proceedings of an International Workshop-Conference on Atherosclerosis held at the University of Western Ontario, London, Ontario, Canada, September 1–3, 1975

Sponsors
Ontario Heart Foundation
Canadian Heart Foundation
University of Western Ontario
European Atherosclerosis Group

Softcover reprint of the hardcover 1st edition 1977
A Division of Plenum Publishing Corporation
227 West 17th Street, New York, N.Y. 10011

DEDICATION

This book is dedicated to the memory of our colleagues and friends who departed since our last large gathering in October, 1973, at the III International Symposium on Atherosclerosis in Berlin. They had been missed by many of those in attendance at the Workshop-Conference at London, Ontario, but in many ways they will always be with us:

1. Mrs. Anna French, Oxford, England, and formerly a member of the Sir William Dunn School of Pathology, a close friend and the wife of our distinguished late colleague, Dr. John French;

2. Dr. John E. Kirk, Washington University, St. Louis, Missouri, a renowned investigator in the field of enzymology of normal and atherosclerotic human arteries, a co-editor of the Series of Monographs on Atherosclerosis (S. Karger, Publisher);

3. Dr. Hugh B. Lofland, Bowman-Gray School of Medicine, Winston-Salem, North Carolina, an outstanding scientist whose animal experimentation contributed much to our understanding of the genetic and biochemical aspect of atherosclerosis;

4. Dr. Barbara Robert, Paris University and "Maitre de Recherche" --CNRS, Paris and Creteil, France, a distinguished scientist who pioneered much of our present day knowledge on several aspects of arterial connective tissues and their reactivity in atherosclerosis; and

5. Dr. Simon Rodbard, City of Hope Medical Center, Duarte, California, a well known and respected investigator who in his life-long career was concerned with the role of biophysical factors in the process of atherosclerosis.

ORGANIZING AND PROGRAMME COMMITTEE

Dr. M. Daria Haust, Chairman

London, Canada

Dr. J.B. Armstrong
Toronto, Canada

Dr. L. Campeau
Montreal, Canada

Dr. K.K. Carroll
London, Canada

Dr. R.W. Gunton
London, Canada

Dr. L. Horlick
Saskatoon, Canada

Dr. J.A. Little
Toronto, Canada

Dr. G.W. Manning
London, Canada

Dr. J.F. Mustard
Hamilton, Canada

Mr. M. Robertson
Toronto, Canada

Dr. C.J. Schwartz
Hamilton, Canada

Dr. B.P. Squires
London, Canada

Dr. Lars A. Carlson
Stockholm, Sweden

Dr. Gotthard Schettler
Heidelberg, Germany

Dr. Günter Schlierf
Heidelberg, Germany

Dr. Gerald Shaper
London, U.K.

Dr. Robert Wissler
Chicago, U.S.A.

LADIES' COMMITTEE

Mrs. R. W. Gunton (Chairman)

Mrs. D. Bocking (Co-Chairman)

Mrs. C. G. Drake (Co-Chairman)

Mrs. H. J. M. Barnett

Mrs. K. K. Carroll

Mrs. J. C. Coles

Mrs. R. A. Goyer

Mrs. R. O. Heimbecker

Mrs. G. W. Manning

Mrs. B. P. Squires

Mrs. A. C. Wallace

Mrs. B. M. Wolfe

ACKNOWLEDGMENTS

The Workshop - Conference was made possible
by the generosity of the following:

AYERST LABORATORIES
(Division of Ayerst,
McKenna & Harrison Ltd.)
Montreal, P.Q., Canada

CANADA PACKERS LTD.
Toronto, Ontario, Canada

CIBA-GEIGY CANADA LTD.
Dorval, P.Q., Canada

CITY OF LONDON
London, Ontario, Canada

GOVERNMENT OF ONTARIO
Toronto, Ontario, Canada

HOECHST PHARMACEUTICALS
(Pharma Division of Canadian
Hoechst Ltd.)
Montreal, P.Q., Canada

HOFFMAN-LaROCHE LTD.
Montreal, P.Q., Canada

LILLY RESEARCH LABORATORIES
(Division of Eli Lilly & Co.)
Indianapolis, Indiana, U.S.A.

LONDON LIFE INSURANCE
COMPANY
London, Ontario, Canada

MERCK FROSST LABORATORIES
Pointe Claire-Dorval, P.Q., Canada

MONARCH FINE FOODS
COMPANY LTD.
(Lever Brothers Ltd.)
Toronto, Ontario, Canada

ONTARIO MILK MARKETING BOARD
Toronto, Ontario, Canada

PFIZER COMPANY LTD.
Montreal, P.Q., Canada

SANDOZ-WANDER INC.
East Hanover, New Jersey, U.S.A.

G.D. SEARLE & COMPANY
OF CANADA LTD.
Oakville, Ontario, Canada

SILVERWOOD DAIRIES
(Division of Silverwood
Industries Ltd.)
London, Ontario, Canada

STANDARD BRANDS CANADA LTD.
Montreal, P.Q., Canada

THE UPJOHN COMPANY
Kalamazoo, Michigan, U.S.A.

PREFACE I

The International Workshop - Conference on Atherosclerosis was held at the University of Western Ontario, London, Ontario, Canada, September 1 - 3, 1975. This book does not represent in a strict sense the entire proceedings of the above Workshop - Conference, but does reflect largely the format and the essential content of the scientific sessions. Thus, each of the three Sections of the book is comprised of the summarized presentations either at the Plenary Sessions (Section I), Proffered Papers (Section II) or Workshops (Section III).

Section I comprises all the presentations of the Plenary Session on September 1 and the first three presentations at the Plenary Session on the last day of the Conference (September 3). The remaining two addresses of the latter Session (Resume of Workshop - Conference and Closing Remarks) follow the Section III at the end of the book. Sections II and III are subdivided into Chapters which correspond to the individual Sessions of Proffered Papers and Workshops, respectively. To facilitate the orientation, particularly for those who attended the Workshop - Conference, a Summary Table of all Sessions of Proffered Papers designated as Chapters in this book, precedes Section II, and a similar Summary Table of Workshops, also designated as Chapters, precedes Section III. The Tables include, in addition, the names of both Chairmen of each Session. The Chairmen whose names do not appear on either Summary Table are those who chaired the two Plenary Sessions, i.e., Dr. S. Wolf, Galveston, U.S.A., and Dr. G. Schettler, Heidelberg, Germany (Plenary Session I) and Dr. J. L. Beaumont, Creteil, France, and Dr. A. Studer, Basel, Switzerland (Plenary Session II).

Only the discussions at Workshop Sessions were recorded at the Conference, and were subsequently transcribed and edited by one or both Chairmen of the appropriate Workshop. This component of the book is not uniform because the format of the submission was left at the discretion of the Chairmen of the individual Workshops. Some Chairmen preferred to summarize the Discussion following each presentation and that of more general nature (at the end of all presentations). Others supplied, whenever possible, a verbatim version. In only two instances the Chairmen of Workshops were unable to provide the Discussion.

The Editors have taken the prerogative of maintaining the tenor of the manuscripts as submitted, and largely only corrections of the typographical and grammatical errors were made.

The Editorial Board was selected in a way to allow to expediate the processing and final editing of the individual Chapters. Thus, almost all members were selected on the "near home basis".

On behalf of both Co-editors sincere thanks are expressed to:

-- all the Chairmen of the Workshop - Conference for receiving from the participants of their respective sessions and pre-editing the manuscripts, and to the Chairmen of the Workshops for transcribing and summarizing the Discussions;

-- the participants in the Workshop - Conference for providing, with a few exceptions, the manuscripts on time and in the format as requested;

-- the members on the Editorial Board for their prompt final reviewing and correcting of the manuscripts prior to publication;

-- the Publishers for the extended support, generosity and continuous cordial co-operation, particularly that of Miss Phyllis Straw and Mr. Stephen Dyer;

-- Mr. Mike Donnelly of the Art Department at the University Hospital, London, for revising the size and printing of the illustrations whenever necessary; and

-- our secretaries, Miss Ruth Watson, Miss Judy Balint and Mrs. Mary-Lou Duffy for their untiring work and invaluable assistance in the preparation of this publication.

G. W. Manning

PREFACE II

During the past decade some Canadian investigators engaged in work on atherosclerosis have been invited to participate in all three International Symposia on that subject (Athens, Greece, 1966; Chicago, U.S.A., 1969; Berlin, Federated German Republic, 1973), and to contribute to numerous other smaller international conferences on similar and related topics. As it was, understandably, the growing desire of the Canadian group to reciprocate the hospitality of so many colleagues throughout the world, an invitation, extended at the Business Meeting of the European Atherosclerosis Group at Berlin's International Symposium in October, 1973, to host a meeting in 1975 in our country, was accepted with pleasure.

The Organizing and Programme Committee was constituted in the late fall of the same year and the first application for support along with a preliminary outline of the proposed Programme was in the hands of the Ontario Heart Foundation for its meeting in the first week of January, 1974. Shortly thereafter copies of the proposal were submitted to other (potential) supporting agencies. Naturally, the originally estimated budget was based on the costs for travel, accommodation and meals as these were operational at the end of 1973. By the time the approval for a nucleus support was granted by late summer and early fall of 1974, the budget rose to almost twice the original estimate; upon the completion of details pertaining to the Programme and local arrangements, all required prior to issuing invitations to potential participants, the budget exceeded well over twice the initially estimated costs. It was therefore essential to indicate in the letter of invitation that the realization of the Conference was contingent upon the self-supporting efforts of as many participants as possible--a step not undertaken lightly by the Committee. The response was remarkable, and we were truly learning by the action and attitude of our colleagues how many friends of Canada there are around the world! Moreover, as the Conference was scheduled for September 1 - 3, i.e., over the Labour Day holiday and this day is jealously guarded as a holy day in the U.S.A., many people doubted whether our American colleagues would be willing to sacrifice it to attend a professional meeting. But they came. Many came by car, travelling great distances and "teaming" up; and some arriving with wives and children. The support of our endeavour was by no means restricted to our colleagues from the U.S.A. but was most generously extended to us by some who came from countries as remote as Japan and Australia. Without the (self-supporting) contributions of all those colleagues, the Conference would not have taken place.

There were several other (than budgetary) "threats" to the Conference, the most serious being our national, extended postal strike just shortly after the written invitations were issued, and communications had to proceed by telephone, telegrams and cables -- thus further impinging upon the budgetary resources. The impending airline strike, just at the time of the scheduled arrival of the participants, was averted, we believe, in part at least owing to the intervention by the good offices of the President of our University, Dr. D.C. Williams.

Not all of our colleagues and friends whom we were hoping to greet here, could be with us. Some, because they departed for ever and this book is, indeed, dedicated to their memory; others, because they had to attend unexpectedly to pressing matters. Of the latter, several donated their energies and support to the Conference nevertheless, and here I wish to mention particularly Dr. William Insull, who was originally scheduled to co-chair one of the Workshops.

There were approximately 450 registrants from twenty two countries at the Workshop-Conference which consisted of two half-day Plenary Sessions (at the beginning and end), sixteen Workshops and fifteen Sessions with (74) Proffered Papers. Half of the afternoon on the second day of the Conference was not scheduled for Scientific Sessions in order to provide for some relaxation prior to embarking upon the bus trip to attend a play ("Saint Joan" by George Bernard Shaw) at the Shakespearean Theatre, Stratford, Ontario.

On behalf of the Organizing and Programme Committee, gratitude is being conveyed to the sponsors of the Conference, i.e., the Ontario Heart Foundation, the Canadian Heart Foundation, the University of Western Ontario (through the generosity of both Dr. D. Carlton Williams, the President, and Dr. Douglas Bocking, Dean of the Faculty of Medicine), and the European Atherosclerosis Group; to the many donors listed separately, whose generosity enabled us to carry on despite the tremendous increases of world travel costs; to all our colleagues and friends who contributed to the scientific aspect of the programme and to those who were generous and understanding in securing the necessary support from other sources; and to the Physical Plant and Food Service Departments of the University of Western Ontario for the excellent facilities, and smooth and competent operation of the many activities often scheduled concurrently. Warm appreciation for hard work, personal sacrifice of time and resources, and excellent results in assuring that the Conference carried an almost personal note of hospitality is expressed to the Ladies' Committee, chaired by Mrs. R.W. Gunton, co-chaired by Mrs. D. Bocking and Mrs. C.G. Drake, and aided by nine other ladies (listed separately). Not only did the ladies organize an interesting programme for the accompanying wives but in addition arranged for the visiting children to be occupied. It is fair to state that the atmosphere of the entire Conference was "induced" by the Ladies' Committee.

It is an almost impossible task to extend my personal appreciation and gratitude to all those, without whose constant and patient help throughout the entire time of preparations for, and at the time of the Workshop - Conference, the efforts would have not succeeded.

I wish to thank all the members of the Organizing and Programme Committee for their devoted work and help in devising the programme, in particular Drs. Carroll, Gunton, Little, Shaper and Wissler; for assisting in obtaining donations, in particular Dr. Schwartz who put into this project much time and energies, and was very successful; for operational aspect of the meetings, in particular Dr. Squires, Chairman of the Local Arrangements Committee who attended to every minute detail and devoted an unlimited amount of his time months prior to, and at every stage of the Conference, both at the level of the scientific and (general) social aspects; and for advising constantly from the overall point of organization of an international meeting, particularly Mr. Murray Robertson of the Ontario Heart Foundation. Sincere appreciation is expressed to Dr. Manning, who graciously accepted the very burdensome responsibility of the Editor of the Proceedings of the Workshop-Conference. Of the Committee members I wish to thank also Dr. Carroll for providing the "steady state" and stabilizing strength throughout the preparations for the Conference. Dr. Carroll was always available for help and advice, be it in scientific or other matters requiring attention.

Personal gratitude is expressed to Miss Evelyn McGloin of the Ontario Heart Foundation (OHF), who, far beyond the call of her duties, selflessly helped in all phases of preparations and execution of the Workshop - Conference, travelled from Toronto to London on several occasions to attend in person to many details, and worked very hard in her quiet, competent and always friendly way. In consultation with Mr. Robertson and aided by a couple of staff members of OHF, she was responsible for the printing and mailing of Programmes, Registration, travel reservations for overseas guests, budget appropriations and other details, too many to be all mentioned.

I wish to thank in a very special way, Mrs. Mary-Lou Duffy, my secretary, for her patience, ceaseless work and as the only person who shared all the concerns that accompany the preparations of a three-day-long scientific endeavour; in helping with the Registration at the Workshop - Conference, Mrs. Duffy was involved from the inception to completion of that Conference.

Finally, I wish to thank all of the numerous people who were helpful, encouraging and understanding, including my colleagues in the department, during the many "taxing" months, particularly those immediately preceding September 1 - 3, 1975.

M. Daria Haust

CONTENTS

Page

ATHEROSCLEROSIS

Metabolic, Morphologic, and Clinical Aspects

(A)

WELCOMING ADDRESS

J. L. A. Colhoun, B.A., M.A., LL.B.
President

Ontario Heart Foundation
Toronto, Canada

Ladies and Gentlemen:

Good morning and a warm welcome to London. We are especially pleased to have so many visitors from abroad at this meeting, and we hope your stay in Canada will be a most pleasant one.

On behalf of the sponsors of this Workshop-Conference I would like, first of all, to express our appreciation to Prof. Daria Haust for her efforts, leadership and expertise in putting together this meeting and, through her, to thank her associates who have participated in the preparation of this three-day programme.

This is truly an international conference with delegates coming from all corners of the world and representing 22 countries. Your programme lists an outstanding group of doctors and scientists as discussion leaders, panelists, and authors of papers. It is indeed a remarkable achievement to gather together such an illustrious group from so many sources. It shows that scientific knowledge and the results of research have no geographical or political barriers or constraints.

I understand that this is the first meeting of the European Atherosclerosis Group in Canada and we welcome you most sincerely.

The Ontario Heart Foundation was established in 1952 to foster research and develop professional and lay education programmes in Ontario on heart disease. Subsequently, the Canadian Heart Foundation was formed with representation from all provinces in Canada.

More recently, those interested in stroke problems have joined the Foundation which seeks to fund research into all diseases related to blood vessels. Since its inception, the Heart Foundation has channeled more than $30 million into research in Canada with about half of that amount coming from Ontario. Over the 5 years ending 1979 we are planning to raise $60 million, of which 77.5% will be directed to research, 6% to professional education, 7% to public education, and 2% to community organization and development.

The funds we have received have allowed our medical colleagues and university teaching hospitals to carry out research over a broad spectrum and have contributed in a significant way to the advances which have been made in the recent past in the diagnosis and treatment (particularly in the field of surgery) of heart and stroke problems. The results of this work have been made known internationally at such meetings as this Workshop.

As research has led to the development of successful techniques to treat valvular and congenital heart defects, our researchers have turned their major attention to the basic causes of atherosclerosis in the hope of making significant contributions to reducing the ravages of cardiovascular disease and stroke. In Canada more than 80,000 persons will die this year from blood vessel diseases, of which heart attacks and strokes will account for more than 65,000. When compared with all other causes of death, this becomes Canada's leading health problem. We are, therefore, glad to have this important conference held here.

Professional education is perhaps the second important objective of the Heart Foundation. As research creates new knowledge, there will arise a great obligation to pass on this knowledge to the medical practitioner so that he can use it as soon as possible in the effective care and treatment of his patients. We believe that this obligation will continue indefinitely and we are delighted that the Foundation can work in concert with you to help us fulfill our obligations in this respect. The publication of the proceedings of this Workshop will provide researchers and practitioners in all parts of the world with an authoritative compilation of the most up-to-date knowledge and thinking on the causes and treatment of atherosclerosis.

It has been a pleasure for the Ontario Heart Foundation to have worked with our co-sponsors, the Canadian Heart Foundation, the University of Western Ontario, and the European Atherosclerosis Group, and I join with them in wishing you well in your deliberations over the next few days.

(B)

INTRODUCTION

M. Daria Haust, M.D.
Department of Pathology, The University of Western Ontario, London, Ontario, Canada

The purpose of this Introduction is to outline briefly the rationale upon which the Programme Committee based its decision regarding the format of the programme for the present International Workshop-Conference.

Prior to proceeding, however, it appears desirable to recall the following:

It has been accepted for over a decade by many investigators that atherosclerosis, with its underlying various forms and stages of arterial lesions, is a complex disease and that any one stage in the disease represents the outcome of an interaction of a multitude of factors (1). It is this feature, indeed, that renders the disease so difficult to "conquer".

The innumerable factors implicated in the etiology and pathogenesis of atherosclerotic lesions have been grouped into those that in some way may relate either to hemodynamics, blood constituents, and/or the artery itself (2). Any factor relating to one of the above three major groups may be involved either in the inception of one of the different forms of the atherosclerotic lesions, in their growth, complications, or in the precipitation of an overt clinical manifestation. Some factors no doubt play a role in the inception of more than one type of lesion and/or may be involved at several levels from the inception to the precipitation of clinical manifestations (3). Of course, information relevant to atherosclerosis is not limited only to that relating to the etiology and pathogenesis (4); other numerous data (5) pertain to prevention and treatment of atherosclerosis, techniques for the study of tissue reactions in vitro, animal experimentation, epidemiology, genetics, the so-called "high risk" factors and others--too many to be mentioned here.

Thus, one of the following two avenues was open to the Committee in considering the programme: either to organize a programme that touched upon all, or at least the major areas of atherosclerosis and would have provided a rather superficial overview of the field or, alternatively, to focus in some depth on a few selected areas only. As is evident from the Programme, the Committee chose the latter avenue. It should be stressed, however, that the areas and topics omitted from the programme were not considered of less importance than those selected. To compensate to a certain degree for the large gaps because of areas omitted, two Plenary Sessions were organized to allow for overviews on such important topics as the place of the aorto-coronary by-pass graft in the treatment of ischemic heart disease; the role of thrombosis in the process of atherosclerosis and myocardial infarction; the effects of drugs on platelets and complications of vascular diseases; the coronary drug project; and the newest developments in the field of plasma lipoproteins. However, other important areas were omitted entirely in order to allow more time for, and study in depth of the subjects selected. It is hoped, indeed, that the next Conference on Atherosclerosis will endeavour to concentrate upon the areas omitted here, such as hemodynamics, genetics, epidemiology, and major risk factors, to name only a few.

Furthermore, the Conference was organized in such a way as to allow for a choice of Workshops to be attended at any given time; for example a clinician concerned largely with the clinical aspect of the disease has a choice on Day I to attend the Workshop on New Therapeutic Approaches to Myocardial Infarction or on Lipid Clinic; a biochemist may choose between "Fate of Lipoproteins", "Regression of Lesions", or "Lipid Clinic"; and a pathologist may be interested in attending the Session on "Regression of Lesions" or on "Myocardial Infarction". Similar multiple choice is available at any time scheduled for the Workshops. With two exceptions the Workshops are interdisciplinary and therefore should provide potentially integrated knowledge on the broad topic of a given Workshop.

Finally, some Workshops were selected to complement the more superficially presented overviews at the Plenary Session. For example, the Workshop on "Endothelium and Permeability" was designed for the study of endothelium as it pertains to permeability alone, thus complementing the presentation at the Plenary Session on the endothelium from a more general point of view.

One of the most important but rather difficult tasks of this Conference was undertaken by Dr. Henry McGill when he kindly agreed (upon "gentle" persuasion) to summarize the Conference in critical terms, and in the following context:

1. what had been learned at the Conference that is truly new?

2. had an agreement been reached on some issues that were controversial, and

3. what are the areas clearly requiring concentrated efforts of enquiry? by what means?

If Dr. McGill, upon his critical analysis, can provide the participants at the Closing Session with at least one concrete answer to the above questions then perhaps each of us would leave this Conference a bit enriched.

REFERENCES

1. Haust, M.D., Injury and repair in the pathogenesis of atherosclerosis. In: Atherosclerosis, pp. 12-20, Jones, R.J.(ed.), Springer-Verlag, Berlin-New York, 1970.

2. Haust, M.D., The morphogenesis and fate of potential and early atherosclerotic lesions in man. Human Pathology 2:1-30,1971.

3. Jones, R.J., Atherosclerosis. Proceedings of the Second International Symposium, Springer-Verlag, New York-Heidelberg-Berlin, 1970.

4. Wissler, R.W., and Geer, J.C., The Pathogenesis of Atherosclerosis, The Williams and Wilkins Co., Baltimore, Md., 1972.

5. Schettler, G., and Weizel, A., Atherosclerosis III, Springer-Verlag, Berlin-New York, 1974.

Section I
Plenary Session

(1)

HIGHLIGHTS OF CURRENT RESEARCH IN ATHEROSCLEROSIS

Dr. G. Schettler

Department of Internal Medicine, School of Medicine

University of Heidelberg, Heidelberg, G.F.R.

During the last 10 years the incidence of coronary heart disease has doubled in West Germany. The incidence of myocardial infarction approximates 250,000 per year. Mortality from myocardial infarction during the period 1952 - 1974 has increased five fold. Even then, the German Federal Republic holds only an intermediate position with regard to the frequency of coronary heart disease.

Finland and United States have the highest death rates from atherosclerotic heart disease. Then follow New Zealand, Scotland, Australia, Canada, England, Israel, while the lowest rates are in Switzerland and Japan. What are the reasons for this? Are there such striking differences between Finland and Switzerland or between Canada and Switzerland? Life conditions in the Federal Republic of Germany and in Switzerland seem to be very similar. It seems to be important to go more into details, to start new field studies and to look for the so-called risk factors. The German Federal Government has just started a field study near Heidelberg. Two communities with 10,000 inhabitants, one more rural and the other more industrial, will be studied by our Infarct-Institut which has now been running for two years.

The object of this study is not only to record the known risk factors but more than this, to look for conditions that can affect the coronary heart diseases and arteriosclerotic complications in other vessel regions. We will attach particular importance to family history and genetic factors and have appointed a large team in order to examine the psychological, psychosocial and socioeconomic stress factors. There are available in the world literature sufficient epidemiological data confirming the significance of risk factors in the atherosclerotic process. Such studies only have value if corresponding well-controlled prevention measures are performed over many years. The work of WISSLER, GEER, ADAMS, THOMAS, DE PALMA, CONNOR and ARMSTRONG supply sufficient evidence for the regression of atherosclerotic lesions in various experimental animals. We should hence seek evidence for the regression of atherosclerosis in man. It is clear that risk factors should be the basis of such an attempt. It is acknowledged that our methods for assessment of the atherosclerotic process are still very incomplete. Neither the invasive nor the noninvasive method are very reliable for recording the clinical manifestations of atherosclerosis, explaining the significance of preclinical findings or to arrive at a prognosis. Although we still have no reliable concept of the pathogenesis of atherosclerosis, as clinicians we cannot wait any longer in the formulation of preventive and therapeutic measures.

Yet the nature of the primary event that initiates atherogenesis continues to elude us. The role of endothelial injury, of blood lipids and lipoproteins, of dietary factors, of muchopolysaccharides etc. continues to receive attention. I am sure we are mistaken if we look for a single initiating factor. I personally favor the lipid infiltration hypothesis. One can produce the disease in experimental animals simply by raising their plasma lipoprotein levels and these experimental lesions are at least partially reversible when lipid and lipoprotein levels are returned to normal. But we must be aware that elevated lipids and lipoproteins represent only one factor in what must be a disease of multifactorial origin. For this reason we have to encourage different disciplines to solve the problem.

We have a long way to go. There are indications that the number of new coronary events is decreasing slightly as a result of preventive measures, but the number of atherosclerotic deaths increases further in most industrial countries. The results of the coronary drug project have given rise to confusion and perplexity, at least in our country. These results should be evaluated very carefully. The laypress has given the study great publicity and interpreted it erroneously. Indeed, like the patients, the government officials responsible were thrown into uncertainty since the side effects of nicotinic acid and clofibrate were brought to the fore and the value of the two substances in prevention and treatment of coronary heart disease was completely ignored. This had the result that hyperlipemic risk patients were extremely disturbed, especially since the value of a prudent diet was completely denied. Absolutely no distinction was made between primary and secondary prevention trials. These differences appear to be highly important both for drug therapy and also for diet. A clarifying statement from those responsible for the coronary drug project appears vitally necessary.

One has to remember that the secondary prevention trials by OLIVER and co-workers in Scotland and by DE WARE and co-workers in England showed positive results. These studies are not totally free of faults (few studies on such a scale can be) and questions have been raised about it by reasonable and responsible critics. This is also the case with the coronary drug project. In these three studies the effect of clofibrate was not well correlated with its lipid-lowering effects. The question has been raised as to whether the protection afforded is actually due to some additional action of clofibrate. As Dr. STEINBERG pointed out some years ago in Chicago it has many mechanisms of action in addition to its effects on lipoprotein metabolism, e.g. there are effects on plasma fibrinogen levels, platelet aggregation, body weight and several other parameters. There might be some other basic primary modes of action which were not yet discovered. They deserve further studies.

Other primary intervention trials should be organized. The elegant cross-over designs used by TURPEINEN, MIETTINEN and co-workers in Helsinki showed that simply changing the nature of the diet lead to the expected lowering of serum cholesterol levels and also to a highly significant reduction of morbidity and mortality from coronary heart disease. This study is not totally free of flaws, but the results seem to be valid, as are the studies by LEREN in Oslo and DAYTON and co-workers in Los Angeles. In my mind it becomes difficult to remain sceptical about the genuine value of low-cholesterol, polyunsaturated fat diet. In all these trials, the lipids and lipoproteins do have a key role. There has been a veritable explosion in the lipoprotein field in the last years. The structure of the plasma lipoproteins has turned out to be much more complex than we believed. There are new results on lipid-protein interactions at a truly molecular level and on lipoprotein secretions and degradation. We are isolating the several enzymes that act on lipoproteins in plasma. The patterns and kinetics of lipoprotein catabolism are important for many cases of hyperlipoproteinemia (HLP) with defects in the removal mechanism. Many patients with elevated lipid levels belong to a genetically determined group. If the disease is monogenetic in many cases and if we can identify the mechanisms involved in lipoprotein removal, we may achieve in the future the ultimate step of identifying specific enzyme defects in certain inherited forms of hyperlipoproteinemia. With respect to the remarkable results of Dr. GOLDSTEIN and Dr. BROWN we hope to complete our knowledge of other forms of primary and secondary hyperlipoproteinemias. As a contribution of our team to these important questions I would like to present the results of Dr. SEIDEL and co-workers, Dr. GRETEN and co-workers, and Dr. HORSCH and co-workers. As you all know, Dr. ZILVERSMIT recently put forward a fascinating theory of atherogenesis according to which not only the beta and pre-beta lipoproteins but also the chylomicrons and their fragments play a role.

In the presence of divalent cations and at physiological salt concentrations heparin and other sulfated polysaccharides cause aggregation of chylomicrons, remnants of chylomicrons and pre-beta lipoproteins, while beta- and alpha-lipoproteins form insoluble complexes with such compounds only at low ionic strength. Heparin also activates lipoprotein lipase. Thus, it is possible that heparin or heparin-like substances act as a bridge which links chylomicrons, pre-beta lipoproteins or remnants and lipoprotein lipase to the vascular endothelium. While adsorbed, the large complexes could be subjected to lipolysis and this lipolytic process at the intimal surface might maintain a very high local concentration of cholesterol-rich lipoproteins and therefore be an important factor in atherogenesis. In this regard, recent studies by BIERMAN and co-workers are relevant; they demonstrated that the uptake of remnant lipoprotein particles by cultured vessel cells was very active, while alpha lipoproteins, for instance, were not taken up by such cells. If remnant particles do indeed possess the postulated association with atherogenesis - a clinical example would by type III HLP - it seems relevant to analyze plasma lipoprotein patterns not only in a fasting plasma but also postprandially with special emphasis on the detection and characterization of such intermediate compounds.

In healthy volunteers we were recently able to identify, isolate and characterize such intermediate particles six hours postprandially from the LDL_1 density class. The particles differ in size, protein-lipid composition and other physicochemical parameters such as precipitation behavior with polyanionic compounds from fasting VLDL, LDL and HDL. They migrate in beta-position on agarose electrophoresis. Using a recently described new technique to visualize lipoproteins by precipitation with polyanionic compounds instead of lipid staining after electrophoresis in agarose gel it is possible to follow the dynamics of these compounds in whole serum. The six-hour-postprandial remnants precipitate with heparin and $MgCl_2$ at physiological salt concentrations of 0.15 M NaCl in contrast to fasting beta- and alpha-lipoproteins which can be precipitated only at lower ionic strength or with dextran sulphate and $CaCl_2$. Further metabolic studies along these lines may yield structurally different intermediate particles in the various forms of hyperlipoproteinemia at different time intervals postprandially and different effects of dietary and drug management. By focusing our attention on the post-prandial plasma we may get new ideas about possible mechanisms of atherogenesis particularly in the large number of patients suffering from atherosclerosis without significant changes of their fasting plasma lipid concentrations.

As you all know, it could be demonstrated that post-heparin plasma lipolytic activity (PHLA) consists of two hydrolytic activities, hepatic triglyceride lipase and lipoprotein lipase, originating respectively from liver and extra-hepatic tissues. These two enzymatic activities could be separated by affinity chromatography on Sepharose with covalently linked heparin and shown to possess different characteristics. LPL requires an apolipoprotein cofactor for full activity and is inhibited when assayed in the presence of protamine sulfate or high salt concentration. H-TGL does not require a cofactor, is not inhibited by protamine sulfate and is maximally active when assayed in solutions containing 0.5 - 1 M NaCl. The separation and partial purification of these two lipases led to the production of specific antibodies which allowed specific measurement of these two enzymes. Applying this new assay system, it could be shown that the hypertriglyceridemia in patients with Type I is entirely due to a lack of lipoprotein lipase, while hepatic lipase was found to be normal. This is also true for at least some patients with Type V lipoprotein pattern. The purification scheme developed by GRETEN, BROWN, EHNHOLM and AUGUSTIN made it possible to study both the molecular properties and the protein and carbohydrate composition of these two key enzymes in lipid metabolism. With the aid of the specific antibodies it should be possible in the near future to localize these enzymes in tissue. This might then help to clarify any possible role of these enzymes in the development of atherosclerosis.

Outlook. It appears important for the future that all medical disciplines cooperate and that, in particular, the psychic and psychosocial factors of coronary heart diseases and disorders of cerebral blood flow are considered. Since atherosclerosis is a systemic disease which begins early in life, preventive measures must be followed throughout life. Genetic factors do not only have a role in the lipid sector and I feel that this requires further work. Particular attention must be given to all cases of coronary heart disease. This applies especially to those cases of sudden unexpected cardiac death in which no single risk factor can be demonstrated anamnestically or catamnestically and where morphological and clinical inflammatory courses are also excluded. Thrombogenesis plays a special role here. The question of when coronary thrombi elicit a heart attack or coronary death is still controversial. It has been proved that coronary thrombosis is the primary cause of myocardial infarction in many cases. There are also many cases of myocardial infarction where the coronary thrombosis has arisen secondarily. It must be asked again and again whether the occluding thrombus can elicit the definitive catastrophe independently of the nature of the primary lesion. In other words, even a thrombus which arises secondarily has clinical consequences. This is extremely important for prophylactic and therapeutic measures. Further investigations should be performed on the role of platelet aggregation and its modification by drugs. The question as to the significance of physical training, the exercise factor in the primary or secondary prevention of coronary heart diseases, always arises. There is no doubt that physical training in appropriate doses has a firm place in the prevention of coronary heart diseases and also of other manifestations of atherosclerosis even if the statistical evidence is not yet sufficient.

A fascinating observation made throughout the world is that the protection of the female sex hormones is being broken through more and more often and that myocardial infarctions in normally menstruating women are becoming more frequent. Cigarette smoking appears to break down the protection; our young female patients with myocardial infarction were almost exclusively heavy cigarette smokers. In my opinion the role of overweight as a single risk factor is still unclear. It should be asked whether there are "low risk" conditions. The combination of underweight, low lipids, non-smoking and physical activity is a favorable profile. However, the role of low blood pressure, particularly in the genesis of the angina pectoris syndrome, must be elucidated further. The angina pectoris syndrome is a chameleon which must be clarified from case to case. In all epidemiological studies of risk constellations we should aim at controlled interventions which should be monitored from case to case by the family doctor, possibly in cooperation with a specialist team. This is very difficult as shown by our investigations in myocardial infarct patients who again smoke more cigarettes year by year after the infarct without affecting the presence or severity of the angina pectoris.

There is no doubt that cooperative studies on an international basis would lead us further. The workshop conference which was so brilliantly prepared by our host Daria Haust illustrates this.

(2)

PLASMA LIPOPROTEINS: RECENT DEVELOPMENTS

Antonio M. Gotto, Jr., M.D., D. Phil and
Richard L. Jackson, Ph.D.

Department of Medicine, Baylor College of Medicine
Houston, Texas, U.S.A.

CLINICAL DEVELOPMENTS

It is less than 50 years since Macheboeuf first isolated and described the plasma lipoproteins (1,2). The reason for the increasing interest in these substances is the evidence associating them to the development of arteriosclerosis (3). Regardless whether or not hyperlipidemia as such is present, the accumulation of lipoprotein-cholesterol in the arterial wall is one of the hallmarks of arteriosclerosis. Hypercholesterolemia is one of the three major risk factors for premature coronary disease (4). The significance of hypertriglyceridemia is less well established. In the past year in the clinical area, we have seen completion of the analysis of the data of the coronary drug project (5). This study showed that lowering triglycerides and the very low density lipoproteins (VLDL) in men who already had a myocardial infarction did not appear to decrease significantly cardiovascular morbidity or mortality. There was some reduction in the incidence of new myocardial infarctions in the subjects treated with nicotinic acid. While an elevation of the low density lipoproteins (LDL) is considered to increase an individual's risk of developing premature coronary disease (3), we still do not know whether or not reduction of the elevation will concomitantly reduce the risk. In the United States, the National Heart and Lung Institute is conducting a nationwide double blind study with cholestyramine to test the hypothesis that reduction of serum cholesterol and LDL will decrease cardiovascular mortality and morbidity. We attribute much of the interest in the diagnosis and management of hyperlipidemia in recent years to three factors: 1) to the known risk of hyperlipidemia in the development of premature arteriosclerosis; 2) to the demonstration that dietary and drug programs of treatment can normalize elevations of plasma lipids in most individuals and 3) to the development and popularization of a simple system of lipoprotein phenotyping that is based largely on the distribution of the plasma lipoproteins (6). There has been a de-emphasis in the last two years in the widespread use of lipoprotein phenotyping including a cautionary note by one of the founders of the classification system. Our own assessment of the current situation is as follows: The basic and most important laboratory measurements to be made are those of the serum or plasma cholesterol and triglyceride. These measurements should not be replaced by lipoprotein electrophoresis or any other procedure. In certain individuals in whom both cholesterol and triglyceride are elevated or the cholesterol value is considered borderline, it may be necessary to measure concentrations of the individual families of plasma lipoproteins in order to establish the phenotype. We have seen a number of individuals in our clinic at The Methodist Hospital in Houston with cholesterol in the range of 260-300 mg% who had elevated levels of HDL and normal levels of LDL. We do not consider this a pathologic condition that requires treatment. Three special problems might be mentioned in connection with lipoprotein phenotyping: 1) the necessity of obtaining some quantitation of LDL in individuals suspected to have type II hyperlipidemia; 2) the requirement of ultracentrifugation to establish the presence of floating β-lipoprotein in type III; and 3) the desirability of measuring postheparin lipolytic activity to distinguish between types I and V. Space does not permit a detailed discussion of the phenotyping of hyperlipidemia (6,7). Suffice it to say that the classification is based largely upon family or families of lipoproteins that are considered to be present in elevated concentrations, thus, the cut-off points and definitions must be somewhat arbitrary. Biochemical markers are actively being sought for the genetic hyperlipidemia, as discussed later.

PHYSIOLOGICAL DEVELOPMENTS

Most of the rest of the presentation will be devoted to recent developments concerning the physiology and chemistry of the lipoproteins and their components, although some aspects of the discussion will touch upon the clinical hyperlipidemias. There are four major families of the plasma lipoproteins: the chylomicrons, which transport the exogenous or dietary triglyceride; the VLDL or pre-β-lipoproteins, which carry the endogenous triglyceride; the LDL or β-lipoproteins, which represent the major transport vehicle for cholesterol; and the high density lipoproteins (HDL) or α-lipoproteins, which some investigators think may protect against arteriosclerosis. High levels of LDL and VLDL have been associated with a high incidence of arteriosclerosis (3).

TABLE I

Human Plasma Lipoproteins

Family	Chylomicrons	VLDL	LDL	HDL
Density Range	<1.006	<1.006	1.019-1.063	1.063-1.210
Major Lipids	Exogenous Triglycerides	Endogenous Triglycerides	Cholesterol Cholesteryl Esters	Phospholipid Cholesteryl Esters
% Protein	2	10	25	50
Major Apoproteins	(Uncertain)	ApoLDL ApoLP-Ser (C-I) ApoLP-Glu (C-II) ApoLP-Ala (C-III) "Arginine rich"	ApoLDL	ApoLP-Gln-I (A-I) ApoLP-Gln-II (A-II)
Minor Apoproteins		ApoLP-Gln-I ApoLP-Gln-II		"Thin Line" (A-III) ApoLP-Ser ApoLP-Glu ApoLP-Ala

Each of these individual families is heterogeneous with respect to both the lipid and the protein or apoprotein components (Table I). There is no universally accepted system of nomenclature for the apoproteins at the present time. Alaupovic has suggested an A,B,C method of classification (8). In this system, the major protein of LDL is called ApoB. There are two major proteins in HDL referred to as ApoA-I and ApoA-II. Each of these contains carboxyl-terminal glutamine. ApoA-I is the predominant component in all HDL species studied thus far. There is a third family, ApoC, which occurs in VLDL and to a lesser extent than HDL. These three contain, respectively, serine, glutamic acid, and alanine as the carboxyl-terminal residues. ApoB or ApoLDL is a major protein constituent in the two atherogenic families, LDL and VLDL. There are other components as well which may be of physiologic importance. The "arginine-rich" protein is as its name implies, rich in arginine (9,10). This protein has been reported to be especially high in concentration in type III hyperlipidemia and in rabbits fed a high cholesterol diet (9,11). It has been suggested that the protein may play a crucial role in cholesterol transport. Another minor apoprotein assigned a trivial name is the "thin-line" protein in HDL (12-14). It may also be found in smaller quantities in VLDL and LDL. One group of investigators has referred to this as ApoD and another group as ApoA-III. One obvious function of the plasma apoproteins is in the solubilization and transport of the plasma lipids, including phospholipid, cholesterol, cholesteryl ester and triglyceride. As knowledge about the apoproteins increases, additional functions have been discovered for the individual components. A few are summarized in Table 2. ApoB in VLDL and LDL may be involved in regulating cholesterol synthesis and its own degradation through an interaction of cells permitting cholesterol uptake into the cell. ApoC-II containing C-terminal glutamic acid is an activator of lipoprotein lipase from adipose tissue (15-17). Brown and Baginsky have presented evidence that ApoC-III is an inhibitor of this enyzme (18). ApoA-I (19,20) and ApoC-I (20) activate lecithin:cholesterol acyltransferase, LCAT. The "thin-line" protein also has been reported to be an activator (21).

The triglyceride-rich lipoproteins, the chylomicrons and VLDL, are probably metabolized by common subcellular pathways. The metabolism of the chylomicrons is summarized in Figure 1. Triglycerides are resynthesized in the intestinal mucosa in the smooth endoplasmic reticulum. ApoB is probably synthesized by the ribosomes of the rough endoplasmic reticulum. Hamilton and Kayden have postulated that ApoB is inserted into a phospholipid-rich plasma membrane fragment to form a phospholipid-ApoB complex (22). This complex would acquire a central core of newly synthesized triglycerides from the smooth endoplasmic reticulum to form a nascent lipoprotein particle which is then released into the plasma space. Redgrave has suggested that the Golgi apparatus

TABLE II

Physiologic Function of Plasma Apolipoproteins

Lipoprotein	Enzyme Regulated
Very Low Density Lp.	
ApoB	HMG-CoA Reductase (?)
ApoC-I	LCAT
ApoC-II	LpLipase (Adipose Tissue)
ApoC-III	
"Arg-Rich"	
Low Density Lp.	
ApoB	HMG-CoA Reductase (?)
High Density Lp.	
ApoA-I	LCAT
ApoA-II	
"Thin-Line"	LCAT (?)

envelopes the fat-containing vesicle of the smooth endoplasmic reticulum and fuses with the plasma membrane at the lacteal cell surface prior to discharge of the chylomicron (23). Newly synthesized intestinal chylomicrons contain ApoB but are devoid of ApoC; when the nascent chylomicrons enter the systemic circulation, a transfer of ApoC, perhaps from HDL, presumably occurs (24). Mahley et al. have proposed that there are two populations of intestinal Golgi apparatus, one involved in chylomicron and the other in VLDL synthesis (25). The hepatic synthesis of VLDL has been extensively studied by Stein and Stein (26) and Hamilton and others (27,28). The lipoprotein particles are thought to be formed in the endoplasmic reticulum, processed in some way in the Golgi apparatus, possibly including attachment of carbohydrate, and transported in vacuoles to the sinusoidal surface of the cell. In abetalipoproteinemia, chylomicrons, VLDL and LDL are all missing from the plasma (29,30).

The chylomicrons and VLDL are both believed to be degraded by the same common mechanism which involves at least two different phases (Fig. 1; 31,32). In phase 1, lipoprotein lipase in peripheral tissues catalyzes the hydrolysis of lipoprotein triglyceride. This enzymic activity is released into plasma from the endothelium of extrahepatic tissues by the administration of heparin. The enzyme has been purified by Bensadoun et al. (33) and

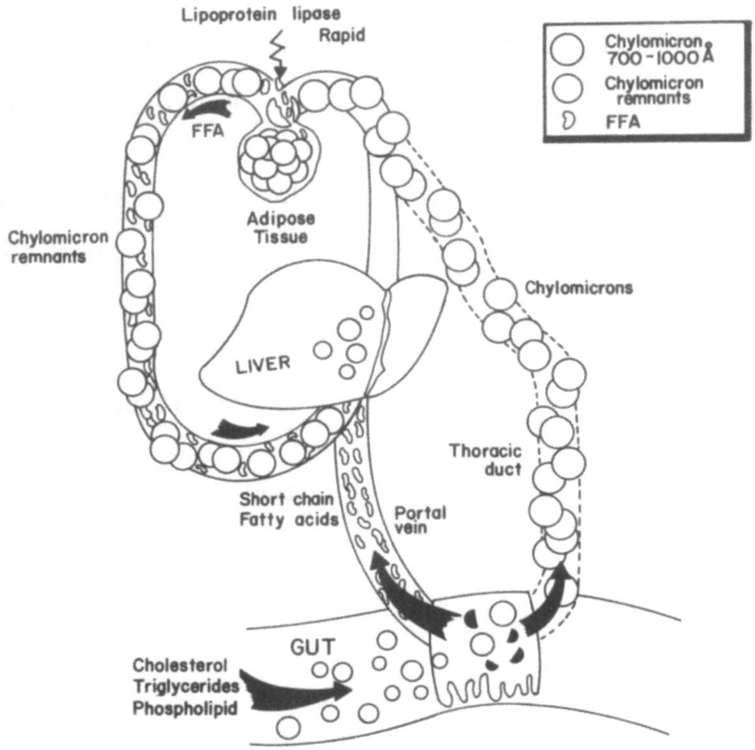

Figure 1

by Greten et al. (34,35). The purified triglyceride lipase requires apoC-II for activation and is inhibited by NaCl or protamine sulfate. Heparin also releases a second triglyceride lipase, this of hepatic origin, which does not require ApoC-II and is not inhibited by NaCl or protamine sulfate (36). The physiologic role of the hepatic triglyceride lipase remains to be clarified.

Removal of the triglyceride in the peripheral tissues produces a triglyceride-poor but cholesterol-enriched particle that has been referred to by Redgrave and others as the "remnant" particle (23). In phase 2, it is believed that the "remnant" particle is taken up and further catabolized by the liver. A similar pathway is envisaged for VLDL (Fig. 2) although the primary source of VLDL is the liver rather than the intestine. The "remnant" particles formed by the partial hydrolysis of VLDL may be either further converted to LDL or catabolized by the liver similar to the chylomicrons. In man, at the present time, VLDL is thought to be the major precursor of LDL (37).

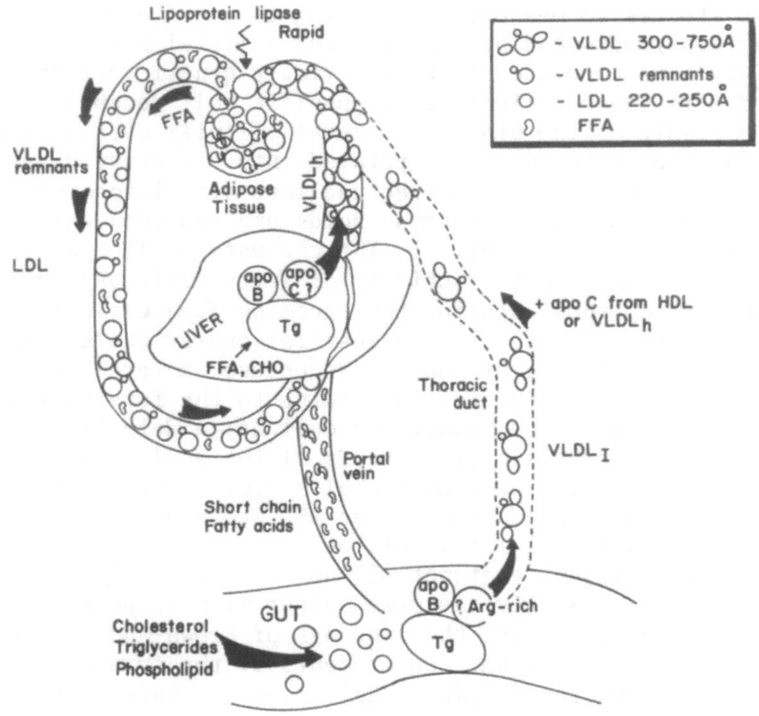

Figure 2

The catabolic fate of LDL is not known. Sniderman _et al._ have presented evidence that LDL catabolism is increased in the hepatectomized pig (38). By implication, this finding suggests that peripheral tissue is the major site of LDL catabolism. Goldstein and Brown have performed an interesting and important series of experiments that may be relevant to LDL catabolism (39,40). They have taken advantage of changes present in the cells of individuals who are homozygous for familial hypercholesterolemia or type II hyperlipidemia. Initially, they showed that cholesterol biosynthesis and HMG-CoA reductase in the fibroblasts of homozygotes were not inhibited to the same extent as normal cells by the addition of whole serum, VLDL or LDL to the culture medium. Fogelman _et al._ observed the phenomenon in the leukocytes of heterozygotes for familial hypercholesterolemia (41). Rothblat (42), Bailey (43), and Williams and Avigan (44) had previously found that cholesterol synthesis in fibroblasts is inversely related to the quantity of cholesterol in the growth medium. Brown and Goldstein carried out studies to measure LDL binding to the fibroblasts of normals, heterozygotes and homozygotes for familial hypercholesterolemia. They have concluded that the primary genetic defect in this disorder is the deficiency of a specific cell receptor for LDL (40). As a result of the binding, several cellular events occur: 1) The surface-bound LDL are incorporated into endocytotic vesicles which eventually become interiorized and fuse with lysosomes. 2) The LDL-protein is degraded to amino acids and peptides which are liberated into the cell medium. 3) The cholesterol liberated from the LDL particle enhances the activity of fatty acyl-CoA:cholesterol acyltransferase, thus, storing the incoming free cholesterol as cholesteryl esters. 4) The free cholesterol and/or cholesteryl esters reduce the activity of HMG-CoA reductase, a rate-limiting enzyme in cholesterol synthesis. According to the interpretation of Brown and Goldstein, the homozygous cell has a defective binding site; as a result, there is oversynthesis of intracellular cholesterol, an increase in intracellular cholesterol esterification and a diminished rate of degradation of the LDL protein, even in the presence of high extracellular levels of LDL. Although is has recently been shown (45,46) that not all homozygotes in Type II fibroblast behave in exactly the same manner with respect to suppression of HMG-CoA activity, the findings of Brown and Goldstein are consistent with the recent measurements of the turnover of [^{125}I] LDL in homozygotes (47,48). Reichl _et al_. have shown that these subjects have a decreased fractional catabolic rate of LDL, a finding shown previously for heterozygotes, and an increased production of LDL (47,48). Alternative interpretations of the findings in familial hypercholesterolemia, other than the deficiency of a specific LDL receptor, have been suggested. Fogelman _et al_. have suggested that the defect lies in the inability of the cell to retain cholesterol (41). The cell compensates for the increased outward flux of cholesterol by oversynthesizing it. While cholesterol is presumed to be the effector of intracellular suppression of HMG-CoA reductase, actually more polar derivatives such as 25-hydroxycholesterol and 7-ketocholesterol are as much as 20 times as effective as cholesterol in suppressing this enzyme and cholesterol biosynthesis (49-51). The significance of the LDL receptor model in regulating cholesterol, LDL and VLDL metabolism in peripheral tissues, the liver and possibly the arterial wall remains to be established. Mechanisms for regulating lipoprotein synthesis and catabolism are complicated and involve different tissues and multiple control points. Recent studies suggest that chylomicrons may play an important role in regulating cholesterol biosynthesis in the liver (52). The specific LDL receptor has thus far been described only in fibroblasts and smooth muscle cells (40).

STRUCTURAL DEVELOPMENTS

The remainder of our discussion will focus on the lipoprotein structure and specifically on the mechanism of lipid-protein binding. For a more detailed treatment, the reader is referred to a recent review (53). While ApoB may be the most important of the apoproteins, less information is available about it owing to its insolubility once it is stripped of its lipid components. Values for the molecular weight of ApoB range from 8,000 to 250,000 with 25,000 being the most common value reported (53). The structure of LDL is also under active investigation. Based on nuclear magnetic resonance spectroscopy (54) or small angle x-ray scattering (55), LDL have been shown to contain protein both in the outer shell of the particle and in the central core. However, in a recent report, Stuhrmann et al. (56) have used neutron scattering techniques to demonstrate that the central core is predominantly occupied by the hydrocarbon chains of the lipid. In the LDL model proposed by Finer et al. (54), the lipid is in the form of a trilayer structure with the neutral lipids packed between the fatty acyl chains of the phospholipid bilayer. Mateu et al. (55) suggest that the lipids are in the form of a bilayer with the neutral lipids packed within the bilayer itself. Further studies are obviously needed to test these different models.

The complete linear amino acid sequences of four of the human plasma apoproteins have been determined. These are ApoC-I, ApoC-III, ApoA-I and ApoA-II. Since these have all been published (57-62), we will not review them here. These are water-soluble proteins and inspection of the primary structure per se does not reveal long sequences of hydrophobic residues. In fact, these molecules contain about the same number of polar and non-polar residues as do the other soluble plasma proteins. Thus, the question arises as to what is the nature of the interaction between these substances and the lipid which they transport in the blood. These apoproteins readily combine with and bind to phospholipids to form stable complexes which can be isolated by density gradient ultracentrifugation and characterized by several different criteria. Very few neutral lipids such as cholesteryl ester and triglyceride are bound. This has led to the conclusion that the primary lipid-protein interaction in the apolipoproteins is between the apoproteins and phospholipid constituents. A variety of methods have been utilized for examination of the apoprotein-phospholipid interaction (Table III). One is an inhibition by the apoprotein of mitochondrial apo-β-hydroxybutyrate dehydrogenase. This apoenzyme has an absolute requirement for phospholipid for reactivation. Thus, an apoprotein or its fragment that binds phosphatidylcholine will competitively inhibit the activation of the enzyme. A second method involves the isolation of the complex, usually by column chromatography or by density gradient

TABLE III

Methods for Studying Protein-Lipid Interactions

1. Inhibition of Apo-β-hydroxybutyrate dehydrogenase
2. Reconstitution and isolation of protein-lipid complexes
3. Changes induced in the CD and fluorescence spectra
4. Formation of stacked discs of phospholipid vesicles

ultracentrifugation. A third approach utilizes the optical methods, circular dichroism and fluorescence, to monitor conformational changes in the protein that occur as a consequence of lipid binding. Since the interaction between apoprotein and phospholipid leads to structural changes in the phospholipid vesicles, a fourth method is to monitor these changes by electron microscopy. Details of the methodology are beyond the scope of this presentation.

When an apoprotein is reconstituted with phosphatidylcholine and with cholesteryl ester, there is a significant increase in the α-helical content as judged by circular dichroism. When phosphatidylcholine is combined with the apoprotein, the change is usually less than when neutral lipids are included. The binding of apoprotein to the phospholipid requires that the fatty acyl chains of the lipid be in the liquid crystalline state (63). There is a remarkable increase in the helicity of ApoC-III when this apoprotein and phospholipid are reconstituted at or near the transition temperature of the phospholipid. Once a complex is formed, lowering the temperature does not reversibly dissociate the complex. We conclude from such observations that binding of the apoprotein to phospholipid occurs maximally at or above the transition temperature at which the phospholipid is transformed into the liquid crystalline state (63).

Other studies have shown that specific regions of the apoprotein molecule appeared to interact preferentially with the phospholipid. For example, the carboxyl-terminal cyanogen bromide fragment of ApoA-II binds phospholipid while the amino-terminal fragment does not (64). The disulfide bond does not appear to be important for phospholipid binding by this apoprotein (65).

ApoC-I or ApoLP-serine contains 57 residues (Fig. 3; 57,58). The longer amino-terminal cyanogen bromide fragment binds phospholipid while the carboxyl-terminal fragment shows only minimal binding activity (66). From three-dimensional models of this apoprotein, there are three regions which may be seen to contain unique structural features (Fig. 4). These regions are

NH_2-Thr-Pro-Asp-Val-Ser-Ser | Ala-Leu-Asp-Lys-Leu-Lys-Glu-Phe | Gly-Asn-Thr-
5 10 15

| Leu-Glu-Asp-Lys-Ala-Arg-Glu-Leu-Ile-Ser-Arg-Ile - | Lys-Gln-Ser-
20 25 30

| -Glu-Leu-Ser-Ala-Lys-Met-Arg-Glu-Trp-Phe-Ser-Glu-Thr-Phe-Gln-Lys-Val-Lys-Glu-Lys-Leu- |
35 40 45 50

Lys-Ile-Asp-Ser-COOH
55

Figure 3. Amino acid sequence of ApoC-I as described by Jackson et al. (57) and Shulman et al. (58).

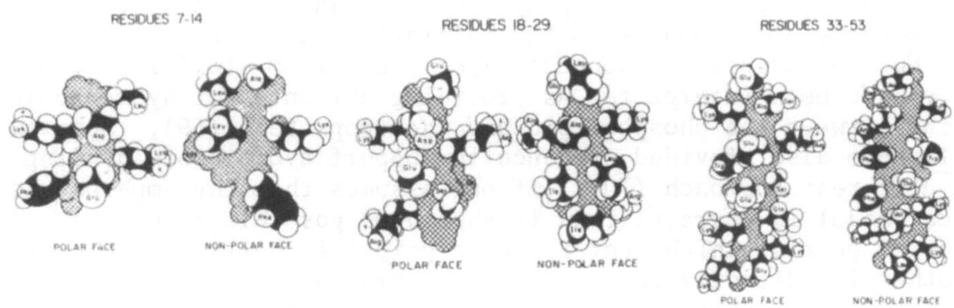

Figure 4. Amphipathic helices of ApoC-I (see text and reference 66 for details).

referred to as amphipathic helices and are believed to represent the phospholipid-binding sites within the apoprotein (66,67). Similar regions occur in all of the apoproteins for which the complete sequence is known. The amphipathic helix contains two faces, a polar and a non-polar one. On the polar face are arranged oppositely charged pairs of amino acids in relatively close topographical arrangement. The distribution of the charged residues along the polar face is such that the negatively charged or acidic aspartic and glutamic acid residues are located in a narrow longitudinal strip in the center of the face while positively charged basic lysine and arginine residues are located in a narrow longitudinal strip to the periphery along the interfacial edge between the polar and non-polar faces. These features are illustrated in Figure 4. Eighteen such amphipathic residues occur in the four apoproteins for which the sequences are known. How can the amphipathic structures account for phospholipid binding in the native HDL molecules? The amphipathic helical regions are envisaged as associating with hydrated phospholipid by half burying at the interface between the hydrocarbon chains and the polar head groups of the phospholipid (Fig. 5). Note that in this model the α-helix lies perpendicular to the axis of the fatty acyl chains of the phospholipid. The main driving force for binding in this model would be the hydrophobic interaction between the non-polar face of the amphipathic helix and the (CH_2) groups of the fatty acyl chains of the phospholipid. The role of the oppositely charged pairs of amino acids are unknown. Nuclear magnetic resonance spectroscopy studies (68,69) have been interpreted as excluding any significant electrostatic interaction between the apoprotein and the phospholipid. If this is, indeed, the case, then perhaps the charged residues play some role in the synthesis of the lipoprotein or perhaps in the initiation of phospholipid binding. Nuclear magnetic resonance experiments from Stoffel's laboratory have been interpreted as providing evidence for hydrophobic binding between the phospholipid and the apoprotein (69). Sparrow et al. have also provided evidence to support hydrophobic binding by a different approach (70). If one assumes that the amphipathic helical model is correct, then it should be possible to devise a synthetic peptide which contains an amphipathic helix but which is not otherwise directly related to any known sequence. Sparrow et al. (70) have synthesized model peptides containing the amphipathic structures described by Segrest et al. (67). Peptide I (Table IV) contains 20 residues and has a hydrophobicity index calculated at 829. Peptide II has 16 residues and a hydrophobicity index of 791. Peptide III has been substituted in residues 7 and 8 by Tyr-Trp for Ala-Ala. Its hydrophobicity index is 1031. While peptides I and II did not bind phospholipid, peptide III did bind (70). Thus, it was possible to convert a non-binding peptide to one that was able to interact with and bind phospholipid though a 2-residue substitution. Peptide III showed the changes in

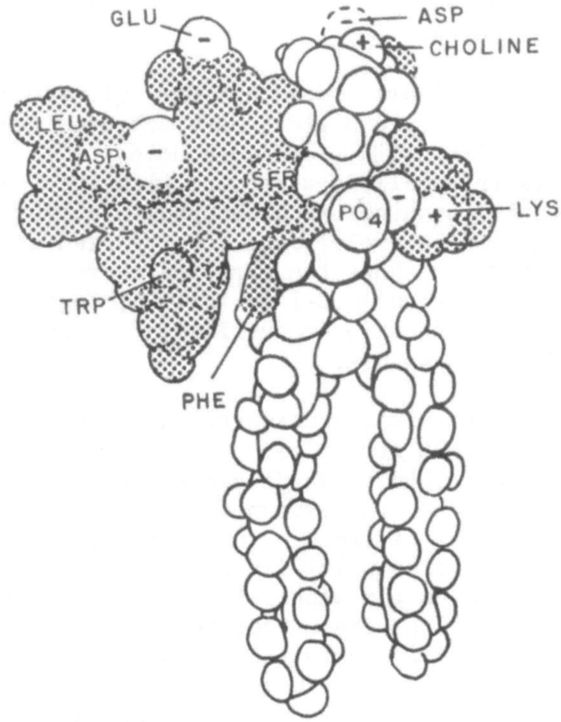

Figure 5. Molecular association of apoprotein and phospholipid.

TABLE IV

Ala-Ser-Leu-Lys-Asp-Ser-Leu-Ser-Asp-Lys-Trp-Lys-Asp-Ser-Leu-Ser-Asp-Lys-Leu-Ser

I

Val-Ser-Ser-Leu-Lys-Asp-Ala-Ala-Ser-Ser-Leu-Lys-Asp-Ser-Phe-Ser

II

Val-Ser-Ser-Leu-Lys-Asp-Tyr-Trp-Ser-Ser-Leu-Lys-Asp-Ser-Phe-Ser

III

physical properties shown by the naturally-occurring apoproteins upon phospholipid binding.

We are pleased to report today that our colleagues in Houston, Drs. James Sparrow and Gerald Sigler, have achieved the complete synthesis of ApoC-I with solid-state methodology (71). The amino acid composition is in excellent agreement with the theoretical. The synthetic material combines with phospholipid, forming a stable complex that can be isolated by density gradient ultracentrifugation. The complex shows the expected increase in α-helical content. Finally, synthetic ApoC-I exhibits biological activity. LCAT activation by the naturally-occurring and synthetic ApoC-I are virtually indistinguishable.

Based largely on physical considerations, a number of models have been proposed for HDL structure. The model of Assmann and Brewer (72) may be described as an "ice-berg" model and is similar to what is thought to occur in membranes. The protein subunits are partially buried in a sea of lipid. In the model of Stoffel et al. (69), the apoprotein is also partially buried in the lipid matrix of the particle. Based on the amphipathic helix, we have suggested a model in which the helical regions of the apoprotein are localized to an outer layer of approximately 14 Å in thickness (73) (Fig. 5). The phospholipid polar head groups and the apoprotein would occupy this region. This model is in good agreement with the measurements obtained from several laboratories by low angle x-ray scattering experiments. Again, the orientation of the phospholipid fatty acyl chains are at right angles to the direction of a helix of the protein. This model can account for the primary interaction in the lipoprotein being the one between the apoprotein and phospholipid. The thickness of an α-helix and the length of the polar head group meet the dimensional requirements to place these structures in an outer shell which would correspond to the high electron dense region observed by x-ray scattering. The fatty acyl groups and the neutral lipids would be localized to the center of the particle. Whether or not any of these models or some other model yet to be postulated will eventually turn out to be correct, one must await further experimentation. The amphipathic helix as well as the other models suggested should be considered as working hypotheses in the current state at the present time.

In conclusion, we have tried to bring together the newest developments in the lipoprotein field. It is not an easy task to achieve both a comprehensive and a comprehensible synthesis of this material. We think that you will conclude with us that information concerning the physiology and the structure of these particles is evolving rapidly and is considerably outstripping the knowledge concerning the diagnosis and management of hyperlipidemia and its relationship to arteriosclerosis.

Acknowledgements. Work from the authors' laboratory described in this review was supported in part by Health, Education and Welfare Grants HL-14194, HL-05435/34 and HL-16512-01. The authors wish to thank Ms. Debbie Mason for assistance in the preparation of the manuscript and to acknowledge our Houston colleagues, Drs. Joel Morrisett, Henry Pownall, James Sparrow, Gerald Sigler and Louis Smith, for their invaluable counsel and discussions. R.L.J. is an Established Investigator of the American Heart Association.

REFERENCES

1. Macheboeuf, M. (1929) Bull. Soc. Chim. Biol. 11:268-293.

2. Machebouef, M. (1929) Bull. Soc. Chim. Biol. 11:485-503.

3. Gofman, J. W., Glazier, F., Tamplin, A., Strisower, B., and De Lalla, O. (1954) Physiol. Rev. 34:589-607.

4. Kannel, B. W., Costelli, W. P., Gordon, T., and McNamara, P. M. (1971) Ann. Int. Med. 74:1.

5. The Coronary Drug Project Research Group. (1975) JAMA 231:360.

6. Beaumont, J. L., Carlson, L. A., Cooper, G. R., Feifer, Z., Fredrickson, D. S., and Strasser, T. (1970) World Health Org. Bull. 43:891.

7. Lees, R. S., Wilson, D. E., Schoenfeld, G., and Fleet, S. (1973) In: Progress in Medical Genetics, Vol. 9. Ed. by A. G. Steinberg and A. G. Bearn, Grunerstratton Publishing, p. 237.

8. Alaupovic, P. (1971) Atherosclerosis 13:141-146.

9. Shore, V. G. and Shore, B. (1974) Biochemistry 13: 1579-1585.

10. Shelburne, F. A., and Quarfordt, S. H. (1974) J. Biol. Chem. 249:1428-1433.

11. Havel, R. J., and Kane, J. P. (1973) Proc. Nat. Acad. Sci. USA 70:2015-2019.

12. Alaupovic, P., Lee, D. M., and McConathy, W. J. (1972) Biochim. Biophys. Acta 260:689-707.

13. McConathy, W. J., and Alaupovic, P. (1973) FEBS Letters 37: 178-182.

14. Kostner, G. M. (1974) Biochim. Biophys. Acta 336:383-395.

15. Bier, D. M., and Havel, R. J. (1970) J. Lipid Res. 11:565-570.

16. Havel, R. J., Fielding, C. J., Olivercrona, T., Shore, V. G., Fielding, P. E., and Egelrud, T. (1973) Biochemistry 12:1828-1833.

17. LaRosa, J. C., Levy, R. I., Herbert, R., Lux, S. E., and Fredrickson, D. S. (1970) Biochem. Biophys. Res. Commun. 41: 57-62.

18. Brown, W. V., and Baginsky, M. L. (1972) Biochem. Biophys. Res. Commun. 46:375-381.

19. Fielding, C. J., Shore, V. G., and Fielding, P. E. (1972) Biochem. Biophys. Res. Commun. 46:1493-1498.

20. Soutar, A., Garner, C., Baker, H. N., Sparrow, J. T., Jackson, R. L., Gotto, A. M., and Smith, L. C. (1975) Biochemistry 14:3057-3064.

21. Kostner, G. (1974) Scand. J. Clin. Lab. Invest. 33, Suppl. 137:19-21.

22. Hamilton, R. L., and Kayden, H. J. (1974) In: The Liver: Normal and Abnormal Functions (Part A) Vol. 5 In The Biochemistry of Disease, Chap. 15. Marcel Dekker, N. Y., pp. 532-372.

23. Redgrave, T. G. (1971) Aust. J. Exp. Biol. Med. Sci. 49: 209-224.

24. Havel, R. J., Kane, J. P., and Kashyap, M. L. (1973) J. Clin. Invest. 52:32-38.

25. Mahley, R. W., Bennett, B. D., Morré, D. J., Gray, M. E., Thistlethwaite, W., and Lequire, V. S. (1971) Lab. Invest. 25:435-444.

26. Stein, O., and Stein, Y. (1967) J. Cell Biol. 33:319-339.

27. Hamilton, R. L. (1972) Advan. Exp. Med. Biol. 26:7-24.

28. Hamilton, R. L., Regen, D. M., Gray, M. E., and Lequire, V. S. (1967) Lab. Invest. 16:305-319.

29. Gotto, A. M., Levy, R. I., John, K., and Fredrickson, D. S. (1971) N. Engl. J. Med. 284:813-818.

30. Scanu, A. M., Aggerbeck, L. P., Kruski, Lim, C. T., and Kayden, H. J. (1974) J. Clin. Invest. 53:440-453.

31. Scow, R. O., Blanchette-Mackie, E. J., Hamosh, M., and Evans, A. J. (1973) Die Lipoproteine des Blutes. Darmstadt, p. 100-114.

32. Simmons, W. J. (1972) In: Blood Lipids and Lipoproteins: Quantitation, Composition, and Metabolism. Ed. by G. J. Nelson, Wiley-Interscience, New York, pp. 705-773.

33. Bensadoun, A., Ehnholm, C., Steinberg, D., and Brown, W. V. (1974) J. Biol. Chem. 249:2220-2227.

34. Greten, H., and Walter, B. (1973) FEBS Letters 35:36-40.

35. Greten, H., Walter, B., and Brown, W. V. (1972) FEBS Letters 27:306-310.

36. Greten, H., Sniderman, A. D., Chandler, J. G., Steinberg, D., and Brown, W. V. (1974) FEBS Letters 42:157-160.

37. Eisenberg, S., and Levy, R. I. Advan. Lipid Res. (In press).

38. Sniderman, A. D., Carew, T. E., Chandler, J. G., and Steinberg, D. (1974) Science 183:526-528.

39. Goldstein, J. L., and Brown, M. S. (1973) Proc. Nat. Acad. Sci. USA 70:2804-2808.

40. Goldstein, J. L., and Brown, M. S. (1975) Amer. J. Med. 58: 14-150.

41. Fogelman, A. M., Edmond, J., Polito, A., and Popjak, G. (1973) J. Biol. Chem. 248:6928-6929.

42. Rothblat, G. J. (1969) J. Cell. Physiol. 74:163-170.

43. Bailey, J. M. (1966) Biochim. Biophys. Acta 125:226-236.

44. Williams, C. D., and Avigan, J. (1972) Biochim. Biophys. Acta 260:413-423.

45. Breslow, J. L., Spaulding, D. R., Lux, S. E., Levy, R. I., and Lees, R. S. New Engl. J. Med. (In press).

46. Avigan, J., Bhathena, S. J., and Schreiner, M. E. (1975) J. Lipid Res. 16:151-154.

47. Reichl, D. Simons, L. A., and Myant, N. B. (1974) Clin. Sci. Mol. Med. 47:635-638.

48. Simons, L. A., Reichl, D., Myant, N. B., and Mancini, M. (1975) Atherosclerosis 21:283-298.

49. Chen, H. W., Kandutsch, A. A., and Waymouth, C. (1974) Nature 251:419-421.

50. Kandutsch, A. A., and Chen, H. W. (1973) J. Biol. Chem. 248: 8408-8417.

51. Kandutsch, A. A., and Chen, H. W. (1974) J. Biol. Chem. 249: 6057-6061.

52. Nervi, F. O., Weis, H. J., and Dietschy, J. M. (1975) J. Biol. Chem. 250:4148-4151.

53. Morrisett, J. D., Jackson, R. L., and Gotto, A. M. (1975) Ann. Rev. Biochem. 44:183-207.

54. Finer, E. G., Henry, R., Leslie, R. B., and Robertson, R. N. (1975) Biochim. Biophys. Acta 380:320-337.

55. Mateu, L., Tardieu, A., Luzzati, V., Aggerbeck, I., and Scanu, A. M. (1972) J. Mol. Biol. 70:105-116.

56. Stuhrmann, H. B., Tardieu, A., Mateu, L., Sardet, C., Luzzati, V., Aggerbeck, L., and Scanu, A. M. (1975) Proc. Nat. Acad. Sci. USA 72:2270-2273.

57. Jackson, R. L., Sparrow, J. T., Baker, H. N., Morrisett, J. D., Taunton, O. D., and Gotto, A. M. (1974) J. Biol. Chem. 249: 5308-5313.

58. Shulman, R. S., Herbert, P. N., Wehrly, K., and Fredrickson, D. S. (1975) J. Biol. Chem. 250:182-190.

59. Brewer, H. B., Shulman, R., Herbert, P., Ronan, R., and Wehrly, K. (1974) J. Biol. Chem. 249:4975-4984.

60. Shulman, R. S., Herbert, P. N., Fredrickson, D. S., Wehrly, K., and Brewer, H. B. (1974) J. Biol. Chem. 249:4969-4974.

61. Baker, H. N., Delahunty, T., Gotto, A. M., and Jackson, R. L. (1974) Proc. Nat. Acad. Sci. USA 71:3631-3634.

62. Brewer, H. B., Lux S. E., Ronan, R., and John, K. M. (1972) Proc. Nat. Acad. Sci. USA 69:1304-1308.

63. Pownall, H. J., Morrisett, J. T., Sparrow, J. T., and Gotto, A. M. (1974) Biochem. Biophys. Res. Commun. 60:779-786.

64. Jackson, R. L., Gotto, A. M., Lux, S. E., John, K. M., and Fleischer, S. (1973) J. Biol. Chem. 248:8449-8456.

65. Jackson, R. L., Morrisett, J. D., Pownall, H. J., and Gotto, A. M. (1973) J. Biol. Chem. 248:5218-5224.

66. Jackson, R. L., Morrisett, J. D., Sparrow, J. T., Segrest, J. P., Pownall, H. J., Smith, L. C., Hoff, H. F., and Gotto, A. M. (1974) J. Biol. Chem. 249:5314-5320.

67. Segrest, J. P., Jackson, R. L., Morrisett, J. D., and Gotto, A. M. (1974) FEBS Letters 38:247-253.

68. Glonek, T., Henderson, T. O., Kruski, A. W., and Scanu, A. M. (1974) Biochim. Biophys. Acta 348:155-161.

69. Stoffel, W., Zierenberg, O., Tunggal, B., and Schreiber, E. (1974) Proc. Nat. Acad. Sci. USA 71:3696-3700.

70. Sparrow, J. T., Morrisett, J. D., Pownall, H. J., Jackson, R. L., and Gotto, A. M. Proceedings of the 4th American Peptide Symposium (In press).

71. Sigler, G. J., Soutar, A. K., Smith, L. C., Gotto, A. M., and Sparrow, J. T. (Submitted to Proc. Nat. Acad. Sci. USA).

72. Assmann, G., and Brewer, H. B. (1974) Proc. Nat. Acad. Sci. USA 71:1534-1538.

73. Jackson, R. L., Morrisett, J. D., Gotto, A. M., and Segrest, J. P. (1975) Mol. Cell. Biochem. 6:43-50.

(3)

ARTERIAL ENDOTHELIUM AND ITS POTENTIALS

M. Daria Haust, M.D.

Department of Pathology
The University of Western Ontario
London, Ontario, Canada

The general arterial endothelial function is threefold: (1) the endothelium, through its selective permeability to basic small-molecular nutrients (glucose, amino acids, electrolytes) supplies the tissues (in this case: the arterial wall) with the necessary provisions for survival; the selective permeability may be, to a certain degree, bidirectional for metabolites and gaseous exchange; (2) it prevents largely the entry of macromolecular (and some other "non-desirable") substances from the blood stream into the arterial wall; and (3) it provides and maintains a surface that prevents thrombosis. To accomplish these tasks, the endothelium must maintain its own integrity and adapt itself to the milieu in which it "operates"; in arteries, this adaptation requires among others, that in systole the endothelium be able to "stretch" along with the other components of the vascular wall. In order that it may carry out its functions and possess the properties required, the endothelium must be appropriately structured.

The purpose of this communication is to review the present status of knowledge of the arterial endothelium in terms of functional morphology; thus, an attempt will be made at relating each of the ultrastructurally delineated components of the endothelial cell to the known function and properties of the endothelium in health, with brief reference to certain disease states, particularly atherosclerosis. This communication does not represent an "all-embracing" review owing to the restrictions of space; reference is made to the now classical monograph of Altschul (1) and to other recently published articles (86, 46, 7, 70) with a somewhat different approach to the reviewing of the subject than that of the presentation to follow.

I. STRUCTURAL SUBSTRATUM OF PROPERTIES AND FUNCTION

In relation to the subject of atherosclerosis, the discussion regarding endothelium should concern itself largely with the endothelial cells of large (elastic) and medium size (muscular) arteries because this disease process affects these vessels. It is known, however, that the endothelium lining the above vessels not only resembles that of all arterial channels, but is of the same, i.e., continuous type, present also in certain capillaries (muscular, myocardial, placental, in smooth muscle layers of the reproductive system) (86). Therefore, some data pertaining to studies carried out on these capillaries, but not available for arteries, will be quoted with reference to arterial structure and function; it is of course possible that such extrapolation is not valid.

A. CELLULAR "EXTERIOR"

1. Luminal Aspect (Surface). The vascular endothelium constitutes a continuous, coherent, innermost cellular monolayer in contact with the blood; it measures 0.5-1.2 micra in thickness, and in large and medium size arteries consists of interlocked flat polygonal cells. The long axis of these cells is parallel to the direction of the blood flow, but this orientation is disarrayed at the origin of the arterial branching and other areas of locally altered hemodynamics, as well as at the sites of lipid deposition in experimental hypercholesterolemia (79). Projecting above the surface into the lumen are cytoplasmic microvilli and marginal folds (the so-called endothelial flaps); the latter represent extensions of the overlapping cellular appositions which are usually oriented in a down-stream direction. The marginal folds may coalesce at times with the cellular membrane enclosing some plasma. It has been suggested that the presence of microvilli might be responsible for the sluggish flow of the cell-free boundary layer of plasma along the endothelial surface. Some investigators believe that this phenomenon facilitates the exchange of metabolites between the arterial wall and the blood (83); it is also possible that the boundary layer prevents certain blood constituents from the contact with the endothelium and potential access into the arterial wall (7). Whether the microvilli play a role in "trapping" of formed blood elements has not been studied closely in arterial endothelium.

Occasionally, typical cilia have been observed to project from the endothelial surface (13). It is unknown whether their function in arteries relates, for example, to the osmolarity (of blood) in analogy to that ascribed to these structures in other tissues, or represents possible endothelial sensors of flow dynamics. Rodbard (71) speculated that such endothelial sensors might exist and it is conceivable that cilia represent the appropriate morphological substratum for such function.

The external (luminal) surface of the endothelium is coated by an ultrathin extraneous polysaccharide layer, the glycocalyx, that when first visualized in the endothelium by Luft (50) was termed "endocapillary layer"; it may be best demonstrated ultrastructurally by the ruthenium red technique (50) or Concanavalin-A reaction (96). Whereas the precise chemical nature of this "glycocalyx" is not known, it is believed to consist, at least in part, of mucopolysaccharides (78). The layer measures up to 1000Å in width (78, 51) and consists of a dense lamina applied closely to the outer leaflet of plasma membrane and an external, less dense, finely fibrillar component.

It is generally assumed that the function of the glycocalyx is linked to the endothelial property of permeability by regulating the access of the various plasma constituents (including lipoproteins) either to the plasmalemmal vesicles involved in transcellular transport, or to the binding sites of the endothelial plasmalemmal membrane. This interpretation is supported by the data indicating that the glycocalyx is thinned in areas of normal arteries known to be subjected to local disturbances in hemodynamics, e.g., those relating to branching (31); such areas exhibit also an increased uptake of a protein-binding dye (56) and of ^{3}H-unesterified cholesterol (84), and an increased permeability to ^{131}I-albumin and ^{131}I-fibrinogen (59, 5). Furthermore, a thinning of the glycocalyx also has been observed in experimental hypercholesterolemia (2) which is accompanied by an increased permeability to albumin (87). Some investigators have reported that this layer increases considerably in thickness in the early stages of experimental hypercholesterolemia (95).

The arrangement, shape, direction and size of the endothelial cells may be best studied by the "en face" technique, particularly by utilizing the Häutchen preparations and aqueous silver nitrate staining (65), because the cells are outlined by distinct black lines. In young animals cell outlines have a regular pattern and each encloses only one nucleus (22). The pattern is irregular in older animals because there may be large, several nuclei-containing cells present (57). Such irregular patterns may be seen more often in advanced age of man and in atherosclerosis (82, 48, 15), and following injury (65).

The silver, interendothelial lines measure over 1 micron in width and whereas in the past they were interpreted as representing many different phenomena, it has become apparent that these correspond to the staining of the intercellular slits at the intricate, complexly arranged junctions between the adjacent endothelial cells (63).

It is less certain, however, what might be the ultrastructural counterpart of the "stomata" and "stigmata" observed on the endothelial surface; these are delineated in the above silver preparations as small loops in areas where the lines fail to enclose a nucleus, or dark spots or deposits in the dark lines themselves, respectively (24). Whereas none of the various interpretations proposed in the past could be substantiated by the ultrastructural studies of the endothelium, it is certain that these features are not representing artifacts; "stomata" and "stigmata" have been consistently observed between two emerging daughter cells in dividing, regenerating venous endothelium (88), and recently were reported to be increased in number in the aortic endothelium at the sites of lipid deposition in hypercholesterolemic animals (rabbits) (79). The latter observation almost certainly rules out the notion that these structures may be related to the permeability because their number and size were found not to be changed in the areas of known increased permeability in normal aortae (see above). It is possible that they reflect discontinuities in the growing endothelium (75), but whether they relate to certain well defined areas of the interendothelial appositions (= junctions) remains to be explored.

Recently, by utilization of several techniques (interference contrast microscopy, histochemistry, scanning electron microscopy) circular flap-like structures measuring 3-5 micra in diameter were observed on the endothelial surface (6). These flaps (or valves) are believed to be attached by a thin stalk to the endothelial cell and to be situated close to the intercellular borders, i.e., junctions. A circular area present beneath the flap and measuring approximately 1 micron in diameter appears to be in continuity with a canal-like structure measuring approximately 5 micra in length and extending from the surface towards the media. The structure was observed in both the areas of increased and normal permeability of normal aortae, and seemed to have an increased permeability to such substances as nigrosin and 0.1-0.2 micra particles of colloidal coal. It was uncertain whether these canal-like structures represented preformed continuous canals. Alternatively, these may represent intercellular regions in which the "tight" junctions are located at the extreme basal parts of the endothelial cells at which the intercellular space (of the junction) forms perhaps a dilated pocket. The authors speculated that the flow through these "canaliculi" may be directed (also?) towards the lumen (6).

The presence of the flaps and canaliculi awaits confirmation from other centres. It remains uncertain in any event whether and in what way these relate to the other enigmatic feature of the endothelial surface, i.e., the "stomata" and "stigmata", and to the other recently proposed transendothelial vesicular pathways (81).

2. Intercellular Junctions. The "interlocking" of the endothelial cells results in a functionally synchronized monocellular

layer; it represents de facto an overlapping of the peripheral cytoplasmic portions of the neighbouring cells, with a total spacing between them in the order of 150-200Å. In developing arteries and regenerating endothelium the intercellular contact is rather straight and perpendicular to the surface. Under these circumstances the contacting cytoplasmic surfaces are arranged rather loosely and form a short interphase (63). In the fully developed arteries and mature endothelium these overlapping appositions are usually complex intricate interdigitations of considerable length and direction that is slanted or tangential to the surface. Moreover, these are highly organized areas that may account on one hand for the cohesiveness of the layer and on the other provide, in addition to the surface microvilli, the structural basis of endothelial capacity for stretching. It has been established that in large arteries (of rat), in analogy to several other vessels, two distinct forms of junctions are identifiable by electron microscopy within the intricate (inter-) endothelial apposition (42):

(1) At sharply localized ("punctate") contacts the two outer plasmalemmal leaflets of adjacent cells appear to be fused, and thus this "tight" junction is represented as a pentilaminar structure. The "tight" junctions form circumferential belts representing (incomplete) zonulae occludens and are local permeability barriers to the passage of protein molecules, by sealing the intercellular space between adjacent endothelial cells.

(2) Other contacting areas of the (same) cellular apposition extend over a considerable length, are not true fusions of outer plasmalemmal leaflets but enclose a regular, 30-40Å wide intercellular space, and appear therefore as septilaminar "gap" junctions. They are believed to play a role in the interendothelial transfer of ions (electronic or ionic coupling) (61, 67) and metabolites (metabolic coupling) (33). Since these gap junctions are plaque-like in shape rather than circumferential belts they are not considered by some investigators to act as permeability seals; this view is supported by experiments in which some small protein molecule tracers reach the subendothelial space passing by these localized gap junctions (43). However, the most recent data based on experiments that were carried out utilizing muscular capillaries and tracer probe molecules of very small dimensions (myoglobin, hemeundecapeptide and hemeoctapeptide) do not support this view (80, 81); the endothelium of these capillaries is of the continuous type and similar to that of aorta and large vessels. It was concluded from these studies that under normal conditions the junctions in the endothelium are not permeable to molecules of size larger than 20Å. Plausible examples in support of each of the two different views have been convincingly cited, and it is possible that the discrepancy results from the structural endothelial differences not only from one vessel to another, but also at different levels of

the same vessel.

How the "stomata" and "stigmata" observed in silver "en face" preparations, and the flap-like structures with associated (trans-endothelial) canaliculi relate to the junctions of endothelial cells has not been established with certainty. It is of interest that in ruthenium red preparations material similar to that of glycocalyx is present in the segments of the intercellular junctions immediately adjacent to the lumen (50, 51). Whether this reflects a true feature or is an artifact of tissue preparation, must await clarification.

The role of the endothelial junctions in the arteries affected by such processes as atherosclerosis and hypertension has been related always, at least in part, to the features of an increased (and indiscriminate?) permeability. An increased permeability that is known to be associated with the intercellular junctions (gaps) has been observed in immature endothelium, and under certain conditions that may apply to the regenerating arterial endothelium (25, 26). In these conditions it might be explained on the basis of prevailing, above-mentioned "loose" and yet unorganized junctions. However, it is not a simple matter to account for similar pathways of increased permeability with respect to the junctions of mature arterial endothelial lining. For this purpose it would be necessary to postulate that the junctions may be temporarily "opened" either by overstretching the surface, as has been proposed for hypertension, or by active contraction of the endothelium, thus permitting an influx of blood constituents through the widened intercellular gaps. Data suggest that under various experimental conditions (11, 12) there is a temporary influx of blood constituents into the subendothelial space through the interendothelial junctions and that this period may be very shortlived (69). It is, however, another matter to assume that these junctions become widened only temporarily and that the opening of the "tight" junctions is a reversible process, as suggested by some investigators (43). Biologically, this would be difficult to explain, since structurally and functionally specialized membranes once lost, must be replaced by a de novo synthesis -- and this requires time. It is probable, however, that the "opening" of the junctions affects the entire circumference of a given cell that becomes "loose" and is "desquamated" into the circulation; by stretching, the neighbouring cells may establish new contacts (between the undamaged cells) and/or initiate immediately the replacement by regenerative process (see below). Recently, the assumed contractile function of the endothelial cells that is allegedly responsible for the temporary opening of the junctions (69, 77), has been questioned (35, 100).

3. Basal Laminal Aspect. The basal aspect of the endothelial cells is intimately associated with a basal lamina (BL) that does

not accompany the cellular contour into the area of junctions. This membrane measures in electron microscopic preparations 500-600Å in width; it consists of a lucent zone immediately adjacent to the endothelial plasma membrane, a moderately electron-dense, finely filamentous mid-zone measuring approximately 300Å in width, and an outer, ill-defined, slightly electron-dense narrow layer. It has been suggested recently that the BL is (at intervals?) attached firmly to the basal endothelial plasma membrane by fibrils varying from 20 to 80Å in diameter, and that the peripheral portions of the cytoplasm facing these attachments are condensed (93).

By histochemical methods and specifically with the periodic acid-Schiff (PAS) reaction the BL appears to be much broader than that visualized by electron microscopy. The PAS-reaction also indicates that the BL contains an ample amount of glycoproteins; some of these might be mucopolysaccharides which are not well demonstrated in conventional stains for electron microscopy.

It has been demonstrated recently, that collagen Type IV constitutes much of the BL (58). Moreover, it has been known for approximately fifteen years that in the developing human aorta the microfibrillar component of the elastic tissue units is closely associated with the endothelial (BL) (36); this suggested that at least the fibrillar element of the elastic tissue may be contributed either by or through the BL. The BL is, of course, an integral, if external, part of the endothelial cells which are instrumental in its genesis. It is therefore reasonable to infer that collagen Type IV (directly) and elastic tissue (perhaps indirectly) both are products of the endothelial cells.

It is believed that the BL has a supportive function for the endothelial lining by providing it with a "firm" base. It is doubtful, however, whether at the same time it provides a restraining means to the cellular extensions of the endothelium, as was believed previously, because in some instances the BL follows the endothelial invaginations into the subendothelial space (30).

In addition to the above functions, the BL may be acting as a coarse filter by retaining large molecules (chylomicra, carbon, mercuric sulfide), at least for a time (53, 14). Experimental evidence suggests that particles larger than 100Å may be retained by the BL (20). In this sense the lamina may play also a role in the permeability. However, the experiments providing the above information on permeability were carried out with various capillaries and no data are available with respect to the arteries.

B. CELLULAR "INTERIOR"

1. Cellular Organelles. The "resting" and mature endothelial cells of artery beyond the childhood are elongated in the direction of the blood flow, flat, polygonal in shape and measure approximately 30x10 micra in the largest and smallest diameter, respectively (21). The cells are dominated by large nuclei that occupy much of the cellular interior and often cause the centricellular slight elevations above the intimal surface. The nucleus is elongated in the long axis of the cell and its chromatin condensed at the periphery; the nucleolus is not overly prominent and is often absent. Several nuclear infoldings may be present, in arteries that were not fixed in situ by pressure perfusion. Until just recently accentuated nuclear infoldings were considered by some investigators as a criterion of an active endothelial contractility (52). The cytoplasm is not abundant; it contains all the usual organelles, but these are few in number. This is interpreted usually as reflecting a low metabolic activity beyond the cell's own primary requirements of maintenance and survival. The few small mitochondria are present usually in the polar perinuclear, or at the basal cellular area; a small Golgi complex, a few, small "empty" profiles or slits of rough surface endoplasmic reticulum (RER), and a small number of cytoplasmic glycogen granules and free ribosomes are present invariably; occasionally, centrosomes may be observed.

In fetal and neonatal arteries and those under various experimental conditions, the endothelial cells are large and cuboidal, have an abundant cytoplasm with a prominent Golgi complex, numerous free ribosomes and glycogen granules, a nucleus with redistributed ("reactivated") nucleoproteins, and many more mitochondria and profiles of RER than those observed in the "resting" cells. The RER is often dilated and contains a variable amount of finely fibrillar floccular material. Recently, structured fibrils with morphological features compatible with those of the 640Å-banded, conventional collagen fibrils were observed within the dilated endothelial cisternae of RER in experimentally produced thickenings of small canine arteries (38). In view of this observation and the discussed relation of the endothelial cell to its own BL (now known to consist biochemically, at least in part, of Type IV collagen); the association of the BL with the microfibrillar component of the newly developing elastic tissue units; and finally, the abundant acid mucopolysaccharides that are present in the immediate subendothelial space, it seems reasonable to conclude that the endothelial cells have the ability and potential to produce all extracellular connective tissue elements during certain stages of vascular development and under experimental conditions.

Cylindrical Weibel-Palade bodies or rods, measuring approximately 0.1 micra in diameter and up to 3 micra in length were first described in the endothelium in 1964 (98). These are limited by a 60-80Å thick unit membrane, and consist of parallel, longitudinally arranged filaments or microtubules (150-200Å in diameter) embedded in a matrix. These structures are not confined to the endothelium as they were observed also in other fluid-exposed, surface-related cells (40). Allegedly, these structures occupy in the aortic endothelium approximately 1 Vol. % of the cytoplasm, a figure perhaps much too high. On the basis of certain structural similarities believed to exist between these rods and the platelets (97), and the reports that following adrenaline administration the aortic wall of the rabbit discharged a clotting-promoting substance into the circulation (76), it has been suggested that there is a relation between these endothelial organelles and the clotting-promoting substance that is released into the blood (27). It is not certain at present how this "clotting-promoting function" relates to the other and overall properties of the vascular endothelium with respect to the blood coagulability, particularly to the antihemophilic factor (45). Cultured endothelium contains the rods (17, 44).

Fine endothelial filaments were described ultrastructurally as early as 1953 (60), and later with the improvement of techniques for electron microscopy were found almost universally. The filaments are often long and most commonly (but not exclusively) appear to be oriented longitudinally; they are most numerous in the basal portion of the cell; at times there is a suggestion that they tend to aggregate into tracks, but this is not a common phenomenon in a resting mature cell. The thin filaments measure approximately 70Å in diameter. In addition, thick (62) and even a striated (32) variety have been observed in endothelial cells at various sites and under a variety of conditions. Renewed interest in the filaments as a potential morphological substratum of a proposed contractile property of the endothelial cells has been stimulated largely by the demonstration of actomyosin antigenically identical to that of smooth muscle cells in the arterial media (4), and by the identification of actin-like filaments with heavy meromyosin (72), in these cells. Moreover, the administration of histamine-type mediators resulted in a swelling and separation of endothelial cells at junctions, and in infoldings in the nuclear membrane, all features considered to be an expression of active endothelial contractility (52). Numerous reports followed the above original observations furnishing supposedly additional evidence for the proposed endothelial contractility; in particular, the concept was ardently employed in support of the thesis that the interendothelial junctions open temporarily as a result of stimuli effecting endothelial contraction and thus, allowing through the widely patent gaps for an influx of blood constituents into the intimal substance (77, 69, 70, 11). Many of these experiments were related specifically to hypertension and atherosclerosis. However, Zeifach expressed the opinion of many other investigators by stating: " ... all-in-all evidence continues to mount against the contractility of vascular endothelium in a functional context." (100). The alternative proposal is that the filaments may represent transitory components of the endothelial cells that appear upon condensation or reorganization of sclero-proteins in response to mechanical stimuli (35), and/or act as a cytoskeleton (68). Indeed, the observations that the filaments are a prominent endothelial feature in hypertension (28), and other conditions (associated with local pressure increases) (39) support the latter contention, particularly in view of the available data that question the relevance of the intercellular junctions in the process of permeability of normal endothelium.

2. Vesicles and Vacuoles. Numerous plasmalemmal vesicles (caveolae intracellulares) measuring approximately 700Å in diameter and limited by a smooth membrane are present in the endothelial cells, particularly along the luminal and basal plasma membranes. They fuse and are in continuity with the cytoplasmic membrane forming flask-shaped structures; the stomal portion communicating with the exterior of the cell measures approximately 300Å in diameter (8, 9). A few vesicles are also present at the cellular junctions. The number of these vesicles varies from one type of endothelium to another but within a given vascular segment they appear to be constant and remain so under a variety of experimental conditions (21, 47, 49). The vesicles are present in the cytoplasm either as a single structure or they may fuse to form rosettes. It has been shown recently that they may also fuse (sequentially) in a row, extending from the luminal to basal portion of the plasma membrane, thus forming a transendothelial channel (80, 81). It is uncertain as yet what, if any, is the relation of this channel formed by the fusion of these vesicles to the proposed endothelial canalicular structures (see above). The ruthenium red stains also the caveolar flasks that are in continuity with, and the vesicles that still contact the external plasmalemmal membrane (78), whereas the intracellular vesicles do not show this reaction. Phosphatase activity also has been demonstrated in the plasmalemmal vesicles (55). Such phosphatases may have an important function in the breakdown of adenosine diphosphate, but this has not been explored in detail with reference to the platelet aggreations in arteries.

On the basis of numerous morphological studies that have utilized tracers of various molecular size and autoradiography, it has been firmly established that the transendothelial transport of proteins takes place via the plasmalemmal vesicles. They represent a dynamic system of transport and it is conceivable that this transport may be bidirectional. Important is to mention the data indicating that in a perfused system and using autoradiography there appears to be a continuous transport of lipoproteins through normal endothelium (90). The HDL-particles appear to pass more readily than the LDL; the slowest is the transport of the VLDL (89). It has been only assumed that this transport takes place via the plasmalemmal vesicles, as autoradiography does not allow for accurate localization because of the size of the marker.

In view of the evidence refuting the belief that the intercellular gaps are also pathways of transport, at least for molecules larger than 20Å in diameter, one would have to ascribe that function exclusively to the plasmalemmal vesicles. It might be expected, therefore, that in conditions of prevailing increased permeability there would be an increased number of these vesicles available for that increased load. Some investigators believe on the basis of their studies that, indeed, conditions such as blood pressure change the vesicular transport (43), whereas other data contradict these observations (29, 74). Assuming that the number of vesicles is constant, the rate of their movement across the cytoplasm would have to increase in conditions of increased permeability and in the presence of undamaged endothelium. The clarification of this problem must await further work.

There are a few profiles of a second type, slightly oblong vesicle in the endothelium; it also fuses with the plasma membrane, and is referred to as a "pit". It measures 800Å-1200Å in diameter, is limited by a membrane that appears internally "spiked" by short ill-defined filaments embedded in a narrow homogeneous coating. The vesicle appears to originate by invagination of a specialized area of the plasma membrane, and is considered to be concerned with selective uptake of substances, particularly proteins, in a variety of cells (73).

The third type of vesicle represents actually a vacuole that may have little in common with the functional aspect of uptake and transport of macromolecules ascribed to the two other types. It may be formed either by a large tubular invagination of, and subsequent detachment from the plasma membrane, or alternatively by fusion of a marginal fold (described above) with the plasma membrane and enclosing the circulating plasma. Uncommon in normal, they have been observed more often in experimentally damaged endothelium (10); in normotensive, hypo-, and hypertensive animals these vacuoles may contain the injected tracers (43).

3. "Bodies and Inclusions". In addition to the above "internal" cellular components, other structures may be present occasionally in the vascular endothelium.

The so-called multivesicular body (MVB) (85) is present at times; its derivation and function is as uncertain in the endothelium, as it is with respect to other cells. These ("true") MVB should not be confused with the structures also designated as such in some studies of experimental hypertension (43), because the former, as defined, represent preformed organized structures, whereas under the above experimental conditions the structures designated as MVB represent inclusions containing the tracer protein.

In normal arteries, but particularly often in disease and under experimental conditions, many forms of "inclusions" may be observed in the endothelium, including those of lipids. Whether these accumulate as the result of a true phagocytic property of the vascular endothelium is not certain; this problem will not be discussed here, and the interested reader is referred to the still valid previous reviews on the subject of endothelial phagocytosis (1, 24). Relevant to the problem of atherosclerosis in addition to the occurrence of lipid droplets in the endothelium are the observations suggesting that the endothelium is capable of engulfing platelets under certain conditions (54).

Dense bodies, lacking internal structure, are present often in the endothelium. These are bounded by a unit membrane and have a size comparable to that of mitochondria. There are some data, based on experiments with injected particulate substances, suggesting that these bodies "correspond" to phagosomes (23), and reference was made to these as being lysosomal in nature (68), but this question has not been clarified entirely for arterial endothelium.

Various pigments and a multitude of "inclusions" of a different type have been described in the vascular endothelium in many so-called storage diseases. Whereas it has not been ruled out that some of these substances may be "taken up" by the endothelial cells from the lumen, it is most probable that these represent secretory products of the metabolically altered endothelial cells.

--- --- --- --- --- --- --- --- --- --- --- ---

Before leaving this section it should be mentioned that certain properties of the endothelium to date have no identifiable structural basis. It is known that the endothelium is the site of: plasminogen activator (92); fibrinolysis inhibitor resembling an antiplasmin (66); antihemophilic factor (factor VIII) (3, 41); activator of Hageman factor (factor XII) (in: 70); major blood group and histocompatibility antigens (3, 44); and has another pro-coagulant activity (94).

It is evident on the basis of the above many different (and seemingly contradicting) functions, including that believed to be associated with the Weibel-Palade granules, that the endothelial lining plays an important role in the maintenance of homeostasis, and thus in several aspects pertaining to atherosclerosis.

II. REGENERATION, PROLIFERATION AND DIFFERENTIATION

Arterial endothelium is remarkably tough despite the fact that it constitutes only a monocellular layer. In health, it remains undamaged for a long time, but it does have a limited life span. It is probable that the renewal proceeds by replacing single rather than groups of cells. Upon the "loosening" at the junctions the cell to be replaced shrinks and is gradually displaced by extensions and later cell divisions of the surrounding endothelium; the process thus avoids the even temporarily area-denuded periods. Studies on DNA-synthesis, using tritiated thymidine and autoradiography showed that even in health there is a continuous renewal of the aortic endothelium, and in the guinea pig the life span was 100-180 days. However, the turnover, while constant for a given area varies even in normal arteries from one segment to another and is particularly increased in areas exposed to greater hemodynamic stresses (bifurcation, branchings); for the latter it was calculated that the life span is 60-120 days. Similar studies carried out in several species and by some modified methods largely confirmed the general principle of renewal in the above terms. It was also demonstrated unequivocally that the endothelium can undergo mitotic division, a property doubted for a long time (for details see: 7, 70).

Effete desquamated endothelial cells may be recovered from the blood in a variety of conditions, and the regeneration of endothelium follows readily upon many forms of injury. Under these conditions the mitosis occurs in the aorta very rapidly. The mode and rate of regeneration depends largely on the extent of denudation; the species of the animal used; the availability of side branches in the vicinity of the damage; and to a certain degree also on nature of the injury (for summary and review see: 7, 70, 99). In regenerating endothelium that follows injury, multinucleated giant cells have been observed in several studies (19, 34). They have been reported to occur in arteries in increased numbers in atherosclerosis (79); it is uncertain whether they represent a truly regenerative phenomenon.

It was shown using tritiated thymidine in vivo that there is a greater DNA synthesis by the endothelial cells of the atherosclerotic lesions than in normal aortas of swine (91). Since this increased rate of DNA-synthesis was not associated with obvious accumulation of the endothelial cells within the lesion, it suggested that there was a rapid turnover rate of these cells. The increased rate of endothelial multiplication in atherosclerosis has been supported by other investigators; recently, a considerable increase in the number of mitotic figures has been observed directly in the aortic "en face" preparation of the endothelium from the sites of lipid deposition in hypercholesterolemic rabbits as compared with controls (79). Just why the endothelial cells over the already established lesions renew themselves so rapidly is a matter of speculation at present.

Proliferation of arterial endothelial cells plays also an important role in the process of organization of mural thrombi; the "growing-over" of the (proliferating) endothelium to cover the thrombus is a prerequisite to the organization. It is not known what precisely the stimulus for this proliferation is. In the experimental arterial thrombosis there is most probably an actual destruction of the underlying endothelium (prior to the thrombus deposition). Since destruction of the endothelium stimulates its proliferation from the edges of viable surrounding cells, these newly proliferating cells grow over the top of the substratum that it now encounters, i.e., the thrombus, as if the thrombus were already a part of the intimal layer. Little is known about the rate of endothelial growth over the thrombus that no doubt depends among others on the size of the latter. Small thrombi that follow, e.g., punctate arterial wounds are covered by endothelium in 6-8 days (16). Variations in the rate of endothelialization of thrombus deposits relative to that of the overall forces of thrombolysis could be a significant factor in rate and amount of incorporation of thrombi into the arterial wall (18). Rapidly proliferating endothelial cells over a thrombus could prevent thrombolysis and be one of the factors determining the original size and subsequent growth of an atherosclerotic plaque. In this context, the proliferating endothelium is related to the process of atherosclerosis.

The regeneration and proliferation of the arterial endothelium may play, in addition, a role in atherosclerosis by differentiating into smooth muscle cells in one form of the lesions, i.e., in the white plaque. The embryological derivation of both cell types, observations in tissue culture, as well as "stepwise" morphogenetic studies in human atherosclerosis (1, 37), all support this concept. The latter does not rule out the probability, that either under certain conditions (64), or to some extent at all times, there may be also a "contribution" to the smooth muscle cell population of the white atherosclerotic plaque from another source.

The proliferative potentials of the endothelium of large and medium size arteries appears to be in some respect at variance with that of the smaller vessels, since no true endothelial tumors of either benign or malignant variety are known to occur in the former. What the possible "restraining" forces for an unlimited proliferation characterizing neoplasms might be in the large arteries, is unknown.

Acknowledgements. Some data included in this presentation are based on work that has been supported by grants-in-aid of research T.3-11 from the Ontario Heart Foundation, Toront, Ontario, and MT-1037 from the Medical Research Council of Canada. The author wishes to thank Mrs. Mary-Lou Duffy for efficient typing of the manuscript.

REFERENCES

1. Altschul, R. Endothelium, Its Development, Morphology, Function and Pathology. The Macmillan Co., New York, 1954.
2. Balint, A., Veress, B., and Jellinek, H. Path. Europ. 9:105, 1974.
3. Becker, C.D., Jaffe, E.A., Nachman, R.L., and Minick, R. In: Atherosclerosis III., Schettler, G., and Weizel, A., eds., pp. 166-169, Springer Verlag, Berlin, 1974.
4. Becker, C.G., and Murphy, G.E. Amer. J. Pathol. 55:1, 1969.
5. Bell, F.P., Gallus, A.S., and Schwartz, C.J. Exp. Molec. Pathol. 20:281, 1974.
6. Björkerud, S., Hansson, H.A., and Bondjers, G. Virchows Arch. Abt. B. Zellpath. 11:19, 1972.
7. Björkerud, S. In: The Smooth Muscle of the Artery. Advances in Experimental Medicine and Biology, Vol. 57, Wolf, S., and Werthessen, N.T., eds., pp. 180-204, Plenum Press, New York, 1975.
8. Bruns, R.R., and Palade, G.E. J. Cell Biol. 37:244, 1968.
9. Bruns, R.R., and Palade, G.E. J. Cell Biol. 37:277, 1968.
10. Buck, R.C. In: Atherosclerosis and its Origin, Sandler, M., and Bourne, G.H., eds., pp. 1-37, Academic Press, New York, 1963.
11. Constantinides, P. In: The Artery and the Process of Arteriosclerosis; Pathogenesis. Advances in Experimental Medicine and Biology, Vol. 16A, Wolf, S., ed., pp. 185-201, and 204-206, Plenum Press, New York, 1971.
12. Constantinides, P., and Wiggers, K.D. Virchows Arch. A Path. Anat. 362:291, 1974.
13. Corbett, W. M.Sc. Thesis, Queen's University, Kingston, Canada, 1961.
14. Cotran, R.S., LaGattuta, M., and Majno, G. Amer. J. Pathol. 47:1045, 1965.
15. Cotton, R., and Wartman, W.B. Arch. Pathol. 71:3, 1961.
16. Crawford, T. J. Pathol. Bacteriol. 72:547, 1956.
17. Csonka, E., Kerenyi, T., Koch, A.S., and Jellinek, H. Arterial Wall 3, No. 1, 31, 1975.
18. Davies, M.J., Woolf, N., and Bradley, J.P.W. J. Pathol. 97:589, 1969.
19. Efskind, L. Acta Pathol. Microbiol. Scand. 18:259, 1941.
20. Florey, H.W. Quart. J. Exptl. Physiol. 49:117, 1964.
21. Florey, H.W. Brit. Med. J. 2:487, 1966.
22. Florey, H.W., Poole, J.C.F., and Meek, G.A. J. Pathol. Bacteriol. 77:625, 1959.
23. French, J.E. In: Evolution of the Atherosclerotic Plaque, Jones, R.J., ed., pp. 15-28, Univ. of Chicago Press, Chicago, Illinois, 1963.

24. French, J.E. Int. Rev. Exp. Pathol. 5:253, 1966.
25. Friedman, M., and Byers, S.O. Brit. J. Exp. Pathol. 43:363, 1962.
26. Friedman, M., and Byers, S.O. Arch. Pathol. 76:99, 1963.
27. Fuchs, A., and Weibel, E.R. Zeitsch. f. Zellforsch. 73:1, 1966.
28. Gabbiani, G., Badonnel, M.-Cl., and Rona, G. Lab. Invest. 32:227, 1975.
29. Garlick, D.G., and Renkin, E.M. Amer. J. Physiol. 219:1595, 1970.
30. Geer, J.C. Amer. J. Pathol. 47:241, 1965.
31. Gerrity, R.G., Richardson, M., and Schwartz, C.J. In: Atherosclerosis, Metabolic, Morphologic and Clinical Aspects, Manning, G.W., and Haust, M.D., eds., Plenum Press, New York, in press, 1976.
32. Giacomelli, F., Wiener, R., and Spiro, D. J. Cell Biol. 45:188, 1970.
33. Gilula, N.B., Reeves, O.R., and Steinbach, A. Nature (Lond.) 235:262, 1972.
34. Gottlob, R., and Zinner, G. Virchows Arch. Pathol. Anat. Physiol. 336:16, 1962.
35. Hammersen, F. In: Proceedings of 7th European Conference on Microcirculation. Part II. Clinical Aspects of Microcirculation, Ditzel, J., and Lewis, D.H., eds., pp. 159-164, S. Karger, Basel, 1973.
36. Haust, M.D., More, R.H., Bencosme, S.A., and Balis, J.U. Exp. Molec. Pathol. 4:508, 1965.
37. Haust, M.D., More, R.H., and Movat, H.Z. Amer. J. Pathol. 35:265, 1959.
38. Haust, M.D., and Trillo, A. unpublished observations.
39. Haust, M.D., and Trillo, A. unpublished observations.
40. Haust, M.D., Wyllie, J.C., and More, R.H. Rev. Can. Biol. 25:117, 1966.
41. Hoyer, L.W., de los Santos, R.P., and Hoyer, J.R. J. Clin. Invest. 52:2737, 1973.
42. Hüttner, I., Boutet, M., and More, R.H. Lab. Invest. 28: 672, 1973.
43. Hüttner, I., Boutet, M., Rona, G., and More, R.H. Lab. Invest. 29:536, 1973.
44. Jaffe, E.A., Nachman, R.L., Becker, C.G., and Minick, C.R. J. Clin. Invest. 52:2745, 1973.
45. Jaffe, E.A., Hoyer, L.W., and Nachman, R.L. J. Clin. Invest. 52:2757, 1973.
46. Jellinek. H. Gazzetta Sanitaria, XLVII-N.1, 22, 1976.
47. Jennings, M.A., Marchesi, V.T., and Florey, H.W., Proc. Roy. Soc. (London) B 156:14, 1962.
48. Lautsch, E.V., McMillan, G.C., and Duff, G.L. Lab. Invest. 2:397, 1953.

49. Luft, J.H. In: Evolution of the Atherosclerotic Plaque, Jones, R.J., ed., pp. 3-14, Univ. of Chicago Press, Chicago, Illinois, 1963.
50. Luft, J.H. Fed. Proc. 25:1773, 1966.
51. Luft, J.H. Anat. Rec. 171:369, 1971.
52. Majno, G., Shea, St.M., and Leventhal, M. J. Cell Biol. 42:647, 1969.
53. Majno, G., and Palade, G.E. J. Biophys. Biochem. Cytol. 11:571, 1961.
54. Marchesi, V.T. Ann. N.Y. Acad. Sci. 116:774, 1964.
55. Marchesi, V.T., and Barrnett, R.J. J. Cell Biol. 17:547, 1963.
56. McGill H.C., Geer, J.C., and Holman, R.L. Arch. Pathol. 64:303, 1957.
57. McGovern, V.J. J. Pathol. Bacteriol. 69:283, 1955.
58. Miller, E.J., and Matukas, V.J. Fed. Proc. 33,5:1197, 1974.
59. Packham, M.A., Rowsell, H.C., Jørgensen, L., and Mustard, J.F. Exp. Molec. Pathol. 7:214, 1967.
60. Palade, G.E. J. Appl. Physiol. 24:1424, 1953.
61. Pappas, G.D., Asada, Y., and Bennett, M.V.L. J. Cell Biol. 49:173, 1971.
62. Phelps, P.C., and Luft, J.H. Amer. J. Anat. 125:399, 1969.
63. Poole, J.C.F. In: The Smooth Muscle of the Artery. Advances in Experimental Medicine and Biology, Vol. 57, Wolf, S., and Werthessen, N.T., eds., p. 237 and p. 239, Plenum Press, New York, 1975.
64. Poole, J.C.F., Cromwell, S.B., and Benditt, E.P. Amer. J. Pathol. 62:391, 1971.
65. Poole, J.C.F., Sanders, A.G., and Florey, H.W. J. Pathol. Bacteriol. 75:133, 1958.
66. Pugatch, E.M.J., Foster, E.A., Macfarlane, D.E., and Poole, J.C.F. Brit. J. Haemat. 18:669, 1970.
67. Revel, J.P., Yee, A.G., and Hudspeth, A.J. Proc. Natl. Acad. Sci. U.S.A. 68:2924, 1971.
68. Rhodin, J.A.G. Physiol. Rev. 42, Suppl. 5, 48, 1962.
69. Robertson, L.A., and Khairallah, P.A. Exp. Molec. Pathol. 18:241, 1973.
70. Robertson, A.L., and Rosen, L.A. Microcirculation, in press, 1976.
71. Rodbard, S. In: The Smooth Muscle of the Artery. Advances in Experimental Medicine and Biology, Vol. 57, Wolf, S., and Werthessen, N.T., eds., pp. 230, 231, Plenum Press, New York, 1975.
72. Rostgaard, J., Kristensen, B.I., and Nielsen, L.E. J. Ultrastruct. Res. 38:207, 1972.
73. Roth, T.F., and Porter, K.R. J. Cell Biol. 20:313, 1964.
74. Schneeberger, E.E., and Karnovsky, M.J. J. Cell Biol. 49:319, 1971.
75. Schoefl, G.I. Ann. N.Y. Acad. Sci. 116:789, 1964.

76. Shimamoto, T., and Ishioka, T. Circ. Res. 7:138, 1963.
77. Shimamoto, T., and Sunaga, T. Proc. Jap. Acad. 48:683, 1972.
78. Shirahama, E., and Cohen, A.S. J. Cell Biol. 52:198, 1972.
79. Silkworth, J.B., McLean, B., and Stehbens, W.E. Atherosclerosis, in press, 1976.
80. Simionescu, N., Simionescu, M., and Palade, G.E. J. Cell Biol. 57:424, 1973.
81. Simionescu, N., Simionescu, M., and Palade, G.E. J. Cell Biol. 64:586, 1975.
82. Sinapius, D. Virchows Arch. Pathol. Anat. Physiol. 322:662, 1952.
83. Smith, U., Ryan, J.W., Michie, D.D., and Smith D. Science 173:925, 1971.
84. Somer, J.B., and Schwartz, C.J. Atherosclerosis 16:377, 1972.
85. Sotelo, J.R., and Porter, K.R. J. Biophys. Biochem. Cytol. 5:327, 1959.
86. Spagnoli, L.G. Gazzetta Sanitaria, XLVII-N.1, 2, 1976.
87. Stefanovich, V., and Gore, I. Exp. Molec. Pathol. 14:20, 1971.
88. Stehbens, W.E. Quart. J. Exptl. Physiol. 50:91, 1965.
89. Stein, O. In: The Smooth Muscle of the Artery. Advances in Experimental Medicine and Biology, Vol. 57, Wolf, S., and Werthessen, N.T., eds., pp. 208-216, Plenum Press, New York, 1975.
90. Stein, Y., and Stein, O. CIBA Fdtn. Symp. 12:165, 1973.
91. Thomas, W.A., Florentin, R.A., Nam, S.C., Kim, D.N., Jones, R.M., and Lee, K.T. Arch. Pathol. 86:621, 1968.
92. Todd, A.S. Atherosclerosis 15:137, 1972.
93. Ts'ao, C., and Glagov, S. Lab. Invest. 23:510, 1970.
94. Tsubohawa, Y. Jap. Circ. J. 34:615, 1970.
95. Weber, G., Fabbrini, P., Figura, N., and Resi, L. Path. Europ. 9:303, 1974.
96. Weber, G., Fabbrini, P., and Resi, L. Virchows Arch. Abt. A Pathol. Anat. Histol. 359:299, 1973.
97. Weibel, E.R. Acta anat. (Basel) 59:390, 1964.
98. Weibel, E.R., and Palade, G.E. J. Cell Biol. 23:101, 1964.
99. Wright, P.H. In: Proceedings of 7th European Conference on Microcirculation. Part II. Clinical Aspects of Microcirculation, Ditzel, J., and Lewis, D.H., eds., pp. 87-91, S. Karger, Basel, 1973.
100. Zweifach, B.W. Microvasc. Res. 3:345, 1971.

(4)

THE CORONARY DRUG PROJECT --- FINDINGS WITH REGARD TO ESTROGEN, DEXTROTHYROXINE, CLOFIBRATE AND NIACIN

JEREMIAH STAMLER, M.D.

Northwestern University Medical School

Chicago, Illinois, U.S.A.

The Coronary Drug Project (CDP) proceeded in the United States from 1966 to 1975 as a collaborative secondary prevention trial supported by the National Heart and Lung Institute (1). It involved 8,341 men age 30 to 64 years on entry in the study, with a documented history of previous myocardial infarction (MI). They participated through 53 clinical centers throughout the country.

Aims

This study from its beginning had three basic objectives: to evaluate long-term therapeutic efficacy post-MI of five pharmacologic regimens influencing serum lipids; to study the clinical course and prognosis of coronary artery disease; and to learn more about the effective conduct of large-scale multicenter trials of treatment for chronic disease.

Design

The main design characteristics of the CDP were (1):

1. Randomized allocation of patients to the five active treatment groups, and to the placebo control group.
2. Double blind design, i.e., the treatment unknown to the patients and the treating physician.
3. A detailed obligatory common protocol.
4. Every patient to be followed for a minimum of five years, and every patient to be followed until all had been observed for at least five years (this was essentially accomplished in the second half of 1974).
5. As part of the common protocol, detailed provisions for

quality control of data through use of a Central Laboratory, a single center for ECG reading by Minnesota Code, a Coordinating Center, and a system of national committees.

The original treatment groups were: Mixed conjugated equine estrogens in two dosage groups, 2.5 and 5.0 mg. per day (ESGI and ESG2); dextrothyroxine, 6.0 mg. day (DT4); clofibrate, 1.8 gm. per day (CPIB); nicotinic acid, 3.0 gm. per day (NICA); and lactose placebo (PLBO). All drugs were packaged in identical capsules and sealed; the common full dosage was nine capsules per day, in a dosage of three t.i.d. For reasons of statistical power, men were randomly allocated to the five active treatment groups and placebo in a ratio of 1 to 1 to 1 to 1 to 1 to 2.5 -- an average of 1,110 patients in each of the five active drug groups and 2,789 in the control group. Randomization was carried out separately for each of the 53 clinics and for two risk groups. Risk Group 1 was made up of patients who had suffered a single uncomplicated infarct; risk Group 2, of patients who had had two or more infarcts or one only with a complicated course (e.g., shock, secondary extension, congestive heart failure, pericarditis, major arrhythmia).

The following conditions for inclusion in the study had to be fulfilled by a potential patient (1):

1. His age on entry had to be between 30 and 64 years.
2. There had to be a qualifying electrocardiogram documenting a past myocardial infarction, with survival for at least three months since most recent MI.
3. He had to be in New York Heart Association functional class I or 11.
4. He must not have had heart surgery.
5. He must have been free of other major life-shortening disease, e.g., cancer.
6. He must not have been on long-term anticoagulants or on lipid-lowering drugs.
7. He must not have been an insulin-dependent diabetic.
8. Also, he had to give his written consent after a thorough explanation of the design of the study and the potential side reactions of the drugs involved. The protocol also provided that throughout the study CDP physicians were to use criteria for best modern medical care as the guiding basis for all treatment decisions concerning all patients.

The rate of recruitment was almost equal over a three-year period between July, 1966 and October, 1969.

The following were among the many clinical events monitored at regular intervals: Death and cause of death, nonfatal cardiovascular complications (e.g., MI, acute coronary insufficiency, angina pectoris, congestive heart failure, ECG abnormalities, stroke, thromboembolic disease), other illnesses; symptoms and signs of possible drug toxicity.

Clinical assessments were performed at the following points in the study: three times in 4-week intervals before entry into the study and then every four months throughout the study. These evaluations were to determine blood lipid levels, to monitor toxicity and side reactions, and to check on adherence to medication. The annual examinations were more extensive than the two nonannual ones which fell in between.

The statistical planning of the study required 8,379 patients (8,341 were actually recruited), based on the following assumptions: Alpha or type 1 error -- the probability that the difference between one of the active treatment groups and the controls was a chance event -- was set at .01; beta or type II error -- the probability that a true difference existed but had been missed by chance -- was set at .05; and the minimal difference in mortality which could be discovered with the assumed alpha and beta levels was .25, i.e., a 25 per cent reduction from an estimated mortality of 30 per cent after five years for the placebo group, i.e., a reduction for a treatment group to 22.5 per cent. The dropout and frank non-adherence rate after five years was estimated at no more than 30 per cent or six per cent per annum for purposes of the sample size calculations. It was assumed that the methods of the study would assure essentially 100 per cent follow-up in terms of the primary mortality end point; in fact, vital status was unknown for only six of the 8,341 men after close-out of the study in February, 1975.

The many quantitative findings available for the CDP patients on entry have been published (1). The following are a few key facts: on the average, the men were 52 years old; one per cent was under 35, 19 per cent between 60 and 64. Two-thirds were in Risk Group 1, i.e., had had only one uncomplicated infarction. Thirty-one per cent had had their most recent MI less than a year before entry; 20 per cent, five or more years before entry; mean time since last MI was 36 months, median time 23 months. Forty-seven per cent had a definite history of angina pectoris prior to entry. Over one-third were still smoking cigarettes, somewhat less than one-half of those who had ever smoked.

As to the distribution of baseline serum cholesterol levels, 48 per cent were in the range equal to or greater than 250 mg./dl., 14 per cent, 300 or greater; the mean value was 251, the median 247; 50 per cent had serum triglycerides of 5.0 m.Eq./L. or greater; 34 per cent of 6.0 or greater; the mean was 6.1* the median 5.0, with marked skewing to the right. As expected, these two lipid variables were significantly correlated (r=0.349).

Detailed univariate and multivariate analyses of a host of baseline characteristics -- demographic, medical historical, medical examination, ECG, X-ray, biochemical -- verified that the randomization procedure had accomplished its purpose of establishing comparability among the six groups at entry.

* 1 mMo 1/L of triglyceride = approximately 30 mg./dl.

TABLE 1

Nonfatal and Fatal Events by Cause, 5.0 mg. Estrogen and Placebo Groups

Event	5.0 mg. Estrogen (1,119 Men)		Placebo (2,789 Men)		RBO+
	No.	%	No.	%	
Definite nonfatal MI‡	63	6.2	82	3.2	0.015
MI incidence (definite nonfatal MI + coronary death	123	11.0	209	7.5	0.13
Definite pulmonary embolism	17	1.5	10	0.4	0.045
Suspect and definite pulmonary embolism or thrombophlebitis	39	3.5	37	1.3	0.004
Coronary death	67	6.0	133	4.8	2.48
Sudden death	48	4.3	76	2.7	0.46
Total mortality--as of February 1, 1970	91	8.1	193	6.9	3.20
Total mortality--as of May 12, 1970	108	9.7	230	8.2	3.38

+RBO signifies relative betting odds (Bayesian approach) (11).

‡MI signifies myocardial infarction. Denominators for nonfatal MI are 1,022 and 2,580 for estrogen and placebo groups, respectively.

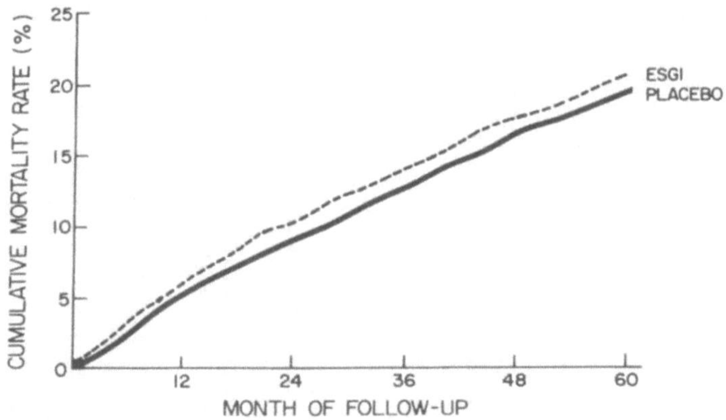

Figure 1 Life table cumulative rates for deaths from all causes for the placebo and lower dose (2.5 mg./day) estrogen group over 60 months of follow-up (8).

TABLE 2
Nonfatal and Fatal Events by Cause, 2.5 mg. Estrogen and Placebo Groups

Event	2.5 mg. Estrogen			Placebo					
	No. of Men	No. with Events	%	No. of Men	No. with Events	%	Z Value	RBO (.25)	RBO (min.)
Death-All Causes	1,101	219	19.9	2,789	525	18.8	0.76	5.82	1.00
Death-All Cardiovascular (CV)	1,101	190	17.3	2,789	481	17.2	0.01	7.61	1.00
Death-All Non-Cardiovascular	1,101	23	2.1	2,789	35	1.1	1.93	0.83	0.83
Death-Cause Unknown	1,101	6	0.5	2,789	9	0.3	1.01	1.09	1.00
Death-All CHD	1,101	162	14.7	2,789	410	14.7	0.01	6.29	1.00
Death-All Sudden CV	1,101	82	7.4	2,789	246	8.8	-1.39	1.77	0.93
Death-All Cancer	1,101	14	1.3	2,789	13	0.5	2.73	0.28	0.09
Death-Lung Cancer	1,101	6	0.5	2,789	4	0.1	2.23	0.72	0.38
Definite Nonfatal Myocardial Infarction (MI)	1,059	121	11.4	2,693	306	11.4	0.05	2.46	0.92
MI Incidence (Definite Nonfatal MI or Coronary Death)	1,101	256	23.3	2,789	652	23.4	-0.08	4.86	1.00
Definite Fatal or Nonfatal Pulmonary Embolism	1,101	17	1.5	2,789	22	0.8	2.13	0.43	0.32
Definite or Suspect Fatal or Nonfatal Pulmonary Embolism or Thrombophlebitis	1,101	52	4.7	2,789	82	2.9	2.75	0.19	0.17

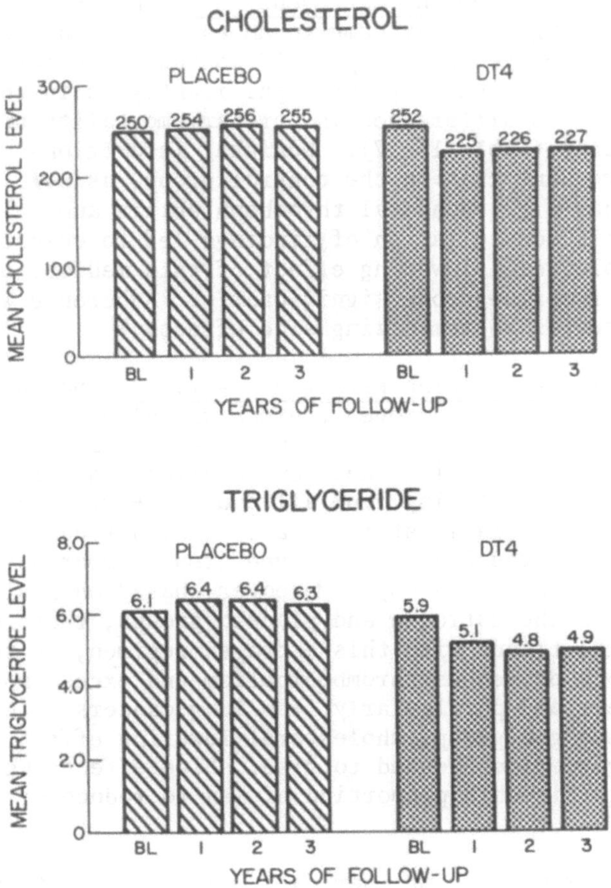

Figure 2 Mean levels of serum cholesterol and fasting triglycerides at baseline and at annual intervals for the dextrothyroxine and placebo groups respectively--cohort of patients completing at least three years of follow-up (9).

Results

Significant results are available in regard to the three major goals of the CDP (2-10). This report summarizes the findings respecting the first objective of the CDP, i.e., assessment of the long-term efficacy of the five drug regimens (7-10).

Mixed conjugated equine estrogens -- 5.0 mg. per day: The group given estrogen 5 mg. per day came to an early termination in May, 1970, after an average follow-up of 18 months. The total mortality experience was negative, but not significantly so in the statistical sense, nor were differences in coronary mortality or sudden death significant (Table 1) (7). Nonfatal infarctions were significantly more frequent than in the control group, as were thromboembolic phenomena (e.g., nonfatal thrombophlebitis and pulmonary embolism) and this constellation of findings led to cessation of this regimen. (Cholesterol-lowering effect of this medication was modest, and serum triglycerides rose significantly. Adherence was poor because of troublesome feminizing side effects.)

Mixed conjugated equine estrogens -- 2.5 mg. per day: Early in 1973, the lower dose estrogen regimen was also discontinued (8). With an average follow-up of 56 months, the data indicated no evidence of an overall positive therapeutic effect in terms of the CDP's primary end point, mortality from all causes (Fig. 1 and Table 2)(8). Rather, there was a small, statistically insignificant excess of total mortality in the 2.5 mg. estrogen group compared to the placebo group (19.9% vs 18.8%). Moreover, based on small numbers of cases in both the estrogen and placebo groups, there were suggestions of adverse trends with this estrogen regimen, in the form of excess incidence of venous thromboembolism and excess mortality from all cancers and particularly from lung cancers. (As with the higher-dose estrogen group, cholesterol-lowering effect was slight and serum triglycerides tended to rise. Side effects were troublesome, leading a sizeable proportion of men to reduce or stop this medication.)

Dextrothyroxine, 6.0 mg. per day: Adherence to this regimen was good. As of February 1, 1970, with an average of 18 months of follow-up, the CDP had recorded evidence suggesting an excess risk of mortality with its dextrothyroxine regimen for a small subgroup of 27 post-MI patients with frequent ectopic ventricular beats in the resting ECG at entry. For this reason, this medication was stopped in 1970 as a precautionary measure for the survivors of this subgroup (7).

In December, 1971 treatment with d-thyroxine 6.0 mg. per day was stopped for all patients, despite sustained reduction in the intermediate end point--serum lipids (Fig. 2) (9). Total mortality was in excess over the control group, reaching almost statistically significant values (Fig. 3 and Table 3). Extensive analyses were

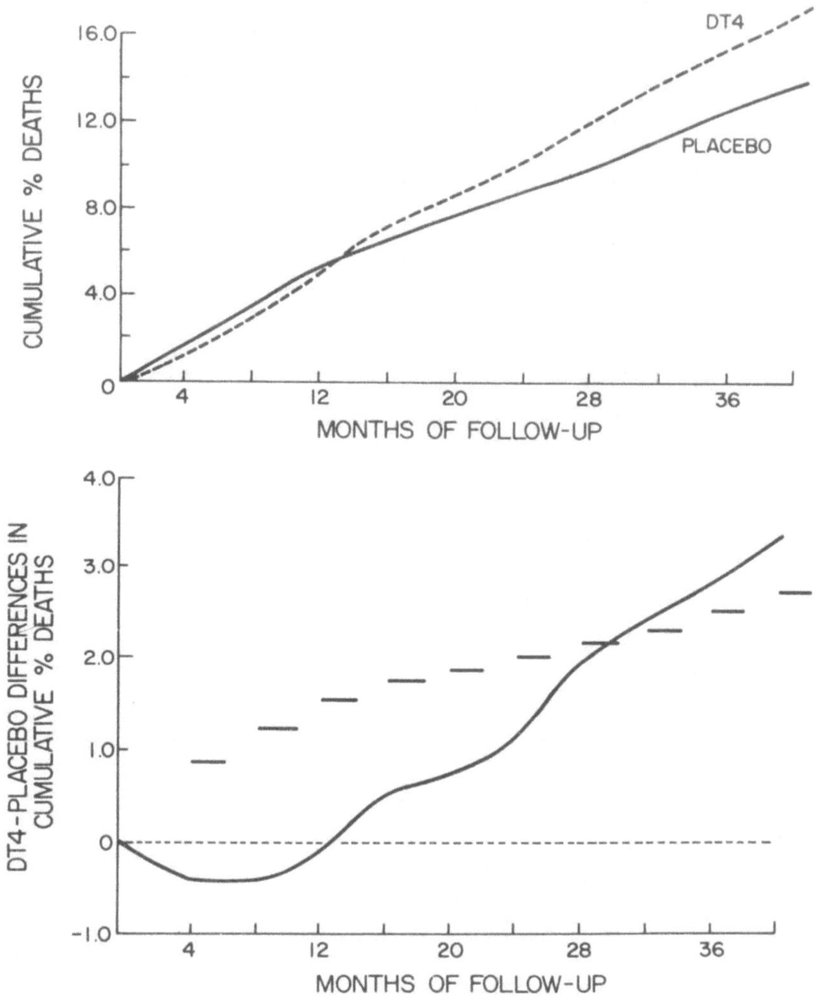

Figure 3 Life table cumulative rates for deaths from all causes for the dextrothyroxine and placebo groups over 40 months of follow-up (upper graph), and the differences between the placebo and dextrothyroxine groups in these cumulative rates (lower graph). Broken lines in the lower graph denote two standard error values at various time points (9).

TABLE 3

Nonfatal and Fatal Events by Cause, Dextrothyroxine and Placebo Groups*

Event	DT4			Placebo			DT4-Placebo	% Difference DT4 - Placebo
	No.of Men	No.of Events	Per-Cent	No.of Men	No.of Events	Per-Cent	S.E.of Diff.	Placebo
1. Death -- All Causes	1,083	160	14.8	2,715	339	12.5	1.88	+ 18.4
2. Death -- All Cardiovascular	1,083	146	13.5	2,715	317	11.7	1.54	+ 15.4
3. Death -- Non-Cardiovascular	1,083	9	0.8	2,715	19	0.7	0.43	**
4. Death -- Cause Unknown	1,083	5	0.5	2,715	3	0.1	2.13	**
5. Death -- All CHD	1,083	119	11.0	2,715	274	10.1	0.82	+ 8.9
6. Death -- Sudden CV	1,083	63	5.8	2,715	162	6.0	0.18	- 3.3
7. Definite Nonfatal MI	1,053	89	8.5	2,618	202	7.7	0.75	+ 10.4
8. Major Coronary Events (Def. Nonfatal MI + CHD Death)	1,083	197	18.2	2,715	449	16.5	1.22	+ 10.3
9. All Suspect or Definite CV Events (Nonfatal or Fatal)	1,083	736	68.0	2,715	1,758	64.8	1.88	+ 4.9

* Excludes 27 DT4 and 74 Placebo patients with frequent ectopic ventricular beats (FEVBs) at entry (1, 7).

**Per cent changes not calculated when per cent deceased was less than 1.0.

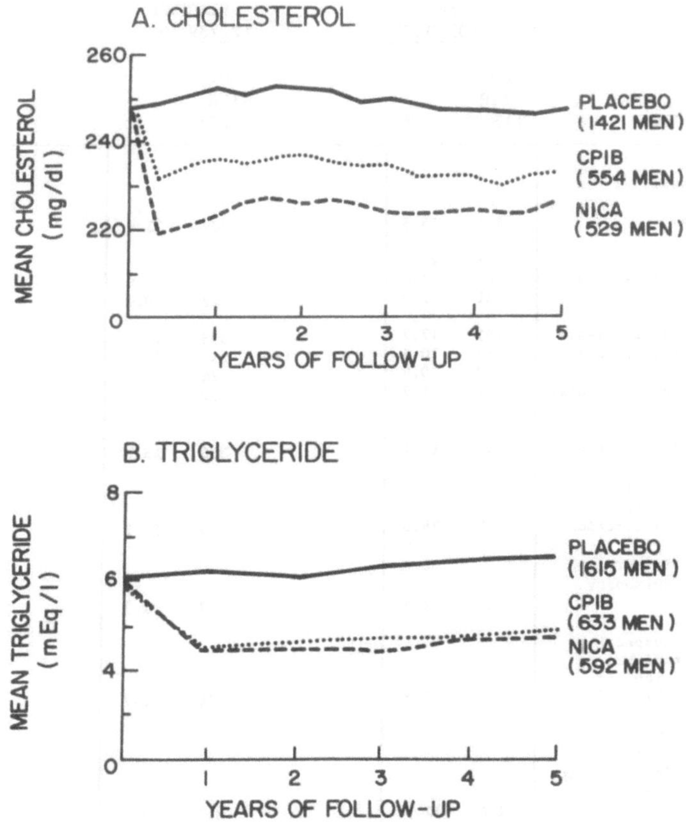

Figure 4 Mean levels of serum cholesterol (in mg/dl) and serum triglyceride (in mEq/l) at baseline and four month (for cholesterol) or annual (for triglyceride) intervals, for the cohorts of men observed for at least five years with no missing determinations (10).

TABLE 4

Death by Cause and Nonfatal Events, Total Follow-Up Experience

EVENT	CPIB (1,103 MEN) NO. WITH EVENT	CPIB %	PLACEBO (2,789 MEN) NO. WITH EVENT	PLACEBO %	Z-VALUES CPIB-PLACEBO*
Death by cause:					
All causes	281	25.5	709	25.4	0.04
All cardiovascular	241	21.8	633	22.7	-0.57
All noncardiovascular	29	2.6	54	1.9	1.35
Cause unknown	11	1.0	22	0.8	0.64
Coronary heart disease	195	17.7	535	19.2	-1.08
Sudden cardiovascular	116	10.5	319	11.4	-0.82
All cancer	10	0.9	24	0.9	0.14
Other noncardiovascular	19	1.7	30	1.1	1.63
Definite, nonfatal myocardial infarction	144	13.1	386	13.8	-0.64
Coronary death or definite, nonfatal myocardial infarction	309	28.0	839	30.1	-1.27
Definite (fatal or nonfatal) pulmonary embolism	26	2.4	37	1.3	2.30
Definite or suspect fatal or nonfatal pulmonary embolism or thrombophlebitis	64	5.8	104	3.7	2.87
Definite or suspect fatal or nonfatal stroke or intermittent cerebral ischemic attack	136	12.3	311	11.2	1.04
Any definite or suspect fatal or nonfatal cardiovascular event	951	86.2	2333	83.7	1.99

* In view of the multiple statistical comparisons made in this study, it is the judgement of the CDP Research Group that a result should not be judged "statistically significant" unless it achieves at least the 1.0% ($p \leq .01$) level of significance ($Z > 2.58$ or $Z < -2.58$) or perhaps even the 0.5% ($p \leq .005$) significance level ($Z > 2.81$ or $Z < -2.81$) (10).

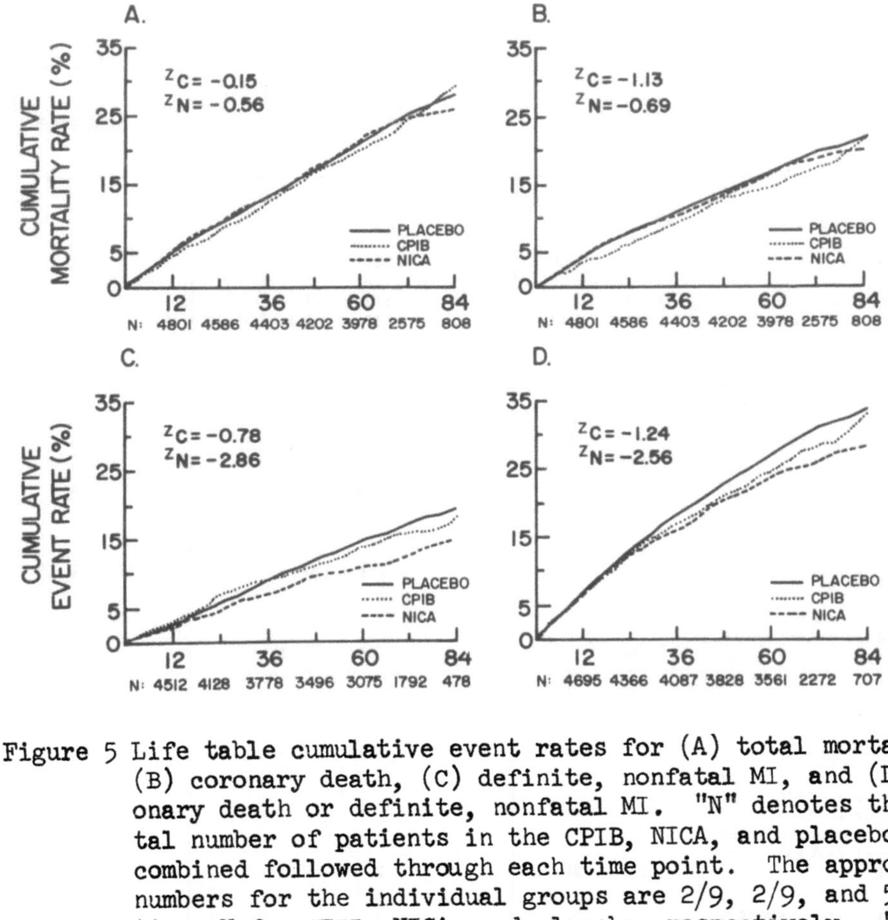

Figure 5 Life table cumulative event rates for (A) total mortality, (B) coronary death, (C) definite, nonfatal MI, and (D) coronary death or definite, nonfatal MI. "N" denotes the total number of patients in the CPIB, NICA, and placebo groups combined followed through each time point. The approximate numbers for the individual groups are 2/9, 2/9, and 5/9 times N for CPIB, NICA, and placebo, respectively. "z_C" and "z_N" denote z-values for the CPIB-placebo and NICA-placebo comparisons, respectively, of the total life table curves (10).

TABLE 5

Deaths by Cause and Nonfatal Events, Five-Year Rates

EVENT	CPIB (1,103 MEN) NO. WITH EVENT	CPIB (1,103 MEN) %	PLACEBO (2,789 MEN) NO. WITH EVENT	PLACEBO (2,789 MEN) %	Z-VALUES CPIB-PLACEBO*
Death by cause:					
All causes	221	20.0	583	20.9	-0.60
All cardiovascular	191	17.3	528	18.9	-1.17
All noncardiovascular	23	2.1	42	1.5	1.27
Cause unknown	7	0.6	13	0.5	0.66
Coronary heart disease	156	14.1	452	16.2	-1.60
Sudden cardiovascular	93	8.4	269	9.6	-1.17
All cancer	7	0.6	16	0.6	0.22
Other noncardiovascular	16	1.5	26	0.9	1.41
Definite, nonfatal myocardial infarction	128	11.6	339	12.2	-0.48
Coronary death or definite, nonfatal myocardial infarction	263	23.8	731	26.2	-1.53
Definite (fatal or nonfatal) pulmonary embolism	20	1.8	30	1.1	1.84
Definite or suspect fatal or nonfatal pulmonary embolism or thrombophlebitis	57	5.2	91	3.3	2.80
Definite or suspect fatal or nonfatal stroke or intermittent cerebral ischemic attack	117	10.6	271	9.7	0.84
Any definite or suspect fatal or nonfatal cardiovascular event	929	84.2	2251	80.7	2.56

* See footnote for Table 4.

TABLE 6

Five-Year Percentages of Deaths by Lipid Findings at Entry

LIPID FINDINGS AT ENTRY		CPIB NO. OF MEN	CPIB % DEATHS	PLACEBO NO. OF MEN	PLACEBO % DEATHS	Z-VALUES CPIB-PLACEBO*
Serum cholesterol						
< 250 mg/dl		573	20.4	1482	19.7	0.36
≥ 250 mg/dl		530	19.6	1307	22.3	-1.25
Serum triglyceride						
< 5 mEq/l		550	18.5	1390	20.9	-1.15
≥ 5 mEq/l		552	21.4	1399	20.9	0.21
Serum cholest. by triglyc.						
< 250 mg/dl	< 5 mEq/l	358	19.0	905	18.5	0.22
< 250 mg/dl	≥ 5 mEq/l	215	22.8	577	21.7	0.34
≥ 250 mg/dl	< 5 mEq/l	192	17.7	485	25.4	-2.13
≥ 250 mg/dl	≥ 5 mEq/l	337	20.5	822	20.4	0.01
Serum cholest. by triglyc.						
< 280 mg/dl	< 6 mEq/l	608	17.4	1458	20.0	-1.36
< 280 mg/dl	≥ 6 mEq/l	224	27.7	640	20.5	2.23
≥ 280 mg/dl	< 6 mEq/l	118	22.0	321	24.9	-0.63
≥ 280 mg/dl	≥ 6 mEq/l	152	17.1	370	21.6	-1.17

* See footnote for Table 4.

done to ascertain subgroups in which this excess mortality might be concentrated. A maximal difference was found for patients who either had had repeated infarcts or had survived one complicated infarct (that is, Risk Group 2 patients), patients who had a definite history of angina pectoris on entry in the study, and patients who on entry had a resting heart rate of 70 or more beats per minute on electrocardiogram. The mortality in the placebo control group for this subgroup was 20.5 per cent while in the DT-4 treated group it was 39.3 per cent.

Among other things, this experience drives home the lesson that benefit: risk ratios for drugs for coronary disease cannot be predicted -- in terms of decisive end points of morbidity and mortality over years -- by their effects on any intermediate end point, e.g., serum lipids. Only that "late painful ordeal", the controlled mass field trial, can give a definitive answer, especially when -- as with drugs -- there is always bound to be some risk.

Clofibrate, 1.8 gm. per day: As reported above, three of the study regimens - 5.0 mg/day of estrogen, 6.0 mg/day of dextrothyroxine sodium, and 2.5 mg/day of estrogen - were discontinued in 1970, 1971,and 1973, respectively, before the scheduled end of the trial in late 1974, because of trends indicative of adverse effect. All patients in the three remaining treatment groups - clofibrate, niacin, and placebo - had their study medication discontinued during June through August 1974 at the planned conclusion of the project. Almost all of the surviving patients in these three groups completed at least five years of follow-up.

Adherence to clofibrate was excellent throughout (10). The drug produced the expected moderate sustained fall in serum cholesterol and marked fall in serum triglycerides (Fig. 4) (10). Nevertheless, no evidence was obtained of significant efficacy of clofibrate with regard to total mortality or cause-specific mortality (Table 4 and Fig. 5) (10). The five-year total mortalities were 20.0% for clofibrate and 20.9% for placebo (Table 5) (10). This small difference does not approach statistical significance. Considering the total follow-up experience - ranging up to 8 1/2 years for some patients - the mortality in the clofibrate group (25.5%) was nearly the same as that in the placebo group (25.4%). No subgroups of the study population were identified in which clofibrate showed clear benefits with regard to mortality. Specifically, no clear cut, consistent significant reduction in mortality was recorded with this drug regimen for men hyperlipidemic at entry (Table 6) (10). There were somewhat - but not statistically significant - lower rates in the clofibrate group with respect to coronary death and the combination of coronary death or definite, nonfatal myocardial infarction. Furthermore, there was a statistically significant excess incidence of thromboembolism, angina pectoris, intermittent claudication and cardiac arrhythmia in the clofibrate group, as well as an excess incidence of the endpoint of any definite or suspected nonfatal cardiovascular event as compared with the placebo group.

TABLE 7

Death by Cause and Nonfatal Events, Total Follow-Up Experience

EVENT	NICA (1,119 MEN) NO. WITH EVENT	%	PLACEBO (2,789 MEN) NO. WITH EVENT	%	Z-VALUES NICA-PLACEBO*
Death by cause:					
All causes	273	24.4	709	25.4	-0.67
All cardiovascular	238	21.3	633	22.7	-0.97
All noncardiovascular	30	2.7	54	1.9	1.45
Cause unknown	5	0.4	22	0.8	-1.17
Coronary heart disease	203	18.1	535	19.2	-0.75
Sudden cardiovascular	133	11.9	319	11.4	0.40
All cancer	9	0.8	24	0.9	-0.17
Other noncardiovascular	21	1.9	30	1.1	1.99
Definite, nonfatal myocardial infarction	114	10.2	386	13.8	-3.09
Coronary death or definite, nonfatal myocardial infarction	287	25.6	839	30.1	-2.77
Definite (fatal or nonfatal) pulmonary embolism	12	1.1	37	1.3	-0.65
Definite or suspect fatal or nonfatal pulmonary embolism or thrombophlebitis	49	4.4	104	3.7	0.95
Definite or suspect fatal or nonfatal stroke or intermittent cerebral ischemic attack	95	8.5	311	11.2	-2.46
Any definite or suspect fatal or nonfatal cardiovascular event	914	81.7	2333	83.7	-1.49

* See footnote for Table 4.

TABLE 8

Deaths by Cause and Nonfatal Events, Five-Year Rates

EVENT	NICA (1,119 MEN) NO. WITH EVENT	NICA (1,119 MEN) %	PLACEBO (2,789 MEN) NO. WITH EVENT	PLACEBO (2,789 MEN) %	Z-VALUES NICA-PLACEBO*
Death by cause:					
All causes	237	21.2	583	20.9	0.19
All cardiovascular	210	18.8	528	18.9	-0.12
All noncardiovascular	24	2.1	42	1.5	1.40
Cause unknown	3	0.3	13	0.5	-0.88
Coronary heart disease	178	15.9	452	16.2	-0.23
Sudden cardiovascular	118	10.5	269	9.6	0.85
All cancer	7	0.6	16	0.6	0.19
Other noncardiovascular	17	1.5	26	0.9	1.59
Definite, nonfatal myocardial infarction	100	8.9	339	12.2	-2.88
Coronary death or definite, nonfatal myocardial infarction	255	22.8	731	26.2	-2.23
Definite (fatal or nonfatal) pulmonary embolism	11	1.0	30	1.1	-0.26
Definite or suspect fatal or nonfatal pulmonary embolism or thrombophlebitis	44	3.9	91	3.3	1.04
Definite or suspect fatal or nonfatal stroke or intermittent cerebral ischemic attack	86	7.7	271	9.7	-1.99
Any definite or suspect fatal or nonfatal cardiovascular event	875	78.2	2251	80.7	-1.78

* See footnote for Table 4.

TABLE 9

Five-Year Percentages of Deaths by Lipid Findings at Entry

LIPID FINDINGS AT ENTRY	NICA NO. OF MEN	NICA % DEATHS	PLACEBO NO. OF MEN	PLACEBO % DEATHS	Z-VALUES NICA-PLACEBO*
Serum cholesterol					
< 250 mg/dl	577	21.5	1482	19.7	0.91
≥ 250 mg/dl	542	20.8	1307	22.3	-0.67
Serum triglyceride					
< 5 mEq/l	530	21.7	1390	20.9	0.40
≥ 5 mEq/l	589	20.7	1399	20.9	-0.12
Serum cholest. by triglyc.					
< 250 mg/dl < 5 mEq/l	346	20.2	905	18.5	0.72
< 250 mg/dl ≥ 5 mEq/l	231	23.4	577	21.7	0.53
≥ 250 mg/dl < 5 mEq/l	184	24.5	485	25.4	-0.24
≥ 250 mg/dl ≥ 5 mEq/l	358	19.0	822	20.4	-0.57
Serum cholest. by triglyc.					
< 280 mg/dl < 6 mEq/l	584	21.1	1458	20.0	0.52
< 280 mg/dl ≥ 6 mEq/l	249	18.9	640	20.5	-0.53
≥ 280 mg/dl < 6 mEq/l	126	25.4	321	24.9	0.10
≥ 280 mg/dl ≥ 6 mEq/l	160	21.9	370	21.6	0.06

* See footnote for Table 4.

A noncardiovascular finding of importance was a more than twofold increase in incidence of gallstones in patients treated with clofibrate (10). The findings of the Newcastle (2) and Scottish (13) clofibrate studies - that clofibrate may be effective in reducing mortality and recurrent myocardial infarction in persons with a prior history of angina pectoris - were not confirmed by the Coronary Drug Project data.

In conclusion, the Coronary Drug Project provides no evidence on which to recommend the use of clofibrate in the treatment of persons with coronary heart disease.

Niacin, 3 gm. per day: Adherence to this regimen was good, and a sizeable sustained fall in serum lipids resulted (Fig. 4) (10). Nevertheless, no evidence was recorded indicating efficacy of niacin with regard to total mortality and cause-specific mortality (Tables 7 and 8, Fig. 5) (10). The five-year total mortality for niacin was slightly higher than that for the placebo group (21.2% vs 20.9%) (Table 8) (10). For the total follow-up experience, the niacin group had a somewhat-but not statistically significant-lower mortality (24.4%) than the placebo group (25.4%) (Table 7) (10). No subgroup of patients was identified in which niacin showed a definite beneficial effect with respect to five-year total mortality. No evidence of significant reduction in mortality was recorded with niacin administration for men hyperlipidemic at entry (Table 9) (10). The niacin group did experience a statistically significant lower incidence of definite nonfatal myocardial infarction than the placebo group; the five-year rates were 8.9% for niacin and 12.2% for placebo, while the incidence for the total follow-up experience was 10.2% for niacin and 13.8% for placebo (Tables 7 and 8, Fig. 5) (10). On the other hand, incidence of atrial fibrillation and of other cardiac arrhythmias was statistically significantly higher among men taking niacin than in the placebo group. Data from this study confirmed previously reported findings of increased incidence of gastrointestinal problems and elevated levels of serum enzymes, serum uric acid, and plasma glucose in men taking niacin (10). The long-term clinical significance of these chemical changes is unknown.

In conclusion, the Coronary Drug Project data yield no evidence that niacin influences mortality of survivors of myocardial infarction; this medication may be slightly beneficial in protecting persons to some degree against recurrent nonfatal myocardial infarction. However, because of the excess incidence of arrhythmias, gastrointestinal problems, and abnormal chemistry findings in the niacin group, great care and caution must be exercised if this drug is to be used for treatment of persons with coronary heart disease.

Discussion

The results of the Coronary Drug Project were consistently negative in regard to ability of any of the five drug regimens to prolong life of middle-aged men recovered from one or more myocardial infarctions. Lack of efficacy with regard to this key and primary end point of the study was recorded although three of the agents -- clofibrate, dextrothyroxine and niacin -- effected a sustained significant reduction in levels of both serum cholesterol and triglycerides. What are the broader implications of these facts, if any?

To address this important question scientifically, other key facts must be considered: In its studies on the natural history of coronary heart disease, utilizing data from the 2,789 placebo patients, the CDP has shown that baseline serum cholesterol (but not triglyceride) levels are independently related to long-term prognosis for men recovered from MI, as they are related to first events (5, 14, 15). While this association is undoubtedly statistically significant for post-MI men, it is a modest one quantitatively. For example, the long-term CDP data yield a slope of only .05 for the unadjusted and adjusted (38 other variables) relationship between baseline serum cholesterol level and five-year mortality from all causes (16). Concretely, this means that for men with mean entry serum cholesterol at about 260 mg./dl., five-year mortality was 21.4 per cent. For men at about 234 mg./dl. (26 mg./dl. or 10% lower), five year mortality was 20.1 per cent, i.e., a mortality rate 6.1 per cent lower. For men at about 208 mg./dl. at entry (52 mg./dl. or 20% lower than 260 mg./dl.), five year mortality was 18.8 per cent i.e., a mortality rate 12.1 per cent lower than that recorded for the men with serum cholesterol of 260 mg./dl. at baseline. This is a modest difference in mortality for a sizeable difference in serum cholesterol -- a difference a good deal greater than effected by any of the drugs used in this study. Thus the original goal set by the CDP in the mid-1960s (before any data of the foregoing type were available), to detect a 25 per cent reduction in mortality possibly related to serum cholesterol reduction, clearly emerges now as unrealistic. Since the CDP data do indicate a relationship between serum cholesterol and long-term prognosis for post-MI men, however modest, the possibility remains that sustained reduction in serum cholesterol by safe means -- e.g., by diet -- can improve life expectancy for such patients. Even a 5 or 10 per cent improvement would be welcome under the circumstances, if possible. Of course, the data from the CDP -- a drug trial -- can throw no light on whether this possibility is real, and a trial to detect a difference in five-year mortality of even 10 per cent would require a very large sample size, much bigger than the CDP, even for a study involving only two groups (diet treatment and control). The likelihood that such a study will be mounted in the foreseeable future is remote. Therefore, physicians have to make a scientific judgment on the best approaches to the treatment of their post-MI patients, based on the available evidence. That evidence indicates the wisdom of reducing serum cholesterol levels by safe -- particularly nutritional -- means.

It should be further clear that the data reported here, from a study of post-MI men, permit no scientific inferences about the value of serum cholesterol reduction -- by drugs and/or diet -- for the prevention of first coronary episodes. The CDP data show very clearly that the factors most powerfully related to long-term prognosis after recovery from MI are not the primary risk factors (hyercholesterolemia, cigarette smoking, hypertension), but rather findings indicative of status of the myocardium -- e.g., ST segment depression on resting ECG, major Q waves, AV conduction disturbances, multiple premature ventricular beats, tachycardia, cardiomegaly on teleroentgenogram (2-5). That is, persons post-MI are very different from persons pre-MI, even very coronary-prone persons. Therefore, extrapolation of CDP findings to the problem of primary prevention of coronary heart disease is unscientific. Every reason remains to continue and extend efforts to achieve the primary prevention of this epidemic disease by use of safe means of control of major risk factors, including hypercholesterolemia (14). In fact, the CDP findings -- by highlighting the impact of residual cardiac damage on prognosis for post-MI patients -- serve to underscore the soundness and importance of a strategy emphasizing primary prevention as the key to controlling this epidemic.

The key bodies of the Coronary Drug Project and their senior staff members are as follows:

Policy Board: Robert W. Wilkins, M.D. (Chairman); Jacob E.Bearman, Ph.D.; Edwin Boyle, M.D.; William M. Smith, M.D., M.P.H.; Christian R. Klimt, M.D., D.P.H. (ex-officio); Jeremiah Stamler, M.D. (ex-officio); Max Halperin, Ph.D. (ex-officio); William J. Zukel, M.D. (ex-officio). Past Member: Louis Lasagna, M.D.

Steering Committee: Jeremiah Stamler, M.D. (Chairman); Kenneth G. Berge, M.D. (Vice-Chairman); David M. Berkson, M.D.; William Bernstein, M.D.; Henry Blackburn,M.D.; Joseph H. Boutwell, M.D.; Jerome Cornfield; Lawrence Friedman, M.D.; Nicholas J. Galluzzi, M.D.; I. Lewis, M.D.; Jessie Marmorston, M.D.; William J. Zukel, M.D. Past Members: Gerald Cooper, M.D.; Milton Nichaman, M.D.; William Parsons, Jr., M.D.; Henry Schoch, M.D.; William Vicic, M.D.

Coordinating Center: Christian R. Klimt, M.D., D.P.H. (Director); Curtis L. Meinert, Ph.D. (Deputy Director); Paul L. Canner, Ph.D.; Sandra Forman, M.S.; Elizabeth C. Heinz; Yih-Min Bill Huang, Ph.D.; Genell L. Knatterud, Ph.D.; William F. Krol, Ph.D. Past Members: David R. Jacobs, Jr., Ph.D.; Suketami Tominaga, M.D.

Central Laboratory: Joseph H. Boutwell, M.D. (Medical Director); Dayton Miller, Ph.D. (Chief); John Donahue, M.S.; James Gill, Jr., M.S.; Sara Gill. Past members: Gerald R. Cooper, M.D.; Eloise Eavenson, Ph.D.; Adrian Hainline, M.D.; Alan Mather, Ph.D.; Margie

Sailors.

ECG Center: Henry Blackburn, M.D. (Director of the Laboratory of Physiological Hygiene); Ronald J. Prineas, M.D. (Director of the ECG Center); Gretchen Newman. Past member: Robin MacGregor.

National Heart and Lung Institute Staff: Thomas Blaszkowski, Ph.D; William Friedewald, M.D.; Lawrence Friedman, M.D.; Max Halperin, Ph.D.; William J. Zukel, M.D. Past Members: Clifford Bachrach, M.D.; Jerome Cornfield; Eleanor Darby, Ph.D.; Michael Davidson, M.D.; Terrance Fisher, M. D.; Starr Ford, Jr., M.D.; William Goldwater, Ph.D.; Richard Havlik, M.D.; Thomas Landau, M.D.; Hubert Loncin, M.D.; Howard Marsh, M.D., Ph.D.; John Turner, M.D.; William Vicic, M.D.

Drug Procurement and Distribution Center: Salvatore D. Gasdia (Officer in Charge)

Editorial Review Board: Jeremiah Stamler, M.D. (Chairman); Kenneth G. Berge, M.D.; Henry Blackburn, M.D.; Jerome Cornfield; William Friedewald, M.D.; Lawrence Friedman, M.D.; Max Halperin, Ph.D., Christian R. Klimt, M.D., D.P.H.; Bernard Tabatznik, M.D.; Robert W. Wilkins, M.D.; Nanette Wenger, M.D.

Data and Safety Monitoring Committee: Jeremiah Stamler, M.D. and Curtis L. Meinert, Ph.D. (Co-Chairman); E.Cowles Andrus, M.D.; Kenneth G. Berge, M.D.; Paul L. Canner, Ph.D.; Thomas Chalmers, M.D.; Jerome Cornfield; William T. Friedewald, M.D.; Lawrence Friedman, M.D.; James Gillette, M.D.; Max Halperin, Ph.D.; Gerald Katskin, M.D.; Christian R. Klimt, M.D., D.P.H.; Robert Levy, M.D.; Dayton T. Miller, Ph.D.; Ronald Prineas, M.D. Past members: Henry Blackburn, M.D.; Fred Ederer; Adrian Hainline, Ph.D.; Elliot Newman, M.D.

Principal Investigators, Clinical Research Centers: Kenneth G. Berge, M.D.; Nicholas J. Galluzzi, M.D.; Jessie Marmorston, M.D.; James A. Schoenberger, M.D.; Samuel Baer, M.D.; Henry K. Schoch, M.D.; J. Richard Warbasse, M.D.; Robert M. Kohn, M.D.; Bernard I. Lewis, M.D.; Richard J. Jones, M.D.; Kenneth H. Hyatt, M.D.; Dean A. Emanuel, M.D.; David Z. Morgan, M.D.; David M. Berkson, M.D.; William H. Bernstein, M.D.; Ernst Greif, M.D.; Richard R. Pyle, M.D.; Ephraim Donoso, M.D.; Jacob I. Haft, M.D.; Gordon L. Maurice, M.D.; Ralph Lazzara, M.D.; Irving M. Liebow, M.D.; Marvin S. Segal, M.D.; Charles B. Moore, M.D.; John H. Morledge, M.D.; Olga M. Haring, M.D.; Robert C. Schlant, M.D.; Joseph A. Wagner, M.D.; Ward Laramore, M.D.; Donald McCaughan, M.D.; Robert W. Oblath, M.D.; Peter C. Gazes, M.D.; Bernard Tabatznik, M.D.; Richard G. Hutchinson, M.D.; Mario Garcia-Palmieri, M.D.; Nathaniel G. Berk, M.D.; Robert L. Grissom, M.D.; Ralph C. Scott, M.D.; Frank L. Canosa, M.D.; Charles A. Laubach, Jr.,

M.D.; Ralph E. Cole, M.D.; Thaddeus E. Prout, M.D.; Bernard A. Sachs, M.D.; Ernest O. Theilen, M.D.; C. Basil Williams, M.D.; Edward L. Michals, M.D.; Fred I. Gilbert, Jr., M.D.; Sidney A. Levine, M.D.; Louis B. Matthews, Jr., M.D.; Irving Ershler, M.D.; Elmer E. Cooper, M.D.; Allan H. Barker, M.D.; Paul Samuel, M.D.

The Coronary Drug Project was carried out as a Collaborative Study supported by research grants and other funds from the National Heart and Lung Institute.

REFERENCES:

1. Coronary Drug Project Research Group, The Coronary Drug Project; Design, Methods and Baseline Results. Circulation, 47, Suppl. 1, 1973.
2. Coronary Drug Project Research Group. The Prognostic Importance of the Electrocardiogram after Myocardial Infarction. Experience in the Coronary Drug Project. Ann. Intern. Med., 77, 677, 1972.
3. Coronary Drug Project Research Group. Prognostic Importance of Premature Beats Following Myocardial Infarction. Experience in the Coronary Drug Project. J.A.M.A., 223, 1116, 1973.
4. Coronary Drug Project Research Group. Left Ventricular Hypertrophy Patterns and Prognosis: Experience Postinfarction in the Coronary Drug Project. Circulation, 49, 863, 1974.
5. Coronary Drug Project Research Group. Factors Influencing Long-Term Prognosis after Recovery from Myocardial Infarction--Three-Year Findings of the Coronary Drug Project. J.Chron. Dis., 27, 267, 1974.
6. Coronary Drug Project Research Group. The Coronary Drug Project--A Secondary Prevention Trial. Schetter, G. and Weizel, A., Eds., Atherosclerosis III, Springer-Verlag, Berlin/New York, p.729,1974.
7. Coronary Drug Project Research Group. The Coronary Drug Project: Initial Findings Leading to Modifications of Its Research Protocol. J.A.M.A., 214, 1303, 1970.
8. Coronary Drug Project Research Group. The Coronary Drug Project: Findings Leading to Discontinuation of the 2.5 mg/day Estrogen Group. J.A.M.A., 226, 652, 1973.
9. Coronary Drug Project Research Group. The Coronary Drug Project: Findings Leading to Further Modifications of Its Protocol with Respect to Dextrothyroxine. J.A.M.A., 220, 996, 1972.
10. Coronary Drug Project Research Group. The Coronary Drug Project: Clofibrate and Niacin in Coronary Heart Disease. J.A.M.A., 231, 360, 1975.
11. Cornfield J., Bayesian Outlook and Its Application. Biometrics, 25, 617, 1969.
12. Physicians of the Newcastle upon Tyne Region. Trial of Clofibrate, in the Treatment of Ischaemic Heart Disease. Brit. Med. J., 4, 767, 1971

13. Research Committee of the Scottish Society of Physicians. Ischaemic Heart Disease: A Secondary Prevention Trial using Clofibrate. Brit. Med. J., 4, 775, 1971.
14. Inter-Society Commission for Heart Disease Resources. Atherosclerosis Study Group and Epidemiology Study Group. Primary Prevention of the Atherosclerotic Diseases. Wright, I.S. and Fredrickson, D.T., Eds., Cardiovascular Diseases--Guidelines for Prevention and Care, U.S. Government Printing Office, Washington, D.C., p. 15, 1974.
15. Stamler, J., Berkson, D.M. and Lindberg, H.A. Risk Factors: Their Role in the Etiology and Pathogenesis of the Atherosclerotic Diseases. Wissler, R.W. and Geer, J.C., Eds., Pathogenesis of Atherosclerosis, Williams and Wilkins, Baltimore, Md., p.14, 1972.
16. Coronary Drug Project Research Group. The Natural History of Myocardial Infarction in the Coronary Drug Project: Prognostic Importance of Serum Lipid Levels, in press.

PRESENTED on behalf of The Coronary Drug Project Research Group

(5)

THE PLACE OF AORTO-CORONARY BY-PASS SURGERY IN THE TREATMENT OF ISCHEMIC HEART DISEASE

LUCIEN CAMPEAU, M.D.

MONTREAL HEART INSTITUTE

5000 East, Belanger Street, Montreal, Quebec, Canada

Our therapeutic approach to ischemic heart disease has undoubtedly changed during the past 8 years since the introduction of aortocoronary bypass surgery. An overview of the objectives and results of this surgery appears necessary before discussing its place in the treatment of the different clinical manifestations of ischemic heart disease. I shall then discuss firstly the indications generally accepted at the present time, and finally uncertain indications which are advocated by some centers but which remain questionable.

The objectives of an ideal mode of therapy should be twofold: improvement of the quality and prolongation of life. This surgery appears to increase the quality of life in most cases and it seems to do so more effectively than medical therapy (1). It relieves effort angina in most patients but it is not certain that it improves heart failure. Whether it prolongs life still remains uncertain. This however is a pertinent question since medical therapy has not been shown effective in that respect, although the preventive effect of the constant use of newer drugs such as the beta-blockers, platelet aggregation inhibitors, the control of known risk factors, and physical training are still unknown.

Quality of life

La "joie de vivre" is a difficult parameter to evaluate but it is nevertheless a real one. After interviewing personally over 800 of these patients 1 to 5 years after surgery, we are convinced that surgery promotes a sense of well being, an emotional state free of the anxiety so common to patients with ischemic heart disease, and confidence in their ability to enjoy a normal life. Their gratitude is extremely rewarding, although occasionally, it has been disquieting when in fact nothing had been done, their grafts being occluded.

Only 58% of our male patients below the age of 65 have returned to a gainful employment, but apparently more resume legitimate recreational activities, including sex. Return to work is a poor criteria for the evaluation of surgical results since it depends on many factors. It was found in our series that failure to return to work was observed more frequently in patients having primary level schooling, no special training nor trade, and having had jobs requiring moderate to heavy exertion. This indeed may suggest that most of these patients did not have a sufficiently good tolerance to exercise to resume these activities although most deny having angina during current activities of life. Many are refused by their employers in spite of a favourable medical report. Some patients prefer off-work social benefits and continue an unofficial job on the side without having to pay income tax as an added bonus. Return to work therefore involves many socio-economical factors in addition to the patient's state of health, and the potential return to work should be analyzed carefully whenever the inability to work is the prevalent indication for surgery.

Relief of effort angina

We have observed among our first 1000 patients having bypass surgery without internal mammary artery implantation, left ventricular wall segmental resection or other non coronary cardiac surgery, that angina has disappeared completely in 70%, decreased in 23% and has remained unchanged or became worst in only 7% at 1 year. Improvement was therefore recorded in 93%. In patients having a follow-up of 3 to 4 years, 48% denied having angina, 41% had less angina, the majority of these being class I to II or IV, and only 11% were not improved. Eighty-nine percent were thus still improved at 3 to 4 years. We are aware of the placebo effect of all interventions in the therapy of angina but it is usually of short duration, and this long term improvement favors a genuine amelioration in the majority of patients, hopefully through increased blood supply to the myocardium. A placebo effect however cannot be ruled out in many cases. We have in fact observed that 41.1% of the angina-free patients had a positive sub-maximal EKG test, at 1 year, as compared to 74.1% of patients who still complained of angina, whether improvement had occurred or not (table 1). Although this difference is significant ($p<0.02$), it is difficult to accept that 41% of angina-free patients had a positive stress test in spite of the known possibilities of false positive tests and also of a positive response in asymptomatic patients with documented ischemic heart disease. Except for three of these patients who had pain during the test and who undoubtedly had not exercised to that degree during their usual activities of life, several are suspected to have myocardial ischemia without pain, possibly through a placebo pain denial phenomenon. It is noted that patients with intraoperative or subsequent myocardial infarction had been excluded from this study knowing that it may be followed by improvement of effort angina. In favor however of a genuine improvement through increased blood supply in many patients is the fact that in our first 105 patients who had angiographic control examinations at one year, as shown in table 2, 88.5% of improved cases, with and without residual angina, had at least one patent graft whereas this was observed in only 11.1% of unimproved patients ($p<0.005$). It is somewhat disquieting however to note that 38.5% (10/26) of cases without a patent graft were nevertheless improved, suggesting a placebo effect at least in these patients.

Table 1: Correlation between the absence-presence of effort angina and EKG stress testing 1 year after aortocoronary bypass surgery

Effort angina	Exercise EKG Neg.	Exercise EKG Pos.
Absent (N 56)	N 33 - 58.9%	N 23 - 41.1%
Present (N 27)	N 7 - 25.9%	N 20 - 74.1%

χ^2_c 6.573 = $p<0.02$

Table 2: Correlation between the course of effort angina and saphenous vein graft patency 1 year after aortocoronary bypass surgery

Effort angina	At least one patent graft	No patent graft
Improved (N 87)	N 77 - 88.5%	N 10 - 11.5%
Unimproved (N 18)	N 2 - 11.1%	N 16 - 88.9%

χ^2_c 43.44 = $p<0.0005$

Cost and duration of symptomatic improvement

The hospital mortality in patients operated for stable angina among our first 1000 patients was 4%. It has decreased to 2.5% in 1974. Complications unrelated to operative deaths are of no consequence except for cerebrovascular accidents which were observed in 4.6% of our patients, and intraoperative myocardial infarction found in 5% of our survivors. Changes in the native circulation and resulting myocardial damage may occur. These complications become significant only when grafts occlude. Changes in grafted coronary arteries may be noted in segments distal or proximal to the graft. The distal segment becomes thrombosed in 20% of arteries in which the graft has occluded before 2 to 3 weeks, but no significant change is observed whenever grafts occlude after that period (2). It is also noteworthy that no significant change occur in the coronary artery segment distal to the graft when it remains patent, as it had been feared at the onset of this surgery, believing that re-establishing normal pressure and flow would step up the progression of atherosclerosis. In fact, the incidence of new obstruction and of significant progression of initial stenoses is not greater at one year in the distal segment of grafted arteries as compared to that of ungrafted arteries. This phenomenon was observed in 8.6% of coronary arteries having patent grafts as compared to an incidence of 13% in ungrafted arteries (2). Progression to complete obstruction of initial or preoperative stenoses in the coronary segment proximal to a graft occurs in 50% of cases. This phenomenon is observed almost exclusively in our experience whenever the initial preoperative stenosis narrows the lumen by at least 75%. It must be stressed that this complication has no consequence whenever the graft remains patent but whenever the graft occludes it is complicated in 50% of cases, by myocardial damage, either localized decreased wall motion or myocardial infarction, the myocardium in that area being supplied only by collateral circulation (3). It is therefore of the utmost importance that grafts remain patent. Graft patency rate at one year in our most recent study carried out in consecutive patients is 85% (4). It should be noted however that the patency rate in grafts with flows measured at surgery below 50 ml/min is 72%, significantly lower than the 90% patency rate obtained in grafts with flows of at least 50 ml/min ($p<0.025$). This suggests that although arteries with a poor distal run-off may be grafted, their chance of remaining patent at one year is significantly less than that expected in grafts to arteries having a good distal run-off. We have also observed that patency rate decreases slightly during the second and third year following surgery, the attrition rate being only 2.5% per year (5). This relatively good long term patency correlates well with the long term improvement observed in patients operated for effort angina.

Survival following surgery

A 4 year survival of 85% was observed in 559 patients operated for stable angina among our first 1000 cases. The hospital mortality was 4% and the late yearly death rate 2.9%. If the expected yearly mortality rate of 4% in unoperated patients is correct (6), surgery does not appear to prolong life in these patients. The striking symptomatic improvement however is not obtained at the expense of a decreased longevity.

It is suggested however that the prognosis may be more closely related to the number of stenosed arteries as well as to the quality of the left ventricular function (7,8). Triple coronary artery disease and left main trunk stenosis are said to be associated with a 8 to 12% annual death rate.

We have compared 44 operated patients having a left main coronary artery stenosis of at least 70% to 27 unoperated patients.

They appeared to be similar in all respects except for the fact that operated patients had more severe angina. The survival curves in these two groups are not different, at 4 years, 75% for the operated patients as compared to 68% for the unoperated patients. The operative mortality rate was 14% and it appears that this high mortality rate was primarily responsible for this lack of improvement. A significant improvement in survival was noted however in the 29 operated patients as compared to 15 unoperated patients when cases having an ejection fraction of at least 0.45 were studied. The operative mortality was only 3% and no late death was recorded, giving a survival rate at 3 years of 97% as compared to a survival of 48% in the nonoperated patients ($p<0.005$).

These observations based on our own experience and that of others are the basis of the following comments and recommendations concerning the place of aortocoronary bypass surgery in the treatment of ischemic heart disease. The priority indication in the first 1000 patients to be operated upon in our institution appears in table 3.

Table 3: Priority indication in the first 1000 patients to have aortocoronary bypass surgery at the Montreal Heart Institute

	NU.
Stable angina	716
Unstable angina	138
Preventive (no to mild angina)	66
Associated to non coronary surgery	58
Heart failure	12
Coronary arteriography complication	5
Arrhythmia	3
Acute myocardial infarction	2
Total	1000

Definite indications

At the present time, the following are considered unquestionable indications: 1) incapacitating effort angina refractory to medical therapy, 2) unstable angina refractory to medical therapy, 3) life threatening ventricular arrhythmias, again refractory to medical therapy. 4) Postmyocardial infarction shock unresponsive to medical therapy.

We do not recommend surgery to all patients with angina pectoris because we still believe that medical therapy is frequently effective. There are also frequent spontaneous remissions. We agree however that medical therapy is fundamentally a negative approach, since all its measures attempt to decrease the oxygen needs of the myocardium. Surgery on the other hand, is a positive step, increasing oxygen supply. This observation in itself has been at times offered as an argument in favor of surgery ... by surgeons of course! Be it as it may, medical therapy may be quite successful when properly conducted. The meaning of incapacitating angina and the lack of response to medical therapy however has changed since this surgery was first introduced. At the onset, it meant that the patient could not carry on necessary activities of life, more specifically at work, and had remained in functional class III to IV, in spite of an optimal medical therapy. We now believe that its interpretation may be extended to include all activities of life, including recreational and other legitimate exertions. Restriction of activities is not always possible nor willingly accepted by patients. To suggest for instance to a patient a sedentary life and cessation of all sports does not appear reasonable when these may be continued following successful surgery. The degree of functional incapacity is also meaningless since a mild angina may be intolerable to a particular patient who does not accept the slightest limitation of activities or who suffers from chronic anxiety because of the occurrence of angina however rare and slight it may be. The unresponsiveness to medical therapy is therefore not only function of the disease itself but it also depends on the physician's willingness and ability to treat adequately, and more importantly, on the patient's compliance to therapy.

Unstable angina refractory to medical therapy is rare in our experience. We believe that at least 85% of patients respond well within 1 to 3 days to in-hospital rest, sedation, beta-blockers, liberal use of Isosorbide dinitrate, and ... intravenous heparin for those who believe in the total package deal! In the others, presenting either recurrent prolonged pains or refractory crescendo angina, surgery appears the only solution. The intra-aortic balloon type assisted circulation, before, during and after coronary arteriography appears to have appreciably decreased the high mortality associated with both angiography and surgery in these most critically ill patients (9).

Thus far, only 6 patients were selected on the basis of recurrent ventricular tachycardia or fibrillation. All had associated left ventricular wall segment resection, all have survived surgery, and all are doing well. It appears to be a rare, but unquestionable indication.

There appears to be no other alternative in cardiogenic shock with a high left ventricular filling pressure which has not responded to medical therapy, nor to the intra-aortic balloon assisted circulation (10,11). However, many of these cases are not amenable to surgery because of extensive, diffuse coronary atherosclerosis and extensive myocardial damage.

Uncertain indications

The followings may be considered: 1) unstable angina during

the acute phase without a medical therapy trial, 2) unstable angina controlled by medical therapy, 3) obstructive coronary disease patterns suspected to have a poor prognosis, 4) acute myocardial infarction with the hope of decreasing infarct size and 5) refractory heart failure.

The surgical treatment of unstable angina during the acute phase irrespectively of its response to medical therapy, is now being tested by a randomized cooperative study in the U.S.A. (12). Thus far, after a mean follow-up of 7 months, it appears that the mortality is not different, 6.8% for the medically treated patients and 9.2% for the surgically treated patients. The incidence of myocardial infarction is less in the medical group, 15% as compared to 29% ($p<0.05$). The surgically treated patients however were markedly improved as far as effort angina and recurrence of unstable episodes, being asymptomatic in 24% as compared to 67% for the medically treated group ($p<0.01$). It does not appear at the present time that surgery is beneficial except for the relief of symptoms. It has been our experience that the operative mortality is significantly less when surgery is carried out several weeks after medical control (13). We now recommend surgery to patients refractory to medical therapy, and to others after several weeks of effective medical therapy whenever they have a triple coronary artery disease, stenosis of the left main or involvement of two major arteries, but always with good distal run-off and a relatively good left ventricular function. One hundred and forty-nine patients operated in these conditions had an operative mortality of 4% and a 4 year survival of 91%. These results suggest that surgery carried out in these conditions may be indicated with the hope of prolonging life, as well as for the purpose of relieving symptoms.

Several centers consider as likely, if not definite indications, with the hope of prolonging life (7,8) significant proximal obstructive disease of three coronary arteries, of the left main trunk, and possibly also of two major arteries, the left anterior descending and either a right-dominant coronary artery or a circumflex of a left-dominant pattern. There appears however to be no indication for surgery as a preventive measure whenever one coronary artery is involved, except possibly in the case of a severe stenosis at the origin of the left anterior descending. These indications may be justified until a definite answer concerning its effect on survival becomes available, most likely from randomized controlled studies. It appears however that it should be advocated only whenever there are ideal conditions as related to a low operative mortality and an expected optimal graft patency rate. It has been shown that an operative mortality of 3% was observed whenever the ejection fraction was at least 0.45 whereas a mortality of 6% was found when the ejection fraction was between 0.25 to 0.45, and finally an operative mortality of 31% in patients with an ejection fraction below 0.20 (14). In our experience in a series of 93 patients having a 3 to 4 year follow-up, the late survival was 77.8% when the ejection fraction was below 0.50 and 98.2% whenever the ejection fraction was above that figure (15).

We have no experience with surgery in acute myocardial infarction but it does not appear from published reports that even early surgery within 2 to 4 hours after the onset of pain prevents infarction, although it may decrease its size and prevent cardiogenic shock as well as more significant long-term sequellae such as heart failure. In practice, it is not a frequent situation since the mean time of hospital admission after the onset of an acute episode is 4 to 8 hours. In most series, patients thus operated upon were already in the hospital, being under investigation, or being treated for ischemic heart disease or for other conditions. Many candidates developed their infarction during coronary arteriography, and many others were physicians who had the good or bad fortune of developing a myocardial infarction while at work. It appears doubtful that this surgery is the proper approach to the therapy of acute myocardial infarction in general, but it may be useful in certain conditions, such as in potentially extensive anterior wall infarction, and postmyocardial infarction angina suggesting an extension.

In our first 1000 patients to have aortocoronary bypass surgery, 32 had refractory heart failure, of whom 12 were operated specifically for that purpose, and 20 because of associated severe angina. The operative mortality was 18% and only 50% were still alive at 3 years. This survival curve is similar to Aldridge's curve found in such patients (16). Furthermore, none of these survivors were improved as far as heart failure was concerned. These patients had diffuse severe asynergy, an ejection fraction in most cases below 0.30, and we do not believe that associated wall resection would have been helpful since the entire left ventricle was severely impaired (17). There is some evidence that aortocoronary bypass surgery improves left ventricular function in some cases (18). It is therefore possible that mild or intermittent heart failure associated with hypokinesia of 1 to 2 wall segments, which is frequently reversible following successful bypass surgery, may be improved by grafting and also by associated segmental wall resection (19).

Conclusion

It appears that aortocoronary saphenous vein graft surgery has thus far been satisfactory. Graft patency rates of 80 to 85% are observed one to 3 years after surgery and it may approach 90% when grafted arteries have a good distal run-off (4,5). Graft alterations occur during the first year and the attrition rate does not appear to exceed 2 to 3% during the succeeding 2 to 5 years. Increased blood supply to the myocardium has been documented by improved EKG stress test, and in a smaller number of patients by normalization of myocardial metabolism and improved left ventricular function (20-22).

The quality of life is definitely improved, although a placebo effect may exist in some patients. Angina disappears in 70% of the cases, and it improves in another 20%. This amelioration persists in the majority for at least 3 to 4 years. It does not cure refractory heart failure. Its role in the treatment of unstable angina and in acute myocardial infarction has not yet been determined, although surgery appears indicated in unstable angina refractory to medical therapy and it seems successful in the therapy of postmyocardial infarction shock particularly when combined with intra-aortic balloon assisted circulation. There is no definite evidence that it prolongs life, but it appears probable that it may do so in certain conditions, triple coronary artery disease and severe left main trunk stenosis, whenever the left ventricular function is still relatively intact.

References

(1) Mathur VS, Guinn GA: Prospective randomized study of coronary bypass surgery in stable angina. The first 100 patients. Circulation **51-52**: 133 (suppl 1), 1975

(2) Bourassa MG, Goulet C, Lespérance J, Campeau L: Progression of coronary arterial disease after aortocoronary bypass grafts. Circulation **127**: 47 (suppl 3), 1973

(3) Bourassa MG, Lespérance J, Campeau L, Saltiel J: Fate of left ventricular contraction following aortocoronary venous grafts: early and late postoperative modifications. Circulation **46**: 724, 1972

(4) Campeau L, Crochet D, Lespérance J, Bourassa MG, Grondin CM: Postoperative changes in aortocoronary saphenous vein grafts revisited. Circulation **52**: 369, 1975

(5) Lespérance J, Bourassa MG, Saltiel J, Campeau L, Grondin CM: Angiographic changes in aortocoronary vein grafts: lack of progression beyond the first year. Circulation **48**: 633, 1973

(6) Kannel WB, Feinleib M: Natural history of angina pectoris in the Framingham study - Prognosis and survival. Amer J Cardiol **29**: 154, 1972

(7) Reeves TJ, Oberman A, Jones WB, Sheffield LT: Natural history of angina pectoris. Amer J Cardiol **33**: 423, 1974

(8) Bruschke AVG, Proudfit WL, Sones FM Jr: Progress study of 590 consecutive nonsurgical cases of coronary disease followed 5-9 years - I. Arteriographic correlations. Circulation **47**: 1147, 1973

(9) Gold HK, Leinbach RC, Sanders CA et al: Intraaortic balloon pumping for control of recurrent myocardial ischemia. Circulation **47**: 1197, 1973

(10) Keon WJ, Bedard P, Shankar KR, Akyurekli Y, Nino A, Berkman F: Experience with emergency aortocoronary bypass grafts in the presence of acute myocardial infarction. Circulation **47-48**: 151 (suppl 3), 1973

(11) Mundth ED, Buckley MJ, Leinbach RC, Gold HK et al: Surgical intervention for the complications of acute myocardial ischemia. Ann Surg **178**: 379, 1973

(12) Conti CR, Gilbert JB,Hodges M et al: Unstable angina pectoris: randomized study of surgical vs medical therapy. National Cooperative unstable angina pectoris study group. Amer J Cardiol **35**: 129, 1975

(13) Théroux P, Campeau L: The influence of timing of surgery on mortality and incidence of myocardial infarction following aortocoronary vein graft surgery in crescendo angina. Amer J Cardiol **31**: 162, 1973

(14) Gott VL: Outlook for patients after coronary artery revascularization. Amer J Cardiol **33**: 431, 1974

(15) Solignac A, Guéret P, Bourassa MG: Influence of left ventricular function on survival 3 to 4 years after aortocoronary bypass. Excerpta Medica **2/4**: 421, 1975

(16) Aldridge HE: Severely dysfunctioning ischemic left ventricle. 5-year follow-up. Circulation **46**: 61 (suppl 2), 1972 (abstr)

(17) Solignac A, Lespérance J, Grondin P, Campeau L: Aorta-to-coronary artery bypass operation for chronic intractable congestive heart failure. Can J Surg **17**: 1, 1974

(18) Campeau L, Elias G, Esplugas E, Lespérance J, Bourassa MG, Grondin CM: Left ventricular performance during exercise before and one year after aortocoronary bypass surgery for angina pectoris. Circulation **49-50**: 103 (suppl 2), 1974

(19) Isom OW, Spencer FC, Glassman E, Dembrow JM, Pasternack BS: Long-term survival following coronary bypass surgery in patients with significant impairment of left ventricular function. Circulation **51-52**: 141 (suppl 1), 1975

(20) Bartel AG, Behar VS, Peter RH, Orgain ES, Kong Y: Exercise stress testing in evaluation of aortocoronary bypass surgery. Report of 123 patients. Circulation **48**: 141, 1973

(21) Mason DT, Amsterdam EA, Miller RR, Hughes JS III, Bonanno JA, Iben AB, Hurley EJ, Massumi RA, Zelis R: Consideration of the therapeutic roles of pharmacologic agents, collateral circulation and saphenous vein bypass in coronary artery disease. Amer J Cardiol **28**: 608, 1971

(22) Chatterjee K, Matloff JM, Swan HJC, Ganz W, Kaushik VS, Magnusson P, Henis MM, Forrester JS: Abnormal regional metabolism and mechanical function in patients with ischemic heart disease. Improvement after successful regional revascularization by aortocoronary bypass. Circulation **52**: 390, 1975

(6)

CURRENT CONCEPTS OF CORONARY THROMBOSIS AS RELATED TO ATHEROSCLEROSIS AND MYOCARDIAL INFARCTION

Robert W. Wissler, Ph.D., M. D.

Department of Pathology
University of Chicago
Chicago, Illinois, U.S.A.

"and the parable of Pedro and the Jackass states that things are not always the way they seem to be"-

INTRODUCTION

On December 7, 1912 a great Chicago physician, Dr. James B. Herrick, published his now famous paper in the JAMA in which he related for the first time the "Clinical Features of Sudden Obstruction of the Coronary Arteries" with an acute heart attack and myocardial infarction (1). This eminent doctor, who also discovered sickle cell anemia, was supported in this study by an almost equally dynamic pathologist, Ludwig Hektoen, who was the first head of pathology at the University of Chicago. Their evidence was good, and for many years there was general acceptance that acute heart attacks were almost always the result of a thrombus in one or more atherosclerotic coronary arteries which, in turn, lead to a myocardial infarct and the signs and symptoms of an acute heart failure.

Then evidence began to accumulate that most of these heart attack victims in big cities like Chicago never make it to the hospital, but rather die suddenly before arrival. When these patients are autopsied - and relatively few of them are - they rarely have an identifiable gross thrombus in a coronary artery, although many of these sudden death victims have severe coronary atherosclerosis (2,3,4) and some of them have subendocardial necrosis.

This paradox has raised the question of whether there may be two or more pathogeneses of fatal acute ischemic heart disease.

HOSPITAL PATIENTS

In fact, these observations may have contributed to the question now frequently voiced of whether coronary thrombosis is really the cause of fatal heart attacks - even in those patients suffering from myocardial infarction who die after several days in a hospital and show recent thrombotic occlusion of a major coronary artery. Is the thrombus instead the result of the infarct (5,6)? This question has naturally produced some consternation in the medical community since much of the modern management of patients who have impending heart trouble has been aimed at preventing coronary arterial thrombosis; and anticoagulants or platelet agglutinin inhibitors certainly would not be very rational preventive medicine under these circumstances, especially since they may carry some threat of hemorrhage. Recently the Council on Thrombosis of the American Heart Association and the Thrombosis Advisory Committee of the National Heart and Lung Institute have collaborated to hold a workshop on this subject (7), and, in so far as one can discern the truth from a workshop, the evidence reported seems to indicate two areas of rather strong concurrence among the experienced participant pathologists and clinicians:
1) Most series of autopsies on patients who have well-developed myocardial infarcts also reveal related thrombosis of a major coronary artery in a very high proportion of the cases (86-95%);
2) In most instances the thrombus is anatomically related to the infarct in such a proximal way as to make it likely that it was the cause of the infarct. They also agreed that almost all of these cases of fatal myocardial infarction had severe coronary atherosclerosis which could very well explain the development of the thrombus.

NON-HOSPITALIZED SUDDEN DEATH PATIENTS

But there is also general consensus that only a small proportion of people who die suddenly at home, on the street, or on the job have demonstrable coronary thrombosis, even though they almost all have very severe stenosing coronary atherosclerosis.

This leaves the question of what is the mechanism of the acute fatal heart attack leading to sudden death? Several possible mechanisms are receiving considerable attention and support.

Fatal arrhythmia without coronary thrombosis or myocardial infarction.
The first of these possible mechanisms is suggested by the first three years of experience of the Seattle "MEDIC I" comprehensive system of resuscitation of human subjects, 823 of whom were unconscious, pulseless and in ventricular fibrillation when medical assistance arrived (8). Of these, 146 were resuscitated from

ventricular fibrillation and subsequently discharged. Out of 95 patients from this group in which adequate ECG and isoenzyme studies were available, more than 50% showed no evidence of myocardial necrosis, and only 17% showed evidence of myocardial infarcts from serial electrocardiograms. These and other observations suggest that many people who collapse on the street, at home or at work are not in the process of developing a classical myocardial infarct and would not necessarily be expected to show a coronary thrombus if they had succumbed and were autopsied.

These studies do not, of course, shed any light on the nature of the trigger mechanism which has produced the ventricular fibrillation. Is it the result of previous ischemic myocardial and conduction system damage from small areas of scarring which were never detected? Or are there other conditions which we do not always recognize which make the heart and its conduction system especially vulnerable to ventricular fibrillation? Schwartz and Gerrity have recently reviewed this subject in depth and have listed a large number of conditions associated with sudden death without demonstrable coronary artery disease (9).

Since a substantial number of the hearts examined from patients who have died suddenly and who have no demonstrable coronary occlusion do exhibit subendocardial necrosis (10), one must at least mention the fact that this pattern of myocardial necrosis is characteristic of patients succumbing after large infusions of catecholamines, such as epinephrine or isoproteronal (11). It is also reported in the hearts of patients who succumb suddenly with pheochromocytomas (12). Can it be that some subjects who die suddenly and who have subendocardial necrosis with no evidence of coronary disease are unusually sensitive to their own catecholamines?

Or, as a second alternative, how many of them may have mild undetected viral myocarditis (13)?

More provocatively, how many unknown pathophysiological mechanisms are there which can lead to subendocardial necrosis and sudden death? Obviously we need more basic research and more knowledge of this process which appears to be responsible for so many deaths.

Coronary platelet microemboli and sudden death.

A second possible mechanism of sudden death accompanied by subendocardial necrosis is better understood in the light of fairly recent investigations of the intramyocardial arterial system (14,15). These studies demonstrate by two different methods the presence of long, penetrating, non-branching terminal arteries which end up as a part of a rather prominent subendocardial network. If something occluded numbers of these arteries almost simultaneously, then one might expect subendocardial necrosis with little other evidence of myocardial damage.

If one puts this anatomical relationship together with the growing body of evidence which indicates that a number of factors in our modern environment may cause "spontaneous" platelet agglutination, then one may have a ready explanation for some of the unexplained sudden deaths which are not necessarily related to severe atherosclerosis of the major coronary arteries.

Much of this evidence has come from the remarkable series of investigations by J. Fraser Mustard and his group in Canada. They have documented in human subjects the effects of hyperlipemia, cigarette smoking and several other factors on platelet agglutination, platelet stickiness and decreased platelet half-life (16). They have also demonstrated in the experimental animal that intracoronary ADP injections will cause massive, but transient platelet agglutination, ventricular fibrillation, sudden death and a reasonably prompt focal myocardial necrosis (17). Other known triggers besides hyperlipemia and cigarette smoking may be circulating antigen-antibody complexes, endotoxins from gram-negative bacilli and excessive quantities of catecholamines.

Although it is very difficult for the pathologist to provide conclusive evidence on this mechanism because of the remarkably transient nature of these clumps of agglutinized platelets, both Jørgensen _et al_, (18) and Haerem (19) have documented their occurrence in the intramyocardial arteries of sudden death victims. However, the absence of such clumps in postmortem material probably does not rule out this mechanism, since they are remarkably labile and may even be lysed at room temperature during the long post-mortem interval which may precede an autopsy in sudden death cases (9).

Platelet aggregates in pulmonary arteries and sudden death.
A disquieting note has been injected into the entire sudden death problem by Pirkle (20). He has enumerated the presence of multiple platelet clumps in small pulmonary artery branches of young people, particularly young women, dying suddenly from no apparent cause. As far as can be ascertained from his report in "Science", he did not rule out the possibility that similar aggregates were being formed in the intramyocardial arteries.

Prostaglandins and platelet aggregation.
An example of a new direction which may provide yet another mechanism for platelet aggregation in relation to sudden death is

the recent report that the intravenous injection of arachidonic acid in small quanitities leads to platelet changes in the blood stream and sudden death in rabbits (21). Apparently, this phenomenon is mediated by the prostaglandins E_2 and F_{2a} from endogenous platelet arachidonic acid (22). To compound the problem there are the striking vasoconstrictive effects of these new prostaglandins which may augment the ischemia produced by the platelet aggregates. All of this suggests that in people who die suddenly one should search for factors stimulating platelet prostaglandin synthesis.

HYPOVOLEMIA

A final classical mechanism that should not be forgotten is the acute myocardial ischemia, ventricular fibrillation and sudden death which may accompany severe internal bleeding or other hidden conditions causing a rapid decrease in blood volume or drop in blood pressure, along with an epinephrine response, platelet agglutination and widespread small artery constriction.

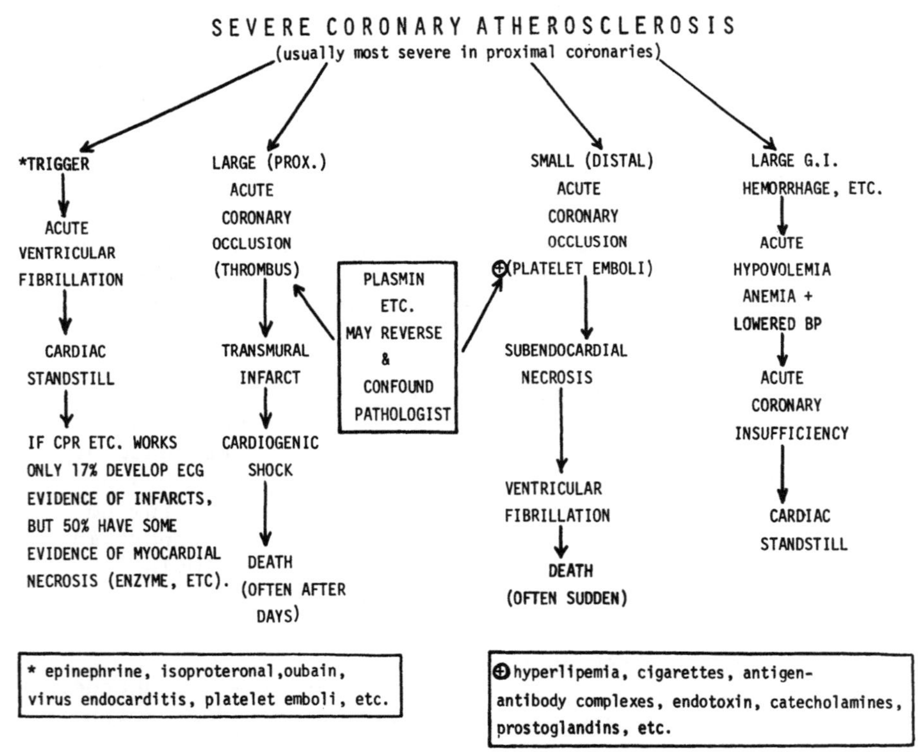

Figure 1.

SUMMARY AND RECOMMENDATIONS

All four of these potential pathogeneses of ventricular fibrillation and sudden death are depicted in diagrammatic form in figure 1. The problem is that at present there is not enough evidence or knowledge about the mechanisms actually involved to really support with any confidence a single approach to prevention or therapy.

The attempts to learn more about the morphological and functional pathology of the conduction system have been frustrating, and progress has been at best painfully slow and tedious. The pathologist's ability to document platelet agglutination as a bona fide mechanism for explaining sudden death does not seem likely to improve greatly in the immediate future. Furthermore, the triggering pathophysiological mechanisms responsible for either a fatal arrhythmia or a fatal platelet agglutination are probably very difficult to identify retrospectively.

Even in the absence of definitive knowledge the following conclusions seem warranted:

1. Attacks of ventricular fibrillation without major coronary artery thrombosis are probably the most common cause of sudden cardiovascular death in the U.S.A.

2. Many of these episodes are probably largely reversible if the victim receives prompt cardiopulmonary resuscitation and emergency medical care, and the successfully resuscitated patient usually does not develop classical myocardial infarction.

3. If these attacks are due to a reversible abnormality of the conduction system without widespread platelet agglutination, then they may be prevented by lidocaine or other similar drugs now available and being developed.

4. If they are triggered by platelet agglutination and transient small intramyocardial artery obstruction, they should be prevented by aspirin or other similar medication.

5. More attention should be focused on the patient's "minor" signs of impending ventricular fibrillation and on cardiopulmonary resuscitation and emergency medical care during the first few minutes following collapse.

Acknowledgements.

The work of the author which has provided material for study and sustained his interest in this subject has been supported through the University of Chicago Myocardial Infarction Unit, and more recently, by the pathological studies supported by the Ischemic Heart Disease Specialized Center of Research at the University of Chicago (NHLI 17648-01). He is also the Director of SCOR-Atherosclerosis at the University of Chicago NHL-15062. The manuscript has been prepared with the help of Elizabeth Anne Wissler and Sharon Stephens whose assistance is gratefully acknowledged.

REFERENCES

1. Herrick, James B.: Clinical features of sudden death obstruction of the coronary arteries. JAMA 59: 2015, 1912.

2. Spain, D.M., Bradess, V.A., Bradess, V.A., Matero, A., Taiter,R: Sudden death due to coronary atherosclerotic heart disease. JAMA 207: 1347, 1969.

3. Friedman, M., Manwaring, J.H., Rosenman, R.H., Donlon, G., Ortega, P., Grube, S.M.: Instantaneous and sudden deaths. Clinical and pathological differentiation in coronary artery disease. JAMA 225: 1319, 1973.

4. Spain, D.M., Bradess, V.A.: Sudden death from coronary heart disease. Survival time, frequency of thrombi and cigarette smoking. Dis. Chest 58: 107, 1970.

5. Meadows, R.: Coronary thrombosis and myocardial infarction. Med. J. Aug. 2: 409, 1965.

6. Roberts, W.C., Buja, L.M.: The frequency and significance of coronary arterial thrombi and other observations in fatal acute myocardial infarction. Am. J. Med. 52: 425, 1972.

7. Chandler, A.B., Chapman, I., Erhardt, L.R., Roberts, W.C., Schwartz, C.J., Sinapius, D., Spain, D.M., Sherry, S., Ness, P.M., Simon, T.L.: Coronary thrombosis in myocardial infarction. Report of a workshop on the role of coronary thrombosis in the pathogenesis of acute myocardial infarction. Am. J. Cardiol. 34: 823, 1974.

8. Baum, Robert S., Alvarez III, Hernan, Cobb, Leonard A.: Survival after resuscitation from out-of-hospital ventricular fibrillation. Circ. 50: 1231, 1974.

9. Schwartz, Colin J., Gerrity, Ross G.: The anatomic pathology of sudden unexpected cardiac death. Circ. 1975 (in press).

10. Miller, R.D., Burchell, H.B., Edwards, J.E.: Myocardial infarction with and without coronary o-clusion. Arch. Int. Med. 88: 597, 1951.

11. Szakacs, J.E., Dimmette, R.M., Cowart, E.C.: Pathologic implications of the catocholamines epinephrine and morepinephrine. U.S. Armed Forces.

12. Kline, I.K.: Myocardial alterations associated with pheochromocytoma. Am. J. Path. 38: 539, 1961.

13. Lisa, J.R., Hart, J.F.: The role of infection in sudden death. New York J. Med. 40: 705, 1940.

14. James, Thomas N., Anatomy of the coronary arteries and veins, chapter 28, pp 630. In: The Heart: Arteries and Veins, Hurst, W.J. and Logue, B.R. eds., Blakiston Division, McGraw-Hill Book Co, New York, 1966.

15. Estes, E.H.,Jr., Dalton, F.M., Entman, M.L., et al.: The anatomy and blood supply of the papillary muscles of the left ventricle. Amer. Heart J. 71: 356, 1966.

16. Mustard, J. Fraser: "latelets and thrombosis in acute myocardial infarction. In: The Myocardium: Failure and Infarction. Braunwald, E. ed. H.P. Publishing Co., Inc., New York, 1974 p. 177.

17. Jørgensen, L., Rowsell, H.C., Hovig, I., Glynn, M.F., Mustard, J.F.: Adenosine diphosphate-induced aggregation and myocardial infarction in swine. Lab. Invest. 17: 616, 1967.

18. Jørgensen, L., Haerem, J.W., Chandler, A.B., Borchgrevink, C.F.: The pathology of acute coronary death. Acta Anaesth. Scand. Suppl. 24: 193, 1968.

19. Haerem, J.W.: Platelet aggregates in intramyocardial vessels of patients dying suddenly and unexpectedly of coronary artery disease. Atherosclerosis 15:199, 1972.

20. Pirkle, Hubert, Carstens, P. : Pulmonary platelet aggregates associated with sudden death in man. Science 185: 1062,1974.

21. Silver, M.J., Hoch, W., Kocsis, J.J., Ingerman, C.M., Smith, J.B.: Arachidonic acid causes sudden death in rabbits. Science 183: 1085, 1974.

22. Hamberg, Mats, Svensson, Jan, Wakabayashi, Toshio, Samuelson, Bengt: Isolation and structure of two prostaglandin endoperoxides that cause platelet aggregation. Proc. Nat. Acad. Sci. U.S.A. 71(2): 345, 1974.

(7)

EFFECT OF DRUGS ON PLATELETS AND COMPLICATIONS OF VASCULAR DISEASE

J. F. Mustard, M. A. Packham and R. L. Kinlough-Rathbone,
Department of Pathology, McMaster University, Hamilton, and
Department of Biochemistry, University of Toronto, Toronto,
Ontario, Canada.

Platelets play a fundamental role in the formation of arterial thrombi. Thrombosis is involved in the development of vascular disease and its complications in at least four ways:

1) Platelets can take part in causing vessel injury. They can increase vessel permeability and they can influence the vessel wall, particularly the smooth muscle cells.

2) Some mural thrombi can become organized and incorporated into the vessel wall.

3) The mural thrombi which form in diseased atherosclerotic vessels may cause clinical complications because of their embolization into the circulation distal to the site of their formation.

4) Thrombi which occlude major arteries in vital organs such as the heart and the brain, cause ischemia, necrosis of tissue, and sometimes death.

Although a number of materials such as fibrin, white blood cells and red blood cells contribute to the formation of thrombi, platelets are one of the main components of arterial thrombi in the early stages of their formation. The response of the blood to vessel injury can be briefly summarized as involving the following mechanisms:

1) Platelets adhere to altered endothelium (4) and to exposed subendothelial structures (5).

2) The coagulation pathway is activated by tissue thrombo-

plastin from damaged cells such as the endothelial cells (6) and by the exposed collagen in the vessel wall (7).

3) Platelet adherence to exposed collagen in the subendothelium and possibly some other subendothelial structures causes the platelets to release ADP from their amine storage granules (5). During this release reaction the platelets form short-lived endoperoxides and related compounds from the arachidonic acid of their phospholipids (8,9). These compounds induce platelet shape change, aggregation and the release of more constituents from the platelet granules.

4) Platelets exposed to released ADP, to thrombin, and to the compounds formed from arachidonic acid, change from their disc shape to spheres with pseudopods and adhere to each other (2). This leads to the formation of a platelet mass at the injury site.

5) When platelets interact with collagen or adhere to each other under the influence of ADP, they promote further activation of the coagulation mechanism by activating factor XI and factor XII (10). In addition, factor V and factor VIII are associated with the surface of the platelets. When the platelet phospholipoprotein (platelet factor 3) is exposed during the release reaction, factors X and II can bind to the platelet surface (11). The platelet surface thus serves as a focus for the localized acceleration of thrombin formation. (There is evidence that platelet factors such as platelet factor 4 inhibit the anticoagulants in blood, thus further enhancing coagulation around the surface of the platelets (12).) The thrombin causes the release of further platelet ADP, and the formation of more short-lived compounds from platelet arachidonic acid. This leads to additional platelet aggregation on top of the initial platelet mass (2). If thrombin reaches an adequate concentration, it will cause the polymerization of fibrinogen to fibrin.

6) The polymerizing fibrin binds strongly to the platelet aggregate (13) and is probably the crucial factor in keeping the platelet mass together since platelet aggregates by themselves are unstable and break up readily (2).

7) If flow is sufficiently slow, polymerizing fibrin will form in the area around the platelet aggregate and the static column of blood may trap red cells and thus create a red thrombus.

8) Vessel wall injury also leads to local activation of the fibrinolytic mechanism by activation of plasminogen to plasmin (14). Thus, while fibrin is forming, fibrinolysis is also taking place (15).

An understanding of the factors governing the formation and dissolution of thrombi at a site of vessel wall injury is essential in understanding the relations among platelets, thrombosis, early vessel wall changes, and the clinical complications of atherosclerosis, and in designing experiments to study these relations. Platelets aggregated by ADP or thrombin, without the binding effect of fibrin, will deaggregate readily. Platelets degranulated by thrombin can be returned to the circulation and survive normally (16, 17). Platelets aggregated by ADP in vivo also deaggregate and return to the circulation with a normal platelet survival (18). Although we do not know whether platelets which have adhered to collagen can return to the circulation, the studies of Baumgartner (19) have shown that after the initial mass of platelets has adhered to a damaged vessel wall, nearly all the material may be dislodged from the injury site within a short time. New material does not seem to adhere readily to the damaged area once the initial thrombus has been dislodged. It therefore appears that when an artery is injured, a mural thrombus will start to form but there will be a balance between the factors promoting its formation and the factors leading to its dissolution. Fragments of the thrombus will break off from time-to-time and shower the distal circulation as platelet emboli.

In addition to the factors already discussed concerning the stability of thrombi and the extent of thrombosis, the conditions of blood flow are also important. The most extensive thrombus formation is likely to occur in areas of disturbed flow (2).

There are a number of drugs which inhibit platelet reactions and thus may have a beneficial effect on vascular disease and its complications. At the present time, the drugs that have been used in man that influence these processes include the following:

(1) Anticoagulants
(2) Non-steroidal anti-inflammatory drugs
(3) Pyrimido-pyrimidines
(4) Clofibrate

Other drugs that can be considered have not been as extensively studied. This subject has been reviewed recently (20, 21, 22).

The anticoagulant drugs act through inhibition of thrombin or its formation. Therefore, they will affect both the coagulation component and the thrombin-induced platelet aggregation and release components of the mechanisms in thrombosis.

The oral anticoagulant drugs such as dicumarol which inhibit the synthesis of factors II, VII, IX and X, are not effective inhibitors of the formation of a platelet mass in response to vascular injury in arteries (23, 24). They do diminish the amount of thrombin formation and hence the thrombin-induced component of the reaction, but they do not have a major effect on the basic mechanisms by which platelets interact with the vessel wall, or on the formation of the initial platelet aggregate. However, heparin, which is an effective inhibitor of thrombin, does reduce the extent of formation of experimental thrombi in arteries (20, 25) and probably does so because it is a powerful inhibitor of the effects of thrombin on both platelets and fibrinogen. In higher doses, heparin reduces the ability of platelets to interact with collagen in the vessel wall (26).

Of more interest lately is the identification of drugs which affect platelet function and therefore, theoretically, may be useful in the management of arterial thrombo-embolic complications. One of the first observations of a drug affecting platelet function, with potential effects on vascular disease complications, was the observation that sulfinpyrazone, a uricosuric agent, prolonged platelet survival and increased platelet turnover in man (27). This observation has been confirmed by Steele et al. (28). It has also been demonstrated that high concentrations of sulfinpyrazone inhibit the platelet release reaction (29) and the response of platelets to subendothelial components of the vessel wall (30). It also inhibits the formation of metabolic products from arachidonic acid (31). However, in the doses used in man, which prolong platelet survival, the drug is not usually found to inhibit in vitro tests of the interaction of platelets with collagen (32). Sulfinpyrazone has been found to inhibit thrombus formation in arterio-venous shunts in subjects on chronic dialysis (33). Detailed analysis of this study in which patients were crossed over from sulfinpyrazone to placebo and from placebo to sulfinpyrazone indicates that the effects of the drug are apparent within one week of starting or stopping the administration of the drug. Sulfinpyrazone also reduced the incidence of transient attacks of cerebral ischemia in patients with carotid artery disease (35), and significantly prolonged longevity in a group of old patients admitted to a chronic care unit with a history of vascular disease complications (36). The drug has also been found to prolong survival in subjects with substitute heart valves (32, 37).

After the observations had been made with sulfinpyrazone, aspirin was found to inhibit the platelet:collagen reaction (38, 39). In tests in vitro, aspirin appears to be a more effective inhibitor than sulfinpyrazone of the reaction of platelets with collagen. It inhibits the release reaction and the formation of metabolites from platelet arachidonic acid (8, 9, 40). This has led to considerable interest in aspirin as a possible anti-thrombotic agent. However, in contrast to sulfinpyrazone, the usual therapeutic doses of aspirin in man do not prolong platelet survival (41), although in samples of platelet-rich plasma prepared from blood taken from these subjects, collagen-induced aggregation and release are inhibited. The difference in the effects of these two drugs on platelet survival may indicate that they act in different ways, and raises the possibility that aspirin and sulfinpyrazone may not have the same effect on arterial thrombo-embolic complications. It has been demonstrated that the combination of aspirin with dipyridamole reduces the dose of dipyridamole required to prolong platelet survival (42). The one prospective study with aspirin that has been reported did not show that aspirin had a significant effect on arterial thrombosis (43). Although the trend was to a decreased mortality in the group of patients given aspirin who had had a myocardial infarction, the difference was not significant. Because of the complexities of such studies and the number of patients required, further trials have been undertaken to examine the effect of aspirin on secondary prevention of myocardial infarction. Aspirin has been reported to reduce the incidence of transient attacks of cerebral ischemia, including amaurosis fugax (44-46). Aspirin has also been found to be effective in preventing thrombosis in Cimino fistulae in uremic patients (47). In contrast to the effect of sulfinpyrazone (36), aspirin was not found to be of benefit in a group of old patients in a chronic care institution (48). It is not certain, however, that the population groups used in the two studies were comparable.

Harker and Slichter (41, 42) have presented evidence that dipyridamole prolongs platelet survival and that it is effective in patients with thrombo-embolic complications associated with cardiac valves. Similar observations have been made by Genton and his associates (49). Perhaps of more interest in terms of the vascular disease aspects of the problem, it has been found that removal of the endothelium from the aorta of baboons shortens platelet survival, and that dipyridamole will restore this shortened survival toward normal (50). Since there is now firm evidence that damage to the endothelium leads to smooth muscle cell proliferation and atherosclerosis (51), and Ross et al. (52) have shown that platelets release a factor which stimulates smooth muscle cell proliferation, the possibility of influencing this process with drugs has arisen. Harker et al. (53) have recently reported that administration of dipyridamole to baboons given homocystine prevents homocystine-induced shortening of platelet survival. The homocystine is believed to cause endothelial injury and loss and this leads to the development of atherosclerotic lesions. Harker et al. (54) have reported that dipyridamole or sudoxicam prevent the intimal lesions caused by homocystine in baboons. This evidence is compatible with the concept that the release of a growth promoting factor from platelets at sites of vessel wall injury plays a critical role in the smooth muscle cell proliferation associated with vascular injury. The observation of Moore et al. (55) that thrombocytopenia prevents the development of atherosclerotic lesions in rabbit arteries exposed to repeated injury, adds further emphasis to the importance of this mechanism. Thus one of the main points that is emerging is the potential effect on vascular disease and its complications of drugs which inhibit the release or secretion of substances from platelets, particularly the material which causes smooth muscle cell proliferation.

Clofibrate was originally developed to lower serum lipids. During the early studies with this drug, it was also found that it had some effect on platelets and, like sulfinpyrazone, prolonged platelet survival and decreased platelet turnover in human subjects (56, 57). The original studies have been confirmed in studies by Genton and his associates (49).

It has been reported from two clinical trials that patients with angina given Clofibrate have a significantly lower incidence of myocardial infarction and sudden death than patients given a placebo compound (58, 59). In these studies, patients with a history of myocardial infarction did not benefit from the administration of Clofibrate. There are some basic problems with the design of these studies which make it difficult to draw firm conclusions (60). A recent study of the American Coronary Drug project (61) on the value of Clofibrate in secondary prevention of myocardial infarction also did not show any beneficial effect in terms of decreased mortality. In this study, subjects with angina did not improve when given Clofibrate. Unfortunately the American and European studies are not comparable. Clofibrate does have an effect on platelet survival but the data from the Clofibrate studies are insufficient to allow one to conclude whether or not Clofibrate affects the mortality of subjects who have had a myocardial infarction.

In considering the effects of platelets on thrombosis and vascular disease, it is important to keep in mind the dietary and environmental factors which are known to affect platelet function. These include: (a) diet, which has been shown to shorten platelet survival and increase platelet turnover if it consists of dairy products and eggs (62). Of interest in this respect are the findings of Renaud et al. (63) and Hornstra (64) that saturated fatty acids in the diet of experimental animals cause the platelets to show an increased sensitivity to aggregating and release-inducing agents, in contrast to platelets from animals given diets rich in polyunsaturated fat. These investigators have also found that these animals showed an increased susceptibility to thrombosis. (b) Smoking, which affects platelet function (65, 66), causes shortened platelet survival and increased platelet turnover (67). In animal experiments, carbon monoxide has been shown to increase vessel injury (68).

(c) Hormones, particularly estrogens, have been found to increase platelet adhesiveness and to enhance the response of platelets to aggregating agents. These effects have been linked to an increased incidence of thromboembolism in subjects taking estrogens. (For review see (20)).
(d) There is also some evidence that stress may cause increased platelet aggregation (69).

If mural thrombi in the coronary circulation which embolize and shower the distal circulation are an important cause of sudden death, then some of these drugs which inhibit platelet reactions may have a significant effect on the sudden death seen with myocardial ischemia. It is important to emphasize that our concepts of thrombus formation now are such that we recognize that thrombi form and undergo dissolution with great frequency and that a mural thrombus can form, break up, and re-form, and again break up. Emboli from it can cause death and there may not be much indication that it was once present on the surface of the coronary artery at the original site of its formation (1, 2). Unless the techniques of pathology can be improved, it may only be possible to establish whether this mechanism is of importance in myocardial ischemia and sudden death by actually carrying out therapeutic trials of primary prevention of myocardial ischemia in individuals at risk.

Even if drugs are shown to be of benefit, they will probably be of little use because of the problem of patient compliance. However, strategies which lead to modification of cigarettes or a reduction in smoking may be of as much use as drugs since stopping smoking appears to have comparable effects to drugs on platelet survival. Furthermore, changing dietary fats from animal fats to vegetable fats produces as great a prolongation of platelet survival as drugs and may be just as effective in preventing atherosclerosis and its complications.

1. Mustard, J.F., Packham, M.A., Moore, S. and Kinlough-Rathbone, R.L. Thrombosis and Atherosclerosis. In: "Atherosclerosis III", eds. G. Schettler and A. Weizel. Springer-Verlag, New York, pp.253-267, 1974.
2. Mustard, J.F., Kinlough-Rathbone, R.L. and Packham, M.A. Recent status of research in the pathogenesis of thrombosis. Thromb. Diath. Haemorrh. Suppl. 59, 157-188, 1974.
3. Mustard, J.F. and Packham, M.A. The role of blood and platelets in atherosclerosis and the complications of atherosclerosis. Thromb. Diath. Haemorrh. 33, 445-456, 1975.
4. Ashford, T.P. and Freiman, D.G. Platelet aggregation at sites of minimal endothelial injury. Am. J. Pathol. 53, 599-607, 1968.

5. Hovig, T. Release of platelet-aggregating substance (adenosine diphosphate) from rabbit blood platelets induced by saline "extract" of tendons. Thromb. Diath. Haemorrh. 9, 264-278, 1963.
6. Nemerson, Y. and Pitlick, F.A. The tissue factor pathway of blood coagulation. In: "Progress in Hemostasis and Thrombosis", Vol.1, ed. T. H. Spaet, Grune and Stratton, New York, pp.1-37, 1972.
7. Niewiarowski, S., Stuart, R.K. and Thomas, D.P. Activation of intravascular coagulation by collagen. Proc. Soc. Exp. Biol. Med. 123, 196-200, 1966.
8. Smith, J.B., Ingerman, C., Kocsis, J.J. and Silver, M.J. Formation of an intermediate in prostaglandin biosynthesis and its association with the platelet release reaction. J. Clin. Invest. 53, 1468-1472, 1974.
9. Willis, A.L., Vane, F.M., Kuhn, D.C., Scott, C.G. and Petrin, M. An endoperoxide aggregator (LASS), formed in platelets in response to thrombotic stimuli - purification, identification and unique biological significance. Prostaglandins 8, 453-507, 1974.
10. Walsh, P.N. The effects of collagen and kaolin on the intrinsic coagulant activity of platelets. Evidence for an alternative pathway in intrinsic coagulation not requiring factor XII. Br. J. Haematol. 22, 393-405, 1972.
11. Jackson, C.M., Dombrose, F.A., Ittyerah, T.R., Gitel, S.N., Esmon, C.T. and Suttie, J.W. Prothrombin binding to phospholipid vesicle surfaces and phospholipid acceleration of prothrombin activation. Proc. Vth Congress of the International Society on Thrombosis and Haemostasis. Paris, France, July, 1975. Abstract 196, p.216.
12. Walsh, P.N. and Gagnatelli, G. Platelet antiheparin activity: Storage site and release mechanism. Blood 44, 157-168, 1974.
13. Niewiarowski, S., Regoeczi, E., Stewart, G.J., Senyi, A., Mustard, J.F. Platelet interaction with polymerizing fibrin. J. Clin. Invest. 51, 685-700, 1972.
14. Nilsson, I.M. and Pandolfi, M. Fibrinolytic response of the vascular wall. Thromb. Diath. Haemorrh. Suppl. 40, 231-242, 1970.
15. Cade, J.F., Hirsh, J., Regoeczi, E., Gent, M., Buchanan, M.R. and Hynes, D.M. Resolution of experimental pulmonary emboli with heparin and streptokinase in different dosage regimens. J. Clin. Invest. 54, 782-791, 1974.
16. Reimers, H.J., Packham, M.A., Kinlough-Rathbone, R.L. and Mustard, J.F. Effect of repeated treatment of rabbit platelets with low concentrations of thrombin on their function, metabolism and survival. Br. J. Haematol. 25, 675-689, 1973.

17. Reimers, H.-J., Cazenave, J.-P., Senyi, A.F., Hirsh, J., Kinlough-Rathbone, R.L., Packham, M.A. and Mustard, J.F. In vivo and in vitro functions of thrombin-treated rabbit platelets. Proc. Vth Congress of the International Society on Thrombosis and Haemostasis. Paris, France, July, 1975. Abstract 445, p.470.
18. Mustard, J.F., Rowsell, H.C., Lotz, F., Hegardt, B. and Murphy, E.A. The effect of adenine nucleotides on thrombus formation, platelet count and blood coagulation. Exp. Mol. Pathol. 5, 43-60, 1966.
19. Baumgartner, H.R. The role of blood flow in platelet adhesion, fibrin deposition, and formation of mural thrombi. Microvasc. Res. 5, 167-179, 1973.
20. Mustard, J.F. and Packham, M.A. Platelets, thrombosis and drugs. Drugs 9, 19-76, 1975.
21. Vermylen, J., de Gaetano, G. and Verstraete, M. Platelets and thrombosis. In: "Recent Advances in Thrombosis" ed. L. Poller. Churchill Livingstone, London, pp.113-150, 1973.
22. Weiss, H.J. The pharmacology of platelet inhibition. In: "Progress in Haemostasis and Thrombosis" Vol.1, ed. T. H. Spaet, Grune and Stratton, New York, pp.199-231, 1972.
23. Merskey, C. and Drapkin, A. Anticoagulant therapy: a critical review. Blood 25, 567-596, 1965.
24. Fulton, G.P., Akers, R.P. and Lutz, B.R. White thromboembolism and vascular fragility in hamster cheek pouch after anticoagulants. Blood 8, 140-152, 1953.
25. Didisheim, P. Animal models useful in the study of thrombosis and antithrombotic agents. In: "Progress in Haemostasis and Thrombosis" Vol.1, ed.T. H. Spaet, Grune and Stratton, New York, pp.165-197, 1972.
26. Rowsell, H.C., Glynn, M.F., Mustard, J.F. and Murphy, E.A. The effect of heparin on platelet economy in dogs. Am. J. Physiol. 213, 915-922, 1967.
27. Smythe, H.A., Ogryzlo, M.A., Murphy, E.A. and Mustard, J.F. The effect of sulfinpyrazone (Anturan) on platelet economy and blood coagulation in man. Can. Med. Assoc. J. 92, 818-821, 1965.
28. Steele, P.P., Weily, H.S. and Genton, E. Platelet survival and adhesiveness in recurrent venous thrombosis. N.Engl.J.Med. 288, 1148-1152, 1973.
29. Packham, M.A., Warrior, E.S., Glynn, M.F., Senyi, A.S. and Mustard, J.F. Alteration of the response of platelets to surface stimuli by pyrazole compounds. J. Exp. Med. 126, 171-188, 1967.
30. Cazenave, J.-P., Guccione, M.A., Packham, M.A. and Mustard, J.F. Inhibition of platelet adherence to damaged vessel wall by drugs. International Workshop - Conference on Atherosclerosis, London, Ont. Sept. 1975. Abstract P.II-3, p.41.

31. McDonald, J.W.D., Stuart, R.K. and Barnett, H.J.M. Effect of aspirin and sulfinpyrazone on platelet prostaglandin synthesis. International Workshop - Conference on Atherosclerosis, London, Ont. Sept. 1975, Abstract P.II-3, p.39.
32. Weily, H.S. and Genton, E. Altered platelet function in patients with prosthetic mitral valves. Effects of sulfinpyrazone therapy. Circulation 42, 967-972, 1970.
33. Kaegi, A., Pineo, G.F., Shimizu, A., Trivedi, H., Hirsh, J. and Gent, M. Arteriovenous-shunt thrombosis: Prevention by sulfinpyrazone. N. Engl. J. Med. 290, 304-306, 1974.
34. Hirsh, J., Gent, M. and Genton, E. The current status of platelet suppressive drugs in the treatment of thrombosis. Thromb. Diath. Haemorrh. 33, 406-416, 1975.
35. Evans, G. Effect of platelet-suppressive agents on the incidence of amaurosis fugax and transient cerebral ischemia. In: "Cerebral Vascular Diseases", Eighth Conference. ed. F. H. McDowell and R. W. Brennan, Grune and Stratton, New York. pp.297-300, 1973.
36. Blakely, J.A. and Gent, M. Platelets, drugs and longevity in a geriatric population. In: "Platelets, Drugs and Thrombosis" eds. J. Hirsh, J. F. Cade, A. S. Gallus and E. Schönbaum. S. Karger, New York, pp.284-291, 1974.
37. Weily, H.S., Steele, P.P., Davies, H., Pappas, G. and Genton, E. Platelet survival in patients with substitute heart valves. N. Engl. J. Med. 290, 534-537, 1974.
38. Evans, G., Packham, M.A., Nishizawa, E.E., Mustard, J.F. and Murphy, E.A. The effect of acetylsalicylic acid on platelet function. J. Exp. Med. 128, 877-894, 1968.
39. Weiss, H.J., Aledort, L.M. and Kochwa, S. The effects of salicylates on the hemostatic properties of platelets in man. J. Clin. Invest. 47, 2169-2180, 1968.
40. Vargaftig, B.B. and Zirinis, P. Platelet aggregation induced by arachidonic acid is accompanied by release of potential inflammatory mediators distinct from PGE_2 and $PGF_{2\alpha}$. Nature [New Biol.] 244, 114-116, 1973.
41. Harker, L.A. and Slichter, S.J. Studies of platelet and fibrinogen kinetics in patients with prosthetic heart valves. N. Engl. J. Med. 283, 1302-1305, 1970.
42. Harker, L.A. and Slichter, S.J. Platelet and fibrinogen consumption in man. N. Engl. J. Med. 287, 999-1005, 1972.
43. Elwood, P.C., Cochrane, A.L., Burr, M.L., Sweetnam, P.M., Williams, G., Welsby, E., Hughes, S.J. and Renton, R. A randomized controlled trial of acetylsalicylic acid in the secondary prevention of mortality from myocardial infarction. Br. Med. J. 1, 436-440, 1974.
44. Harrison, M.J.G., Marshall, J., Meadows, J.C. and Russell, R.W.R. Effect of aspirin in amaurosis fugax. Lancet, 2, 743-744, 1971.

45. Mundall, J., Quintero, P., Von Kaulla, K., Austin, J. and Harmon, R. Transient monocular blindness and increased platelet aggregability treated with aspirin. A case report. Neurology (Minneap.) 22, 280-285, 1972.
46. Dyken, M.L., Kolar, O.J. and Jones, F.H. Differences in the occurrence of carotid transient ischemic attacks associated with anti-platelet aggregation therapy. Stroke 4, 732-736, 1973.
47. Andrassy, K., Ritz, E., Schoeffner, W., Hahn, G. and Walter, K. The influence of acetylsalicylic acid on platelet adhesiveness and thrombotic fistula complications in hemodialysed patients. Klin. Wochenschr. 49, 166-167, 1971.
48. Heikenheimo, R. and Järvinen, K. Acetylsalicylic acid and arteriosclerotic-thromboembolic diseases in the aged. J. Am. Geriatr. Soc. 19, 403-405, 1971.
49. Genton, E. (Personal communication).
50. Harker, L.A. and Slichter, S.J. Arterial thromboembolism - quantitation and prevention. Proc. IVth International Congress on Thrombosis and Haemostasis, Vienna, Austria, June, 1973, Abstract 136, p.170.
51. Moore, S. Thromboatherosclerosis in normolipemic rabbits: a result of continued endothelial damage. Lab. Invest. 29, 478-487, 1973.
52. Ross, R., Glomset, J., Kariya, B. and Harker, L. A platelet-dependent serum factor that stimulates the proliferation of arterial smooth muscle cells in vitro. Proc. Natl. Acad. Sci. U.S.A. 71, 1207-1210, 1974.
53. Harker, L.A., Slichter, S.J., Scott, C.R. and Ross, R. Homocystinemia : vascular injury and arterial thrombosis. N. Engl. J. Med. 291, 537-543, 1974.
54. Harker, L.A., Ross, R. and Slichter, S.J. Chronic endothelial cell injury and platelet factor-induced arteriosclerosis. Proc. Vth Congress of the International Society on Thrombosis and Haemostasis, Paris, France, July 1975, abstract 38, p.56.
55. Moore, S., Friedman, R.J., Singal, D.P., Gauldie, J. and Blajchman, M. Inhibition of injury-induced thromboatherosclerotic lesions by anti-platelet serum in rabbits. Proc. Vth Congress of the International Society on Thrombosis and Haemostasis, Paris, France, July 1975, abstract 39, p.58.
56. Gilbert, J.B. and Mustard, J.F. Some effects of Atromid on platelet economy and blood coagulation in man. J. Atherosclerosis Res. 3, 623-633, 1963.
57. Glynn, M.F., Murphy, E.A. and Mustard, J.F. Effect of Clofibrate on platelet economy in man. Lancet 2, 447-448, 1967.
58. Arthur, J.B. et al. Five year study by a group of physicians of the Newcastle upon Tyne region: Trial of Clofibrate in the treatment of ischaemic heart disease. Br. Med. J. 4, 767-775, 1971.

59. Oliver, M.F. Ischaemic heart disease: a secondary prevention trial using Clofibrate. Report by a research committee of the Scottish Society of Physicians. Br. Med. J. 4, 775-784, 1971.
60. Feinstein, A.R. Clinical Biostatistics: XVIII. The Clofibrate trials: Another dispute about contratrophic therapy. Clin. Pharmacol. Ther. 13, 953-968, 1972.
61. The Coronary Drug Project Research Group. Clofibrate and niacin in coronary heart disease. JAMA 231, 360-381, 1975.
62. Mustard, J.F. and Murphy, E.A. Effect of different dietary fats on blood coagulation, platelet economy, and blood lipids. Br. Med. J. 1, 1651-1655, 1962.
63. Renaud, S., Kinlough, R.L. and Mustard, J.F. Relationship between platelet aggregation and the thrombotic tendency in rats fed hyperlipemic diets. Lab. Invest. 22, 339-343, 1970.
64. Hornstra, G. Dietary fats and arterial thrombosis. Haemostasis, 2, 21-52, 1973-74.
65. Hawkins, R.I. Smoking, platelets and thrombosis. Nature 236, 450-452, 1972.
66. Levine, P.H. An acute effect of cigarette smoking on platelet function. A possible link between smoking and arterial thrombosis. Circulation 48, 619-623, 1973.
67. Mustard, J.F. and Murphy, E.A. Effect of smoking on blood coagulation and platelet survival in man. Br. Med. J. 1, 846-849, 1963.
68. Thomsen, H.K. Carbon monoxide-induced atherosclerosis in primates, an electron-microscopic study of the coronary arteries of Macaca irus monkeys. Atherosclerosis 20, 233-240, 1974.
69. Haft, J.I. and Fani, K. Intravascular platelet aggregation in the heart induced by stress. Circulation 47, 353-358, 1973.

Section II
Proffered Papers

SECTION II - (PROFERRED PAPERS)

SUMMARY TABLE

DAY I September 1 P.M.	CHAPTER 1 (PI-1) Clinical Epidemiology Dr. W.F. Connell, Canada Dr. J.M. Beveridge, Canada	CHAPTER 2 (PI-2) Myocardial Infarction Dr. G.W. Manning, Canada Dr. S.P. Ahuja, Canada	CHAPTER 3 (PI-3) Fate of Lipoproteins Dr. J. Renais, France Dr. W.L. Holmes, U.S.A.	CHAPTER 4 (PI-4) Aortic Glycosaminoglycans, Gangliosides and Glycolysis Dr. H. Hauss, Germany Dr. R.A. Goyer, Canada	CHAPTER 5 (PI-5) Hemodynamics Dr. H. Jellinek, Hungary Dr. A.C. Wallace, Canada
DAY II September 2 A.M.	CHAPTER 6 (PII-1) Hyperlipidemia in Man and Treatment Dr. J. Davignon, Canada Dr. J.O. Parker, Canada	CHAPTER 7 (PII-2) Atherosclerosis and Childhood Dr. C.J. Miras, Greece Dr. W.D. Bocking, Canada	CHAPTER 8 (PII-3) Fibrinolytic Activity; Platelets Dr. J.R. Hampton, England Dr. H.J.M. Barnett, Canada	CHAPTER 9 (PII-4) Permeability; Tissue Culture Dr. T. Shimamoto, Japan Dr. S. Moore, Canada	CHAPTER 10 (PII-5) Experimental Models of Hyperlipidemia Dr. C.B. Taylor, U.S.A. Dr. S. Fedoroff, Canada
DAY III September 3 A.M.	CHAPTER 11 (PIII-1) Experimental Hypercholesterolemia Dr. P.J. Lupien, Canada Dr. G. Steiner, Canada	CHAPTER 12 (PIII-2) Lipid Composition and Metabolism in Man Dr. A. Angel, Canada Dr. L. Lewis, U.S.A.	CHAPTER 13 (PIII-3) Metabolic Control in Animal Tissues Dr. E. Morrison, U.S.A. Dr. A. Kuksis, Canada	CHAPTER 14 (PIII-4) Experimental Lesions - Morphology Dr. J. Roland, France Dr. R.M. O'Neal, U.S.A.	CHAPTER 15 (PIII-5) Surgical Techniques, Investigation and Treatment Dr. C.G. Drake, Canada Dr. D.R. Wilson, Canada

CHAPTER 1
CLINICAL EPIDEMIOLOGY

(1)

HYPERLIPOPROTEINEMIA IN CHRONIC HEMODIALYSIS PATIENTS AND LONG-TERM RENAL TRANSPLANT RECIPIENTS

R.A. Bear, M.D., F.R.C.P.(C), R. Lee, M.D., F.R.C.P.(C), Z. Shainhouse, M.D., G. Buckley

St. Michael's Hospital and The University of Toronto, 30 Bond Street, Toronto, Ontario, Canada

INTRODUCTION: Since 1968 (1) it has been known that lipoprotein abnormalities often develop in patients on maintenance hemodialysis (2,3) and in recipients of successful renal homo-transplants (3). As high as 50% mortality from premature cardiovascular disease has been reported in chronic dialysis patients. This report documents the incidence, type and natural history of hyperlipoproteinemia (HLP) occurring in patients on hemodialysis and with renal transplants.

METHOD: Fifty-seven patients with chronic renal failure ranging in age from 20 to 52 years were studied for serum lipid abnormalities during maintenance hemodialysis therapy and/or following successful renal transplantation. 35 patients were renal transplant recipients on varying doses of prednisone (15-40 mg) and azothioprine (50-150 mg). 33 patients were on chronic hemodialysis. 11 of these patients were followed through renal transplantation.

Laboratory procedures were as follows: cholesterol by the method of Carr and Drekter (4), triglyceride by Bucolo and David (5), and lipoprotein paper electrophoresis by Frederickson, Levy and Lees (6). LDL and HDL cholesterol were determined after ultracentrifugation. The diagnosis and typing of HLP was according to Frederickson and Levy (7).

RESULTS: 48% of 33 chronic hemodialysis patients, average age 36 yr. and average duration of dialysis 16 months, had HLP Type IIB (6%) and Type IV (42%), Table I.

TABLE I - MEAN SERUM CHOLESTEROL AND TRIGLYCERIDE IN 33 CHRONIC HEMODIALYSIS PATIENTS

TYPE	NUMBER (m/f)	%	CHOL	TRIG
Normal	10/7	52	172	98
I	0	0	-	-
IIA	0	0	-	-
IIB	2/0	6	331*	167*
III	0	0	-	-
IV	6/8	42	188	202*

* Significantly different from normal ($p < .001$), remainder not significant.

The incidence and type of lipoprotein abnormalities in 35 long-term renal transplant patients, average age 40, average months post-transplantation 19, average prednisone dose 18 mg, is detailed in Table II.

TABLE II - MEAN SERUM LIPIDS AND LIPOPROTEINS IN 35 LONG-TERM RENAL TRANSPLANT RECIPIENTS

TYPE	NUMBER (m/f)	%	CHOL	TRIG	LDL CHOL	HDL CHOL
Normal	13/4	49	230	112	154	48
I	0	0	-	-	-	-
IIA	2/4	17	274**	116	223**	51
IIB	1/1	6	407**	403**	363**	29
III	0	0	-	-	-	-
IV	7/3	28	222	167**	140	38

** Significantly different from normal ($p < .001$), remainder not significant.

Note that whereas the LDL cholesterol may be elevated in renal transplant patients, HDL cholesterol remains normal.

Eleven patients were followed through renal transplantation. Six (4 normal, 2 type IV) had no change in lipoprotein pattern. Two changed from IIB to normal, 2 from IV to IIA, and 1 from normal to IIA.

DISCUSSION: Although chronic hemodialysis therapy has been successful in prolonging the lives of patients with end stage kidney disease, it is well known that such patients often develop HLP (1,2,3) and that mortality from premature cardiovascular disease among hemodialysis patients approaches 50% (8). The present study confirms the previous observations of a 40% incidence of Type IV HLP in these patients (3). We have shown after transplantation half the patients have a change in lipid levels and lipoprotein types.

The elevation of triglyceride in hemodialysis patients has been related to decreased lipoprotein lipase activity leading to decreased triglyceride catabolism (6). Others suggest increased insulin levels may promote increased hepatic VLDL production (1). Another cause of triglyceridemia may be the high carbohydrate diet, plus the carbohydrate from the dialysis bath.

51% of 35 long-term renal transplant recipients had HLP. Although Type IV HLP was most frequent (28%) it was less frequent than in hemodialysis patients (42%) ($p = .05$). Our results in renal transplant recipients are similar to those of Lazarus et al (3) except for a slightly higher incidence of Type IV in our patients (16% vs 28%).

A number of factors have been implicated in the pathogenesis of the HLP of renal transplant recipients (3) including dietary abnormalities, corticosteroid medication, increased plasma insulin, glucagon, and parathormone levels and even the presence of chronic viral infection.

Cardiovascular disease is the most common cause of death in hemodialysis patients and aside from rejection and infection is also the leading cause of death among long-term renal transplant recipients (2,3). Although factors such as hypertension and hyperparathyroidism may contribute to vascular disease, it is likely that HLP plays a role. Therefore, it is important that these patients at risk be identified and treated.

1. Bagdade, J.D., et al, New Engl. J. Med. 279:181, 1968
2. Bagdade, J.D., Ked. Int. 7:S-370, 1975
3. Lazarus, J.M., et al, Ked. Int. 7:S-167, 1975
4. Carr, J., Drekter, J., Clinical Chemistry 2, Oct 1956
5. Bucolo, G., David, H., Clinical Chemistry 19, p476, 1973
6. Frederickson, D., et al, New Engl. J. Med. 276, p34, 1967
7. Frederickson, D., et al, Adv. Exper. Med. Biology 4:307, 1969
8. Brunner, F.P., et al, Proc. Europ. Dialysis Trans. Assoc. 9:3, 1972

(2)

CHOLESTEROL TRACKING; PREDICTION OVER TIME OF SERUM CHOLESTEROL IN EVANS COUNTY. GA.

G. Heiss, H.A. Tyroler, C. Hames

Department of Epidemiology, School of Public Health

University of North Carolina, Chapel Hill, North Carolina, U.S.A.

Fasting serum cholesterol was determined in 1960 and 1967 on 2530 subjects representing the biracial community of Evans County, under C.D.C. laboratory control and employing the Abell-Kendall method (1). For each age-race-sex cohort, mean serum cholesterol increased over the seven years of follow-up, as a function of age and body mass (exemplified for males in Figure 1).

In males, increases of cholesterol occurred predominantly in the younger cohorts, while females experienced an almost uniform rate of increase at all ages. Black examinees showed a larger overall increase when compared to white subjects (2).

Within age-race-sex cohorts, each subject's serum cholesterol intake was highly predictive of his cholesterol value seven years later. The Pearson product moment correlation between the two cholesterol measurements in each subject was of the order of 0.70 irrespective of race, age, sex, body mass, and social class, each of which is a determinant of the level of serum cholesterol (Table I).

In addition, the similarity in the ranking of subjects at the two examinations, seven years apart, was not influenced by the initial level of serum cholesterol (Figure 2) (3).

These observations, derived from a total, biracial community, suggest that individual cholesterol values are set as early as 15 years of age. Despite the known individual variability, subjects generally retain their cholesterol "position" within their cohorts over time, in the presence of factors shifting the population distribution.

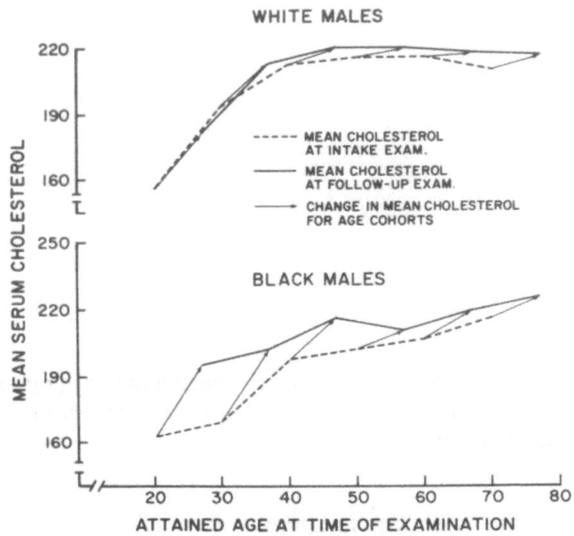

Figure 1. Change in mean serum cholesterol over seven years of follow-up, for cohorts identified by age at examination in 1960. Evans County Cardiovascular Survey.

Table I. Intra-individual correlation of serum cholesterol measurements in 1960 and 1967. Evans County Cardiovascular Survey.

Race/Sex Group	N	Cholesterol in 1960 Mean	(S.D.)	Cholesterol in 1967 Mean	(S.D.)	Change of Cholesterol Mean	(S.D.)	Correlation Cholesterol 1960, 1967
White Males	697	202.6	(42.5)	212.7	(39.2)	10.1	(30.7)	0.72
White Females	785	217.8	(50.1)	229.8	(57.7)	12.0	(44.9)	0.66
Black Males	309	200.3	(40.3)	212.6	(42.3)	12.3	(33.7)	0.68
Black Females	424	210.4	(44.0)	228.1	(50.7)	17.7	(39.2)	0.67
Total Population	2215	209.2	(42.6)	221.8	(49.7)	12.6	(38.3)	0.69

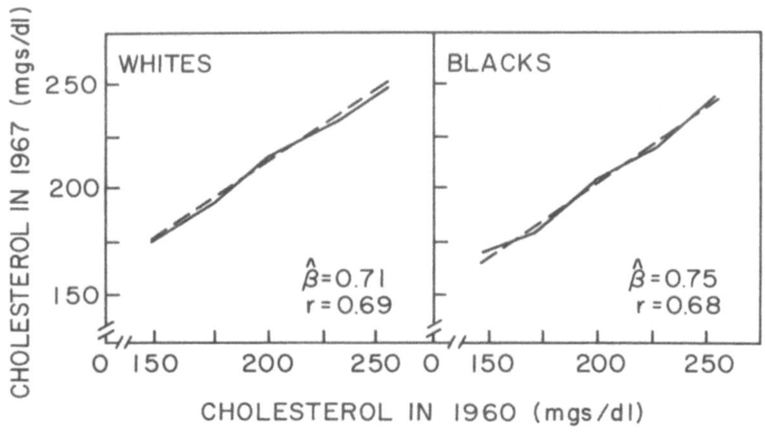

Figure 2. Simple linear and piece-wise regression (by quartiles) of cholesterol in 1967 on cholesterol in 1960, by race. Evans County Cardiovascular Survey.

REFERENCES

1. McDonough, J.R. et al.: Coronary heart disease among Negroes and white in Evans County, Ga. J. Chronic Dis. 18:443-468, 1965.
2. Tyroler, H.A. et al.: Black-White differences in serum lipids and lipoproteins in Evans County. Prev. Med. (in press).
3. Gardner, M.J., Heady, J.A.: Some effects of within-person variability in epidemiological studies. J. Chronic Dis. 26:781-795, 1973.

(3)

CORONARY HEART DISEASE PROFILE IN AUSTRALIAN MEN AND SOME FACTORS INFLUENCING SURVIVAL

Palmer, J., Leelarthaepin, B., McGilchrist, C., Blacket, R.

Departments of Medicine and Statistics,

University of New South Wales, Sydney, Australia

Australia is an affluent country with a high mortality from coronary disease. Before 1966 no systematic study of the coronary profile of Australians had been made. In that year our group began a study of the effect of dietary modification in secondary prevention. We present here data on entry characteristics and survival in relation to them.

ENTRY CHARACTERISTICS

Entry characteristics of coronary men (CM) have been compared with those of healthy men in the contemporaneous Busselton population survey (BM). In three decades from 30 to 59 the numbers were for CM 46, 190 and 222 and for BM 242, 256 and 242. Eighty-six percent of CM had survived myocardial infarction and 14% had newly diagnosed angina pectoris. Nationality and occupation showed no relevant differences. Marital disruption was somewhat more common in CM.

There was a significant preponderance of heavy smokers in CM ($P < 0.01$) most striking in the younger men where there were very few non-smokers and a large excess of heavy smokers ($P < 0.001$). In the later decades smoking was much less significant. Among smokers the duration of cigarette smoking was also greater in CM than BM.

Height of CM was 1.70 metres and of BM 1.74 metres ($P < 0.001$). At infarction CM weighed 78.0 Kg. Mean weight for BM was 75.2 Kg. ($P < 0.001$). Body mass index (W/H^2) of CM at infarction was 27.0.

For BM it was 24.8 ($P < 0.001$). When compared by decade this was due to the greater body mass of CM under 40.

Despite mean weight loss of 4.8 Kg. since infarction CM had higher serum cholesterol levels than BM in each decade. The overall means were 282 mg./100 ml. and 251 mg./100 ml. ($P < 0.001$). The most striking difference was at age 30-39 where the means were 301 mg./100 ml. and 242 mg./100 ml. CM were also hypertriglycerid-aemic. The means for each decade were 247, 288 and 175 mg./100 ml. When four subjects with serum triglyceride levels greater than 800 mg./100 ml. were deleted the means were not much altered. Mean serum urate levels for CM were 6.7 mg./100 ml. and for BM 5.9 mg./100 ml. ($P < 0.001$). No changes with age were noted. There were no apparent differences in blood sugar one hour after a glucose load in BM and CM. The mean systolic blood pressure in CM was 137 mm.Hg. and in BM 130 mm.Hg. ($P < 0.001$). The difference was most marked in CM under 50. Although these differences may be real, a number of factors make the comparison of doubtful validity. Nevertheless it agrees with the experience of others. Similar differences were noted in diastolic pressure.

Thus the coronary profile of Australian men is similar to that of Americans. Coronary men tend to be shorter than average, overweight, hyperlipidaemic, hyperuricaemic, excessive cigarette smokers and have higher blood pressure than those who remain healthy up to age 60.

SURVIVAL IN RELATION TO ENTRY CHARACTERISTICS

Mean age at entry was 48.9 years. 276 men had had no previous symptoms of CHD while 182 gave a history of previous infarction or angina. After initial investigation they were randomly allocated to two groups. All subjects were advised to lose weight if necessary. In one group there was no further dietary intervention, while the other group was advised to adopt a low fat, low cholesterol, high polyunsaturated diet. The present analysis takes no account of the dietary or any other interventions practised.

Overall five year survival was 81%. Survival was better in men under 45 than in those 45 to 59 but this was not significant. As recorded at entry the site of infarction classed as either anterior or inferior by ECG had no influence on survival. Systolic blood pressure, serum lipid levels, smoking habit, glucose tolerance and family history of CHD likewise had no prognostic influence.

By univariate analyses each of the following factors had an unfavourable prognostic influence: any previous manifestation of CHD, severe infarction, any grade of angina pectoris or dyspnoea at entry, ST-T changes with or without Q waves, cardiomegaly, high relative body weight and hyperuricaemia.

Each of the following was associated with five year survival in the range 84 percent to 91 percent: absence of previous CHD, mild or moderate infarction, absence of angina or dyspnoea, ECG normal or with T wave abnormalities only, normal heart size, relative body weight below the first quartile of the distribution. In contrast severe infarct was associated with only 50 percent survival after five years, grade II or more angina at entry sixty-five percent survival after five years and cardiomegaly fifty-eight percent survival after five years.

We have not assessed the influence on prognosis of reduction of risk factors after infarction. The findings so far emphasize the critical importance of the structural and functional integrity of the myocardium in determining survival. It would appear that standard clinical examination provides some very useful signposts to prognosis. A similar conclusion has emerged from the American Coronary Drug Project.

Reference: Coronary Drug Project Research Group. J. Chron. Dis. 1974, 27, 267.

(4)

EXERCISE ST SEGMENT DEPRESSIONS IN ASYMPTOMATIC HYPERLIPOPROTEINAEMIA AND ITS RELATION TO VARIOUS LIPOPROTEIN CLASSES

Anders G. Olsson

King Gustaf V Research Institute, Karolinska Hospital,

S-104 01 STOCKHOLM, Sweden

PURPOSE OF STUDY

To determine the frequency of ST segment depressions during exercise in asymptomatic men with different types of hyperlipoproteinaemia (HLP) and to study the dependence of this finding on the concentrations of various lipoprotein (LP) classes.

MATERIAL AND METHODS

Serum cholesterol and triglyceride (TG) concentrations were determined in 12 000 men attending a health control centre. Asymptomatic subjects with serum cholesterol above 350 mg/100 ml and/or TG above 3.50 mmol/l were studied further with 1. quantitative LP analysis in the preparative ultracentrifuge with estimation of very low (VLDL), low (LDL) and high (HDL) density LP classes, LP paper electrophoresis and typing of HLP (1) and 2. resting ecg and exercise ecg to near maximal heart rate. All subjects with overt atherosclerotic disease, hypertension, electrolyte disturbances or other conditions possibly influencing the interpretation of the ecg were excluded. An age matched control group with normal serum lipid concentrations coming from the same health control centre was offered identical investigations.

RESULTS

Normal resting ecgs were most often seen in the control groups. ST segment depressions at rest were rare in both control and HLP groups. The number of subjects and frequencies of ST depressions during and/or after exercise in the different types of HLP are given in Table I. The frequency of ST depressions increased with age. In all types of HLP the frequency of ST depressions was higher than in the control groups. The frequency of the more pronounced ST

Table I. Percentage of subjects with ST depressions 4-1-4.4 (Minnesota code (1)) during and/or after exercise in different types of HLP and in controls. n=number of subjects.

Age, yrs	36-50		>50		All ages	
	n	%	n	%	n	%
Controls	26	8	23	26	49	16
II A	11	45^{x}	15	53	26	50^{xx}
II B	6	50	8	75^{x}	14	64^{xx}
III	3	0	6	100^{xx}	9	67^{xx}
IV	47	32^{x}	34	50	81	40^{xx}

x, xx indicate significant difference against control groups on the 5 and 1 per cent level.

depressions (i.e. 4.1 and 4.2) was distributed between the different HLP types approximately as the frequency of 4.1-4.4.

The relation between ST depressions and HLP was also studied by multiple regression technique using the different LPs and other factors as independent variables.

Age was invariably the most significant determinant for exercise ST depression ($p<0.001$). Adding singly LPs upon age, LDL cholesterol was the most significant determinant to ST depression ($p<0.001$), followed by LDL TG ($p<0.05$) and VLDL TG ($p<0.05$). Adding LPs and other factors (blood pressure, glucose tolerance, smoking, weight-height index etc.) upon age and LDL cholesterol only resulted in a furhter significance for VLDL TG ($p<0.05$). By using the three significant terms age, LDL cholesterol and VLDL TG tables were then constructed predicting the probability for ST depression during exercise.

CONCLUSION

A considerable body of evidence indicates that the ST depressions of this magnitude are ischaemic in origin in subjects without hypertension, digitalis treatment or electrolyte disturbances (e.g. 3). One of the most important causes of myocardial ischaemia is coronary atheromatosis. Therefore, a probable reason for the increased frequency of ST depressions in HLP is a greater amount of coronary atheromatosis in this condition. Also, it is plausible that the increased LP concentrations - or some closely related mechanism - are responsible for this. The regression analysis showed that not only the concentration of LDL but also VLDL are of importance in the development of exercise ST depressions. These findings therefore suggest that elevation of both LDL and VLDL - alone or in combination - promote the development of ST depressions during exercise probably through an increase of coronary atherosclerosis.

REFERENCES

1. Fredrickson, D.S., Levy, R.I. and Lees, R.S.: Fat transport in lipoproteins - an integrated approach to mechanisms and disorders. New Engl. J. Med. 276:34, 94, 148, 215 and 273, 1967.

2. The Scandinavian Committe on ECG Classification. The "Minnesota code" for ECG classification. Adaption to CR leads and modification of the code for ECGs recorded during and after exercise. Stockholm 1967.

3. Mattingly, T.W.: The postexercise electrocardiogram. Its value in the diagnosis and prognosis of coronary arterial disease. Am. J. Cardiol. 9:395, 1962.

(5)

ATHEROSCLEROTIC CARDIOVASCULAR MORTALITY IN THE ISLAND OF CRETE STUDY

Christ Aravanis, M.D., and A. Corcondilas, M.D.

Faculty of Medicine, Athens University

Athens, Greece

The aim of epidemiological studies in Greece, as part of an international co-operative program, was to 1) examine a definite group of middle age men living under similar conditions, 2) to follow the subsequent disease experience of these men and 3) to discover possible relationships between the pre-disease characteristics and the incidence of the disease, notably cardiovascular (CVD), resulting from atherosclerosis.

This report presents data in one of the population samples in the rural area of Crete, Greece fully examined nearly 15 years ago and followed since. The island of Crete is situated in the southern part of Greece, is mountainous and is known since the Minoic civilization 4000 years ago; it is agricultural and the inhabitants are small farmers. The first study started in 1960 and covered 686 men aged 40-59 years in prescribed villages. Characteristics of the examined sample were: co-operation, stability in residence, occupation and diet, no sharp contrasts in economic standards and no sharp retirement with age. Parameters taken into consideration were: body weight, body fatness, blood pressure, physical activity, electrocardiographic findings at rest and after exercise, serum cholesterol, smoking habits, lung function and diet.

Entry and follow-up data have shown that prevalence and incidence of overweight and obesity are low; with a subcutaneous fat thickness of 5 mm, less than 3% of the Cretans are obese. Hypertension is also less frequent particularly for men over 50 years of age; 12% of the men had high blood pressure greater than 150/90 mm Hg.

In regard to serum cholesterol, men in Crete had a low cholesterol with a mean value of 202 mg per 100 ml. More than 93% of the people are physically very active with a sustained endurance type of habitual activity; this results from the fact that agriculture is underdeveloped and work is arduous due to the lack of mechanized farming. People are poor peasants and small land-owners, who walk daily long distances to work.

In regard to smoking habits people tend to smoke rather heavily and more than one-third of them smoke more than 20 cigarettes daily.

The diet of this population is of special interest, since it is simple and plain although nutritionally good; it is remarkable for being high in total fats exclusively arriving from olive oil which provides more than one-third of the daily calories, but very low in animal fats; saturated fatty acids provide about 8% of dietary calories. Intake of animal proteins also is low. The daily caloric intake of 2750 calories consists mainly of bread, pulses, vegetables, potatoes, olives, olive oil and fruits in varying proportions around the year, but without considerable seasonal differences.

Morbidity and mortality from CVD is low and cases of myocardial infarction and angina pectoris are rare in a population aged now 54 to 73 years. During the 14-year period of follow-up 5 people died from coronary heart disease and another 5 from cerebral vascular accidents, an incidence of 5.2 per year per 10.000. Peripheral arterial diseases are practically nonexistent. Total all-causes death rate reflects the low death rate from CVD with the result to be lower, in the order of 64 cases per year per 10.000.

From the presented data one can conclude that CVD, a sequela of atherosclerosis, is rare among the farmers in Crete and in comparison with many other Western countries.

Whatever mechanisms may account for the remarkably low prevalence and incidence of CVD among Cretans, there is no question that their way of life and habits of eating act probably as very important factors in keeping these people free of risk factors and thus relatively "immune" from the number one killing diseases of today, i.e., atherosclerotic cardiovascular diseases.

REFERENCES

Aravanis, C., et al., On the study of ischaemic heart diseases on the islands of Crete and Corfu, Greece. Prog. Bioch. Pharm. 4: 12, 1968.

Aravanis, C., et al., Rural populations in Crete and Corfu, Greece. Ed. A. Keys. Acta Med. Scandin., Suppl. 460, p. 209, 1967.

Aravanis, C., et al., The islands of Crete and Corfu. Ed. A. Keys, Circulation, Suppl. 41, 1: 88, 1970.

CHAPTER 2
MYOCARDIAL INFARCTION

(1)

NON-OBSTRUCTIVE MURAL CORONARY THROMBOSIS IN SUDDEN DEATH

R.J. Frink, MD

Mercy General Hospital, Cardio-Pulmonary Dept.

1004 J Street, Sacramento, California, U.S.A.

Instantaneous death (death within seconds to a few minutes) in patients considered to be healthy and without a history or clinical evidence of cardiac disease is commonly believed to be due to a disturbance in heart rhythm.[1,2] Post-mortem examination usually reveals the presence of coronary arteriosclerosis.[1-3] The rhythm disturbance is often explained on the basis of phasic changes in already compromised coronary blood flow.[3] The resulting ischemia is thought to precipitate the lethal arrhythmia. Another possible mechanism is the obstruction of the micro-circulation secondary to embolization of platelet or fibrin aggregates from a thrombus situated upstream in the main epicardial coronary branches.[4-7] A considerable amount of evidence, both in animals and in humans has been accumulated which demonstrates a relationship between platelets, arterial thrombosis and sudden death.[3,4,6]

This report deals with five males, ages 32 - 44, without prior history of heart disease, all of whom died an instantaneous death. One died during a noon time nap at work; one died while swimming across a pool; another died while resting on the living room couch; one collapsed in the men's room at work and a fifth developed gas pains while mowing the lawn and expired shortly thereafter.

All hearts were obtained fresh and intact at the autopsy table. The coronary arteries were injected with a different colored barium gelatin mass[8] and then the heart was fixed in formalin. The arteries were dissected free from the external surface of the heart, decalcified, cut at 2 - 3 mm intervals and each section mounted for histologic study. Each heart was bread-loafed from apex to near the base of the heart with multiple myocardial sections taken for histologic study. The sinus node and A-V node blocks were cut at 2 - 3 mm intervals and each section mounted for histologic examination. All myocardial and A-V node sections were stained with hemotoxylin and eosin (H & E), Masson's trichrome stain, phosphotungstic acid hemotoxylin (PTAH) and hemotoxylin-basic Fuchsin-picric acid (HBFP) stain. The HBFP stain was used to identify early ischemic changes in the myocardium and in the conduction system. Appropriate X-rays and photographs were taken at all stages of the examination used with each heart.

All patients had some degree of coronary arteriosclerosis but all major arteries were patent. All exhibited at least one non-obstructive mural coronary thrombus in a major epicardial branch. In three of five cases, the thrombus was in the proximal LAD. No acute or old infarction was evident grossly or microscopically. The blood supply to the sinus node was intact in all five cases. The microscopic blood supply to the A-V node and His Bundle was normal in four cases. One case had significant disease of the A-V node artery. A definite downstream fibrin/platelet embolus could be found in two cases. A portion of the His Bundle and/or bundle branch system stained positive with the HBFP stain in four of the five cases.

DISCUSSION

A non-obstructive mural thrombus is an acute active lesion. Sudden, unexpected death is certainly an acute event. Circumstantial evidence relates these two acute problems as cause and effect. The finding of definite downstream platelet/fibrin emboli plus possible early myocardial ischemia suggests obstruction to the micro-circulation. Animal experiments clearly relate cardiovascular collapse and rhythm disturbances, particularly ventricular fibrillation to obstruction of the micro-circulation by platelet aggregates.[9] We can assume the mechanism of death in these five cases was either ventricular fibrillation or cardiac arrest. The great majority of these cases die as a result of ventricular fibrillation.[1] The evidence suggests repeated embolization of platelet/fibrin emboli from an upstream thrombus, which obstructs the micro-circulation and thus precipitates a lethal arrhythmia, probably ventricular fibrillation. The positive HBFP stains of the His Bundle and/or bundle branches suggest that the conduction system may play an integral part in lethal arrhythmias.

REFERENCES

1. Liberthson RR, Nagel EL, Hirschman JC, Nussenfeld SR, Blackborne BD, Davis JH; Pathophysiologic observations in prehospital ventricular fibrillation and sudden cardiac death. Circ 49:790-798 1974

2. Friedman M, Manwaring JH, Roseman RH, Donlon G, Ortega P, Grube

SM; Instantaneous and sudden deaths. Clinical and pathological differentiation in coronary artery disease. JAMA 225:1319-1328 1973

3. Roberts WC, Buja LM; The frequency and significance of coronary arterial thrombi and other observations in fatal acute myocardial infarction. Amer J Med 52:425-443 1972

4. Mustard JF; Platelets and thrombosis in acute myocardial infarction. Hosp Pract 7:115, 1972

5. More RH, Haust MD; The role of thrombosis in occlusive disease of coronary arteries. In: Anticoagulants and Fibrinolysis. Eds. MacMillan RL, Mustard JF; Philadelphia, Lee and FeBiger, p143, 1961

6. Jørgensen L, Haerem J, Chandler AB, Borchgrevink CT; The pathology of acute coronary death. Acta Anaesth Scand Suppl 29:193, 1968

7. Ehrlich JC; Shinohara Y; Low incidence of coronary thrombosis in myocardial infarction. A restudy by serial block technique. Arch Path 78:432, 1964

8. Frink RJ, James TN; Normal blood supply to the human His Bundle and proximal bundle branches. Circ 47:8-18 1973

9. Jørgensen L, Rowsell HC, Hovig T, Glynn MD, Mustard JF; Adenosine diphophate induced platelet aggregation and myocardial infarction in swine. Lab Invest 17:616, 1967

(2)

IMPROVED BIOCHEMICAL DETECTION OF MYOCARDIAL ISCHEMIC INJURY.

Robert Roberts, M.D., FRCP(C) and Burton E. Sobel, M.D., FACC

Department of Medicine, Washington University

St. Louis, Missouri, U.S.A.

Elevated serum CPK activity is an extremely sensitive index of acute myocardial infarction, but false positives occur with a frequency of around 15%. (1) CPK exists as three isoenzymes, MM, MB and BB, analysis of which should enhance diagnostic specificity. Until recently, quantification of individual serum CPK isoenzyme activity was inadequate due to imprecision in assay procedures. Recently, we have described a kinetic and fluorometric assay which is linear with respect to time and isoenzyme activity, having a sensitivity of .001 IU/ml with reproducibility $\pm$ 3%. (2) Utilizing this assay, the present study was designed to determine the sensitivity and specificity of serum CPK isoenzymes in the diagnosis of myocardial infarction.

To determine the sensitivity of MB CPK, CPK isoenzymes were analyzed in serum samples obtained every two hours from 100 patients admitted to the Cardiac Care Unit with definite acute myocardial infarction. Total serum CPK activity was elevated in all cases with a mean peak of 0.852 IU/ml. All patients exhibited elevated MB CPK isoenzyme activity with a mean peak serum level of 0.089 IU/ml. Thus, elevated MB CPK is a sensitive index of acute myocardial infarction, a finding in agreement with that of others. (3)

The specificity of elevated MB CPK as an index of myocardial injury in conditions with injury to organs other than the heart has not been thoroughly elucidated. To evaluate specificity, two types of information are required: 1) is MB CPK present in human tissues other than the heart; and 2) is its release responsible for elevations in serum MB CPK. CPK isoenzyme activity was quantified in fresh human tissue biopsies obtained at the time of surgery. Tissues were homogenized in a sucrose medium containing 1 mM mercaptoethanol buffered at a pH of 7.4. Results of CPK isoenzyme assays performed on human biopsies are shown below. All assays were performed in triplicate.

Tissue	CPK (IU/g)	MM	MB	BB
Muscle	3200 ± 200	3200 ± 200	0	0
Heart	680 ± 60	584 ± 40	96 ± 5	0
Brain	180 ± 30	0	0	180 ± 30
GI Tract	140 ± 20	0	0	140 ± 20
Lung	13 ± 2	1 ± .2	0	12 ± .5
Kidney	9 ± 1.5	1 ± .1	0	8 ± .5

To determine whether serum MB CPK is elevated following surgery, serial serum samples were obtained from 100 post-operative patients. Surgical procedures included thoracotomy (30); laparotomy (70) with GI tract procedures (38), GU (22), and GYN (10). Total serum CPK activity increased in all patients (260 ± 61 (SD) mIU/ml). However, serum MB CPK activity was not elevated in any. None of these patients exhibited clinical or electrocardiographic evidence of myocardial damage.

The false positives seen with total serum CPK activity are due to CPK predominantly from skeletal muscle. If MB formed even a small fraction of the total CPK activity in skeletal muscle, its activity could be significant since skeletal muscle contains 300% more CPK than myocardium. Other studies have been performed evaluating CPK isoenzymes in skeletal muscle but were performed on tissues obtained at necropsy. (3,4) MB that may have been present could have been overlooked because of its lability. Since the present study utilized tissue biopsies processed immediately, artifact of this type could be excluded. The possibility that different muscles have different CPK isoenzyme profiles has not been adequately excluded in the past. Since more than 200 individual muscles exist in man, we examined this problem by selecting post-operative patients such that the surgical procedures involved injury to a large variety of muscles, including those of the thorax, abdomen, thigh, leg and hand. Under no circumstances did serum MB CPK activity increase.

In conclusion, of the human tissues examined in this study, the only tissue containing significant amounts of MB CPK was the heart. Serum obtained from 100 patients after surgery exhibited no elevation of MB CPK. Serum from patients with acute myocardial infarction consistently exhibited elevated MB CPK activity. Thus, elevated serum MB CPK is both a sensitive and a specific index of myocardial injury.

REFERENCES

1. Goldberg, D.M., Windfield, D.A.: Diagnostic accuracy of serum enzyme assays for myocardial infarction in a general hospital population. Brit. Heart J. 34: 597, 1972.

2. Roberts, R., Henry, P.D., Witteveen, S.A.G.J., Sobel, B.E.: Quantification of serum creatine phosphokinase (CPK) isoenzyme activity. Amer. J. Cardiol. 33: 650, 1974.

3. Konttinen, A., Somer, H.: Determination of serum creatine kinase isoenzymes in myocardial infarction. Amer. J. Cardiol. 29: 817, 1972.

4. Smith, A.F.: Separation of tissue and serum creatine kinase isoenzymes on polyacrylamide gel slabs. Clin. Chim. Acta. 39: 351, 1972.

(3)

MYOCARDIAL PERFUSION ASSESSED BY DIRECT CORONARY ARTERIAL INJECTION OF RADIOLABELLED PARTICLES

W.J. Kostuk, M.D., F.R.C.P.(C)

Dept. of Medicine, University Hospital, University of Western Ontario, London, Ontario, Canada

Full assessment of coronary atherosclerotic disease necessitates not only the determination of symptoms, but also the coronary anatomy, collateral circulation patterns and left ventricular function. The coronary arteriogram does not measure regional myocardial perfusion at the capillary level, while the left ventricular angiogram cannot distinguish between reversible and irreversible myocardial dysfunction. Such evaluation is becoming more important as the number of patients being considered for aorto-coronary by-pass surgery increases. The delivery of additional blood to heavily scarred myocardium is a needless procedure. Myocardial perfusion as measured by the labelled albumin particle method (1, 2) is a promising technique which appears to be capable of distinguishing between scarred myocardium and ischemic, yet viable, myocardial tissue. We have assessed this technique in patients undergoing diagnostic coronary angiography and would like to present the results in our first 400 patients.

METHOD

All patients had cardiac catheterization including left ventricular and selective coronary angiography. Following the latter, particles of human serum albumin labelled with either Iodine^{131} or Technetium^{99} were injected selectively into each coronary artery. The particles are 20-30μ in diameter and have a biological half life of 3-5 hrs. The dose range for ^{99m}Tc microspheres was 300 μCi consisting of 20-30,000 particles; 150 μCi of I^{131} macroaggragated albumin were used with similar number of particles. Following completion of the invasive cardiac procedure, the patient was transferred to the Nuclear Medicine Laboratory for myocardial imaging. Scans were obtained in the anterior and 45° left anterior oblique position (LAO) with a rectilinear scanner. The scanner is connected to a computer which permits a colour coded pictorial display as well as allowing differentiation of radioactivity in the appropriate count range.

RESULTS

The myocardial perfusion images of each patient were analyzed and compared with the coronary arteriograms, left ventricular angiograms and electrocardiograms. Each patient was classified into one of four groups on the basis of their coronary artery anatomy and the myocardial perfusion scans.

GROUP	DESCRIPTION *	NO.
A	NCA/NMP	127
B	NCA/AMP	74
C	CAD/NMP	100
D	CAD/AMP	99

*Abbreviations: NCA = Normal coronary arteries, NMP = Normal myocardial perfusion, CAD = Coronary atherosclerotic disease, AMP = Abnormal myocardial perfusion.

The normal myocardial perfusion anatomy correlated with normal coronary anatomy seen angiographically. The distribution of the radioactive particles injected into the left coronary artery corresponds to the area outlined by the left anterior descending (LAD) and left circumflex branches seen in the same projections. The distribution of the radioactive particles injected into the right coronary artery demonstrates intense activity inferiorly but little activity anteriorly as seen in the LAO view; this indicates the predominant perfusion being in the distribution of the posterior descending and posterolateral branches of the right coronary artery with minimal perfusion of the right ventricular wall. The LAO position is a valuable one in that it provides the best delineation of abnormality. In this view, the left anterior descending coronary arterial distribution is visualized anteriorly, the circumflex distribution posterolaterally and the right coronary artery distribution inferiorly. In those individuals with a nondominant right coronary artery, the distribution of the posterolateral branch of the right coronary artery occurs more proximally and can usually be distinguished from that associated with right coronary artery occlusion.

Group A had both normal coronary arteries and myocardial perfusion. The coronary arteries were considered to be normal even in the presence of a minor degree of plaque formation and sites of noncritical stenosis ($<$75%).

Group B patients had normal coronary arteries but abnormal myocardial perfusion. Seven of the 74 patients in this group exhibited a flow defect; invariably this was associated with the presence of a short, left main stem coronary artery such that the selective catheter tended to enter either the LAD or circumflex branch. Twenty-four patients had a cardiomyopathy. Indeed, almost all patients with congestive cardiomyopathy whom we have studied by this technique showed abnormal scans of a diffuse, patchy nature. In patients with hypertrophic obstructive cardiomyopathy, on the other hand, the abnormality tended to be localized to the thickened ventricular septum (3). In 35 patients, myocardial perfusion abnormalities were noted in patients with valvular heart disease in the presence of normal coronary arteries. The degree of abnormality appeared related to the severity of the valvular dysfunction. Individuals with predominant mitral stenosis, showed augmented perfusion of the right ventricle, whereas, those with an incompetent mitral valve in addition, showed an abnormality in their left ventricular myocardial perfusion. With aortic incompetence the overall heart size was increased together with a decrease in left ventricular perfusion. On the other hand, with an obstructive aortic valve lesion, normal perfusion was often observed in spite of a severe degree of obstruction.

In Group C, in spite of a critical stenosis or a complete occlusion of a coronary artery, the combined right and left myocardial perfusion scans were normal, indicative of good collateral perfusion.

Group D exhibited perfusion defects in association with the critical stenosis or occlusion seen angiographically. Such defects were associated with an abnormality of left ventricular contraction. Conversely, over 50% of patients with CAD who exhibited localized hypokinesis on the left ventricular angiogram had a normal myocardial perfusion scan indicating ischemic, but viable myocardial tissue. On the other hand, a dilated, diffusely hypokinetic left ventricle invariably showed large perfusion defects indicative of extensive scarred myocardium. Likewise, the presence of akinesis and/or dyskinesis on the left ventriculogram was often, but not invariably, associated with a perfusion defect.

The electrocardiographic finding of Q waves or bundle branch block, is usually associated with a perfusion defect, although 25% of such patients (usually inferior wall infarction) showed overall normal myocardial perfusion. On the other hand, 25% of patients who do not exhibit ECG evidence of previous myocardial damage showed an abnormal myocardial perfusion scan.

Initial postoperative studies in 65 patients (not included in this series) have shown that only 10% of patients with normal myocardial perfusion scans pre and postoperative continue to have significant angina. On the other hand, approximately 55% of those with an abnormal perfusion image 2 weeks postoperatively have continued with their symptoms.

Myocardial perfusion imaging in conjunction with coronary and left ventricular angiography is a valuable diagnostic tool in the evaluation of regional myocardial perfusion in patients with coronary atherosclerotic disease. The labelled albumin particle technique is capable of distinguishing between scarred, nonviable myocardium and ischemic, but viable myocardium. This difference is important if aorto-coronary by-pass surgery is being contemplated.

REFERENCES

1. Ashburn, W.L., Braunwald, E., Simon, A.L., Peterson, K.L., and Gault, J.H.: Myocardial perfusion imaging with radioactive labelled particles injected directly into the coronary circulation of patients with coronary artery disease. Circulation 44:851-865, 1971.

2. Jansen, C., Judkins, M.P., Grames, G.M., Gander, M., and Adams, R.: Myocardial perfusion color scintigraphy with MAA. Radiology 109:369-380, 1973.

3. Kostuk, W.J. and Chamberlain, M.J.: Abnormal myocardial perfusion in patients with cardiomyopathy. Annals of The Royal College of Physicians and Surgeons of Canada 8:12, 1975.

This work was supported by the Ontario Heart Foundation.

(4)

CONTROLLED TRIAL OF A CARDIAC AMBULANCE SERVICE MANNED BY AMBULANCE PERSONNEL

J. R. Hampton, M.D.,
Department of Medicine
University of Nottingham and General Hospital
Nottingham, England

Ambulances manned by specially-trained crews and equipped for the resuscitation of patients with arrhythmias have been claimed to reduce the mortality of heart attacks. While there can be no doubt that such services have saved lives, no comparisons have been made between these and routine ambulance services. In Nottingham a special cardiac ambulance manned by trained ambulance personnel was established in 1973 and as it proved impossible to man the special service continuously, it was decided to conduct a trial of the efficacy of the new service by comparing the mortality of patients brought to hospital by the cardiac ambulance with that of patients brought in by the routine ambulance service.

During one year, the cardiac ambulance was sent out to 502 calls, of which 112 proved to be for patients with heart attacks. The overall mortality in this group (including patients dead on arrival in hospital and patients dying in hospital) was 40%.

During the same period the Nottingham City routine ambulance service brought to hospital 396 patients with heart attacks. Of these, 324 were transported at times when the cardiac vehicle was not available, and in this group the overall mortality was 51%. Transport by the cardiac ambulance therefore appears to be associated with a significantly ($p < 0.05$) lower mortality than transport by the routine ambulance service at times when the cardiac vehicle was not available.

However, in the group of patients with heart attacks transported by the routine ambulance service at times when the cardiac vehicle was available but for some reason was not used, the overall mortality was 68%, which is significantly higher than in either the group of patients carried by the cardiac ambulance or in the group carried by the routine ambulance service at times when the cardiac vehicle was not available.

Thus, the routine ambulance service seems to have been associated with a much higher mortality when the cardiac vehicle was available (68%) than when it was not (51%). Since the routine vehicle had the same personnel and equipment whether the cardiac vehicle was available or not, it seems intrinsically unlikely that the routine service will actually have been worse just because a cardiac vehicle was available. The only logical deduction is that there must have been inadvertent selection of low-risk cases for transport by the cardiac ambulance, with an undue proportion of high-risk cases being transported by the routine service. This is supported by comparing the mortality at times when the cardiac vehicle was not available so that the routine service had to be used (51%) with the total mortality at times when the cardiac vehicle was available (patients carried by the cardiac vehicle plus patients carried by the routine service) - the total mortality at these times again being 51%.

The patients in the different groups were found to be similar in terms of age, sex, in numbers with previous heart attacks, and in their clinical state on arrival at hospital. However, in the group of patients brought to hospital by the routine service at times when the cardiac vehicle was available, there was a higher proportion with a short (less than 30 minutes) duration of symptoms, more had had their attack away from home, and more had called for an emergency ambulance directly rather than first calling their General Practitioner. Patients carried by the cardiac ambulance tended to have a longer duration of symptoms before the arrival of the ambulance, were more likely to have had their attack at home, and were more likely to have called their General Practitioner first.

REFERENCES

Adgey, A.A.J., Allen, J.D., Geddes, J.S., James, R.G.G., Webb, S.W., Zaidi, S.A., and Pantridge, J.P. Lancet 2:501, 1971.

Dewar, H.A., McCollum, J.P.K., and Floyd, M. Brit. Med. J. 3:226, 1969.

Gearty, G.F., Hickey, N., Bourke, G.J., Mulcahy, R. Brit. Med. J. 3:33, 1971.

Liberthson, R.R., Nagel, E.L., Hirschman, J.C., Nussenfeld, S.R. New Eng. J. Med. 291:317, 1974.

Rytand, D.A. Arch. Int. Med. 88:207, 1951

White, N.M., Parker, W.S., Binning, R.A., Kimber, E.R., Ead, H.W., and Chamberlain, D.A. Brit. Med. J. 3:618, 1973.

(5)

THE HEPARIN NEUTRALIZING ACTIVITY TEST IN THE DIAGNOSIS OF ACUTE MYOCARDIAL INFARCTION (MI)

O'Brien, J.R., Etherington, M.D., Jamieson, S., Lawford, P. and Sussex, J.
Portsmouth & S.E. Hampshire District Pathology Service, Central Laboratory, St. Mary's General Hospital, Portsmouth, England

INTRODUCTION

We have previously shown that the test for heparin neutralizing activity (HNA) shows a significant increase in HNA in patients long after recovery from a myocardial infarct (post-MI) (O'Brien 1974; O'Brien et al. in the press). There is also increasing evidence that HNA in platelet poor plasma usually reflects platelet factor 4 (PF4) presumably derived from platelets broken down or undergoing release in the circulation. Accordingly it seemed appropriate to study this test in the acute disease (ac-MI). Abnormal tests long after the event may reflect a predisposition to MI: they are unlikely to be the result of the MI. Changes found immediately after the acute event are much more likely to be the result of the episode.

THE TESTS

Citrated blood is centrifuged at 3500 rpm for 10 mins to produce platelet poor plasma (PPP). To 0.1ml PPP is added 0.1ml heparin 0.8 U/ml and 20 secs later thrombin 0.1ml 10 U/ml: clotting is carried out in duplicate in glass tubes at 37°C. Because the patient's plasma is used as substrate in the HNA test, the patient's reaction to thrombin must be shown to be normal. Thus 0.1ml PPP + 0.1ml thrombin 1 U/ml is clotted. This must - and in this study did - give the standard time of 23 ± 2 secs before the HNA result can be accepted. Aliquots of a frozen control were also tested daily. Platelet counts were by Coulter Model B 70μ aperture and the mean platelet volume estimated by the MCV Computer standardized with latex beads 2.02μm diameter.

THE PATIENTS

Eighty-eight patients admitted to hospital with suspected MI were studied. The tests were carried out as soon as possible, usually on the second day after the episode and often serially. Twelve patients were studied up to 3 m. The diagnosis of acute MI was only established after a full work up; 54 patients were accepted as having true MI. The rest, called "chest pain", did not have MI and the final diagnosis was usually acute angina but other diagnoses occurred. Patients studied 3 m - 5 yr after the episode, called post-MI, have been previously reported (O'Brien et al. in the press). Controls were of the same age and sex and gave no abnormal history.

RESULTS

There was virtually no overlap in HNA clotting times between the ac-MI and the chest pain: 49 of the ac-MI results were <16 secs while 5 were from 19-28 secs and lie in the post-MI and normal range. Of the 34 chest pain results, 32 were >16 secs. The platelet count and volume of the ac-MI were also very significantly different from the controls ($P = 0.01$ and 0.001 respectively). The chest pain group had large platelets but the HNA time was barely abnormal ($P < 0.1$).

The 12 patients studied serially for 1-3 m showed a slight, but insignificant, prolongation of the HNA time by 11-15 days. By 1-3 m the time was as long (mean 20 secs) as that of the post-MI group who were studied 3 m - 5 yr after the infarct. Thus it takes about 6 weeks for this test to reach the seemingly static post-MI range.

UNITS	Acute MI	Chest pain	Post MI	Controls
NUMBER	54	34	39	74
HNA CLOTTING TIME : SECS	12.8 ± 6.98	25.1 ± 13.5	20.9 ± 9.56	28.2 ± 12.02
PLATELET COUNT $\times 10^9 l$	189 ± 92	216 ± 122	211 ± 163	230 ± 126
MEAN PLATELET VOLUME	9.64 ± 3.04	9.65 ± 2.69	8.56 ± 1.30	8.00 ± 1.44

CONCLUSIONS

This test is non-specific and HNA is raised in diffuse intravascular coagulation, by acute DVT*to a lesser extent, by pregnancy and by operations. However if these conditions can be excluded and the patient is admitted with chest pain and this HNA test is short - a result that can be obtained in 15 mins from collecting the blood - it is extremely likely that the patient has had an MI. A test in the normal range does not exclude the diagnosis but makes it very unlikely. The count and the size, while showing significant differences from normal, do not help discriminate.

If excess HNA truly indicates excessive platelet involvement, then this finding together with that of fewer, larger platelets, are all compatible with an increase in platelet turnover with excess of young, large platelets. At least in post-MI we have evidence of increased activity, since the bleeding time is short (O'Brien et al. 1973). Presumably these changes found after an acute episode follow, and are the result of, the episode. It seems unlikely, but can not be excluded, that they precede the episode and so may be related to the cause.

* = deep vein thrombosis

REFERENCES

O'Brien, J.R. (1974): Anti-thrombin III and heparin clotting times in thrombosis and atherosclerosis. Thrombosis et Diathesis Haemorrhagica, 32:116.

O'Brien, J.R., Etherington, M.D., Jamieson, S. and Klaber, M.R. (1973): Stressed template bleeding time and other platelet function tests in myocardial infarction. Lancet, 1:694.

O'Brien, J.R., Etherington, M.D., Jamieson, S., Lawford, P., Lincoln, S.V. and Alkjaersig, N. (in the press): Blood changes in atherosclerosis and long after myocardial infarction and venous thrombosis. Thrombosis et Diathesis Haemorrhagica.

CHAPTER 3
FATE OF LIPOPROTEINS

(1)

CHYLOMICRON REMNANT PARTICLE FORMATION *IN VIVO* IN HEPATECTOMISED RAT.*

A. Vost, D. M.-E. Pocock and S. Pleet

McGill University Medical Clinic
The Montreal General Hospital
Montreal, Que., Canada

The triglyceride-rich lipoproteins, chylomicrons and very low density lipoproteins, are initially catabolised by enzymatic removal of part of their triglyceride mass in extrahepatic tissues (1). Subsequently the cholesteryl esters and part of the cholesterol retained in the chylomicron remnant particles are cleared from plasma by liver; in the hepatectomised rat chylomicron triglyceride is cleared but chylomicron cholesterol and cholesteryl esters accumulate in plasma in particles with an apparent mean diameter approximately half that of their precursor chylomicrons (2).

Chylomicrons of diameter >1200 A° were prepared by ultracentrifugation of lymph from rats with cannulated thoracic ducts fed ^{3}H-glycerol and ^{14}C-cholesterol by intraduodenal tube. ^{3}H-triglyceride formed >90% of ^{3}H-lipid and 70% of ^{14}C-cholesterol was esterified in these chylomicrons. Rats with indwelling polythene cannulas in the right jugular vein and carotid artery were functionally hepatectomised by removal of the gastrointestinal tract between diaphragm and rectum and their plasma volume was restored by 2 mls rat serum. Chylomicrons were injected as an intravenous bolus and serial arterial blood samples taken for 90 min. Serum lipids were extracted and chromatographed by conventional techniques. In sham operated rats chylomicron ^{3}H-triglyceride had a $T\frac{1}{2}$ of 3.5 min and 50% of the ^{14}C-lipid was cleared from plasma in 15 min; in 4 hepatectomised rats ^{3}H-triglyceride was cleared but no significant disappearance of ^{14}C-cholesterol or its esters was observed between 10 and 60 mins after injection of chylomicrons if excess hemodilution from sampling was avoided. From 10 to 90 min, ^{14}C-cholesterol and ^{14}C-cholesteryl esters showed identical percentage changes with time in 2 experiments. These findings are consistent with the hypothesis that cholesteryl esters in triglyceride-depleted chylomicron remnant particles are cleared by liver in the intact rat; they indicate, however, that chylomicron free cholesterol clearance from plasma is also dependent on the presence of liver.

To investigate the possibilities of production of more than one form of chylomicron remnant particle and of participation of other lipoproteins in transport of chylomicron cholesterol, serum lipoproteins were examined by agarose bead column chromatography. 90 minute serum containing <6% of labeled lipid in intact chylomicrons was applied to Bio Gel A-5 m (Bio-Rad Labs. Calif.) columns (3) and 90% of ^{3}H-lipid and 80% of ^{14}C-lipid were recovered in lipoproteins larger than low density lipoproteins (LDL) and 20% of ^{14}C-lipid was recovered in the elution volume of LDL and high density lipoproteins (HDL). By using Bio Gel A-150 m, the major lipoprotein peak (on A-5 m columns) was separated into two peaks, Peak I and Peak II (Fig 1); Peak III contained LDL and HDL.

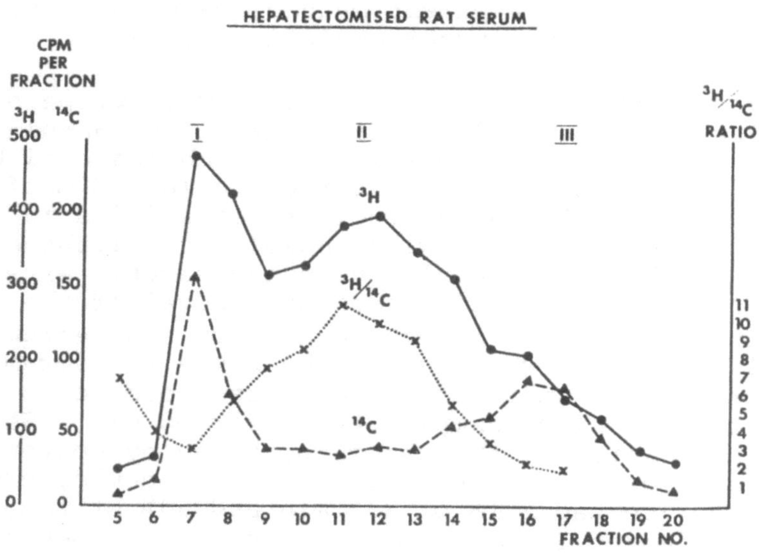

Fig. 1

In injected chylomicrons 70% of ^{3}H and ^{14}C-lipid were recovered in Peak I. By 90 min the $^{3}H/^{14}C$ ratio in Peaks I and II had fallen to 20% or less of their ratio at 20 and 30 minutes (n = 2) indicating continued formation of ^{3}H-triglyceride depleted particles in both Peaks I and II. The $^{3}H/^{14}C$ ratio in these two peaks differed significantly (Fig 1). At 20, 30 and 90 mins ^{14}C-cholesterol in Peaks I and II was 75% esterified but in Peak III only 37% was esterified. Immediate addition of lecithin-cholesterol acyltransferase inhibitors after plasma sampling did not alter the proportion of ^{14}C-cholesterol esterified in plasma.

These experiments indicate that both free and ester cholesterol in chylomicrons are equally dependent on the presence of the liver for plasma clearance. The results also suggest the possible formation of 2 distinct forms of triglyceride-depleted remnant particles from injected chylomicrons but this requires further investigation.

(1) HAVEL, R. J. In Handbook of Physiology, Section 5, American Physiological Society, Washington D. C., 499-507 (1965).

(2) REDGRAVE, T. G., J. Clin. Invest. 49, 465-471 (1970).

(3) RUDEL, L. L., J. A. LEE, M. M. MORRIS and J. M. FELTS, Biochem. J. 139, 89-95 (1974).

*This work was supported by M.R.C. Operating Grant #MA-3900.

(2)

USE OF ESTERIFIED RETINOL TO TRACE THE DEGRADATION OF CHYLOMICRONS IN CHOLESTEROL-FED RABBITS *

A. Catharine Ross† and D. B. Zilversmit ‡

Division of Nutritional Sciences and Section of
Biochemistry, Molecular and Cell Biology
Cornell University, Ithaca, New York, U.S.A.

In the normal rat (1) and dog (2) chylomicron triglyceride (TG) is rapidly hydrolyzed in peripheral tissues. Partially degraded chylomicrons containing intestinal cholesteryl esters are subsequently taken into liver parenchymal cells (1). Cholesteryl esters may be recirculated in hepatogenous very low density lipoproteins (VLDL). Dietary retinyl esters are co-transported with esterified cholesterol in chylomicrons and are also removed by the liver (3). However, esterified retinol is not recirculated in hepatic VLDL. Esterified retinol may therefore be useful as a specific marker for tracing the degradation of TG-rich VLDL of intestinal origin.

Cholesterol feeding in rabbits produces a rapid elevation in the concentration of plasma VLDL having a high content of esterified cholesterol and relatively little TG. Hypercholesterolemic VLDL could be either partially degraded chylomicrons or hepatic VLDL of modified composition. To test the hypothesis that cholesterol feeding in rabbits produces an imbalance between production and clearance of intestinal lipoproteins, and therefore results in an elevated concentration of circulating chylomicron remnants, we have measured the clearance from plasma of lymph chylomicrons labeled with [^{14}C] cholesteryl esters and [^{3}H] retinyl esters.

METHODS

Doubly labeled chylomicrons, $S_f > 400$, were isolated from thoracic duct lymph of cholesterol-fed rabbits given [^{14}C] cholesterol and [^{3}H] retinyl acetate § intraduodenally. The chylomicron dose for injection into recipients contained 19-23 mg TG/kg bodyweight; more than 86% of the ^{14}C and 92% of the ^{3}H activity was esterified.

Recipients were female New Zealand white rabbits fed a chow diet supplemented daily with 2.7 g cottonseed oil with or without 500 mg cholesterol; all rabbits were conscious and absorptive. Serial plasma samples were analyzed for TG content and for radioactivity in cholesteryl and retinyl esters after partition of lipids into hexane (4) and separation of esters by Al_2O_3 column chromatography (4). In some cases, aliquots of plasma were separated by salt gradient centrifugation (5) into lipoproteins of S_f>400, 100-400, 20-100, and S_f<20.

RESULTS AND DISCUSSION

Cholesterol feeding for only 3 days produced plasma cholesterol concentrations of 157-371 mg/dl compared to 31-108 mg/dl in controls. No difference in plasma TG concentration or in the rate of removal of TG mass following chylomicron injection has been observed (6), therefore chylomicron remnant formation is equally rapid in normal and cholesterol-fed rabbits. Fig. 1a illustrates the disappearance of labeled cholesteryl and retinyl esters from whole plasma of control rabbits: both ^{3}H and ^{14}C esters were rapidly removed for 20-25 min. In 5 rabbits, half-times for removal of esterified retinol and cholesterol equalled 9-14 min. After 25 min, the fractional removal rates became slower. Cholesterol-fed rabbits cleared both retinyl and cholesteryl esters much more slowly than controls (Fig. 1b). Ultracentrifugation of plasma showed that control rabbits, injected with labeled chylomicrons of S_f>400, rapidly formed and removed labeled lipoproteins of S_f 100-400 and S_f 20-100 (Fig. 2a). Cholesterol-fed rabbits, in contrast to controls, formed and retained doubly labeled plasma lipoproteins of S_f 100-400 and S_f 20-100. These results indicate that partially degraded chylomicrons accumulate in the form of plasma VLDL in the cholesterol-fed rabbit.

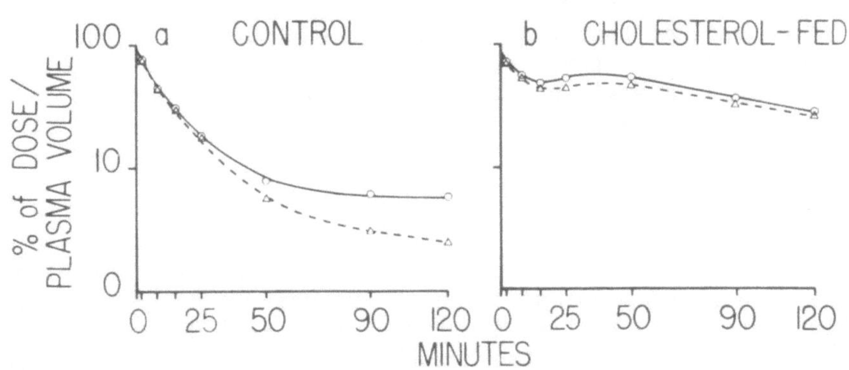

Fig. 1. Removal from plasma of chylomicron cholesteryl esters —o— and retinyl esters --Δ--.

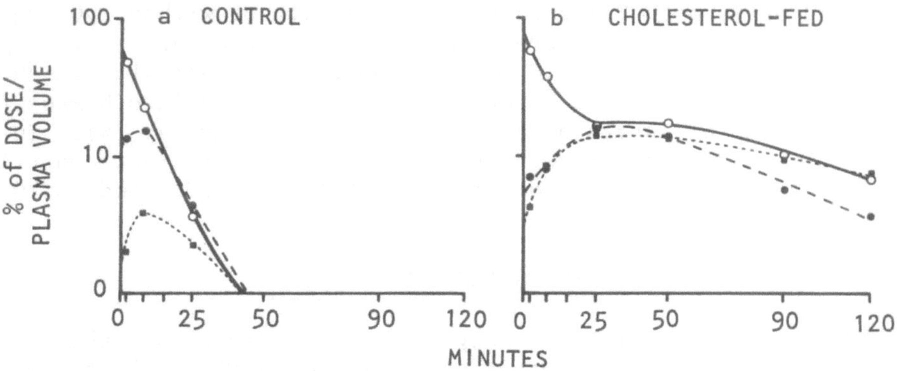

Fig.2. [^{14}C] cholesteryl ester activity in lipoproteins of S_f>400 —o— , S_f 100-400 - -•- -, and S_f 20-100 ---■--- .

In both control rabbits after 25 min and cholesterol-fed animals, the decrease of plasma [^{3}H] retinyl esters exceeded that of plasma [^{14}C] cholesteryl esters. Fractionation of plasma showed that only lipoproteins of S_f<20 contained more labeled esterified cholesterol than esterified retinol. This relative increase in esterified cholesterol could be due either to recirculation of labeled cholesteryl esters in endogenous lipoproteins, or to an intravascular transfer of chylomicron esterified cholesterol to plasma lipoproteins having a slower fractional turnover rate than chylomicrons or their degradation products. The possibility of cholesteryl ester transfer was investigated by in vitro incubation of doubly labeled chylomicrons with unlabeled normal or hypercholesterolemic plasma. After incubation at 37°C for 25 or 60 min, 9 and 16%, respectively, of the labeled esterified cholesterol was found in lipoproteins of S_f<20; however, transfer of labeled retinyl esters was less than 3%. These in vitro observations suggest that the increase in [^{14}C] cholesteryl esters relative to [^{3}H] retinyl esters seen in 2 hr studies is due to intravascular transfer of a small portion of chylomicron cholesteryl esters to lipoproteins of S_f<20.

SUMMARY

Moderately hypercholesterolemic rabbits hydrolyzed chylomicron TG at the same rate as normal animals, but were found to accumulate partially degraded intestinal lipoproteins of S_f 100-400 and S_f 20-100. These results support the hypothesis that the hypercholesterolemia induced by cholesterol feeding results at least in part from an inability to clear chylomicron remnants in proportion to the rate of their formation.

REFERENCES

1. Redgrave, T. G. J. Clin. Invest. 49: 465, 1970.
2. Bergman, E. N., and R. J. Havel, B. M. Wolfe, T. Bøhmer. J. Clin. Invest. 50: 1831, 1971.
3. Goodman, D. S., and H. S. Huang, T. Shiratori. J. Lipid Res. 6: 390, 1965.
4. Thompson, J. N., and P. Erdody, R. Brien, T. K. Murray. Biochem. Med. 5: 67, 1971.
5. Minari, O., and D. B. Zilversmit. J. Lipid Res. 4: 424, 1963.
6. Ross, A. C., and D. B. Zilversmit. Fed. Proc. 34: 939, 1975.

---

* Supported by N.I.H. grant HL 10933.

† N.I.H. Predoctoral Trainee (GM 00824).

‡ Career Investigator, American Heart Association.

§ Kindly provided by Dr. W. E. Scott of Hoffman-LaRoche, Nutley, N. J.

(3)

POSTHEPARIN PLASMA LIPOPROTEIN LIPASE AND HEPATIC LIPASE IN NORMAL HUMAN SUBJECTS: RELATIONSHIP TO AGE, SEX AND TRIGLYCERIDE METABOLISM

Huttunen, J.K., Ehnholm, C., Kekki, M. and Nikkilä, E.A.

Third Department of Medicine, University of Helsinki

Finland

Lipoprotein lipase (LPL) is assumed to have a key role in serum triglyceride removal. The total lipolytic activity of postheparin plasma (PHLA) has been widely used to measure tissue LPL until it was demonstrated that at least two separate triglyceride lipases are present in the circulation after heparin administration. One of these activities resembles adipose tissue LPL in being inhibited by 1 M NaCl and by protamine sulphate and activated by serum (Ehnholm et al. 1974, Krauss et al. 1974). The other enzyme is similar to a lipase present in the liver with activation by 1 M NaCl and without serum requirement.

We have recently developed and validated an immunochemical method for the separate assay of postheparin lipoprotein lipase (LPL) and hepatic lipase (HL) (Huttunen et al. 1975). Here we report the activities of postheparin plasma LPL and HL in normal human subjects with particular emphasis on their relationship to age, sex and triglyceride metabolism. The studies were carried out in healthy normoglyceridemic subjects (47 males and 35 females), aged from 22 to 67 years. Postheparin plasma lipases were measured after i.v. administration of heparin, 1 mg/kg b.w. Measurement of LPL was carried out in the presence of HL antiserum at 0.1 M NaCl and with added serum. In the assay of HL the activity of LPL was inhibited by 1 M NaCl and by omitting the serum activator. Measurement of plasma triglyceride turnover was carried out by endogeneous labeling of total plasma triglyceride with glycerol-2-^{3}H and subsequent assay of the decay of radioactivity during 24 hrs (Nikkilä and Kekki 1971).

Postheparin plasma lipase activities in males and females under and over 45 years are shown in Table 1. The activity of LPL decreased with age in both sexes ($r = -0.45$, $p < 0.001$ for males, $r = -0.39$, $p < 0.01$ for females). No significant age variation was observed in the activity of HL. The mean activity of LPL was higher in females than in males in both age groups, whereas the activity of HL showed an opposite sex ratio.

Table 1. Postheparin plasma lipase activities in normal subjects

Sex	Age	No	Lipoprotein lipase	Hepatic lipase
			μmol FFA/ml plasma/hr	
Males	20-70	47	18.6 ± 6.2	26.8 ± 9.9
	<45	25	21.3 ± 5.4	26.6 ± 10.9
	>45	22	15.4 ± 5.7	27.0 ± 8.7
Females	20-70	35	25.8 ± 9.3	18.6 ± 7.5
	<45	19	28.3 ± 9.9	18.6 ± 7.0
	>45	16	22.8 ± 7.6	18.6 ± 9.6

Mean ± SD

A composite of the correlations between the activity of postheparin lipases and different parameters of triglyceride metabolism is shown in Table 2. A highly significant inverse correlation was observed between the fasting plasma triglyceride and the activity of postheparin plasma LPL in both sexes, whereas no relationship was present between the plasma triglyceride concentration and the activity of HL. A significant positive correlation was found between the activity of LPL and the fractional turnover of triglycerides both in males and in females. The activity of HL did not correlate with the fractional turnover. No relationship was found between either postheparin plasma lipase and the absolute turnover rate of plasma triglycerides.

Table 2. Correlations between the activities of postheparin plasma lipases and various parameters of plasma triglyceride metabolism

x	y	r	p
Lipoprotein lipase	Plasma TG	-0.54	<0.001
Lipoprotein lipase	FTR of plasma TG	+0.61	<0.001
Lipoprotein lipase	TR of plasma TG	-0.11	NS
Hepatic lipase	Plasma TG	+0.01	NS
Hepatic lipase	FTR of plasma TG	+0.29	NS
Hepatic lipase	TR of plasma TG	+0.25	NS

FTR = fractional turnover; TR = turnover, NS = nonsignificant

These results are compatible with the hypothesis that postheparin plasma LPL reflects the removal efficiency of VLDL triglyceride and suggest that the removal rate regulates the plasma triglyceride concentration at physiological range. Thus, the decrease of postheparin plasma LPL activity with age is consistent with the age-related increase of serum triglyceride level. Furthermore, the high activity of LPL in females in comparison to males is in agreement with the higher removal rate of endogeneous plasma triglycerides in females than in males (Nikkilä and Kekki 1971). The activity of postheparin HL was not correlated with any of the parameters of triglyceride metabolism in this study. The role of this enzyme in lipoprotein metabolism remains unknown.

REFERENCES

Ehnholm, C. et al., in Atherosclerosis III. Springer-Verlag, 1974, 557.

Huttunen, J.K. et al., Clin.Chim.Acta, 1975, in the press.

Krauss, R.M. et al., J.Clin.Invest. 54, 1974, 1107.

Nikkilä, E.A., Kekki, M., Acta Med.Scand. 190, 1971, 49.

(4)

LIPOPROTEIN LIPASE AND HEPATIC LIPASE ACTIVITY IN POST-HEPARIN PLASMA OF PATIENTS WITH HYPERTRIGLYCERIDEMIA

Esko A. Nikkilä, Jussi K. Huttunen and Christian Ehnholm

Third Department of Medicine
University of Helsinki
Helsinki, Finland

The postheparin plasma contains two separate triglyceride lipases of which the lipoprotein lipase is responsible for the primary removal of circulating triglycerides in peripheral tissues. The exact function of the other enzyme, hepatic lipase, is still unknown but it might be active in the elimination of triglycerides contained in "remnant particles" and LDL. A primary defect in the triglyceride removal as a cause of elevated plasma triglyceride level has been demonstrated only in the rare Type I hyperlipoproteinemia whereas in the common forms of hypertriglyceridemia the total postheparin plasma lipolytic activity (PHLA) is either normal or only moderately decreased. As the two enzymes which contribute to the PHLA are not regulated in a parallel fashion and may even be selectively influenced, e.g., by drugs (Ehnholm et al. 1975) it is possible that subtle changes in the activities of these enzymes which are not detectable by total PHLA assay might underlie the common types of hypertriglyceridemia. This possibility has been examined in the present study.

MATERIAL AND METHODS

The lipoprotein lipase and hepatic lipase were assayed by an immunochemical method (Huttunen et al. 1975) in plasma taken 15 minutes after intravenous injection of heparin (1 mg/kg). The material consisted of 30 untreated patients with Type IIb, IV or V hyperlipoproteinemia.

RESULTS AND DISCUSSION

All three patients with Type V disorder had postheparin

lipoprotein lipase activity below the normal range. On the other hand, most of the patients with increased VLDL concentration (Type IV) and all the subjects with a combined elevation of VLDL and LDL (Type IIb) had lipoprotein lipase activity within normal range. However, the mean lipoprotein lipase activity of Type IV patients was significantly decreased in comparison with the controls ($p<0.005$). There was no correlation between the individual plasma triglyceride and lipoprotein lipase values.

In contrast to lipoprotein lipase the activity of hepatic lipase was not decreased in any of the patients with elevated plasma triglyceride level. On the contrary, it was clearly evident that many patients had high normal or even elevated postheparin hepatic lipase activity, even though the mean value of all patients or of Type IV cases was not significantly increased above that of controls. No correlation was present between the plasma triglyceride concentration and the postheparin hepatic lipase activity. The patients who had elevated hepatic lipase values were more obese than those with normal hepatic lipase activity. Preliminary data suggest that elevated postheparin hepatic lipase activities are associated with high turnover (production) or plasma VLDL triglyceride.

Our results differ from those published recently by Krauss et al. (1974). Using protamine inhibition of lipoprotein lipase for selective assay of the two postheparin plasma lipases these authors did not find any significant differences in the activity of either lipase between control subjects and patients having Type IIb, IV or V hyperlipoproteinemia. On the other hand, Böberg (1972) and Persson (1973) have been able to show a significant inverse correlation between plasma triglyceride concentration and PHLA or adipose tissue lipoprotein lipase activity. In our series such a correlation was not evident but there was a significant decrease of average lipoprotein lipase activity in patients with elevated VLDL concentration. This finding is best compatible with a hypothesis that hypertriglyceridemia is primarily caused by an increased production of VLDL and the people having lipoprotein lipase activity in the lower normal range are more sensitive to develop elevated plasma triglyceride level than the others. The present results do not support the concept that hepatic lipase is involved in the removal of VLDL triglycerides but the preliminary data rather suggest that this enzyme might have some function in the secretion of triglycerides into plasma.

REFERENCES

Boberg, J.: Acta Med. Scand. 191:97 (1972)

Ehnholm, C., Huttunen, J.K., Kinnunen, P.J., Miettinen, T.A. and Nikkilä, E.A.: New Engl. J. Med. 272-1314 (1975)

Huttunen, J.K., Ehnholm, C., Kinnunen, P.K.J. and Nikkilä, E.A.:

Clin. Chim. Acta 63:335 (1975)

Krauss, R.M., Levy, R.I. and Fredrickson, D.S.: J. Clin. Invest. 54:1107 (1974)

Persson, B.: Acta Med. Scand. 193:447 (1973)

(5)

AUTOIMMUNE HYPERLIPIDEMIA IN THE NEPHROTIC SYNDROME

BEAUMONT J.L., ANTONUCCI M. and BERARD M.

Unité de recherches sur l'Athérosclérose de l'INSERM

Hôpital Henri Mondor, 94010 Créteil, France

In a previous report (1), two cases (Ler... and Lac...) in which a nephrotic syndrome was associated with an IgG λ monoclonal gammopathy and a marked hyperlipidemia were studied.
- When purified and activated, the IgG λ Ler... was found to react with human LDL and the IgG λ Lac... with human VLDL and HSA. On the other hand, in the whole plasma no activity was detected against these macromolecules. According to the data, it was concluded that these IgG λ behaved like auto-antibodies which are blocked by the circulating antigens. Also it was suggested that the associated hyperlipidemia may be induced by these autoantibodies.
- Autoimmune hyperlipidemia (AIH) may be induced by a variety of antibodies which inhibit various stages of the complex lipolytic process by which the lipid load is removed from the circulating lipoproteins (2,3).

Since the last report, the mechanism of AIH was demonstrated in case Lac... which is characterized by a major hypertriglyceridemia and a type IV lipoprotein pattern :
- In vivo , it was found that the plasma post-heparin lipase activity was reduced.
- In vitro, it was demonstrated that the purified and activated IgG λ Lac... was able to inhibit the release of fatty acids from a human serum activated C^{14} triolein substrate by the following lipases : whole human plasma post-heparin lipase; human hepatic lipase, after blocking the plasma post-heparin lipase by protamine sulfate ; rat plasma port-heparin lipase. On the other hand, the pancreatic lipase activity was not or only a little inhibited (Figure). The inhibition of adipose tissue lipase activity is under study.

In these experiments, nearly a 100% inhibition of the fatty acid release is obtainable with 50 µg of purified IgG λ and a 50% inhibition with 5 to 10 ug in a 1 ml total volume.

Thus it is obvious that the IgG λ Lac... blocks the lipolysis of the triglycerides in this system. Furthermore it is likely that this blocking is the result of the binding of the IgG λ to the substrate at a site which is necessary for its attack by the lipases. However we do not know yet the exact structure which is involved in this binding. It is present in VLDL, HDL and serum albumin preparations and may be an apolipoprotein. On the other hand, a binding of the IgG with the lipase or with a complex of the substrate and the lipase can not be completely excluded.

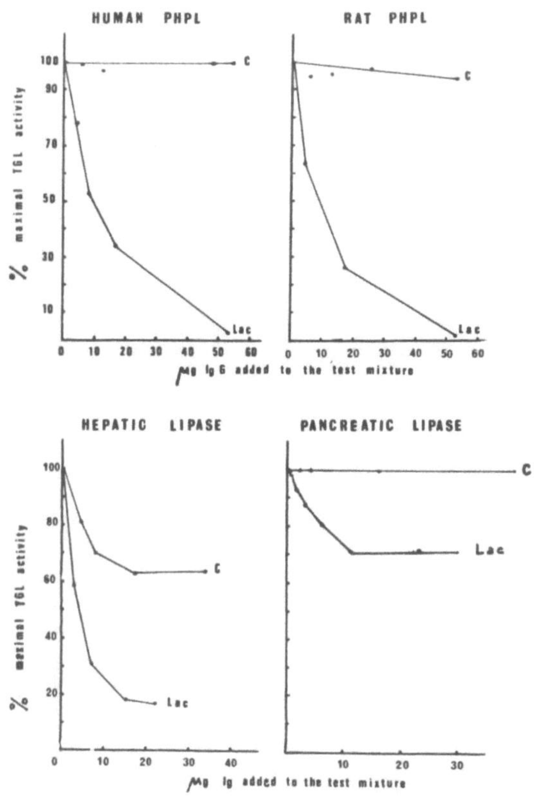

FIG. 1. EFFECTS OF IgG LAC. ON TRIGLYCERIDE LIPASE ACTIVITY

Fatty acid release after 15 min incubation in a mixture of a human serum activated C12 + C14 triolein substrate and several lipases with preincubated added IgG λ Lac or normal human pooled IgG (IgG C.)

REFERENCES

1- BEAUMONT J.L., ANTONUCCI M., LAGRUE G., GUEDON J. and PEROL R.- Nephrotic syndrome, monoclonal gammopathy and autoimmune hyperlipidaemia. - CLIN. EXPER. IMMUNOL., 1974, 18, 225

2- BEAUMONT J.L., - L'hyperlipidémie par auto-anticorps anti-bêtalipoprotéines. Une nouvelle entité pathologique. - A.R. ACADEMIE DES SCIENCES PARIS Série D, 1965, 21, 4563

3- BEAUMONT J.L. - Autoimmune hyperlipidemia. An atherogenic metabolic disease of immune origin. EUROP. J. CLIN. BIOL. RES., 1970, 15, 1037

CHAPTER 4
AORTIC GLYCOSAMINOGLYCANS, GANGLIOSIDES AND GLYCOLYSIS

(1)

FURTHER STUDIES ON GLYCOSAMINOGLYCAN -- LIPOPROTEIN INTERACTIONS

S.R. Srinivasan, B. Radhakrishnamurthy and G.S. Berenson

Louisiana State University Medical Center
Department of Medicine
1542 Tulane Ave., New Orleans, Louisiana, U.S.A.

The complexing of glycosaminoglycans (GAG) with serum low density lipoproteins (LDL) in the presence of certain cations are used to quantitate serum lipoproteins (LP). Further, LP-GAG complexes have been isolated from atherosclerotic lesions (1) thereby establishing a role of these complexes in the pathogenesis of atherosclerosis. Although the nature of interactions between LP and other sulfated polyanions in the absence of metal cations is fairly well understood, information about the specificity and nature of interaction in the presence of metal ions is scanty. These studies describe the LP-heparin interactions, using immobilized heparin (2) as a model system, in the presence of Ca^{++}, Mg^{++} and Mn^{++}.

METHODS

Heparin was coupled to 1,4-diaminobutane sepharose 4B derivative (3) and the heparinated gel was equilibrated with LDL, very low density (VLDL) and high density (HDL) lipoproteins at pH 7.4 in the presence of varying concentrations of metal ions. The contents were then centrifuged and the supernatant analyzed for cholesterol as a measure of unreacted LP. LDL was acetylated and treated with phospholipase C as described previously (2,4) and the acetylated LP and phospholipase C treated LP studied for interaction with heparin. LP-GAG complexes were isolated from human fatty streak and fibrous plaque lesions as described previously (1) and were analyzed as a corollary to the study of in vitro complexing.

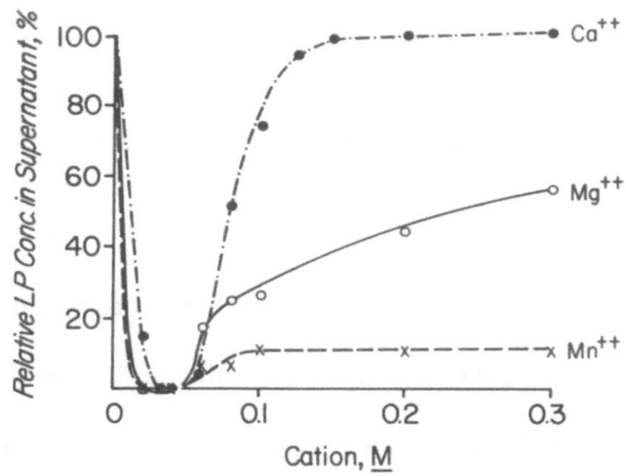

Figure 1: Interaction between LDL and heparin-substituted agarose gel in the presence of varying concentrations of Ca^{++}, Mg^{++} and Mn^{++}.

RESULTS

The LDL-heparin interaction in this system was found to be quantitative within a narrow and critical range of metal ion concentration, 0.02 to 0.04 M (fig. 1). Above this range of metal ion concentration the interaction became reversible to varying degrees depending upon the nature of the metal ion. The reversibility of 0.3 M cation concentration was 100%, 60% and 10% with Ca^{++}, Mg^{++} and Mn^{++}, respectively, indicating an influence of specific metal ions in the relative stability of the complexes. Furthermore, complexes obtained with 0.03 M Ca^{++}, Mg^{++} and Mn^{++} dissociated by different amounts after addition of increasing molarity of NaCl; the NaCl concentration required for 50% dissociation of the complexes was 0.03 M, 0.09 M and 0.19 M in the case of Ca^{++}, Mg^{++} and Mn^{++}, respectively. Experiments performed with VLDL and heparinated gels indicated that VLDL behaved very similar to LDL with respect to its binding capacity in the presence of these metal ions.

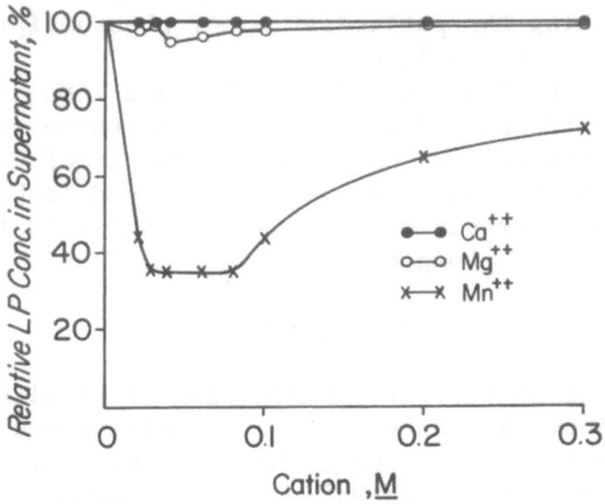

Figure 2: Complex formation between HDL and heparin-substituted gels in the presence of varying concentration of Ca^{++}, Mg^{++} and Mn^{++}.

Similar interaction studies with HDL (fig. 2) indicated no observable interaction between HDL and heparinated gel in the presence of Ca^{++} or Mg^{++}; in contrast about 60% of HDL interacted with heparin in the presence of Mn^{++} at a concentration of 0.025 M to 0.075 M. This observation is important since Mn^{++} is being widely used for the selective precipitation of VLDL and LDL for isolation and quantitation of LP. In order to evaluate the degree of insoluble complex formation in a HDL-Mn-heparin system, HDL and its subfractions HDL_2 and HDL_3 were treated with Mn^{++} and free heparin under the conditions used for serum LP precipitation (5). Based on these results, about 25% of HDL, 40% of HDL_2 and 10% of HDL_3 precipitated as insoluble complexes.

Studies with modified LDL indicated that about 95% of the acetylated LDL interacted with heparinated gel in the presence of Ca^{++}, suggesting that the free amino groups are not essential for LDL-heparin interaction in the presence of divalent metal ions.

Phospholipase C treated LDL was mixed with free heparin and Ca^{++} and the degree of insoluble complex formation was measured in terms of turbidity as described previously (6). Insoluble complex formation decreased as the amount of phospholipids hydrolyzed increased, indicating the participation of phospholipids in the formation of insoluble complexes.

Since similar LP-GAG complexes of LDL and VLDL have been isolated from fatty streaks and fibrous plaques, these were analyzed for Ca^{++} and phospholipids. Significant amounts of Ca^{++} (8-38 moles Ca^{++}/10 moles phospholipids) were observed to be part of the complexes, and considerable variations were noted in the relative proportions of Ca^{++} to phospholipid.

DISCUSSION

The studies of an in vitro interaction of LP with the GAG heparin clearly show that there are marked differences in the stability and specificity of the LP-heparin complexes formed in the presence of Ca^{++}, Mg^{++} and Mn^{++}, and they show the need to use properly metal ions for selective and quantitative precipitation of certain fractions of lipoproteins. It is suggested that the interaction of LDL with polyanions in the absence of metal ions is considered an electrostatic phenomenon and the positive charges on LDL necessary for the interaction are contributed by basic amino groups. However, since heparin forms insoluble complexes only in the presence of certain metal ions indicates a different kind of reaction mechanism noted for soluble complexes. Amenta and Waters (7) postulated an electrostatic bonding mechanism involving Ca^{++} as a cation bridging the sulfate groups of GAG and the anionic groups of phospholipids of LDL. Our observations seem to support their concept. The specificity of Ca^{++} for interacting with only LDL and VLDL in vitro and its presence in significant amount in the LP-GAG complexes isolated from arterial lesions suggest that the formation of LP-Ca^{++}-GAG complexes is a possible mechanism for the accumulation of VLDL and LDL in the arterial wall. This type of complexing would not involve HDL and in fact in the isolation of LP-GAG from atherosclerotic lesions no HDL is observed (1).

REFERENCES

1. Srinivasan, S.R., Dolan, P., Radhakrishnamurthy, B. and Berenson, G.S. Atherosclerosis 16, 95 (1972).

2. Iverius, P-H. J. Biol. Chem. 247, 2607 (1972).

3. Cautrecases, P. J. Biol. Chem. 245, 3059 (1970).

4. Nishida, T. and Cogan, N. J. Biol. Chem. 245, 4689 (1970).

5. Burstein, M. and Samaille, J. Clin. Chem. Acta 5, 609 (1960).

6. Srinivasan, S.R., Lopez-S.A., Radhakrishanmurthy, B., and Berenson, G.S. Atherosclerosis 12, 321 (1970).

7. Amenta, J.S. and Waters, L.L. Yale J. Biol. Med. 33, 112 (1960).

Acknowledgement

Supported by funds from the National Heart and Lung Institute of the USPHS (HL 02942), the Specialized Center of Research--Arteriosclerosis (HL 15103) and the American Heart Association.

(2)

INTERACTIONS OF GLYCOSAMINGLYCANS WITH COLLAGEN AND ELASTIN IN BOVINE AORTA

B. Radhakrishnamurthy, H. Ruiz and G. S. Berenson

Louisiana State University Medical Center
1542 Tulane Ave., New Orleans, Louisiana, U.S.A.

At the present time little is known about the biologic role of glycosaminoglycans (GAG) in cardiovascular tissues or the role they play with other connective tissue components in cardiovascular tissues. Elucidation of the interactions between GAG and the fibrous proteins would aid in the understanding of the molecular organization within cardiovascular structure. In earlier studies of the aorta (1) proteoglycans (GAG with covalently bound proteins) were extracted by several dissociative solvents. These studies indicate that about half of the total uronic acid contained in the tissue was isolated. The uronic acid material extracted by dissociative methods is part of a proteoglycan containing both chondroitin sulfates (CS) and dermatan sulfate (DS). No heparan sulfate (HS) was obtained although aorta contains considerable amount of this GAG. In an attempt to understand the nature of the non-extractable GAG and their relation to fibrous proteins, bovine aorta was selectively hydrolyzed with elastase and collagenase and GAG were isolated from the hydrolyzates, characterized and quantitated.

EXPERIMENTAL

Digestion of aorta by elastase-Pulverized dry-defatted bovine aorta (1 g) was digested with 320 units of elastase (swine pancreas, chromatographically purified, 80 units/mg, Worthington Biochemical Corp., Freehold, N.J.) at 37° for 48 h. in Tris-HCl buffer, pH 8.8, 0.2 M. A small amount of thymol was added to inhibit bacterial activity. Since elastase is known to possess some proteolytic activity it was inhibited by soybean trypsin inhibitor as described by Walford and Kickhofen (2). A blank extraction without the enzyme was simultaneously carried out.

Digestion of aorta with collagenase - Digestion of aorta with 100 units of collagenase (Cl. histolyticum, chromatographically purified, 200 units/mg, Worthington) was carried out in Tris-HCl buffer, pH. 7.5, 0.05 M containing 0.36 mM $CaCl_2$. The conditions of hydrolysis were similar to those described for elastase. Since the collagenase preparation did not demonstrate any detectable proteolytic activity no protease inhibitor was used.

Similar hydrolysis with the enzymes were carried out on the residual tissues after extraction with 0.15 M NaCl and 3.0 M $MgCl_2$.

Isolation and characterization of GAG -- The digestion mixture after enzyme hydrolysis was centrifuged and from the supernatant GAG were isolated by the usual procedure (3). Briefly, this consisted of treatment of the supernatant with 0.1 N NaOH at 5° for 18 h., precipitation of peptide material with trichloroacetic acid, filtration through celite, dialysis, concentration to a small volume and determination of uronic acid. The GAG mixture was then fractionated on a Dowex-1 Cl^- column eluting with a stepwise increasing concentration of NaCl 0.5 to 4.0 M. The fractions were extensively analyzed for characterization and quantitation.

RESULTS AND DISCUSSION

The composition of GAG isolated from the aorta by digestion with the enzymes is shown in Tables I and II. Elastase digestion of the aorta without protease inhibitor released about 90% of the total hexuronate from the tissue and the composition of individual GAG is shown in Table I. Elastase in the presence of protease

TABLE I

ISOLATION OF GAG FROM BOVINE AORTA BY DIGESTION WITH ELASTASE AND COLLAGENASE

ENZYME	HA	Chon	HS	CS-A/C	DS	Hep†
			(μg uronic acid/g tissue)			
Elastase	398	52	378	668	115	50
Elastase + Protease Inhibitor*	360	46	360	325	124	--**
Collagenase	415	50	26	590	38	46
Blank (no enzyme)	280	52	18	348	--	--

* Maximum Inhibition

--** Not detected--within 5%

† Abbreviations -- Hyaluronic acid (HA), Chondroitin (Chon), Chondroitin sulfate (CS), dermatan sulfate (DS), heparan sulfate (HS), Heparan (Hep).

inhibitor released most of the GAG except 50% of CS. Collagenase digestion gave 15% more hyaluronic acid (HA) and 70% more CS, lesser amounts of HS and DS. It is interesting to note that 75% of HA, 40% of CS and all chondroitin (Chon) can be extracted by Tris buffer alone.

Since some GAG from aorta can be easily extracted with 0.15 M NaCl and 3.0 M $MgCl_2$ the tissue was first extracted repeatedly with these salt solutions and the residual tissue then digested with the enzymes to find out what specific GAG could be solubilized with these enzymes. The composition of GAG isolated from these digests is shown in Table II. The residual tissue contained considerable amount of HA which could be obtained by digestion of the tissue with the enzymes. All HS in the tissue was solubilized by elastase but not by collagenase. A greater amount of DS was obtained by elastase hydrolysis than by collagenase. Collagenase, on the other hand, solubilized more CS than elastase.

It is evident from these studies that all proteoglycans cannot be extracted with dissociative solvents like 3.0 M $MgCl_2$. Since aorta contains 60-70% elastin, solubilization of elastin is

TABLE II

ISOLATION OF GAG FROM BOVINE AORTA AFTER 0.15 M NaCl and 3.0 M $MgCl_2$ EXTRACTION FOLLOWED BY DIGESTION WITH ELASTASE AND COLLAGENASE

ENZYME	HA	Chon	HS	CS-A/C	DS	Hep
			(μg uronic acid/g tissue)			
NaCl						
Elastase + Protease Inhibitor*	110	--	320	40	105	--**
Collagenase	130	--	--	310	20	36
Blank (no enzyme)	46	--	--	34	--	--
$MgCl_2$						
Elastase + Protease Inhibitor*	178	--	366	28	92	--
Collagenase	126	--	--	184	16	--
Blank (no enzyme)	--	--	--	24	--	--

* Maximum Inhibition

--** Not detected--within 5%

necessary for the extraction of the remainder of the uronic acid material from the tissue. These findings suggest further that in aorta HS and DS, at least in part, are firmly bound to elastin and CS to collagen, although the precise nature of binding is not known. It is possible that these GAG are entrapped in the network of collagen and elastin fibers (4) or that the sulfate groups of GAG react with collagen and elastin through Ca^{++} forming stable complexes in the aorta (5,6).

REFERENCES

1. Ehrlich, K., Radhakrishnamurthy, B., Ruiz, H., and Berenson, G.S. Fed. Proc. 33:1557, 1974.

2. Walford, R.L. and Kickhofen, B. Arch. Biochem. Biophys. 98:191, 1962.

3. Roden, L., Baker, J.R., Cifonelli, J.A. and Mathews, M.B. Methods in Enzymology, 28:73, 1972.

4. Mathews, M.B. Biochem. J. 96:710, 1965.

5. Srinivasan, S.R., Lopez-S.A., Radhakrishnamurthy, B., and Berenson, G.S. Atherosclerosis 12:321, 1970.

6. Urry, D.W. Adv. Exp. Med. Biol. 43:211, 1974.

Acknowledgement

Supported fy funds from the National Heart and Lung Institute of the USPHS (HL 02942), the Specialized Center of Research--Arteriosclerosis (HL 15103) and the American Heart Association.

(3)

STRUCTURAL CHARACTERIZATION OF GANGLIOSIDES FROM NORMAL AND ATHEROSCLEROTIC HUMAN THORACIC AORTAS

W. Carl Breckenridge

Lipid Research Clinic

University of Toronto, Toronto, Ontario, Canada

A proliferation of cells, with characteristics of medial smooth muscle cells, occurs in the intimal region of the artery wall and has been considered important in the early phases of atherosclerosis (1,2). In addition, it has been claimed that cells on the surface of advanced lesions appear to be of monoclonal origin and different from the same cells in the media of adjacent normal tissue (3). These observations suggest that some form of alteration or transformation of the medial smooth muscle cell may occur in the atherosclerotic lesion.

In addition to various enzyme alterations many transformed cells often show changes in glycolipids and gangliosides (4) which are considered important in cell-cell communication (5). Since a migration and proliferation of cells appear to be a feature of the process of atherogenesis investigations have been undertaken to assess the composition of gangliosides in human aortas.

In a recent report (6) we noted that 2-4 fold increases in ganglioside N-Acetyl neuraminic acid were observed in aortas showing extensive involvement with fatty streaks and/or raised yellow fibrous lesions. Gangliosides were also isolated from plasma lipoproteins but at concentrations much lower than the aorta. In order to assess the possible contribution to aoritc gangliosides from plasma we have assessed the structure of gangliosides in plasma and intima-media preparations of normal and abnormal thoracic aortas.

Gangliosides were isolated from chloroform-methanol extracts of homogenized tissue by aqueous partition. Following saponification and repartition they were isolated by thin layer chromatography. The monosaccharides, fatty acids and sphingosine bases were analyzed by gas liquid chromatography following methanolysis.

The major component in all preparations was GM_3, a monosialyl ganglioside containing equi molar amounts of glucose, galactose and sialic acid. It had a mobility on thin layer chromatography similar to GM_3 isolated from dog erythocytes. While this component accounted for 90-95% of the ganglioside sialic acid in plasma or normal tissue, two additional components corresponding to GM_1 and GD_1 gangliosides were present in abnormal aortas and contributed about 15-20% of the sialic acid. However, they contained N-Acetyl glucosamine in addition to the monosaccharides listed above. A minor very polar component was also noted in the abnormal tissue.

The fatty acid composition of the GM_3 component showed some differences in the three preparations. The major normal fatty acids were C16:0; C18:0; C22:0; C24:0; C24:1. As shown in the Table, proportionally higher amounts of C24:0 and C24:1 were found in the aorta tissue as compared to those from plasma. In contrast to the tissues, the plasma gangliosides contained more stearic than palmitic acid. The presence of hydroxy fatty acids was assessed by thin layer chromatography. Small amounts were detected only in the abnormal tissue.

Analyses of the amino bases as trifluoroacetates indicated C18 sphingosine was the major component. They were also analyzed as N-Acetyl trimethyl silyl ethers and possessed retention times similar to _threo_ and _erythro_ forms of sphingosine and dihydrosphingosine. No major differences were noted in the three preparations.

In general, the composition of the ceramide portion is similar in some respects to previous reports for fatty acids of cerebrosides (7) and sphingosine bases from aorta (8). Although the data would be compatible with the idea that part of aortic gangliosides may arise from plasma infiltration, not all the material results from

Fatty Acid Composition of Gangliosides

Fatty Acid	Plasma	Normal Aortas (%)	Abnormal Aortas
16:0	13.9	25.9	24.5
17:0	1.7	0.5	0.7
18:0	24.8	13.0	13.7
18:1	4.6	1.6	1.5
20:0	6.2	4.5	4.0
22:0	19.0	14.4	13.3
23:0	5.0	3.1	1.9
24:0	12.9	17.1	18.7
24:1	11.9	19.2	21.8

such a process since the fatty acid composition is different and two additional gangliosides are found in the abnormal tissue. Furthermore, the process of infiltration would need to be rather specific since the tissue levels are much higher than plasma on a wet weight basis.

The ganglioside patterns do not follow trends noted in many transformed cells. Usually the complex pattern noted in the normal cell is greatly simplified in the transformed cell consisting mainly of GM_3. In the present study GM_3 is the major component in both the normal tissue and the diseased areas while more complex species appear in the diseased tissue.

1. Wissler, R.W. J. Atheroscler. Res. 8: 201 (1968)
2. Ross, R. and J.A. Glomset. Science 180: 1332 (1973)
3. Benditt, E. and J.M. Benditt. Proc. Natl. Acad. Sci. U.S.A. 70: 1753 (1973)
4. Hakamori, S. and W.T. Murakami. Proc. Natl. Acad. Sci. U.S.A. 60: 300 (1968)
5. Roth, S., E.J. McGuire and S. Roseman. J. Cell. Biol. 51: 536 (1971)
6. Breckenridge, W.C., J.L. Halloran, K. Kovacs and M.S. Silver. Lipids 10: 256 (1975)
7. Foote, J.L. and E. Coles. J. Lipid Res. 9: 482 (1968)
8. Panganamala, R.V., J.C. Geer and D.G. Cornwell. J. Lipid Res. 10: 445 (1969)

(4)

STUDIES ON THE ROLE OF INCREASED ARTERIAL GLYCOLYSIS IN ATHEROGENESIS

Zemplenyi, T., Blankenhorn, D. H., Rosenstein, A.J., and Alexander, N.

USC School of Medicine
Los Angeles, CA, U.S.A.

Aerobic glycolysis is a comparative rarity in normal tissues, whereas it is almost the hallmark of neoplastic tissue (1), and it also appears to be a characteristic of arterial metabolism. The question arises whether the high rate of arterial glycolysis is in any way related to atherogenesis. The conclusions from different lines of investigations appear to shed some light in this regard.

A. In aortic homogenates of perinephritic hypertensive rabbits, we measured mainly the activity of glycolytic enzymes, Krebs cycle enzymes and enzymes of the ATP cycle. The results were always calculated on the protein, DNA and fat-free dry weight bases (Figure). The activity of the glycolytic enzymes aldolase and lactate dehydrogenase was significantly elevated in the hypertensive animals and the phosphofructokinase and α-glycerophosphate dehydrogenase activity also showed a trend in this direction. On the other hand, the activity of ATPase, creatine phosphokinase and adenylate kinase manifested a tendency toward decreased activity in the aortas of hypertensive animals. Of special interest was the comparatively high activity of glycerokinase, the enzyme which catalyzes the phosphorylation of glycerol into glycerophosphate, a precursor of triglycerides and phospholipids.

B. Although the connection between experimental diabetes and atherosclerosis is not as unequivocal as in the case of hypertension, it is noteworthy that the activity of glycerokinase was again significantly elevated in the diabetic animals as compared with controls, and the activity of aldolase,

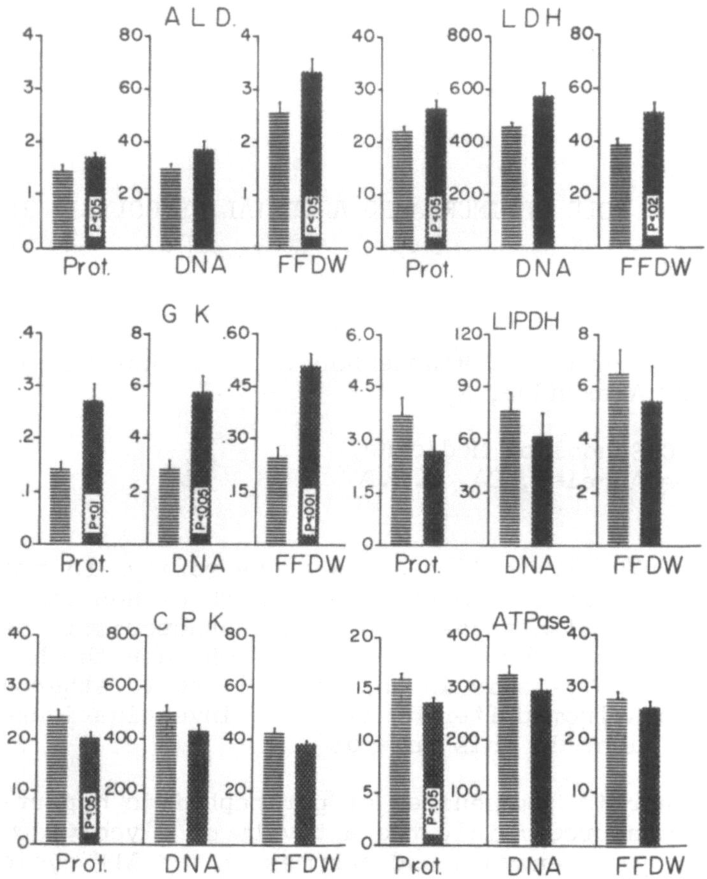

Figure. Comparison of enzyme activities in aortas from control and hypertensive rabbits (first and second bar in each doublet). Activities are expressed in nanomoles of substrate converted by the enzyme per minute and calculated on the extract protein. DNA and fat free dry weight bases. Upright lines on bars = SEM. For other details see text.

and other glycolytic enzymes (phosphofructokinase, pyruvate kinase) exhibited a similar general tendency.

C. In very young pigeons the activity of arterial phosphofructokinase, which catalyzes one of the essential regulatory steps of glycolysis, as well as the activity of aldolase is significantly higher in the more atherosclerosis-susceptible White Carneau (WC) strain than in the resistant Show Racer (SR) strain. In contrast, the activity of malate dehydrogenase and lipoamide dehydrogenase is lower in the WC than SR arteries (2). The latter enzyme is a component of the pyruvate dehydrogenase complex which regulates the conversion of pyruvate to oxaloacetate and consequently the utilization of glucose (and some amino acids) by the Krebs cycle. All the above evidence strongly suggests a shift toward a rise in the rate of glycolysis in the atherosclerosis-susceptible WC arteries. However, it is impossible to definitely conclude from differences in enzyme activities alone, whether they are functionally effective. Therefore, in subsequent experimental series, we measured the in vivo concentrations of metabolic intermediates using a freeze-clamping technique with liquid N_2. Practically all intermediates of glycolysis, as well as some Krebs cycle intermediates and energy rich compounds were determined.

Comparison of the aortas of young SR and WC pigeons revealed a lower concentration of malate, ATP and ADP in the White Carneau arteries. The level of glucose-6-phosphate and fructose-1,6-diphosphate was higher in the aortas of Show Racer pigeons. As glucose-6-phosphate is the common intermediate of both glycolysis and glycogenolysis, we also calculated the ratio of lactate to glucose-6-phosphate in each aorta separately. In the aortas of WC pigeons this ratio was significantly higher than in the SR aortas. A similar trend was found for the ratios of lactate to fructose-1,6-diphosphate. If we assume that the diffusion of lactate from the aortas was not different in the two pigeon strains then the data are in accordance with a more efficient rate of glycolysis in the WC aortas. Furthermore, in related studies by Kalra and Brodie (3), in which surviving arteries of young pigeons were incubated with $[^{14}C]$ glucose, the steady-state level of lactate and the ratio of α-glycerol phosphate to dihydroxyacetone phosphate were significantly higher in the WC than in the SR arteries.

It has to be added that human and animal arteries are characterized by a predominance of the anaerobic lactate dehydrogenase fractions (4). The same applies for arteries of hypertensive and diabetic animals.

One possible interpretation of all the data could be that the elevated rate of glycolysis is secondary to a relative hypoxia of the vessel wall. In view of the delicate nourishment of the arterial wall through the vasa vasorum and/or diffusion, this may be a plausible explanation. Hypoxia could also favor synthesis of fibrotic tissue and perhaps also of lipids (4).

However, another explanation might also be considered in view of the recent elegant and provocative studies by the Benditts (5). They assume that intimal cells exist for years unexpressed in a "subthreshold neoplastic state". We mentioned before that aerobic glycolysis is a hallmark of tumor cells. It is tempting to speculate that the increased rate of glycolysis in preatherosclerotic arteries may be as well an expression of such a subthreshold neoplastic state.

REFERENCES

1. Gregg, C. T. (1972). Some aspects of the energy metabolism of mammalian cells. In "Growth, Nutrition, and Metabolism of Cells in Culture", G. H. Rothblat and V. J. Cristofalo, (Eds.), Academic Press, New York and London, Vol. I, p. 83.

2. Zemplenyi, T., and Rosenstein, A. J. (1975). Arterial enzymes and their relation to atherosclerosis in pigeons. Exp. Mol. Pathol. 22, 225.

3. Kalra, V. K. and Brodie, A. F. (1974). Metabolic differences between the arteries of atherosclerosis susceptible and resistant pigeons. Biochem. Biophys., Res. Commun. 61, 1372.

4. Zemplenyi, T. (1975). Vascular Metabolism, Vascular Enzymes, and the Effect of Drugs. In "Pharmacology of Hypolipidemic Agents", Handbook of Exp. Pharmacology, Springer-Verlag, Berlin, Heidelberg, New York, Vol. 41.

5. Benditt, E. P. and Benditt, J. M. (1973). Evidence for a monoclonal origin of human atherosclerotic plaques. Proc. Nat. Acad. Sci. U.S.A. 70, 1753.

(5)

INFLUENCE OF GLYCOSAMINOGLYCAN CONTENT ON DIFFUSIVE TRANSPORT OF CALCIUM AND WATER ACROSS THE IN VITRO ARTERY WALL

Charles E. Glatz*, Louise C. Tortorelli, & Thomas A. Massaro
Chemical Engineering Department, Univ. of Wisconsin
Madison, Wisconsin, USA, 53706
* Iowa State University, Ames, Iowa, U.S.A.

Previous work has associated the glycosaminoglycan (GAG) content with mass transfer behavior of a number of systems. In the present research, GAG content and mass transfer measurements were carried out on the same sections of porcine thoracic aorta. The results demonstrate that naturally occurring changes in GAG content can account for observed differences in arterial permeability.

MATERIALS AND METHODS

Tissue was obtained at slaughter from each of seven sibling Yorksire barrows, age 35-38 wks. One inch adventitia-free sections were placed in a standard two compartment diffusion cell. Both compartments were filled with Hanks' solution while only the upstream one was initially charged with the isotopic tracers $^{45}Ca^{++}$ and ^{3}HHO. Appearance of tracer on the downstream side was followed by liquid scintillation counting.

The effective membrane diffusion coefficient $\bar{D}_{eff,i}$ was calculated as

$$\bar{D}_{eff,i} = \frac{d}{(c_i' - c_i'')} \frac{V''}{A} \frac{\Delta c_i}{\Delta t}$$

where d is the tissue thickness; A, the flow cross-section; c_i' and c_i'', the upstream and downstream concentrations; and $\Delta c_i''/\Delta t$, the steady state change of downstream concentration with time t. The subscript "eff" refers to the use of bulk concentrations rather than the true concentrations within the membrane, and V'' is the downstream concentration.

Following the diffusion experiment the tissue section was analyzed for GAG content by the procedure of Svejcar and Robertson (1). This gave a GAG distribution of five fractions, nominally hyaluronic acid (HA), heparan sulfate (HS), chondroitin 4-sulfate (CS-4), chondroitin 6-sulfate (CS-6), and dermatan sulfate (DS). Keratan sulfate and heparin were not found.

For each animal GAG distributions and $\bar{D}_{eff}$ of Ca^{++} and H_2O were measured at two thoracic aorta locations. A linear regression analysis was done for $\bar{D}_{eff, Ca}$ and $\bar{D}_{eff, H_2O}$ against the five GAG fractions and separately vs. total GAG. The analysis was then repeated using only those fractions with statistically significant ($p < 0.1$) regression coefficients in the initial regression.

RESULTS AND DISCUSSION

The linear regressions:

$$\bar{D}_{eff, Ca} = \text{constant} - 10.8\, C_{HA} + 1.35\, C_{CS-4} + 5.49\, C_{DS} \quad (p<0.01)$$

$$\bar{D}_{eff, H_2O} = \text{constant} - 7.16\, C_{HA} + 1.33\, C_{CS-4} + 6.53\, C_{DS} \quad (p<0.05)$$

were obtained. They correlate an increase in arterial permeability with a decrease in the content of hyaluronic acid relative to CS-4 and DS. i.e. the increase in arterial diffusive permeability to Ca^{++} and H_2O correlates with a decrease in the ratio of non-sulfated to sulfated GAG. A comparison with literature results (2-5) for changes in GAG content with artherosclerosis shows the predominate trend during early artherosclerotic involvement to be a decrease in non-sulfated:sulfated GAG which would result in an increase in arterial permeability to Ca^{++} and H_2O.

The lack of any observed effect of total GAG content on diffusive transport may be the result of the small range of total GAG encountered. The range was 50% of the lowest value relative to ranges of 100-300% for the individual fractions. It may be that large enough changes in total GAG to effect permeability do not occur.

This work was supported in part by a research grant from the United States Public Health Service (HL-13954) and by Fellowship support for C. E. G. from the National Science Foundation.

REFERENCES

1. Svejcar, J., and W.V.B. Robertson, Anal. Biochem., 18 333-50 (1967).

2. Adams, C. W. M., Vascular Histochemistry, Lloyd-Luke Ltd., London (1967).

3. Kumar, V. et al., J. Atherosler. Res., 7, 573-581 (1967).

4. Murata, K. and Y. Oshima, Atherosclerosis, 14, 121-129 (1971).

5. Vijayakumar, S. T. et al., Atherosclerosis, 21, 1-14 (1975).

CHAPTER 5
HEMODYNAMICS

(1)

INTERRELATIONSHIP OF HYPERTENSION AND ATHEROSCLEROSIS IN A SUBHUMAN PRIMATE MODEL

Hollander W, Madoff IM, Paddock J and Kirkpatrick J

Boston University Medical Center

75 East Newton Street, Boston, Ma., U.S.A.

Hypertension is recognized as one of the major precursors of atherosclerotic vascular disease (Kannel et al. Dis. Chest. 56:43, 1969). There is evidence in man and experimental animals that a sustained elevation of arterial blood pressure regardless of its cause aggravates and accelerates atherosclerosis (Page & McGubbin Renal Hypertension. Chicago, Year Book Medical Publishers, 1968; McGill Lab. Invest. 18:463, 1968). The actual mechanism by which hypertension aggravates atherosclerosis has not been established. It also is not clear that hypertension per se, in the absence of other atherogenic factors can cause atherosclerosis. The present study was undertaken to clarify some of the interrelationships of hypertension and atherosclerosis in a subhuman primate model with hypertension.

Hypertension was produced in the cynomolgus monkey by surgically coarcting the mid-thoracic aorta. The same surgical procedure was used previously to produce aortic coarctation in the dog (Hollander et al. J. Clin. Invest. 47:1221, 1968). As a result of coarcting the aorta, the blood pressure in the arteries proximal to the coarctation rises whereas the blood pressure in the arteries distal to the coarctation remains relatively normal. This experimental form of hypertension appears to be useful in studying the mechanical effects of hypertension on the arteries as well as evaluating the possible role of humoral factors on arterial wall function.

Two groups of monkeys were studied for 6 months. One group included normotensive and coarcted hypertensive monkeys fed a standard diet and the second group included normotensive and hypertensive monkeys fed an atherogenic diet consisting of 2% cholesterol and 10% butter. The serum cholesterol and lipoprotein levels were not significantly different in the normotensive and hypertensive monkey fed the standard diet or the atherogenic diet (Table 1). During the atherogenic diet, serum cholesterol rose to about 525 mg% in both groups and this was associated with significant increases in the low density and very low density lipoproteins and a decrease in the high density lipoprotein fractions.

Table 1

SERUM CHOLESTEROL & LIPOPROTEIN LEVELS IN THE CYNOMOLGUS MONKEY (mg/100 ml)

	Standard Diet		Atherogenic Diet	
	Normo-tensive	Hyper tensive	Normo-tensive	Hyper-tensive
Cholesterol	145	142	524	532
VLDL	35	32	148	143
LDL	132	137	763	750
HDL	307	298	113	121

The hypertension produced in the cynomolgus monkey appears to run a clinical course similar to that observed in hypertensive man. Some of the hypertensive complications observed included enlargement of the heart, congestive heart failure, hypertensive retinopathy and electrocardiographic signs of left ventricular hypertrophy. In addition, the pathologic findings in the heart and arteries of the hypertensive monkey appear very similar to that reported in hypertensive man (Vlodaver et al. Circulation 38:449, 1968). The hypertensive coarcted monkey fed an non-atherogenic diet consisting of Purina monkey chow for six months did not develop complicating atherosclerosis. However, the hypertensive coarcted monkey fed an atherogenic diet consisting of 2% cholesterol and 10% butter for 6 months developed severe and extensive fibrofatty plaques of the main coronary arteries and their extramural and intramural branches. Almost all the coronary arteries examined had atherosclerotic lesions (table 2). The narrowing of the arterial lumen caused by the atherosclerosis varied from 65 to 100%. In marked contrast to these findings the non-coarcted monkey fed the same atherogenic diet developed some "fatty streaks" in the main coronary arteries but without involvement of the small coronary branches. The maximal narrowing of the lumen of the coronary arteries produced by the foam cell lesions was about 15% and only 1 of 5 coronary arteries examined was involved (table 2). It was concluded from these findings that hypertension markedly accelerated and aggravated coronary atherosclerosis.

Table 2

THE EFFECT OF HYPERTENSION ON CORONARY ATHEROSCLEROSIS IN CYNOMOLGUS MONKEYS FED AN ATHEROGENIC DIET FOR 6 MONTHS

	Atherogenic Diet	Atherogenic Diet + Hypertension
No. of coronary arteries involved	1.0 ± 0.08	4.7* ± 0.4
Average degree of narrowing (%)	8 ± 7.8	74* ± 15.0

*$p < 0.01$

Hypertension also appeared to exert a powerful effect on the development of cerebral atherosclerosis. The hypertensive coarcted monkey fed the atherogenic diet developed moderate to severe cerebral atherosclerosis while the normotensive monkey fed the same atherogenic diet showed no atherosclerotic involvement of the cerebral arteries.

Although hypertension *per se* did not appear to cause athero-' sclerosis, it did appear to produce intimal lesions that had some similarities to those of atherosclerosis. The hypertensive coarcted monkey fed an non-atherogenic diet developed focal intimal lesions as well as marked thickening of the musculo-elastic media. These changes occurred in the arteries proximal to the coarctation but not distal to the coarctation suggesting that a high level of pressure with resulting increase in tangential stress on the arterial wall is responsible for these changes. The intimal lesions of hypertension and atherosclerosis appear to be similar in that the lesions are focal and are characterized by proliferation of cells, connective tissue and acid mucopolysaccharides. One of the major differences between the intimal disease appears to be the presence of lipid in atherosclerotic lesions and the absence of lipid in hypertensive lesions.

The present findings support earlier observations (Hollander et al. J.Clin.Invest. 47:1221, 1968; Wolinsky. Circ. Res. 26:507, 1970; Hollander. Circulation 48 1112, 1973), that hypertension has a major effect on the metabolism of the acid mucopolysaccharides and connective tissue proteins of the arteries without necessarily altering the metabolism of lipids. These changes are likely due to a direct mechanical effect of the hypertension on the smooth muscle cell and/or endothelial cell resulting in the multiplication of these cells and an augmented synthesis of AMPS, collagen and elastin. It also appears likely that the acceleration and aggravation of atherosclerosis by hypertension is related to the stimulatory effects of the hypertension on the proliferation of cells and connective tissue in the intima.

(2)

ALTERED RENAL FLOW IN THE LOCALIZATION OF SUDANOPHILIC LESION IN RABBIT AORTAS

Margot R. Roach, M.D., Ph.D. & Joan Fletcher, R.T., A.H.T.

Departments of Biophysics and Medicine, University of Western Ontario, London, Canada

In the past five years several laboratories have begun work to try to demonstrate what flow factors are involved in the localization of atherosclerotic lesions. If flow is important, then to determine its effect one must use an animal with relatively constant flow throughout the experimental period. For this reason we chose to use rabbits whose cardiac output does not alter appreciably if they remain in cages.

One of the major unsolved problems in hemodynamic investigations of atherosclerosis is the fact that all available probes are large, and so cannot be used biologically without distorting the flow. Thus, any analysis of flow factors must be based on careful mapping of lesions combined with model studies.

Cornhill and Roach (1974) pointed out the importance of polar coordinate mapping to assess how flow into a branch off the aorta modifies the size and shape of a lesion on the aortic wall near that orifice. All of their lesions, except those around the coronary ostia, were distal to the orifices. They found (in press) that the lesions were consistent in shape, but varied in size with the size of the branch and with the time of hypercholesterolemia.

To demonstrate that altered flow can alter the localization of lesions in the cholesterol-fed rabbit, we decided to do unilateral nephrectomies, leaving the renal artery as a blind stump in which there would be some flow. Four groups of six rabbits each were operated on under nembutal anaesthesia. These included those with right or left nephrectomies, and right or left sham operations. The rabbits were allowed to recover for one week and

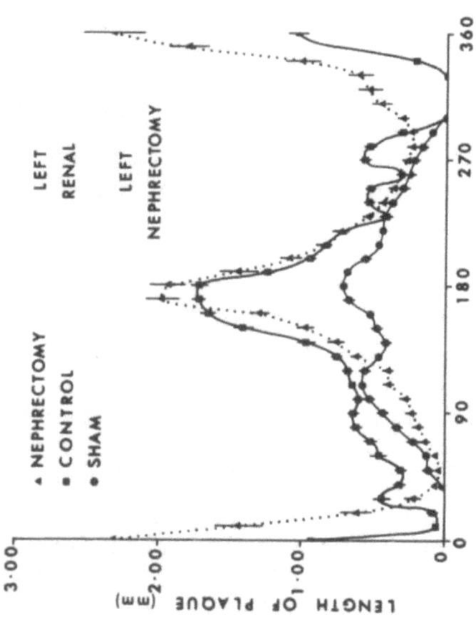

Fig. 1

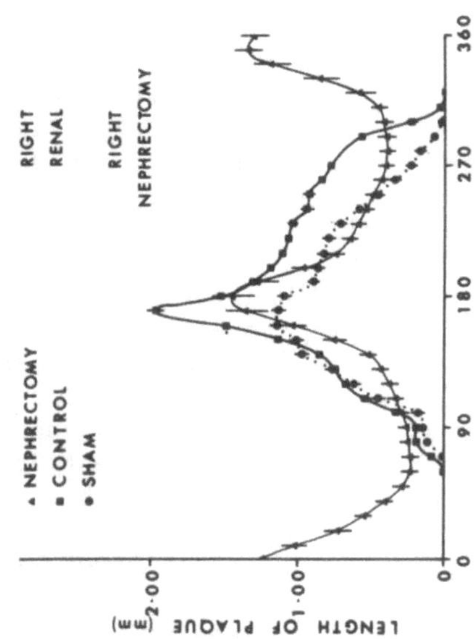

Fig. 2

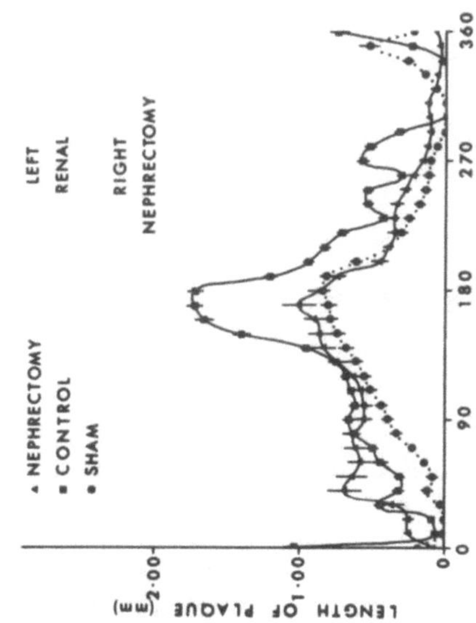

Fig. 3

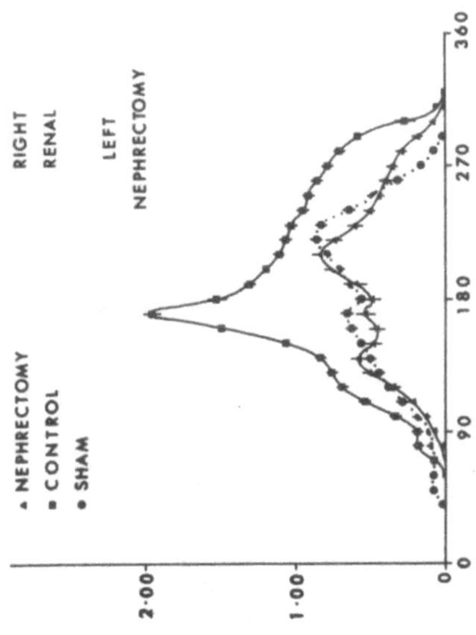

Fig. 4

were then fed a diet of 2% cholesterol and 6% corn oil (Kritchevsky et al. 1962) well mixed with ground rabbit pellets for four weeks. The results were compared with those in rabbits fed the same diet for the same period. Six animals were included in each group.

The results are summarized in Figures 1-4. The most striking differences are around the blind stump which shows the development of proximal as well as distal peaks. In addition, the left periorofificial lesion is altered by right nephrectomy while the right one is unaffected by left nephrectomy. Most operated groups show a decrease in the distal peak compared to the control. We presume this is due to altered tethering, although more experiments are required to prove this.

REFERENCES

Cornhill, J.F., Roach, M.R. Quantitative method for the evaluation of atherosclerotic lesions. Atherosclerosis 20:131-136, 1974.

Cornhill, J.F., Roach, M.R. A quantitative study of the localization of atherosclerotic lesions in the rabbit aorta. Atherosclerosis (in press).

Kritchevsky, D., Tepper, S.A., Langdon, J. Cholesterol vehicle in experimental atherosclerosis. Part IV. Influence of heated fat and fatty acids. J. Atheroscler. Res. 2:115-122, 1962.

(Supported by the Ontario Heart Foundation)

(3)

THE HEMODYNAMIC BASIS OF ATHEROSCLEROSIS

Meyer Texon, M. D.

New York University Medical Center

520 First Avenue, New York, N. Y., U.S.A.

The laws of fluid mechanics apply to the natural conditions in the circulatory system as they apply to any hydraulic system. The effect of the laws of fluid dynamics is considered the primary factor in the development of atherosclerosis because it alone can account for the localization and progressive development of atherosclerotic lesions at specific areas of predilection characterized by curvature, branching, external attachment, or tapering. While such vascular configurations occur in many variations of geometry or anatomical pattern with corresponding variations in patterns of blood flow, their common feature is the production of localized segmental zones of diminished lateral pressure. The diminished lateral pressure or suction effect which occurs in some phase of pulsatile flow in the cardiac cycle is the initial stimulus which produces intimal proliferation as the first change in the progressive development of atherosclerosis. Atherosclerosis may therefore be considered the reactive biological response of blood vessels to the effect of the laws of fluid mechanics at sites of predilection determined by local hydraulic conditions in the circulatory system.

The statistical association of age, sex, race, diet, cholesterol, exercise, occupation, emotional stress, hypertension, smoking and obesity, or so called risk factors with atherosclerosis does not constitute scientific proof of a causative mechanism. A primary causative factor or mechanism for atherosclerosis must determine its presence as well as its absence in all cases and in every given case.

Atherosclerosis occurs not at random locations but rather at specific sites of predilection which can be precisely defined, predicted, and produced. The Hemodynamic Basis of Atherosclerosis is supported by all the correlated data adduced from human autopsy specimens, the laws of fluid mechanics, mathematical computer analysis and animal experiments in which atherosclerosis was consistently produced by altering vascular configurations in dogs fed a normal diet.

A normal or ideal range of blood volume for a given blood vessel requires a range of pressure and velocity of blood flow which minimizes intimal proliferation due to either excessively high blood velocity or excessively low blood velocity. Atherosclerotic lesions reflect the local increase in blood velocity and local decrease in lateral pressure or tensile force. Occlusive endothelial and fibroblastic proliferation in bypass grafts represent the reparative obliteration of the vessel due to diminished blood flow.

Since blood flow is necessary for life and blood flow inherently causes atherosclerosis, the best we can hope to achieve is to minimize or retard the development of atherosclerosis by modifying or controlling the relevant hydraulic specifications which cause atherosclerosis.

Modification of the features of pulsatile flow which may be expected to retard the development of atherosclerosis are 1) a slower pulse rate, 2) a lower rate of change of blood velocity from minimum to maximum, 3) a decreased peak blood velocity, 4) a decreased mean velocity, and 5) a smaller range of blood velocity.

REFERENCES

1) Texon, M.: A Hemodynamic Concept of Atherosclerosis With Particular Reference to Coronary Occlusion. A.M.A. Arch. Int. Med. 99:418-427, 1957.

2) Texon, M., Imparato, A. M., and Helpern, M.: The Role of Vascular Dynamics in the development of atherosclerosis. J.A.M.A., 194, 1226-1230, 1965.

3) Texon, M.: The Role of Vascular Dynamics (Mechanical Factors) in the Development of Atherosclerosis. In Russek, H. I. and Zohman, B. L., Eds.: Coronary Heart Disease. Philadelphia, J. B. Lippincott Co., 1971, pp. 121-136.

4) Texon, M.: The Hemodynamic Basis of Atherosclerosis. Further Observations. Bull. N. Y. Acad. Med. 48:733-740, 1972.

5) Texon, M.: Atherosclerosis, Its Hemodynamic Basis and Implications. Med. Clinics of North America. 58, 257-268, 1974.

(4)

CITY - WIDE SCREENING FOR DETECTION OF HYPERTENSION

Donald S. Silverberg, M.D., M.Sc., F.R.C.P. (C)

University of Alberta Hospital

Edmonton, Alberta, Canada

We have screened 65,000 people in Edmonton for hypertension. Screening has taken place in shopping centres, drug stores, businesses, government offices, high schools and universities. Of those over the age of 18, 3.3% were found to be normotensive and taking antihypertensive medication. Another 8.8% were found to have elevated blood pressure. The criteria below were used for hypertensives. Of this group 34.5% had been previously unaware of their condition, 18.7% had never received medication, 18.2% had received medication in the past but had discontinued it, 26.1% were still on medication and 2.5% were not taking any antihypertensive medications and were uncertain if they had ever done so. 88 % of the hypertensives not on treatment went to their physician. Of this group 41% received medication. By examining the physicians' readings of hypertensive people, it was found that physicians treated systolic hypertension in 32% of cases, mild diastolic hypertension (up to 104 mm Hg) in 46%, moderate diastolic hypertension (105 to 114 mm Hg) in 85% and severe diastolic hypertension (more than 114 mm Hg) in 100%.

Hypertensive Values (in mm Hg) According to Age

	Under 40	40 - 64	65 and over
Systolic	$\geq$ 155	$\geq$ 160	$\geq$ 165
Diastolic	$\geq$ 95	$\geq$ 95	$\geq$ 100

In an 18 month follow-up of the group that received medication, 15% had their medication discontinued by their physician. Of the group that was to stay on medications, 8.6% stopped them on their own, 65.1% have achieved a normal blood pressure ($<$160/95 mm Hg), 13.8% have achieved blood pressures of 160 - 169/95-99 mm Hg, 8.6% have lower pressures than at the onset but above 169/99 mm Hg and 3.9% are higher now than at onset of treatment.

The degree of blood pressure control did not seem to be related to age, sex, initial blood pressure level or previous awareness of the presence of hypertension. Diuretics were used initially in 93.5% of cases. Potassium sparing diuretics were always used in combination with thiazides.

Screening for hypertension in this survey appeared to be associated with a high degree of patient compliance.

CHAPTER 6
HYPERLIPIDEMIA IN MAN AND TREATMENT

(1)

LIPID-PROTEIN PROPORTIONATE AND DISPROPORTIONATE VARIETIES OF LIPOPROTEINEMIA

J. Edwards, Thos. J. Muckle, C. J. Schwartz

Chedoke Hospital and McMaster University Medical Centre

Hamilton, Ontario, Canada

Although usually designated "serum lipoprotein electrophoretic analysis", in reality the conventional versions of the original Lees and Hatch (1963) technique represent something much nearer to electrophoretic serum lipid analysis. It is the lipids which are demonstrated in the technique, and commonly no direct attention is given to the corresponding apolipoproteins. It seemed possible that closer attention to the apolipoproteins and their quantitative relationship with carried lipids might provide information which could be usefully applied to subclassification of varieties of dyslipoproteinemia. Lipoprotein lipid and protein were therefore estimated and compared in a series of serum specimens. This paper presents some preliminary results of this investigation.

Materials and Methods

Sera from fasting patients were used fresh or after a single freezing at -70°C. These included specimens from 25 normal persons, and 165 abnormals including 36 Type II hyperlipoproteinemia, 81 Type IV, 19 Type V, and 29 which showed abnormalities which did not fall clearly into one or other of the types of the hyperlipoproteinemia classification of Fredrickson and Lees (1965). Immunoelectrophoresis was carried out by the micromethod of Scheidegger (1955) using 1% Oxoid Ionagar No. 2 in aqueous barbitone buffer of ionic strength 0.05 and pH 8.5 $\pm$ 0.1. Preparations were stained either with 100 mgm.% each Nigrosin and Ponceau S in 2% aqueous acetic acid, or 100 mgm.% Sudan Black B in aqueous ethanol for demonstration of lipid after the method of Uriel (1964). Polyacrylamide gel disc electrophoresis was carried out after the method of Narayan et al (1965), using the

Ames Company Quick-Disk QDL Reagent Kit which involves prestaining of lipids by Sudan Black B in ethylene glycol as originally described by McDonald and Ribeiro (1959). Radial immunodiffusion was carried out after the method of Mancini et al (1965). Commercial antisera were used for immunoelectrophoresis and radial immunodiffusion. Precision with these methods was achieved by meticulous attention to the technique and maintenance of standards.

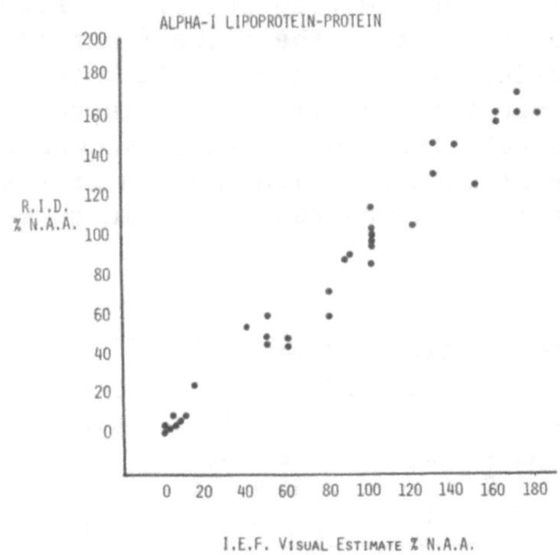

FIGURE 1

Estimation of the amount of specific protein and lipid in the particular fractions as revealed in these preparations was carried out by visual inspection of the patterns. This proved to be a better tool than we had expected, since the values for lipid and protein so obtained correlated well with the values provided by other techniques of estimation. (For example Fig. 1 for alpha-1 lipoprotein.) The data were analysed according to type of hyperlipoproteinemia, electrophoretic fraction, and the three lipid-protein proportionate relationships.

Results

No disproportion between lipid and protein was found in any of the three major electrophoretic fractions in any of the normal sera.

Table I

APPROACH BY TYPE			
LIPOPROTEIN	TYPE II (n=36)	TYPE IV (n=81)	TYPE V (n=19)
Beta	33 (92%) L = P↑	40 (49%) L = P↓	14 (75%) L = P↓
	0 P > L	39 (48.6%) P > L	5 (26%) P > L
	3 (8%) L > P	2 (2.5%) L > P	0 L > P
Prebeta	no notable disproportions	55 (68%) L = P↑	15 (80%) L = P↑
		0 P > L	0 P > L
		26 (32%) L > P	4 (20%) L > P
Alpha	28 (78%) L = P N ↑ or ↓	11 (14%) L = P↓ or N	5 (26%) L = P↓ or N
	8 (22%) P > L	70 (86%) P > L	14 (74%) P > L
	0 L > P	0 L > P	0 L > P

Table I shows the data relating to the hyperlipoproteinemia examples. The underlining of three sets of characters is simply to indicate the proportionate increase of lipid and protein in the particular lipoprotein characteristic of each of the three varieties. It can be seen that Type II sera showed very few cases with disproportionately excess lipid in the beta, none of any sort in the prebeta, and about a fifth of the total number in the alpha showed disproportionate lipid reduction. In Type IV lipid and protein were proportionate in beta, prebeta and alpha fractions in respectively half, two-thirds and one-sixth. Disproportion manifest in the alpha fraction was lipid reduction, in the prebeta fraction lipid excess, while both forms occurred in the beta fraction. In Type V a quarter showed disproportionate excess of the protein in the beta fraction, a fifth showed disproportionate excess of lipid in the prebeta fraction, and an impressive three-quarters in the alpha fraction showed reduced lipid relative to protein.

Table 2

APPROACH BY ELECTROPHORETIC FRACTIONS n = 165			
LIPOPROTEIN	L = P	P > L	L > P
Beta	110 = 66%	49 = 30%	6 = 4%
Prebeta	104 = 63%	0	61 = 37%
Alpha	50 = 30%	115 = 70%	0

Table 2 summarises the data arranged for electrophoretic fractions and the three lipid-protein proportionate variants. It can be seen that lipid and protein in the beta and prebeta fractions were proportionate in two-thirds of the cases, while in contrast only one-third of the alpha fractions were equivalent. In approximately one-third of the beta fractions there appeared to be a disproportionate excess of protein over lipid, while in about a third of the prebeta fractions the converse was true. Over two-thirds of the alpha fractions showed a relative excess of protein over lipid. Finally, note that no prebeta fraction was found with an obvious excess of protein over lipid and, vice versa, no alpha fraction was found to show apparent excess of lipid over protein.

The disproportion most frequently found was in the alpha fraction, so an attempt was made to correlate these changes with clinical conditions. Figure 2 shows that low alpha lipid with low alpha-1 apolipoprotein consistently accompanied hepatic parenchymal cellular dysfunction, while low alpha-1 lipid accompanied by normal or raised level of alpha-1 apoprotein was peculiar to the hyperlipoproteinemias, mainly Types IV and V.

Discussion

The findings suggest that the amount of lipid associated with serum apolipoproteins of these three major lipoproteins may vary to a substantial degree. The interrelationship seems to differ among the three. Thus excess of lipid over protein was never found in the

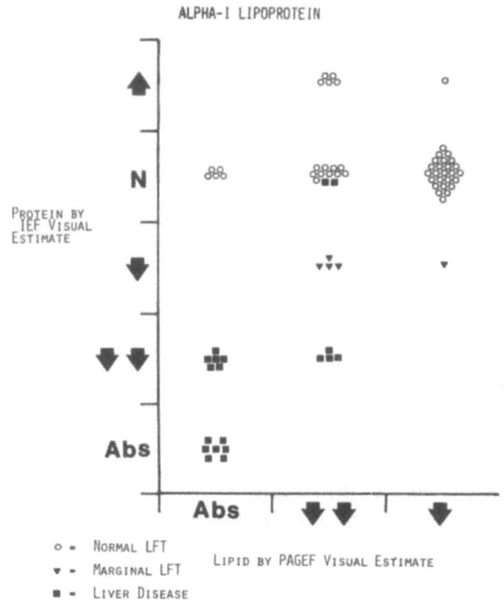

FIGURE 2

alpha fraction, although the converse was frequently observed. On the other hand, the opposite was true of the prebeta fraction. Here protein proportionately greater than lipid was never found, while almost a third of the samples showed an excess of lipid over protein. Last, both forms of disproportion were found to occur in the beta fraction, although most of these were of the protein-in-excess-of-lipid variety.

In summary, by comparing the results of lipid and protein analyses of serum it has been possible to further subdivide the classical hyperlipoproteinemia Types II, IV and V on the basis of the relative proportions of stainable lipid and antigenically ordinary protein demonstrable in the three major serum lipoprotein electrophoretic classes. The clinical relevance of these subclasses is presently under study.

References

1. Lees, R.S. and Hatch, F.T. 1963 J. Lab. Clin. Med. 61; 518.
2. Fredrickson, D.S. and Lees, R.S. 1965 Circulation 31; 321-327.
3. Scheidegger, J.J. 1955 Int. Arch. Allerg. 7; 103-110.
4. Uriel, J. 1964 in "Immunoelectrophoretic Analysis" edited by Grabar, P. and Burtin, P. pp 30-57, Elsevier, Amsterdam.
5. Narayan, K.A., Narayan, S. and Kummerow, F.A. 1965 Nature 205; 246-248.
6. McDonald, H.J. and Ribeiro, L.P. 1959 Clin.Chim.Acta 4; 458-459.
7. Mancini, G., Carbonera, A.O. and Heremans, J.F. 1965 Immunochemistry 2; 235-254.

(2)

METABOLIC EFFECTS OF THE BILE ACID SEQUESTRANT POLIDEXIDE (SECHOLEX[R]) IN MAN

L. A. Simons, N. B. Myant

Department of Medicine
University of NSW, Sydney, Australia, and
MRC Lipid Metabolism Unit, Hammersmith Hospital
London, U.K.

Cholestyramine has an accepted place in the treatment of hypercholesterolemia, acting as a non-absorbable bile acid sequestrant. Although it is effective and safe during long-term administration, its use has been complicated by gastro-intestinal side-effects and by the occasional development or aggravation of hypertriglyceridemia.

The present study was designed to evaluate the new anion-exchange resin polidexide (also known as Secholex ®, DEAE-Sephadex and PDX-C1), in relation to its effects on plasma lipids and on cholesterol and bile salt metabolism.

Experimental Design and Methods: Six subjects (2 normals, 2 type IIa and 2 type IIb hyperlipidemics) were treated with increasing doses of polidexide, 3-30 g/day, for 56 to 123 days. Five of these subjects were alternatively treated with cholestyramine 16-28 g of base/day. Plasma cholesterol, triglycerides and apolipoprotein-B were measured serially before and during therapy. Fecal bile acids were measured by gas-liquid chromatography and endogenous neutral steroids by the isotopic balance method, using a preliminary I.V. pulse injection of ^{14}C-cholesterol.

Results: There was a significant reduction in plasma cholesterol concentration in all subjects treated with polidexide. Control mean cholesterol was 317±40 mg/100 ml (SEM) compared with treatment mean 256±34mg/100 ml ($P < 0.002$). Plasma apolipoprotein-B levels behaved

<u>Table 1</u>: Endogenous Fecal Steroid Excretion During Therapy with Polidexide or Cholestyramine [a].

No.	BILE ACIDS (mg/day ± 1SD)			ENDOGENOUS NEUTRAL STEROIDS(mg/day ± 1SD)		
	CONTROL	POLIDEXIDE	CHOLESTYR.	CONTROL	POLIDEXIDE	CHOLESTYR.
1	277 ± 92	$1429 \pm 69^{**}$	$2615 \pm 31^{**,**}$	-	-	-
2	300 ± 36	$1599 \pm 188^{**}$	$2008 \pm 172^{**,++}$	-	-	-
3	203 ± 89	$851 \pm 180^{**}$	$1289 \pm 437^{**,NS}$	371 ± 62	499 ± 169^{NS}	$499 \pm 57^{++,NS}$
4	301 ± 25	$1504 \pm 120^{**}$	-	484 ± 48	$601 \pm 84^{+}$	-
5	310 ± 44	$1954 \pm 212^{**}$	$3136 \pm 540^{**,*}$	811 ± 53	664 ± 67^{NS}	$724 \pm 119^{NS,NS}$

a. Mean values during the control period and during the periods of therapy at maximum dose level. Polidexide was compared with control, and cholestyramine with control and polidexide results respectively, using Student's t-test:

** $P < 0.001$ ++ $P < 0.02$ NS not significant

* $P < 0.01$ + $P < 0.05$

in a parallel fashion (control 189±49 mg/100ml compared with treatment 161±41 mg/100ml, P< 0.02). In subjects with fasting plasma triglyceride concentrations< 100 mg /100ml, no significant change in triglyceride concentration occurred. Two subjects with control values > 130 mg/100ml showed increases in triglycerides (135±27 to 174±20 mg/100ml and 190±69 to 224±39 mg/100ml). Approximately equivalent responses were noted with cholestyramine therapy.

Measurement of endogenous fecal steroids was possible in 5 subjects on polidexide and in 4 of them on cholestyramine. The overall changes in fecal steroids are summarised for all subjects in Table 1. There was an average 5.3 fold increase in bile acid excretion on 15-30 g/day of polidexide, and an average 8.1 fold increase in bile acid excretion on 20-28 g/day of cholestyramine. Bile acid excretion was significantly higher with cholestyramine than with polidexide at comparable doses. There was a small but significant increase in endogenous neutral steroid excretion in 1 out of 3 subjects treated with polidexide or cholestyramine.

CONCLUSIONS:

Polidexide is an effective cholesterol-lowering agent but it is likely to aggravate a pre-existing hypertriglyceridemia. Its use is not associated with a large change in endogenous neutral steroid excretion. This suggests (but does not prove) that there may be little change in the amount of cholesterol absorption. Polidexide appears to act essentially as a bile acid sequestrant, but is less efficient at stimulating bile acid production than is cholestyramine. Despite this difference, both resins have a similar effect on blood lipids at comparable doses.

(3)

COLESTIPOL HYDROCHLORIDE, A NEW HYPOLIPIDEMIC DRUG: A TWO-YEAR STUDY - SUMMARY

Elmer E. Cooper, M.D. and A. M. Michel, BSMT

Santa Rosa Medical Centre,

San Antonio, Texas, U.S.A.

Colestipol* Hydrochloride is an insoluble, nondigestible, nonabsorbable, tasteless, odorless copolymer of polyethylenepolyamine and epichlorhydrin. It sequesters bile acids in the intestinal tract by its capacity to bind cholates through anion exchange and by its permeability to micellar aggregates of bile acids. The product is then excreted in the feces. When cholesterol formation in vivo is insufficient to compensate for the amount of cholesterol removed for bile acid synthesis, a net decrease in plasma concentration will result.[1,2] Therefore, this synthetic organic polymer provides an attractive pharmacotherapeutic approach to decreasing plasma and tissue cholesterol pools in hyperlipidemic patients.

Bile acids are formed in the liver by degradation of cholesterol and are secreted into the bile. After ingestion of a meal, bile is secreted into the intestine where it plays an important role in facilitating the absorption of dietary lipids. The bile acids are then absorbed from the small intestine(ileum) and returned via the portal blood back to the liver where they are resecreted into the bile. Each day a small pool of bile acids, approximately 2-4 gm is cycled through the intestine from six to ten times, and only a minimal amount, approximately 0.6 gm, is lost in the feces. An amount of bile acid equivalent to the daily loss is synthesized from cholesterol by the liver to maintain a pool of constant size.

Bile acids thus serve two useful functions: first, they are the end products of the metabolism of cholesterol by the liver and, since the nonrecirculated bile acids are eliminated in the feces, account for much of the cholesterol turnover. Second, the bile acids are concerned with the absorption of lipids from the intestinal contents into the intestinal mucosa and they regulate metabolic processes within the absorptive cell.[3] When bile acids are sequestered from the lumen of the gastrointestinal tract,[4] cholesterol ester hydrolysis and cholesterol absorption will be impeded. Sequestering bile acids by colestipol enhances conversion of hepatic cholesterol into bile acids and the loss of a portion of the bile acids in the feces further interferes with cholesterol absorption. Both of these biologic phenomena lower the cholesterol pool.

A randomized, placebo-controlled, single-blind study was done using 60 subjects with cholesterol levels of over 250 mg/100 ml for 104 weeks. Patients with normal phenotypes, types 2, 3, and 4, were given 5 gm 3 times daily and experienced an average drop of 40 mg/100 ml (14%). While patients with types 2, 3, and 4 hyperlipidemia responded effectively, cholesterol levels in type 2 patients dropped earliest and most consistently with an average decrease of 50 mg/100 ml (19%). A comparable group of patients with hyperlipidemia taking the placebo (Avicel) showed on average no change in serum cholesterol. Serum triglyceride values were not altered significantly. The patients in both groups came for office visits every month during the first year and bimonthly thereafter, were interviewed, examined, and weight and blood pressure were recorded. They were questioned concerning possible side effects. Cholesterol, triglycerides, glucose, bilirubin, creatinine, calcium, phosphorus, sodium, chloride, potassium, uric acid, and SGOT were assayed monthly in a central laboratory. Hct, Hgb, WBC, differential, platelet count, prothrombin time, and urinalysis were determined in our laboratory at the same intervals. Phenotyping was done on these subjects. Eighty-six of the entire group of the 189 were type 2; 42 were type 4; 5 were type 3; and 55 had normal patterns. Of these 189 patients qualified, 152 were randomized; 76 were assigned to the placebo group and 76 to colestipol. 30 patients were purposely placed on the colestipol regimen because of multiple atherosclerotic risk factors or family histories of early coronary deaths. 7 hyperlipidemic patients with prior diagnoses of cholesterol gallstones were treated as in the patients with atherosclerotic risk factors. 99 patients have completed the 2 year study. Within this group 60 were treated with colestipol. Collectively in these subjects the serum cholesterol decreased from a pretreatment value of 300 mg/100 ml to 250 mg/100 ml after one month, to 267 mg/100 ml after 6 months, 262 mg/100 ml after one year and 279 mg/100 ml after 2 years of medication. The serum cholesterol level changed little in the 39 randomized placebo group. No direct effects on serum enzymes or on liver or kidney function occurred. This may be further evidence to substantiate the impression that colestipol is nonabsorbable and indigestible. Blood chemistries, hematology, and urinalyses showed no abnormalities. Body weights remained stable. The drug appeared to be well tolerated. There was no steatorrhea, constipation, or marked change in stool pattern. Several patients initially complained of fullness, bloating and rectal irritation, but soon even these side effects disappeared. There was no evidence of bleeding tendencies. Prothrombin times were not prolonged. There was no indication of fat-soluble vitamin interference, nor was it expected in the dosage range used in our colestipol study.

The work of Admirand & Small[5], Vlahcevic & colleagues[6], Danzinger and others[7], has shown recently that patients with cholesterol cholelithiasis have a diminished bile acid pool. In order to determine the possibility of the production of lithogenic bile during the use of bile acid sequestering agents, most of the patients had gallbladder visualization before the study, and all had it at the end of the 24 months. During this interval there was no evidence of cholelithiasis formation in any of the patients in either group. The 7 patients with known cholesterol cholelithiasis at the onset of the study, who it is assumed, had the lithogenic bile, were followed furing the 2 years of their colestipol therapy to determine if the resin did indeed render the bile more lithogenic. X-ray film studies taken at 6-month intervals during the 2 years disclosed no evidence of increase or decrease in the number or the size of the stones.

The evidence to date indicates that during the 2 years of our bile acid sequestration study, the drug effectively depressed cholesterol but the hepatic synthesis of bile apparently compensated for the lowering of the total bile acid pool. Therefore, no lithogenic milieu was produced. Conclusive long-term studies of this resin must be done to preclude the remote possibility of the production of lithogenic bile and cholelithiasis.

REFERENCES

1. Parkinson, TM., Gundersen, K., Nelson NA.: Effects of colestipol, (U-26,587A), a new bile acid sequestrant, on serum lipids in experimental animals and man. Atherosclerosis 11: 531-537, 1970.
2. Chobanian, AV., Hollander, W.: Body cholesterol metabolism in man. I. The equilibration of serum and tissue cholesterol. J. Clin. Invest. 41:1732-1737, 1962.
3. Schiff, L., Carey, JB. Jr., Dietschy, JM. (eds): Bile Salt Metabolism. Springfield, Ill., Charles C. Thomas Publisher, 1969.
4. Moore, RB., Crane, CA., and Frantz, ID. Jr.: Effect of cholestyramine on the fecal excretion of intravenously administered cholesterol- 4-14C and its degradation products in a hypercholesterolemic patient. J. Clin. Invest. 47:1664-1671, 1968.
5. Admirand, WH., Small, DM.: The physiochemical basis of cholesterol gallstone formation in man. J. Clin. Invest. 47: 1043-1052, 1968.
6. Vlahcevic, ZR., Bell, CC., Buhac, I., Farrar, JT., and Swell, L.: Diminished bile acid pool size in patients with gallstones. Gastroenterology 59:165-173, 1970.

7. Danzinger, RG., Hofmann, AF., Schoenfield, LJ., and Thistle, JL.: Dissolution of cholesterol gallstones by chenodeoxycholic acid. N. England J. Med. 286:1-8, 1972.

*Colestid, The Upjohn Company

(4)

DIETARY INFLUENCE ON MOLECULAR DISTRIBUTION OF SERUM LIPOPROTEINS IN SUBJECTS WITH PROVEN CORONARY ARTERY DISEASE

Robert C. Bahler, M.D., Jan J. Opplt, M.D., Ph.D.

Case Western Reserve University, School of Medicine
and Cleveland Metropolitan General Hospital
3395 Scranton Road, Cleveland, Ohio, U.S.A.

Levels of some lipoprotein classes are well known to be responsive to dietary alterations. Nevertheless, there is a need for the further explanation of mechanisms resulting in these changes in patients with proven coronary artery disease (CAD). In particular, the question of whether qualitative changes in serum lipoproteins can occur secondary to dietary intervention has not been examined. One of us developed a new technique of molecular distribution of serum lipoproteins[1], a method which separates lipoproteins on the basis of their particle size. It provides an important new approach to the study of lipoprotein metabolism during dietary interventions.

METHODS

The 15 male patients (mean age 43) selected for study were characterized by angiographically confirmed CAD, abnormal routine lipid screening studies, absence of clinical diabetes, and normalglycemia. Serum samples were obtained after a 14 hour fast. Total plasma lipoproteins were studied by analytical ultracentrifugation and by paper and agarose-gel electrophoresis. Plasma levels of cholesterol and triglycerides were measured. Plasma lipoproteins were isolated as a total moiety by preparative ultracentrifugation at a density of 1.21. The flotant was subjected to molecular filtration on a pretreated Sepharose - 6B column. Very precise standard conditions were maintained. Each subfraction obtained was characterized by its elution volume, electrophoretic mobility in agarose-gel, flotation rate, and immunochemical identification of its corresponding apoproteins. The molecular sizes in each subfraction were studied by electronmicroscopy and a light scattering method using a laser as the light source. These studies were completed before and after three months of dietary intervention. "Type" specific dietary instructions (based on USPHS dietary manuals) were supervised by a clinical nutritionist.

RESULTS AND CONCLUSIONS

Using the conventional classification (analyses of serum cholesterol and triglycerides, agarose-gel electrophoresis and ultracentrifugal flotation), we classified ten subjects as Type IV -dyslipoproteinemia, two subjects as Type IIB, and one as Type IIA. Two other patients revealed minimal changes in lipids and lipoproteins. This report represents our preliminary experience with the first group of ten patients characterized by Type IV dyslipoproteinemia.

The serum triglyceride level fell in all subjects (233 $\pm$ 28 to 177 $\pm$ 33, p=0.01). Mean cholesterol levels were unchanged (232 $\pm$ 27 to 222 $\pm$ 26) although there were three subjects with a greater than 30 mg.% decline. The decrease in total triglyceride levels was not clearly reflected in the agarose-gel electrophoretic patterns, although the electrophoresis revealed the tendency of α-lipoproteins to increase and the pre-β - lipoproteins to decrease. The analytical ultracentrifuge showed a near significant decrease in the standard lipoprotein class of very low density lipoproteins, characterized by -S 400 to -S 70. No other significant changes in the ultracentrifugal pattern were observed.

The mechanism of dietary changes in serum lipoproteins was revealed by the study of their molecular distribution. The common response (in nine of ten patients) was characterized by quantitative changes in the area of very-low-density lipoproteins although qualitative changes, in particle size of the individual fractions, were not observed. The above mentioned changes consist in decreasing quantities of lipoprotein molecular associations (representing the subfractions II and III -Fig.1,2). Subfractions II and III are relatively diffuse (elution volume 150-170 ml.), seldom forming a discrete peak. This broad band corresponds to a broad spectrum of lipoprotein molecules. The size of these lipoprotein molecules varies between 1000 Å - 600 Å (Fig.3,4) which qualifies them as associations of large molecules of very-low density lipoproteins. The distribution of these lipoproteins in a gravitational field, according to their specific densities, reveals lipoprotein - classes of -2700 S to -400 S and, in lesser amounts, classes of -400 S to -75S. Their mobility in an electric field, measured in agarose-gel, is always close to the mobility of the pre-β -fraction of serum lipoproteins. These molecular associations are characterized by a typical multiband of VLD-apolipoproteins, isolated by delipidation and then separated electrophoretically in polyacrylamide gel. Type IV subjects were found, by the laser-light scattering technique, to have lipoprotein particles which tended to be larger than those seen in similar fractions from normal subjects . Dietary therapy did not significantly alter the particle size of any individual fractions, nor of the quantitatively lowered subfractions II and III.

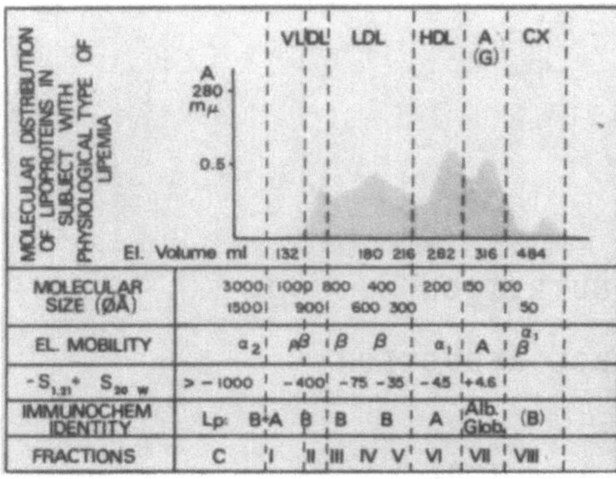

Fig. 1

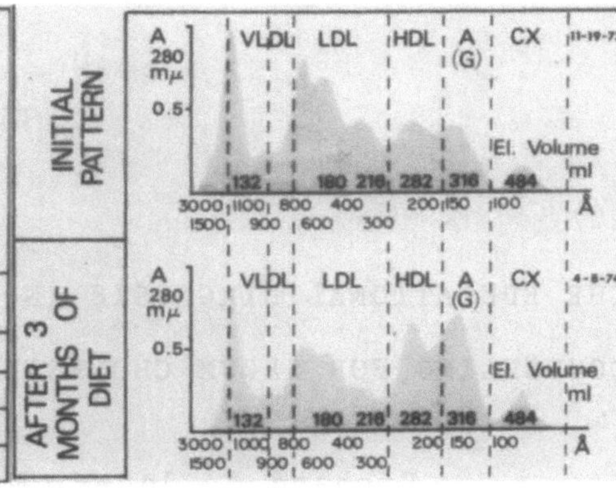

Fig. 2

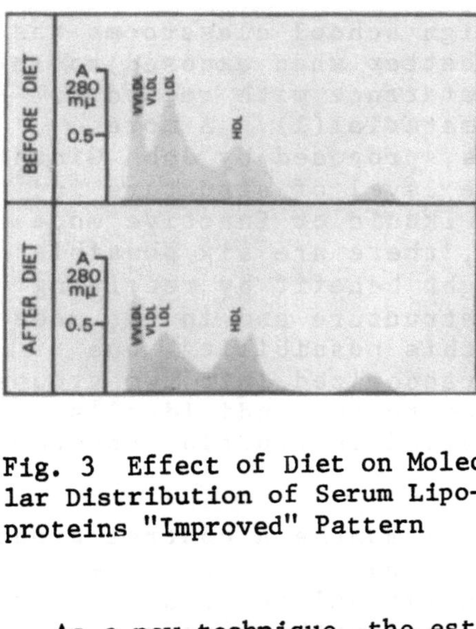

Fig. 3 Effect of Diet on Molecular Distribution of Serum Lipoproteins "Improved" Pattern

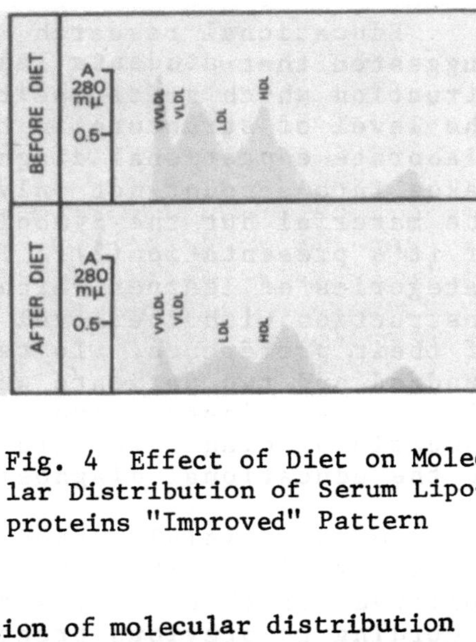

Fig. 4 Effect of Diet on Molecular Distribution of Serum Lipoproteins "Improved" Pattern

As a new technique, the estimation of molecular distribution of serum lipoproteins permits the detection of changes in concentration, as well as changes in formation of molecular associations of lipoprotein subclasses. These changes may not be well reflected in other currently utilized techniques.

1. Opplt Jan J., Opplt, M.A.: Separation of plasma lipoproteins according to molecular size. Clin Chem 20:906, 1974.
2. Opplt Jan J., Simic Glavaski B., Bahler R.C., Opplt M.A.: Molecular Distribution of Plasma Lipoproteins in Type IV Hyperlipoproteinemia. Clin Chem 21:990, 1975.

(5)

THE EDUCATIONAL DIAGNOSIS IN NUTRITION COUNSELING FOR SERUM CHOLESTEROL REDUCTION

Richard J. Jones, M.A., M.D.,
Dorothea Turner, M.A., Linda A. Slowie, M.A.

Department of Medicine, University of Chicago
950 E. 59th Street, Chicago, Illinois, U.S.A.

Educational research in high school classrooms has suggested that students learn better when exposed to instruction which suits their preference with regard to the level of structure in the material(1). A more elaborate educational diagnosis, proposed by John Ginther, takes into account not only the level of structure in the material but the Symbolic, Ikonic or Enactive mode of it's presentation(2). Thus, there are six possible categories of learner which might benefit by receiving instruction with the level of structure and in the mode of their preference. To test this possibility, one hundred and two patients were randomized into two groups: IIa received instruction matched to the individual's educational diagnosis, IIb received instruction counter to the educational diagnosis.

For an initial period of six months a control group I was enrolled. This included 67 patients who were followed for three months of individualized instruction according to previous precepts, and without regard to their educational diagnoses. Their mean cholesterol level was reduced by 31.8mgm% or 11.3% after three months of dietary instruction and reached a maximum reduction of 14.4% at nine months. Serum triglyceride reduction was 14.8% and body weight loss 4.6% at three months. The dietary intake, as recorded, showed a mean change at three months of -9.9% calories, -7.4% total fat, -27.0% saturated fatty acid glycerides and -35.0% dietary cholesterol with +131% polyunsaturated fatty acid glycerides.

The patients in group II were instructed in the American Heart Association diet by nutritionists, who were blindly given their assigned modes and levels of structure, which either matched or did not match their educational diagnosis as determined by two questionnaires. The nutritionists pursued a course of six lessons in the assigned mode and level of structure. Many original materials were devised to round out the teaching armamentarium for certain learner categories. The level of structure was determined largely by the nutritionist as she carried out the interview and/or manipulated the teaching devices.

Randomization was successful in that no clinical differences were apparent between IIa and IIb. Serum cholesterol reduction averaged only 14mg% (4.7%) at three months when the course of instruction was completed. The extent of serum cholesterol reduction was quite comparable in these two groups at two months. At the three month visit, the serum cholesterol level of group IIb returned virtually to base-line levels while the maximum cholesterol reduction for IIa was maintained and continued until the six month visit when the difference between the two groups was statistically significant.

Diet records reported at three months after the onset of instruction showed a 19.2% caloric reduction in IIa, but only a 12.6% reduction in IIb respectively. At three months, the reduction in saturated fat was 43% and 38%, in cholesterol intake was 43% and 36%, and the increase in polyunsaturated fatty acid glycerides was 82% and 105% in IIa and IIb respectively. The 3 month change in the "diet factor", Φ, of Keys, Anderson, and Grande(3), was about the same in both groups. Except for the greater reduction in caloric intake seen in group IIa, none of the dietary differences was statistically significant.

When patients were categorized according to the preferred level of structure and mode, and the cholesterol reduction averaged, or if the reduction was arbitrarily considered fair to good if equal to or more than 25mg% and poor if less than 25mg%, there was no difference in the rate of success of achieving such a reduction in the two groups. If success was defined as a reduction in serum cholesterol or a reduction in serum triglyceride of 25mg% or a loss of body weight of 5 pounds or more, the rate of success was a little better in Group IIb than in Group IIa, although this was not statistically significant.

In conclusion, we have suggestive evidence that those patients receiving instruction matched to their preference, did show a more sustained reduction in their cholesterol level than the counter group. There is evidènce that true cognitive learning is more lasting than short term learning and is better measured sometime after the acquisition period (4). Modern psychological theory suggests two or three memory compartments, with at least a long and short term memory, each of which may require different factors for their intensification. Since it is the long term memory that we wish to influence in regard to dietary management of hypocholesteremia it is not inconsistent with present psychological theory that the measure of our influence upon the patient's learning will appear sometime after the educational experience is completed as occurred here.

1. Berlin,B.M. "The Learning Experiences of Students" PhD dissertation. Department of Education. University of Chicago 1965.

2. Ginther,J. Educational Diagnosis of Patients. J. Am. Diet. Assoc.59:560 (1971).

3. Keys, A., Anderson,J.T. and Grande,F. Prediction of Serum Cholesterol Responses of Man to Changes of Fat in the Diet.Lancet II:959 (1957).

4. Greeno,J.G. The Structure of Memory and the Process of Solving Problems. Solso,R.L.(Ed.) "Contemporary Issues in Cognitive Psychology". New York: John Wiley and Sons 1973 p.112.

(1)

METABOLIC RESPONSE TO INTRALIPID INFUSIONS IN THE NEONATAL PERIOD

REID, W.D., M.D., F.R.C.P. (C);
ROBINSON, Halina, Chem. Eng.
Department of Paediatrics
University of Western Ontario
London, Ontario, Canada

The lipid profile in neonates receiving an intravenous infusion of intralipid during the first week of life was studied. Twenty infants of mean gestational age 34 weeks (28-40) and mean birth weight 2243 grams (1000-3800) were studied. A 10% solution of intralipid was infused at a dosage of 4 k/Kg over a four-hour period. The remainder of the caloric intake was supplied by an aminoacid and glucose solution. All fluids were given by scalp vein.

Blood samples were drawn before the infusion of intralipid began and at zero, 1 and 3 hours after the infusion had been completed, on the first, third and fifth day of alimentation. The concentration of total lipid and triglycerides are reported from this study. Twenty infants were initially studied, but this was reduced to 15 infants on the third day and 12 on the fifth day as some infants had their intravenous alimentation discontinued due to neonatal complications not related to the intralipid infusion.

The highest recorded total lipid concentration was 3.668 gm%. On the first day 12 out of 20 infants had total lipid levels exceeding 1.5 gm% at the end of the infusion. Although the levels gradually fell during the first three hours after infusion, two infants had total lipid levels exceeding 1.5 gm% at three hours after infusion. On the third day 8/15 and 2/15 had total lipid greater than 1.5 gm% at zero and 3 hours after infusion respectively. On the fifth day of infusion 10/12 and 3/15 had greater than 1.5 gm% of total lipid at zero and 3 hours.

Triglyceride levels exceeded 1.5 gm% at the end of the infusion in 6/20, 1/15 and 3/12, on the first, third and fifth day respectively. All patients had triglyceride levels below 1.5 gm% by 3 hours after the infusion.

TABLE I

TRIGLYCERIDE LEVELS GREATER THAN 1,500 mgm%		
Day	End of Infusion	3 Hrs. After
1st	6/20 (30%)	0/20 (0%)
3rd	1/15 (6.6%)	0/15 (0%)
5th	3/12 (25%)	0/12 (0%)

The baseline total lipid level was significantly higher before the infusion of the third day, as compared to the infusion on the first day (p less than 0.01) and tended to remain elevated at the fifth pre-infusion day as well. There was no significant elevation of the baseline triglyceride level on the third or fifth day as compared to the pre-infusion level on the first day.

TABLE II

TOTAL LIPID (mgm%)				
Day	Before (Mean)	0 (Mean)	1 Hr. (Mean)	3 Hrs. (Mean)
1st	492	2057	1797	1253
3rd	693	1703	1421	1025
5th	612	2034	1550	1081

TABLE III

TRIGLYCERIDES (mgm%)				
Day	Before (Mean)	0 (Mean)	1 Hr. (Mean)	3 Hrs. (Mean)
1st	106	1116	1006	434
3rd	107	738	732	313
5th	75	1002	693	277

Conclusions and Summary:

No clinical deterioration occurred in our infants during periods of severe hyperlipemia. Nevertheless, it cannot be assumed that such hyperlipemia is safe without long-termed follow-up. In order to infuse an adequate caloric intake in a small premature infant, the total intralipid infusion could be extended over a more prolonged period than four hours. One attractive alternative is to mix the glucose-aminoacid solution with the intralipid. This mixture could then be infused over a 24-hour period. The rate of infusion may be more important than the total amount infused per kilogram per 24 hours.

No triglyceride accumulation was noted between the first pre-infusion day and that of the third or fifth day, although this represents a short period of study. The baseline elevation of the total lipid level on the third pre-infusion day as compared to the first pre-infusion sample may represent a developing intolerance.

(2)

SERUM CHOLESTEROL AND TRIGLYCERIDE LEVELS IN CHILDREN FROM A BIRACIAL COMMUNITY--THE BOGALUSA HEART STUDY

Ralph R. Frerichs, Sathanur R. Srinivasan, Larry S. Webber, and Gerald S. Berenson
Specialized Center of Research--Arteriosclerosis
Louisiana State University School of Medicine
New Orleans, Louisiana, USA

INTRODUCTION

The need to recognize Coronary Artery Disease (CAD) risk factors at an early age is becoming increasingly important. Serum cholesterol has long been known to be a major independent risk factor for CAD in adults (1). More recently, the level of serum triglycerides has been incriminated as a CAD risk factor independent of cholesterol (2) although the evidence for independence is not conclusive (3).

During the 1973-1974 school year, 3,524 children, ages 5 through 14 years residing in Bogalusa, Louisiana, were examined as part of the Bogalusa Heart Study. This population represents 93% of the 3,786 children eligible, of whom 37% are blacks and 63% whites. Due to a policy of limiting venipuncture to two attempts, no blood samples were obtained from 78 children (2.2%). Each child was asked to fast for 12-14 hours before venipuncture; compliance was determined by interview on the morning of the examination. Of the 3,446 samples, only 263 (7.6%) were obtained from nonfasting children.

MATERIALS AND METHODS

Total serum cholesterol and triglycerides were analyzed simultaneously in a Technicon Auto-Analyzer II (AAII) according to the protocol developed by the Lipid Research Clinics in collaboration with the Center for Disease Control (CDC), Atlanta, Georgia. Our laboratory has passed the final phase of the standardization and control program of the CDC. A serum calibrator, provided by the CDC, was used during every analytical run to convert the cholesterol values obtained by the AAII to the standard reference method of Abell-Kendall. The CDC also provided cholesterol and triglyceride (triolein) standards.

Every day of screening, an extra blood sample was collected as a blind duplicate on a random selection of approximately 12% of the children for assessment of measurement errors. New names and new identification numbers were placed on the duplicate samples to ensure blind analyses. Based on 431 duplicate samples, the standard deviations of the measurement errors for serum cholesterol and triglycerides were 9.14 mg% and 9.66 mg% respectively; the coefficients of variation of the measurement errors were 5.5% and 13.3%. These values represent not only the error in laboratory analyses of two independent samples but also the error associated with the collection and processing of samples before they arrive at the laboratory.

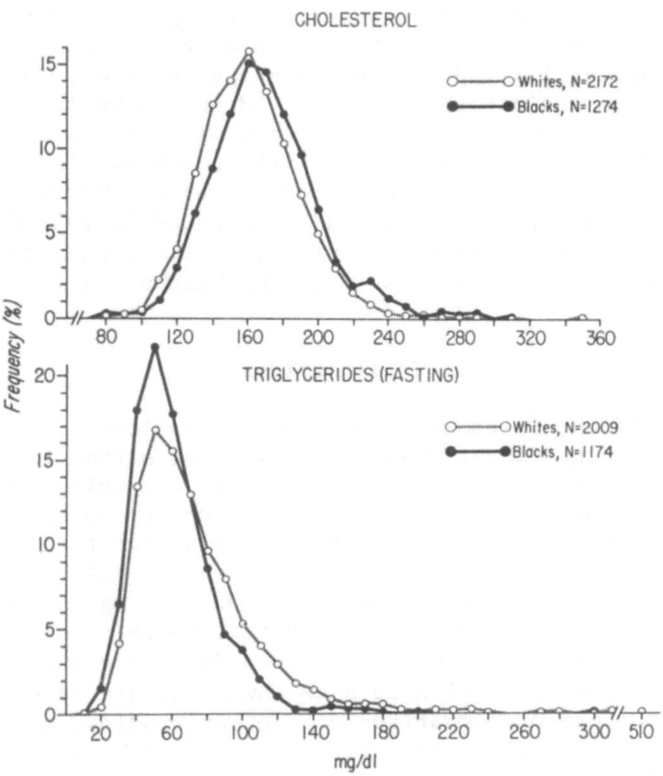

Figure 1: Distributions of total serum cholesterol and triglycerides by race in children, ages 5 through 14 years.

RESULTS

In order to determine the effect of a 12- to 14-hour fast on lipid levels, a comparison was made of blood samples from the 3,183 fasting children and the 263 nonfasting children. There was no statistically significant difference between mean serum cholesterol levels in fasting and nonfasting children (165.3 mg% for fasting versus 162.7%, $p < .16$) whereas the mean level of serum triglycerides is significantly lower in fasting children (68.7 mg% for fasting versus 87.2 mg%, $p < .0001$). Therefore, for cholesterol, the values reported are for both fasting and nonfasting children whereas for triglycerides, only values from fasting subjects are presented.

Total Serum Cholesterol

Black children had significantly greater levels of serum cholesterol than white children (fig. 1) (mean of 170 mg% versus 162 mg%, $p < .001$). No uniform differences were observed in cholesterol levels between boys and girls in either racial group. Ninety percent of the blacks had values between 126 mg% (5th percentile) and 226 mg% (95th percentile) while 90% of the whites were between 121 mg% (5th percentile) and 210 mg% (95th percentile). Due to a slight decrease in cholesterol levels in 13 and 14 year old children, there is a negative correlation of cholesterol with age for this decade of observation. However, the slight negative slope is statistically significant only in white boys (-.89 mg% per year, $p < .01$). Values greater than 200 mg% were found in 13% of the black children and 9% of the white children while concentrations exceeding 230 mg% were found in 4.1% of the blacks and 1.5% of the whites.

Serum Triglycerides

White children, in contrast to the observations of cholesterol noted above, had significantly greater levels of serum triglycerides (fasting) than black children (means of 71 mg% for whites versus 61 mg%, $p < .001$; median of 63 mg% in whites versus 55 mg%) (fig. 1). In addition, in both racial groups girls have higher triglyceride levels than boys (64 mg% for black girls versus 59 mg%, $p < .001$; 77 mg% for white girls versus 69 mg%, $p < .001$; 77 mg% for white girls versus 69 mg%, $p < .001$). All statical tests of serum triglycerides were performed on transformed data (log 10) since the distributions exhibited a definite skew toward higher values. However, for the purpose of comparison with other studies, we are reporting the means of the untransformed data. With age, triglyceride values increase in all children although the slope was not significant in black girls. Ninety percent of the white children have values between 36 mg% (5th percentile) and 136 mg% (95th percentile) whereas the values for the same percentage of black children are between 32 mg% (5th percentile) and 105 mg% (95th percentile). Concentrations greater than 140 mg% were found in 4.3% of the whites and 1.4% of the blacks.

Interrelationship between serum cholesterol and serum triglycerides

The correlation of serum cholesterol and serum triglycerides in blacks and in whites was tested to determine if the correlation coefficients are from the same underlying population. The correlation in children 5 though 14 years old is significantly higher in whites than in blacks for both boys (whites, $r = .27$; blacks, $r = .14$; $p < .01$) and girls (whites, $r = .24$; blacks, $r = .11$; $p < .02$).

DISCUSSION

The levels of both serum cholesterol and serum triglycerides are highly variable within a population and require large numbers of people before subtle differences become statistically significant. Our mean lipid levels are relatively close to values found in the literature although the recently reported Muscatine study (4) is a notable exception with a mean serum cholesterol level 20 mg% higher than in our comparable population of white children (Bogalusa, 162 mg%; Muscatine, 182 mg%).

The racial difference noted in the correlation coefficients of serum cholesterol with serum triglycerides is most likely due to the differences between the races in the levels of the lipoprotein macromolecules, primarily the α-lipoproteins since black children within the same community have higher levels than whites (5).

Acknowledgement

Supported by funds from the National Heart and Lung Institute of the USPHS (HL 02942), the Specialized Center of Research--Arteriosclerosis (HL 15103) and the American Heart Association.

REFERENCES

1. Stamler, J. Med. Clin. North Am. 57:5046, 1973.
2. Carlson, L.A. and Bottiger, L.E., Lancet 1, 865, 1972.
3. Kannel, W.B., Castelli, W.P., Gordon, T. and McNamara, P.M. Ann. Intern. Med. 74:1, 1971.
4. Lauer, R.M., Connor, W.E., Leaverton, P.E., Reiter, M.A. and Clarke, W.R., J. of Pediatrics 86:697, 1975.
5. Srinivasan, S.R., Frerichs, R.R. and Berenson, G.S., Clin. Chim. Acta, in press, Dec. 1975.

(3)

IDENTIFICATION AND MANAGEMENT OF THE CHILD AT RISK FOR ATHEROSCLEROSIS

V Rose,* MB, BS, FRCP(C); DM Allen, RN, PHN; RG Pearse, MB, B.Chir; & JE Chappel, BA.Sc.
* Assistant Professor, Department of Paediatrics, University of Toronto; Staff Physician, Division of Cardiology, The Hospital for Sick Children, Toronto, Ontario, Canada.

There is much pathological and epidemiological evidence[1-5] of an association between personal characteristics, environmental factors, and premature development of atherosclerosis (AS), which is a complex multifactorial disease. Clinical manifestations of AS are very rare in the first 2 decades of life, but risk factors and early arterial changes are identifiable in childhood. The management of hyperlipidemia in children poses multiple problems.[6]

In 1972 we established a clinic for identifying and treating children at risk for AS, 1) to define hypercholesterolemia in various age groups and to screen children with a family history of premature coronary artery disease, particularly hyper-β-lipoproteinemia; 2) to institute dietary changes to reduce serum cholesterol levels; and 3) to assess effects and side-effects. We defined normal ranges of cholesterol values up to 3 mo, 4-12 mo, and for 5-yr periods up to 20 yr, in 1232 inpatients with conditions unlikely to cause 2° hyperlipidemia, 936 healthy ambulant children, and 1935 with congenital heart disease (CHD). Mean levels and upper normal limits were unstable during childhood and were lowest in the 1st yr of life (Fig.1), with no significant sex-related difference. Means were lower in inpatients possibly reflecting diet and/or iv medication, and were significantly lower in children with cyanotic CHD than normals or acyanotic disease (Fig.2). Analysis of cholesterol levels in CHD vs cyanosis, O_2 saturation, congestive heart failure and recent heart surgery showed a significant shift toward lower levels (Table). Primary hyper-β-lipoproteinemia was found[7] in 16 of the 4103 children screened (1:256), in 12 of their siblings, and in 14 children of known at-risk families. Six of these 42 patients had CHD, cyanotic in 2. Screening of parents of the 16 index patients identified 9 fathers and 2 mothers affected, and a positive history in 4 families; the 16th patient had been

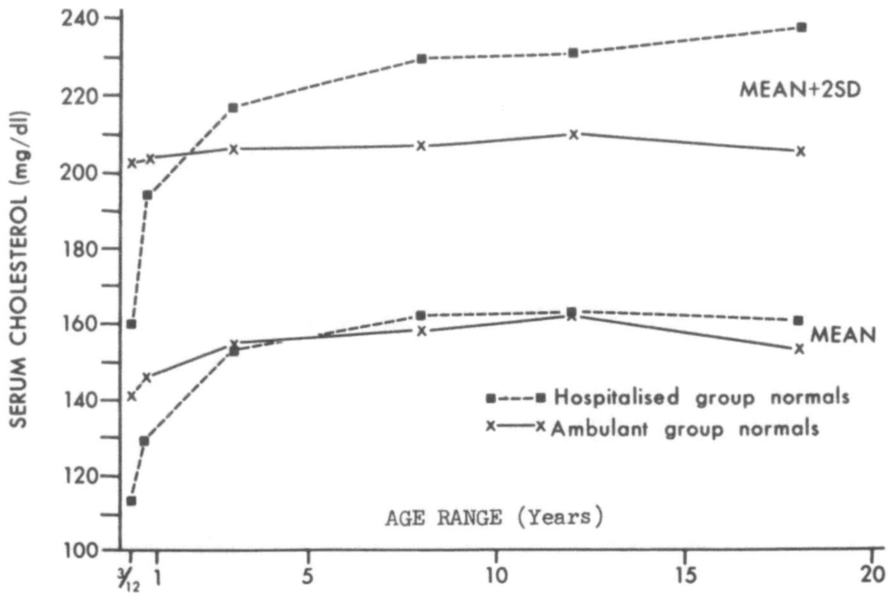

FIG.1 - Mean serum cholesterol values vs age in normal children

adopted. One large kindred was detected by routine screening of a child at follow-up of PDA ligation: 6 of her 9 siblings (and many 2nd-degree relatives) had the lipid disorder, and their father had died of coronary disease at age 39.

The nutrition protocol provides calories and protein adequate for growth and development, lower cholesterol intake, high polyunsaturated:saturated-fat ratio, and much practical advice. As little is known of long-term effects of prolonged dietary and drug therapy in growing children, we limit the treatment of hypercholesterolemia to children of high-risk families. Since lipid values in the 1st yr of life are greatly influenced by the type of dietary fat,[8] in borderline cases we defer treatment decisions until 1 yr of age, when cows' milk and mixed diet are established. Cholestyramine is reserved for older children unresponsive to dietary therapy.

TABLE. Mean serum cholesterol values (mg/dl) in CHD

	Cyanosis		O_2 saturation		Digoxin		Surgery	
	Yes	No	<89.9%	96-100%	Yes	No	<1 mo.	No
Mean	129.5	142.6	124.6	135.8	121.4	143.9	124.7	140.9
SD	33.4	29.1	35.1	31.2	33	28.3	29.1	29.6
P	<0.002		<0.002		<0.002		<0.01	

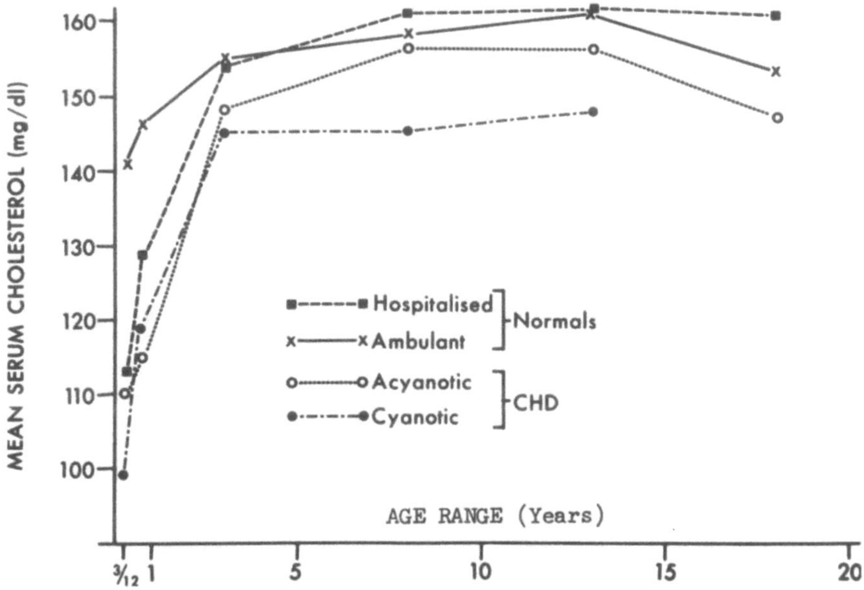

FIG. 2 - Mean serum cholesterol values in healthy children and children with CHD vs age

We are following 12 children closely; family doctors instruct and care for the others. Response appears better in the young (Fig. 3) but is less readily achieved when initial cholesterol value is high. Cholesterol reduction has averaged 20%; in 3 of the 12, the level is below upper normal limit (<200 mg/dl) and in a further 3 is <200 mg/dl.

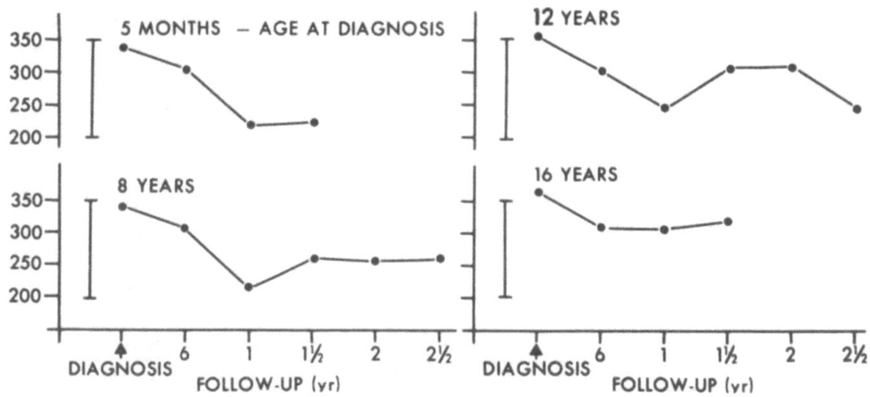

FIG. 3 - Effect of diet on serum cholesterol level in primary hyper-β-lipoproteinemia

REFERENCES

1. JP STRONG & HC McGILL. J. Atheroscler. Res. 9:251-65, 1969.
2. Z VLODAVER, HA KAHN & HN NEUFELD. Circulation 39:541-50, 1969.
3. D JAFFÉ, SW HARTROFT, M MANNING & G ELETA. Acta Paediat. Scand.: suppl. 219:1971, pp 1-28.
4. WB KANNEL, WP CASTELLI, T GORDON & PM McNAMARA. Annals of Int. Med. 74, 1-12, 1971.
5. WC ROBERTS, VJ FERRANS, et al. Am. J. Cardiol. 31:55-7, 1973.
6. JK LLOYD. Brit. Heart J. 37:105-14, 1975.
7. RI LEVY & BM RIFKIND. Am. J. Cardiol. 31:547-56, 1973.
8. WK SCHUBERT. Am. J. Cardiol. 31:581-87, 1973.

(4)

A STUDY OF THE DOSE-EFFECT RELATIONSHIP OF CHOLESTYRAMINE IN CHILDREN WITH FAMILIAL HYPERCHOLESTEROLEMIA

J. Ramsay Farah, M.D., Peter O. Kwiterovich, M.D., Catherine A. Neill, M.D.

The Johns Hopkins University

Department of Pediatrics, Johns Hopkins University
Baltimore, Maryland, U.S.A.

Premature atherosclerosis is a major public health problem in the United States. Points at issue for the pediatrician are, for example: what is the appropriate age to identify various risk factors associated with early cardiovascular disease; what preventive measure should be implemented, and what really is the role of the pediatrician in such a task? Although it is not proven that reduction in plasma cholesterol will lower the incidence of coronary artery disease, most pediatricians agree that children that have inherited high cholesterol levels represent a group of sufficiently high risk to warrant identification and treatment.

Type II hyperlipoproteinemia is a heterogeneous group of disorders characterized by increased plasma concentrations of total cholesterol and low density (beta) lipoproteins (1). The latter, measured in terms of their cholesterol content, shall be referred to simply as LDL. One genetic form of type II hyperlipoproteinemia is familial hypercholesterolemia, the most commonly recognized form of familial hyperlipoproteinemia in childhood (2). Familial hypercholesterolemia is completely expressed at birth and in the first year of life (3,4). Elevations in plasma LDL and cholesterol are extreme; the criteria for abnormality in this study were an LDL of 170 mg% and a cholesterol of 230 mg%. The clinical phenotype consists of premature coronary heart disease and xanthomas, which may start as early as the second decade and progressively increase into adulthood. The biochemical phenotype, as recently described by Brown and Goldstein (15), includes a deficiency in the binding of LDL to the plasma membrane of the cell with a resultant defect in the regulation of the rate limiting enzyme of cholesterol biosynthesis (HMG CoA Reductase). The treatment in the pediatric age group basically rests on diet and drugs. A significant fall in LDL may occur with diet alone. Many children, however, will also require medication.

A drug which has been effective in lowering LDL and cholesterol is cholestyramine. This anion exchange resin is insoluble in water and not absorbed by the gastrointestinal tract upon ingestion. Cholestyramine ionically binds bile salts, thereby interfering with their enterohepatic recirculation. Moreover, with the unavailability of the free bile acids, micellar formation may be disrupted. Dietary and gut cholesterol are less available for absorption and may get eliminated with the cholestyramine-bile salt complex in the stools. The overall net effect is a reduction in plasma cholesterol and LDL.

Several groups of investigators have described significant drops in LDL and cholesterol in children with familial hypercholesterolemia treated with cholestyramine (6,7). However, relatively little information is available on the dose-effect relationship of cholestyramine. The objectives of this study were therefore:

(1) to determine the optimal dose of medication required in children to significantly lower their LDL and cholesterol;
(2) to relate this dose to their body weight and pre-treatment levels of LDL and cholesterol;
(3) to study the effectiveness of a dose given twice daily; and
(4) to monitor for potential side-effects, such as, fat soluble vitamin malabsorption.

Twenty children and young adults heterozygous for familial hypercholesterolemia were identified through screening children of affected parents followed at the Lipid Research Clinic. Their mean age was 15 years. The mean baseline cholesterol and LDL before dietary treatment were 312 and 251 mg% respectively. Following treatment as outpatients with a cholesterol lowering diet for one to twenty-four months, mean cholesterol and LDL fell to 273 and 222 mg % respectively, which represented a mean drop of 11%.

Thirteen patients were studied on Protocol 1. The patients were maintained on an outpatient isocaloric diet, consisting of less than 200 mgs. of cholesterol with a polyunsaturated to saturated fat ratio of 2.0. The same diet was continued for the 21 days during their admission to the metabolic unit. Following 5 days of adaptation and baseline evaluation, cholestyramine was started at an initial dose of 1 gram per day and was progressively increased by 1 gram daily up to a total of 16 grams per day given twice daily.

All patients except one had a dose response curve which may be summarized as follows: namely, after a stable baseline period, the elevated cholesterol and LDL decreased rapidly as the cholestyramine was progressively increased by 1 gram per day. The levels of cholesterol and LDL fell into the normal range and then reached a plateau, after which additional cholestyramine was ineffective. In one patient, who had the highest level of LDL (290 mg/100 ml), 16 grams of cholestyramine was insufficient to normalize LDL and cholesterol, which were still falling during the last day on the metabolic ward.

In summary, the results of Protocol 1 showed that the mean dose of cholestyramine needed to normalize LDL was 7 grams per day and that a plateau for LDL (mean 128 mg/100 ml) was reached at a mean dose of 11 grams per day. The total mean % decrease at plateau of plasma cholesterol was 32% and LDL 43%.

West and Lloyd (16) have expressed the dose of cholestyramine on a body weight basis; however, in studying the dose of cholestyramine needed to normalize LDL, we found it to have no correlation with the body weight of the children. Similarly, there was no correlation between the baseline LDL and body weight, indicating that the heavier children did not have a high LDL. There was, however, a significant correlation between the post dietary plasma LDL and the dose of cholestyramine needed to normalize LDL. The correlation coefficient was 0.93 with a high degree of significance. ($p < 0.001$).

This regression line was next used to test the hypothesis that we could predict the amount of cholestyramine required to normalize LDL, based on the post diet level of LDL in a child. The predicted amounts were: for a post dietary plasma LDL of 200 mg% or less, up to 4 grams; for an LDL between 200 and 240 mg% up to 8 grams; for an LDL between 240 to 280 mg% up to 12 grams; and, for an LDL above 280 grams %, 16 grams i.e., an adult dose.

To test the above hypothesis, seven patients were studied on Protocol II, the first part of which consisted of the same dietary treatment and adaptation period as in Protocol I. Each patient was then started on the dose of cholestyramine predicted by the regression equation to normalize his LDL and cholesterol. After 8 days the dose was increased to the next level.

The LDL fell below normal in each child, at a mean of 4 ($\pm$ 2) days. For example, one patient, with an LDL of less than 200, was given 4 grams of cholestyramine daily in 2 equal doses. The LDL level rapidly decreased to normal, continued to fall, and then leveled off. The increase in cholestyramine from 4 to 8 grams per day did not lower the LDL further, an observation similar to that found in Protocol I. The same plateau effect was observed in the children studied by both protocols.

None of our patients on the dose of cholestyramine used in either protocol demonstrated any significant side-effects such as fat-soluble vitamin malabsorption.

In conclusion, the appropriate dosage of cholestyramine in a child with familial hypercholesterolemia is related to pre-treatment levels of LDL, dosage appears predictable and should be individualized. A nadir of LDL exists, after which cholestyramine is ineffective. The drug can be conveniently and effectively given twice daily.

1. Fredrickson, D.S. & Levy, R.I. Familial Hyperlipoproteinemia. In The Metabolic Basis of Inherited Disease. ed. Stanbury,J.B. Wyngaarden, J.B. & Fredrickson, D.S. 3rd Edn. Ch.26, New York: McGraw-Hill, p. 545-614. 1972.

2. Kwiterovich, P.O., Fredrickson, D.S. & Levy, R.I. Familial hypercholesterolemia (One form of familial type II hyperlipoproteinemia). A study of its biochemical, genetic and clinical presentation in childhood., J. Clin. Invest. 53:1237-1249, 1974.

3. Kwiterovich, P.O., Levy, R.I. & Fredrickson, D.S. Neonatal diagnosis of familial type II hyperlipoproteinemia. Lancet 1:118-122, 1973.

4. Glueck, C.J., Hickman, F., Schoenfeld, M., Steiner, P & Pearce, W. Neonatal familial type II hyperlipoproteinemia: Cord blood cholesterol in 1880 births. Metabolism 20:597-608, 1971.

5. Brown, M.S. and Goldstein, J.L. Familial Hypercholesterolemia: Defective binding of lipoproteins to cultured fibroblasts associated with impaired regulation of 3 Hydrozy 3 Methyl Glutaryl Coenzyme A Reductase activity. Proc. Nat. Acad. Sci. 71:788-792, 1974.

6. Glueck, C.J., Fallat, R. & Tsang, R. Pediatric familial type II hyperlipoproteinemia: therapy with diet and cholestyramine resin. Pediatrics 52: 669-679, 1973.

7. West, R.J. & Lloyd, J.K. Use of cholestyramine in treatment of children with familial hypercholesterolemia. Arch. Dis. Childh. 48:320-374, 1973.

(5)

HYPERLIPIDAEMIA AND WEIGHT GAIN AFTER MATURITY

Blacket, R.B., Woodhill, J M , Palmer, A.J., Leelarthaepin, B., McGilchrist, C.A.

Department of Medicine, Prince Henry Hospital, Little Bay, N.S.W. 2036, AUSTRALIA

In affluent western societies average weight gain in males over the two decades after maturity is of the order of 9-12 kg Increase in total plasma lipids over this period tends to parallel increase in body weight but whether there is a causal relationship is not clear. One approach to the problem is to use the tool of weight reduction; this is the subject of this paper.

We studied two distinct groups of patients. The first comprised 12 men with type 2a hyperlipidaemia and 10 with type 2b. Their mean age was 49 years. Nearly all of them had survived myocardial infarction and were moderately obese. Controls for this group were 28 survivors of infarction of similar age and relative body weight (RBW) who were a mixture of type 2a and type 2b. The second group of patients were healthy blood donors mean age 40 years chosen at random because they had type 4 hyperlipidaemia on screening They should reflect the common variety of type 4 in this community. Both groups were evaluated nutritionally and then took a standard high protein, minimum carbohydrate diet of approximately 1600 calories. When weight had ceased to fall they continued an isocaloric diet calculated as approximately 2300 calories The details are reported elsewhere.[1,2] Both groups and the type 2 controls who failed to lose weight were followed for a minimum of 12 months

Changes in body weight and serum lipids appear in table 1. In both type 2a and type 2b relative body weight (RBW) declined from 117 to 100 and there was a very significant fall in both serum cholesterol (SC) and serum triglyceride (STG). There was a 24.8% drop in serum cholesterol. 13 of the 22 men now had "normal"

	TYPE 2a (N = 12)		TYPE 2b (N = 10)		TYPE 4 (N = 20)	
	$\bar{X}$	S.D.	$\bar{X}$	S.D.	X	S.D.
BODY WEIGHT (kg)						
ENTRY	87.6	9.1	88.5	12.7	76.8	7.9
NADIR	74.9	8.5	75.0	7.0	68.7	6.8
STEADY STATE	75.9	8.9	75.8	7.6*	67.6	6.1***
BODY MASS INDEX						
ENTRY	28.1	2.7	28.4	3.5	26.1	1.1
NADIR	23.9	2.3	24.0	1.7	23.3	0.9
STEADY STATE	24.3	2.4***	24.3	2.1**	22.9	0.5***
RELATIVE BODY WEIGHT %						
ENTRY	117	10	117	15	107	5
NADIR	99	9	99	7	95	4
STEADY STATE	100	9***	100	8**	94	3
SERUM CHOLESTEROL mg/100 ml						
ENTRY	309	27	340	46	245	37
NADIR	238	39	259	50	227	44
STEADY STATE	239	30***	249	22***	226	30
SERUM TRIGLYCERIDE mg/100 ml						
ENTRY	136	26	249	83	273	81
NADIR	94	26	163	52	112	35
STEADY STATE	97	31**	139	35***	126	26***

TABLE 1. BODY WEIGHT, INDICES OF OBESITY AND SERUM LIPIDS. MEANS AND STANDARD DEVIATIONS

Starred probability values refer to within type comparisons between entry and steady state *$p < 0.05$, **$p < 0.01$, ***$p < 0.001$

lipid patterns in which SC was less than 260 mg/100 ml and STG less than 160 mg/100 ml. In the 28 controls with initial RBW of 118, and SC of 284 mg/100 ml., who failed to lose weight on a modified fat diet SC declined by only 6.3% and STG by 5.2% ($p < 0.001$). Stepwise regression analysis showed that Δ SC correlated most strongly with Δ body weight and only weakly with delta dietary fat. Daily calorie intake at steady state was 18% lower than on entry. In 9 men at steady state lower weight distribution of the nutrients was normal and P/S was 0.43; in 11 P/S ratio was 1.95. ΔSC did not differ significantly in these two subgroups.

The type 4 men were not obese when compared with age matched controls but had gained on average 5.9 kg. since age 20. Over 4.4 months on the reducing diet RBW declined from 107 to 95 and remained there over the next 10 months. 17 men now had "normal" lipid levels. Mean reduction in STG was 54% from 273 to 126 mg/100 ml. Daily calorie intake was now 26% lower, carbohydrate 39% lower and saturated fat 28% lower than on entry. Carbohydrate now accounted for 32% of calories, alcohol for 4.8% and fat for 44%. Changes in dietary cholesterol and polyunsaturated fatty acids were not significant. There was only a weak correlation between delta STG and delta body weight. Thus the most common mild to moderate form of type 4 appears to be a metabolic disorder brought out by no more than average weight gain in subjects taking a normal diet. It can usually be suppressed by reduction to truly ideal weight with modest restriction of carbohydrate and alcohol.

We conclude that weight gain after maturity is an important factor in causing hyperlipidaemia in those who develop it. Maintenance of ideal body weight throughout life should reduce the three common forms of hyperlipidaemia that is, type 2a, type 2b and type 4 without changes in dietary fat and cholesterol. To achieve very low risk levels of SC, that is, below 200-220 mg/100 ml., reduction in dietary saturated fat and cholesterol appears mandatory in some.[1]

References

1. Leelarthaepin, B., Woodhill, J.M., Palmer, A.J , Blacket, R.B. Lancet 1974, ii, 1217.
2. Blacket, R.B., Woodhill, J.M., Leelarthaepin, B., Palmer, A.J. Lancet 1975, ii In the press.

CHAPTER 8
FIBRINOLYTIC ACTIVITY; PLATELETS

(1)

ASSOCIATIONS BETWEEN FIBRINOLYTIC ACTIVITY AND OTHER VARIABLES IN AN INDUSTRIAL POPULATION

T. W. MEADE, R. CHAKRABARTI AND W. R. S. NORTH

MRC-DHSS EPIDEMIOLOGY AND MEDICAL CARE UNIT

NORTHWICK PARK HOSPITAL, HARROW, HA1 3UJ, ENGLAND

Fibrinolytic activity (FA) is one of a number of measures of haemostatic function being carried out in a prospective study of clinical thrombotic disease, including ischaemic heart disease (IHD), in an industrial group in North-West London (Meade, 1973). FA is measured by the dilute blood clot lysis time of Fearnley et al. (1962), and is expressed as 1/lysis time in hours x 100. Recruitment into the study is in a random order from a nominal roll; the response rate is about 80%. All participants working on days are seen between 0900 and 1030 hours. Venepuncture is performed without compression of the arm after a 10-15 minute period of rest; participants in whom venipuncture was difficult have been excluded from the analyses which follow. FA is significantly greater in black men than white men (but there is no difference between black and white women); results from black participants have therefore also been excluded. Findings deal with 625 day-men aged 18-64, and 290 day-women aged 18-59; of the women, 43 were on oral contraceptives when recruited.

Figure 1 shows that in men, FA decreases significantly with age; most of the fall occurs at a steady rate before the age of about 45. At 30-34, for example, mean FA in men is about 32.0, while from 50 to 64 it is about 27.0 (a difference in lysis time, at this range of FA, of about half an hour). There is no significant alteration in FA with age in women not on oral contraceptives, in whom FA is about 31.0. Neither the menstrual cycle nor the menopause appear to affect FA. However, FA is significantly higher (39.8) in women on oral contraceptives than in those not; this increase is associated with coagulation, lipid and blood pressure changes that would be expected to favour thrombogenesis (Meade et al, 1975).

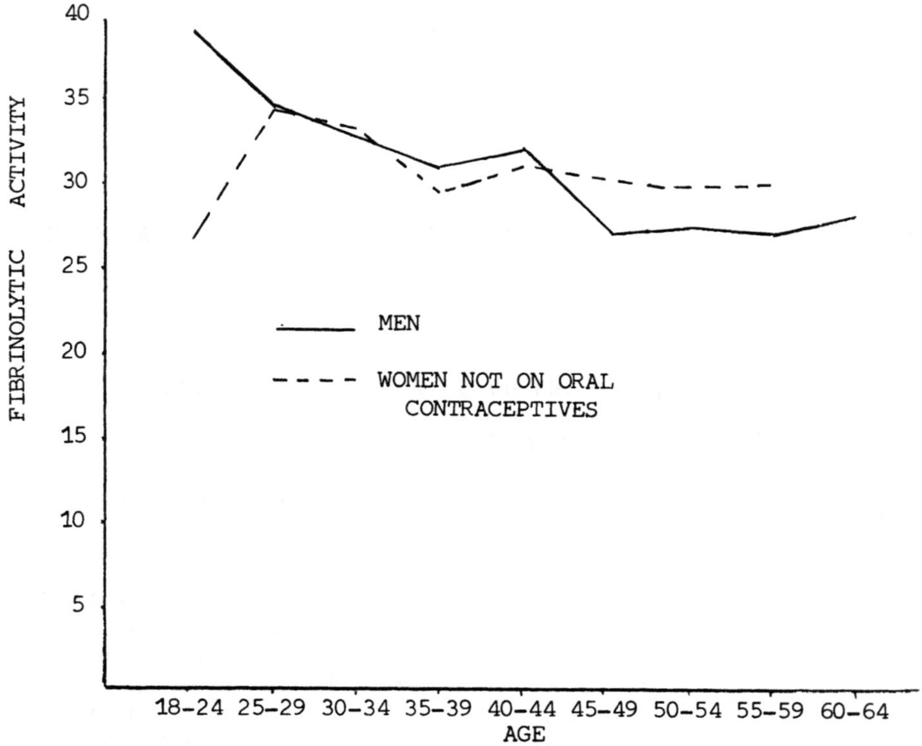

FIGURE 1. FA AND AGE. DECREASE WITH AGE IN MEN: $P < 0.001$
NO SIGNIFICANT CHANGE WITH AGE IN WOMEN.

TABLE 1. CORRELATION COEFFICIENTS (r) BETWEEN FIBRINOLYTIC ACTIVITY (FA) AND BLOOD PRESSURE, SUPRA-ILIAC SKINFOLD THICKNESS, BLOOD CHOLESTEROL AND SERUM TRIGLYCERIDES

	Correlations† of FA with: Men	Women
Blood pressure		
Systolic	-0.026	0.067
Diastolic	-0.107*	0.058
Supra-iliac SF	-0.212**	-0.165*
Cholesterol	-0.119*	-0.097
Triglycerides	-0.195**	-0.148*

† corrected for changes with age in FA and other variables shown.

* $P < 0.01$ **$P < 0.001$

Table 1 shows the correlations between FA on the one hand, and blood pressure (systolic and diastolic), supra-iliac skinfold thickness, blood cholesterol and serum triglycerides on the other. With the exception of systolic blood pressure, these correlations are statistically significant in the men, but only those with triglycerides and supra-iliac skinfold thickness are significant in the women. The true correlations are likely to be higher than those shown, possibly substantially, because of the effects of laboratory error and other sources of variability.

As expected, there is a very marked and immediate increase in FA after exertion (stepping on and off a chair 20 times in about a minute), this increase averaging about 20% of the resting level.

FA is significantly less in cigarette smokers than in non-smokers; in day-men, for example, FA values (adjusted to age 40) are 28.3 and 30.9 respectively. Among smokers, however, there is no evidence for a trend of decreasing FA with increasing cigarette consumption. It will be necessary to see whether the difference in FA between non-smokers and smokers persists when associations of FA with other variables have been allowed for. FA is not affected by habitual alcohol intake.

Mean FA in the first ten men who had had a definite myocardial infarct (WHO criteria) when recruited into the study was 19.4, compared with 27.4 for men of the same age free of IHD when first seen.

These findings are all consistent with the hypothesis that FA plays a role, possibly a major one, in determining the onset of clinical thrombotic disease, including IHD; the results of the prospective part of this study will clarify this point. Although there are associations between FA and more generally recognized IHD "risk factors", FA is probably largely independent of these other factors, and its measurement may thus improve the accuracy of the prediction of individual chances of IHD; in this event, it would be necessary to consider modifying FA as well as, or instead of, other postulated causes and mechanisms in IHD.

Fearnley, G. R., and Chakrabarti, R. (1962). Lancet, 2, 128.

Meade, T. W. (1973). Thrombosis et Diathesis Haemorrhagica, Supplement 54, 317.

Meade, T. W., et al. (1975). Work in progress.

(2)

EFFECTS OF ASPIRIN AND SULFINPYRAZONE ON PLATELET PROSTAGLANDIN SYNTHESIS

J.W.D. McDonald, R.K. Stuart and H.J.M. Barnett

Depts. of Medicine and Clinical Neurological Sciences, Univ. of Western Ontario
London, Canada

Antiinflammatory drugs may prevent thrombosis by inhibiting platelet prostaglandin (PG) synthesis. We have studied: 1. the effects of aspirin (ASA) and sulfinpyrazone (SPZ) *in vitro* on platelet PG synthesis. 2. PG synthesis *in vitro* using platelets from patients with transient cerebral ischemic attacks (TIA) who are receiving either placebo (PLC), ASA (1200 mg daily) or SPZ (800 mg daily). 3. the platelet release reaction (PRR) using platelets from PLC and SPZ-treated TIA patients. 4. PRR using platelets from control subjects in the presence and absence of added SPZ.

METHODS

Tris-saline suspensions of washed platelets were lysed by freeze-thawing, equilibrated for 7 min. at 37°C, preincubated in the presence or absence of inhibitors for 2 min., and incubated with arachidonic acid-^{14}C (AA) for one minute. ^{14}C-labelled PGs were extracted successively in ethanol and chloroform and then chromatographed on mini-columns of silicic acid. Following elution of AA with chloroform-methanol (CM) (98:2), PGs were eluted with CM (94:6). The latter fraction contained a compound which chromatographed on TLC with carrier PGD_2 and a second unidentified product. Since synthesis of both compounds was inhibited equally by ASA, PG synthesis was expressed in terms of total counts per minute eluted in CM (94:6) from silicic acid.

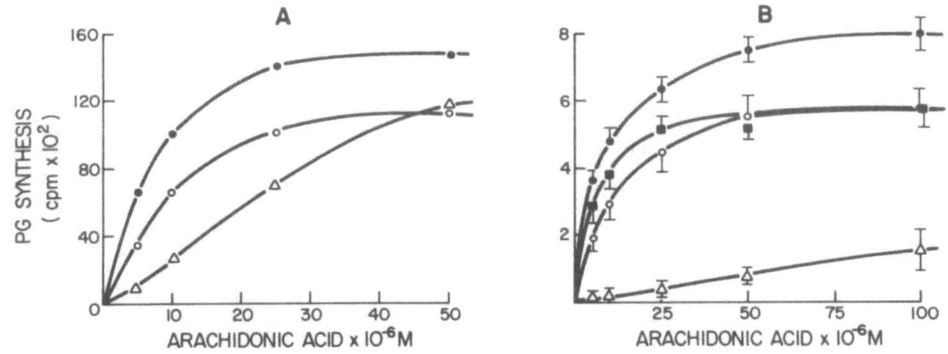

Figure 1: PG Synthesis from AA-^{14}C.
A. Preincubation of 3×10^8 platelets in saline (●). SPZ, 50 μM (○) or 500 μM (△). AA-^{14}C S.A. = 8 μc/μmole.
B. Platelets from control subjects (● N=6) or TIA patients treated with PLC (■ N=5), SPZ (○ N=5), or ASA (△ N=4). PG synthesis expressed as cpm/10^8 platelets. AA-^{14}C S.A. = 1.6 μc/μmole.

RESULTS

ASA inhibited platelet PG synthesis *in vitro* (not shown) as reported by others. We found that SPZ is also a potent inhibitor (Fig. 1A). Kinetic analysis showed that inhibition by SPZ is competitive with respect to AA. Platelets from TIA patients receiving PLC appeared to synthesize PGs (Fig. 1B) less actively than those from young healthy controls. PG synthesis from ASA-treated patients was strongly inhibited at all AA concentrations. However, platelets from SPZ-treated patients resembled the PLC group, with the possible exception of synthesis at lower AA concentrations.

PRR in platelets from controls was inhibited by SPZ added *in vitro* (Fig. 2A) when the stimulus (collagen concentration) was sufficiently low. Similarly, PRR induced by dilute collagen was inhibited in platelets from SPZ-treated patients (Fig. 2B).

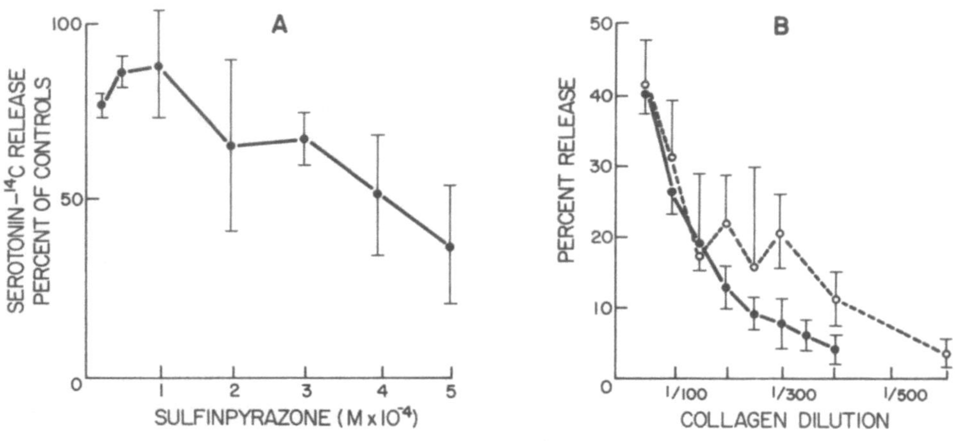

Figure 2: Effect of SPZ on Release of Serotonin-^{14}C by Collagen
A. SPZ was incubated in PRP for 2 min. prior to induction of 5-24% release by dilute collagen (N=4).
B. Platelets from TIA patients receiving SPZ (● N=7) or PLC (o N=5).

CONCLUSIONS

SPZ, like ASA, inhibits platelet PG synthesis. Unlike ASA which exhibits an irreversible effect on platelets, SPZ must be present in the system. Inhibition by SPZ is competitive with respect to AA and therefore is best demonstrated at low AA concentrations. Platelet release of serotonin in response to dilute collagen *in vitro* is inhibited in patients receiving SPZ or by SPZ added *in vitro*. It is suggested that higher concentrations of collagen *in vitro* may result in formation of free AA in concentrations sufficiently high to relieve SPZ inhibition in studies in which lack of effect of SPZ is reported. Release and aggregation induced *in vitro* by weak stimuli, and PG synthesis at low AA concentration may be similar to *in vivo* conditions. There is no reason to suppose that intense release and aggregation stimulated by concentrated collagen preparations, or the more rapid synthesis of PGs at high AA concentration resemble these conditions more closely. Clinical efficacy of SPZ (and ASA) may relate to inhibition of platelet PG synthesis.

(3)

INCREASE IN PLATELET FACTOR 4-LIKE ACTIVITY IN THE INITIAL STAGES OF ATHEROSCLEROSIS IN PIGEONS

V. Fuster, B. A. Kottke, C. E. Ruiz, J. C. Lewis, and E. J. W. Bowie

Mayo Clinic and Mayo Foundation

Rochester, MN., U.S.A.

The concept that platelets, by adhering to a damaged endothelial surface and releasing platelet factors, may play a role in the initiation of atherosclerosis has recently received further support by the group of Russell Ross and L.A. Harker (1). They have demonstrated that a heat stable, non-dializable low molecular weight protein released from platelets and detectable in serum may be implicated in the stimulation of the intimal cell proliferation at the initial stages of atherosclerosis. Because the known properties of this protein may be consistent with platelet factor 4, we decided to study the relationship between changes in platelet factor 4-like activity in serum and the development of atherosclerosis in two interesting species of pigeons: the white Carneau species that we call atherosclerosis-susceptible because they develop spontaneous atherosclerosis, first grossly apparent at 9 months of age and the show Racer species that we call atherosclerosis-resistant because they do not develop atherosclerosis.

A chronological relationship between platelet factor 4-like activity levels in serum (heparin neutralizing activity of serum heated at 60° C) and the development of atherosclerotic lesions was first studied in 9 atherosclerosis susceptible pigeons grouped in different ages: 3 pigeons were 6 months old, 3 were 1 year old and 3 were 3 years old. The pigeons of 1 year of age and the older showed marked elevated levels of platelet factor 4-like activity in serum when compared with the 6 month-old group ($p < 0.001$). Such a rise, which seemed to occur between 6 months and 1 year of age coincide chronologically with the development of the early

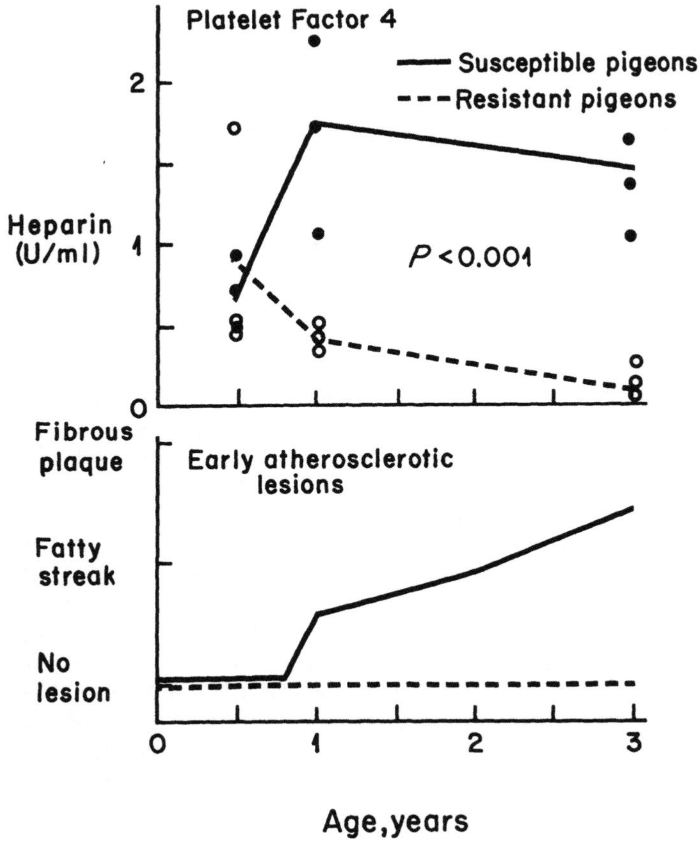

Fig. 1. Atherosclerosis Susceptible and Resistant Pigeons. Closed circles - susceptible pigeons; Open circles - resistant pigeons.

atherosclerotic lesions in this species of pigeon (Fig. 1).

By contrast, we performed the same study in 9 **atherosclerosis** resistant pigeons and, apart of 1 of the pigeons 6 months old that had elevated serum platelet factor 4-like activity, all the other pigeons had low levels. This coincides with the lack in development of atherosclerosis at different ages in this species of pigeon (Fig. 1).

We tried to answer the question of whether or not the high level of platelet factor 4-like activity in serum of the atherosclerotic susceptible pigeons derives from the thrombocytes or nucleated platelets. So, when thrombocytes from thrombocyte rich plasma were damaged or destroyed by Triton X or by clotting, platelet factor 4-like activity were found to be very high only in the atherosclerosis-susceptible pigeon. By contrast, the plasma made poor in thrombocytes and also treated with Triton X or clotting, showed no platelet factor 4-like activity in any of the two pigeons. This suggests that the active substance we detect in the serum of the atherosclerosis-susceptible pigeons is mainly liberated from the thrombocytes.

Preliminary studies on thrombocyte count, and in thrombocyte size and ultrastructure by transmission electromicroscopy did not show obvious differences between the two species of pigeons. However, studies by scanning electromicroscopy of thrombocyte adhesiveness to a glass surface showed that thrombocytes from the atherosclerosis susceptible pigeons have only few pseudopods. However, thrombocytes from the atherosclerosis resistant pigeons show numerous pseudopods. Such differences in the surface of thrombocytes between the two species of pigeon became first apparent at one year of age, coinciding chronologically with the development of the aortic lesions in the atherosclerosis susceptible pigeons.

In summary, the changes in platelet factor 4-like activity in serum and in the response of thrombocytes to a glass surface, both coincide chronologically with the development of the early atherosclerotic lesions in the pigeon. This opens the question of whether such changes precede and cause the lesions or follow the development of such lesions. This is a question that at present we are actively investigating.

REFERENCE:

1. L. A. Harker, R. Ross and S. J. Slichter: Chronic endothelial cell injury and platelet-factor induced arteriosclerosis. Proceedings Vth Congress of the International Society on Thrombosis and Haemostasis. Paris, 1975, p. 56.

(4)

INHIBITION OF PLATELET ADHERENCE TO DAMAGED VESSEL WALL BY DRUGS

J.-P. CAZENAVE, M.A. GUCCIONE, M.A. PACKHAM, and J.F. MUSTARD
Department of Pathology, McMaster University, Hamilton, and Department of Biochemistry, University of Toronto, Toronto, Ontario, Canada.

Adherence of platelets to subendothelial structures of damaged vessel walls is involved in several aspects of vascular disease; (a) the adherence of platelets to the vessel wall leads to the development of arterial thrombi and thromboembolic complications of atherosclerosis; (b) platelets release a factor which promotes the growth of smooth muscle cells (1) and fibroblasts (2) and thus could be involved in the development of atherosclerotic lesions; (c) platelets also release or form elastase (3), collagenase (4) and materials which increase vascular permeability (5).

To measure platelet adherence to subendothelial structures, everted segments of rabbit aortas were mounted on rods, scraped to expose the subendothelium and rotated in a suspension of rabbit platelets labelled with ^{51}Cr (6). The suspending medium was Tyrode solution containing either 0.35% or 4% bovine serum albumin and apyrase.

We first examined the effect of drugs (acetylsalicylic acid (ASA) and sulfinpyrazone) used in humans to prevent complications of atherosclerosis. In vitro, ASA (10 μM) decreased the adherence of platelets by 63 ± 5%. In other experiments, ASA was given orally to rabbits (25 mg/kg), the blood was collected 1 or 17 hr later and the platelets were isolated and resuspended; adherence was reduced by 78 ± 3% compared with control platelets. Thus inhibition of these platelets by ASA could not be removed by washing the platelets. We also showed that ASA did not affect the vessel wall. These results are in contrast to those of Baumgartner and Muggli (7) who did not find that ASA inhibited the adherence of platelets in citrated whole blood to the damaged vessel wall.

Sulfinpyrazone (100 μM) inhibited adherence of platelets to the damaged aorta by 50 ± 2%. When sulfinpyrazone was given orally to rabbits (150 mg/kg) and the platelets harvested 2 hr later and washed, platelet adhesion was not inhibited, indicating that sulfinpyrazone had to be present to have an inhibitory effect. Sulfinpyrazone has been shown to increase platelet survival (8,9) and to reduce thromboembolic complications (10).

Because penicillin G and cephalothin have been reported to cause bleeding in man (11,12) we examined their effects on platelet adherence. In vitro incubation of washed platelets with penicillin G or cephalothin (1.5 to 15 mM) inhibited platelet adhesion to damaged aorta segments by 50 to 70%. Inhibition persisted despite further washing of the platelets. Reserpine inhibits the interaction of platelets with collagen and has been shown to inhibit the development of cholesterol-induced atherosclerosis in rabbits (13). In vivo administration of reserpine (5 mg/kg) to rabbits 18 hr before preparation of a platelet suspension, or in vitro addition of reserpine (2 to 10 μM) to a platelet suspension, diminished adhesion by 80%. Thus ASA, sulfinpyrazone, penicillin G, cephalothin or reserpine inhibit platelet adherence to subendothelial structures. Thus these or related drugs may be of value in the management of atherosclerosis and its thromboembolic complications.

References

1. Ross, R., Glomset, J., Kariya, B., and Harker, L.: A platelet-dependent serum factor that stimulates the proliferation of arterial smooth muscle cells in vitro. Proceedings of the National Academy of Sciences, U.S.A., 71, 1207, 1974.

2. Kohler, N., and Lipton, A.: Platelets as a source of fibroblast growth-promoting activity. Experimental Cell Research, 87, 297, 1974.

3. Robert, B., Robert, L., Legrand, Y., Pignaud, G., and Caen, J.: Elastolytic protease in blood platelets. Series Haematologica, 4, 175, 1971.

4. Chesney, C.M., Harper, E., Colman, R.W.: Human platelet collagenase. Journal of Clinical Investigation, 53, 1647, 1974.

5. Packham, M.A., Nishizawa, E.E., and Mustard, J.F.: Response of platelets to tissue injury. In: Biochemical Pharmacology, Suppl., p. 171, Pergamon Press, Oxford, London, 1968.

6. Cazenave, J.-P., Packham, M.A., Guccione, M.A., and Mustard, J.F.: Inhibition of platelet adherence to damaged surface of rabbit aorta. Journal of Laboratory and Clinical Medicine (in press).

7. Baumgartner, H.R., and Muggli, R.: Effect of acetylsalicylic acid on platelet adhesion to subendothelium and on the formation of mural platelet thrombi. Thrombosis et Diathesis Haemorrhagica, Suppl. 60, 345, 1974.

8. Smythe, H.A., Ogryzlo, M.A., Murphy, E.A., and Mustard, J.F.: The effect of sulfinpyrazone (anturan) on platelet economy and blood coagulation in man. Canadian Medical Association Journal, 92, 818, 1965.

9. Steele, P.P., Weily, H.S., Davies, H., Genton, E.: Platelet survival in patients with rheumatic heart disease. The New England Journal of Medicine, 290, 537, 1974.

10. Kaegi, A., Pineo, G.F., Shimizu, A., Trivedi, H., Hirsh, J., Gent, M.: Arteriovenous-shunt thrombosis: Prevention by sulfinpyrazone. The New England Journal of Medicine, 290, 304, 1974.

11. Fleming, A., and Fish, E.W.: Influence of penicillin on the coagulation of blood with especial reference to certain dental operations. British Medical Journal, 2, 242, 1947.

12. Raccuglia, G., and Watermann, N.G.: Anticoagulant effect of sodium cephalothin (Keflin). American Journal of Clinical Pathology, 52, 245, 1969.

13. Carrier, O., Clower, B.R., and Whittington, P.J.: Inhibition of cholesterol-induced vascular lesions by dietary reserpine. Journal of Atherosclerosis Research, 8, 229, 1968.

(5)

EXPERIMENTAL MODIFICATION OF PLATELET SURVIVAL

H.J. REIMERS, J. GREENBERG, J.-P. CAZENAVE, M.A. PACKHAM AND J.F. MUSTARD
Department of Pathology, McMaster University, Hamilton, and Department of Biochemistry, University of Toronto, Toronto, Ontario, Canada

Shortened platelet survival and increased platelet turnover in subjects who have had clinical manifestations of atherosclerotic vessel disease have been demonstrated by a number of investigators (1-4). Several drugs such as sulfinpyrazone, persantin, and clofibrate which lengthen platelet survival also appear to decrease the incidence of thromboembolic complications (for review see (5)). Thus it seems important to determine the factors that influence platelet survival. We have investigated the effects on platelet survival of agents that alter the platelet surface, some of which also cause the release of platelet granule contents. It was demonstrated previously that the survival of platelets in vivo was unchanged in animals into which ADP was infused to cause transient platelet aggregation (6).

We have now investigated the survival of platelets exposed to thrombin in vitro (7). Washed rabbit platelets labelled with ^{14}C-serotonin and ^{51}Cr released 90% of their ^{14}C upon exposure to 0.5 units/ml thrombin. The resuspended platelets aggregated upon addition of collagen and low concentrations of ADP. Upon infusion into thrombocytopenic animals, they shortened the bleeding time from a punctured vein from 668 ± 46 sec to 228 ± 63 sec ($p < 0.001$). The survival of thrombin-degranulated platelets injected into rabbits was 98.5 ± 0.9 hr (control platelets 98.5 ± 1.2 hr, $p = 1$). These findings indicate that platelets that have been aggregated and have undergone the release reaction in response to thrombin are functionally intact and viable.

Similar observations have also been made with platelets treated in vitro with plasmin (0.5 g/l) (8). These platelets released 30% of their ^{14}C-serotonin and upon resuspension and infusion into rabbits, their survival time was the same as that of platelets that had not been exposed to plasmin.

These experiments demonstrate that platelets aggregated by ADP, thrombin or plasmin survive normally in vivo, even if they have lost a large portion of their granule contents in response to these proteolytic enzymes.

In contrast, removal of 12 to 15% of the total platelet sialic acid from the platelet surface by treatment with purified neuraminidase in vitro, results in rapid removal of rabbit platelets from the circulation of the animals into which they are infused (9). The neuraminidase-treated platelets showed little change in their response to aggregating and release-inducing agents. To explore further the role of surface glycoproteins in platelet survival, platelets were incubated with sodium periodate (0.5 to 1 mM for 10 minutes), washed and resuspended (10). Upon infusion into rabbits, these platelets were also rapidly cleared from the circulation. The response of these platelets to aggregating agents was less than that of control platelets. These results indicate that alteration of the surface glycoproteins may determine the length of time that platelets survive in the circulation.

Although thrombin (11) and plasmin (12) alter platelet surface glycoproteins, the changes they cause do not shorten platelet survival. Thus, exposure of platelets to thrombin and plasmin during thrombus formation and dissolution in vivo probably does not alter them in such a way that their survival is shortened.

References

1. Murphy, E.A., and Mustard, J.F.: Coagulation tests and platelet economy in atherosclerotic and control subjects. Circulation, 25, 114, 1962.

2. Abrahamsen, A.F.: Platelet survival studies in man, with special reference to thrombosis and atherosclerosis. Scand. J. Haematol., Suppl. 3, 1968.

3. Harker, L.A., and Slichter, S.J.: Arterial and venous thromboembolism: Kinetic characterization and evaluation of therapy. Thromb. Diath. Haemorrh. 31, 188, 1974.

4. Steele, P.P., Weily, H.S., Davies, H., Genton, E.: Platelet function studies in coronary artery disease. Circulation, 48, 1194, 1973.

5. Mustard, J.F., and Packham, M.A.: Platelets, thrombosis and drugs. Drugs, 9, 19, 1975.

6. Mustard, J.F., Rowsell, H.C., Lotz, F., Hegardt, B., and Murphy, E.A.: The effect of adenine nucleotides on thrombus formation, platelet count and blood coagulation. Experimental and Molecular Pathology, 15, 43, 1966.

7. Reimers, H.-J., Cazenave, J.-P., Senyi, A.F., Hirsh, J., Kinlough-Rathbone, R.L., Packham, M.A., and Mustard, J.F.: In vivo and in vitro functions of thrombin-treated rabbit platelets. Abstract 445, Vth Congress of the International Society on Thrombosis and Haemostasis, Paris, July, 1975.

8. Cazenave, J.-P., Reimers, H.-J., Greenberg, J., Niewiarowski, S., Packham, M.A., and Mustard, J.F.: Modifications of platelets that affect platelet adherence to collagen or damaged aorta and platelet survival. Abstract 406, Vth Congress of the International Society on Thrombosis and Haemostasis, Paris, July, 1975.

9. Greenberg, J., Packham, M.A., Cazenave, J.-P., Reimers, H.J., and Mustard, J.F. Effects on platelet function of removal of platelet sialic acid by neuraminidase . Laboratory Investigation, 32, 476, 1975.

10. Cazenave, J.-P., and Mustard, J.F.: Modification of platelet function by sodium periodate. Federation Proceedings, 34, Abstract 3597, 1975.

11. Phillips, D.R., and Agin, P.P.: Thrombin substrates and the proteolytic site of thrombin action on human platelet plasma membranes. Biochimica et Biophysica Acta, 352, 218, 1974.

12. Matsuda, S., Muraki, H., Ando, Y., and Hasegawa, M.: Action of plasmin on plasma membranes of human platelets. Abstract 505, Vth Congress of the International Society on Thrombosis and Haemostasis, Paris, July, 1975.

CHAPTER 9
PERMEABILITY; TISSUE CULTURE

(1)

HYPERREACTIVE ARTERIAL ENDOTHELIAL CELLS IN ATHEROGENESIS

Effect of Smooth Muscle Relaxants

Takio Shimamoto, M.D., Kinya Moriya, D.V.M., Masahiko Kobayashi, Ph.D., Takeo Takahashi, Ph.D., Fujio Numano,M.D.
Institute of Japan Atherosclerosis Research
Sugayama-Bldg., 2-23, Kanda-Awaji-Cho, Chiyoda-Ku,
Tokyo, Japan

We have reported on the contractile and phagocytic properties of the arterial endothelial cells and regard these properties to be important in atherogenesis (Jap. Heart J. 13:573, 1972). The endothelial contractility may be induced by various atherogenic stimuli, and results in the entry of LDL and VLDL into the arterial wall and intimal edema (J. Atheroscl. Res. 3:87, 1963). Robertson and Khairallah also reported on the contractile property of the arterial endothelial cells and its significance in atherogenesis (Circ. Res. 31:923, 1972).

We employed intravenous injections of carbon particles measuring 200-700 Å (Perikan ink) in the study of the transendothelial transport in different segments of the arterial tree and in various species, and observed that such transport took place in animals susceptible to atherosclerosis and in areas of predilection for the development of lesions (Jap. Heart J. 16:76, 1975). The carbon particles were not transported across the arterial endothelial cells of normotensive rats; in the aortas of dogs and rhesus monkeys the transport was minimal, but it was considerable in the large arteries of rabbits and chicks, and in the spontaneously hypertensive rats. In the latter this phenomenon was also observed in the small caliber arteries (Circle of Willis). Once in the subendothelial space the carbon particles were observed by electron microscopy to accumulate along the internal elastic lamina (IEL) being "stagnated" here temporarily, while the smaller (125 Å in diameter) ferritin particles passed through the IEL. This implies that the IEL may serve as a barrier to particles beyond a certain size. This was also indicated by our immunofluorescent studies which showed that in the aorta of rhesus monkeys HDL passed freely through the IEL whereas the LDL and particularly the VLDL were prevented from passing at least for 24 hours; the entry of the carbon particles into the subendothelial space was always accompanied by the entry of LDL and occasionally also by VLDL.

To elucidate the role of actomyosin in the transendothelial transport of LDL, 120 adult rabbits were used in a series of experiments. The animals received one of the following compounds: ATP-increasing substance: pyridinolcarbamate (1-10 mg/kg p.o., 0.1-1 mg /kg i.v.); actomyosin-deranging substances: Vinblastine (0.1-1 mg/kg i.v.) and Colchicine (0.1-1 mg/kg i.v.): Ca-permeability inhibiting substance: iproveratril (0.1-1 mg/kg i.v.); and cyclic AMP-phosphodiesterase inhibitor: phthalazinol (EG626) (0.1-1 mg/kg p.o. and i.v.).

Following this "pretreatment" the animals received an intravenous injection of carbon particles (50% solution of Perikan ink diluted in saline, 5 ml/kg) and of angiotensin II (1 µg/kg) as a challenge (Jap. Heart J. 16:76, 1975). Two hours later all animals were sacrificed for light and electron microscopic examination of the arteries. The infusion of 500 ml of saline mixed with heparin through a catheter inserted into caval veins followed by an in situ fixation with 10% buffered formaldehyde solution.

RESULTS

In the aortas of the control (placebo) animals, the carbon particles were distributed diffusely in the intima of the entire aorta. The accumulation was spotty and streaky but considerable in marginal areas of orifices of the aortic branches. In these locations, particularly in the downstream areas from the branching points, the distribution resembled that of early stages of fatty spots and streaks.

In aortas of animals pretreated with pyridinolcarbamate (5-10 mg/kg p.o., 1 mg/kg: i.v.), phthalazinol (0.1 mg/kg p.o. and i.v.), iproveratril (0.5-1 mg/kg i.v.), Colchicine (o.5-1 mg/kg i.v.), and Vinblastine (0.5-1 mg/kg i.v.), the transendothelial entry of carbon particles was significantly reduced as compared with that of the placebo control group. The number of carbon particles was not only reduced in the intima of the entire thoracic aorta, but also in the marginal areas of the orifices to aortic branches. In animals pretreated with pyridinolcarbamate combined with phthalazinol, the carbon entry was strikingly inhibited in the entire aortic intima and the carbon particles were scarce in marginal areas of the branching points. There were fewer carbon particles observed in the intima under these experimental conditions than found when either of the two compounds was administered alone.

DISCUSSION

The above results show that the endothelial cell relaxants have an inhibitory effect upon the transport of the carbon particles by hyperreactive arterial endothelial cells. The relaxants probably inhibit the contractile and phagocytic activity of these cells by different mechanisms, e.g., an increased production of ATP by pyridinolcarbamate; an increase of cAMP-level by phthalazinol; the calcium

Inhibitory Effect of Endothelial Cell Relaxants on Carbon-entry

Drugs / No. of Animals	Placebo	PDC	EG626	PDC + EG626		Ipro-veratril	Col-chicine	Vin-blastine
		10 mg/kg p.o.	10 mg/kg p.o.	10 mg/kg p.o.	1 mg/kg i.v.	1 mg/kg i.v.	1 mg/kg i.v.	1 mg/kg i.v.
1	+++	++	+	+	±	+	++	++
2	+++	++	+	+	±	+	++	+
3	+++	+	+	±	-	+	+	+
4	++	+	+	±	-	+	+	+
5	++	+	+	±	-	+	+	+
6	++	+	+	±		±	+	±
7	++	±	±	±		±	±	±
8	++	±	±	±		±	±	±
9	++	±	±	-		±	±	±
10	++	±	±	-		±	±	±

+PDC-pyridinolcarbamate, EG626-phthalazinol
+The grade of quantity of carbon particles entered the intima as shown in this table.

permeability - inhibition by iproveratril; and the derangement of actomyosin by Colchicine and Vinblastine. With the exception of iproveratril and Vinblastine all were known to have a preventive effect upon experimental atherosclerosis in cholesterol-fed rabbits. Of particular interest with respect to atherosclerosis is the highly effective combination of the ATP-increasing and cAMP-increasing drugs.

Conclusion. Pyridinolcarbamate, phthalazinol, iproveratril, Colchicine, and Vinblastine signficantly reduced or prevented the transendothelial transport of carbon particles from the blood stream into the subendothelial space of aortas through the hyperreactive, arterial endothelial cells in rabbits.

(2)

THE EFFECT OF MODERATE INCREASES IN SERUM CHOLESTEROL ON THE BLOOD-ARTERY CHOLESTEROL TRANSFER BARRIER

Bondjers,G., Hansson,G., Brattsand,R., and Björkerud,S.

Department of Internal Medicine I, University of Göteborg

S-413 45 Göteborg, Sweden

Atherosclerotic arterial disease has been related to hypercholesterolemia both in clinical and in experimental studies. However, the effect of hypercholesterolemia on cholesterol transfer and retention in relationship to the major blood-artery transfer barrier, the intact endothelium, is little known.

MATERIAL AND METHODS

Moderate hypercholesterolemia (up to 700 mg%) was induced in male, albino rabbits by cholesterol supplement to the diet. Serum cholesterol was maintained on constant, and individually different levels by individual dosage of cholesterol to each rabbit (0.1 - 0.3 gms. daily). The serum cholesterol levels were controlled every second week. 24 hrs before killing the animals, the lipoproteins of a serum aliquot were labelled *in vitro* and reinjected intravenously. After killing the animal, non-atherosclerotic tissue was sampled with respect to endothelial integrity after visualization of regions with defective endothelium with the Evans blue dye exclusion test (1). Free and esterified cholesterol in the tissue samples was determined with a fluorometric ultra micro method, and radioactivity with liquid scintillation counting.

RESULTS AND DISCUSSION

In samples from regions with intact endothelium, the content of free cholesterol remained constant, when serum cholesterol increased from normal up to 400 mg % (fig. 1A). On the other hand, we have observed that the uptake of free cholesterol from serum in these regions increases with increasing serum cholesterol (2). This suggests control of the cholesterol levels in the tissue by increasing elimination of cholesterol. Above 400 mg% the elimination capacity may be exceeded. Such a suggestion is compatible with the observation that HDL-bound cholesterol increased with increasing serum cholesterol

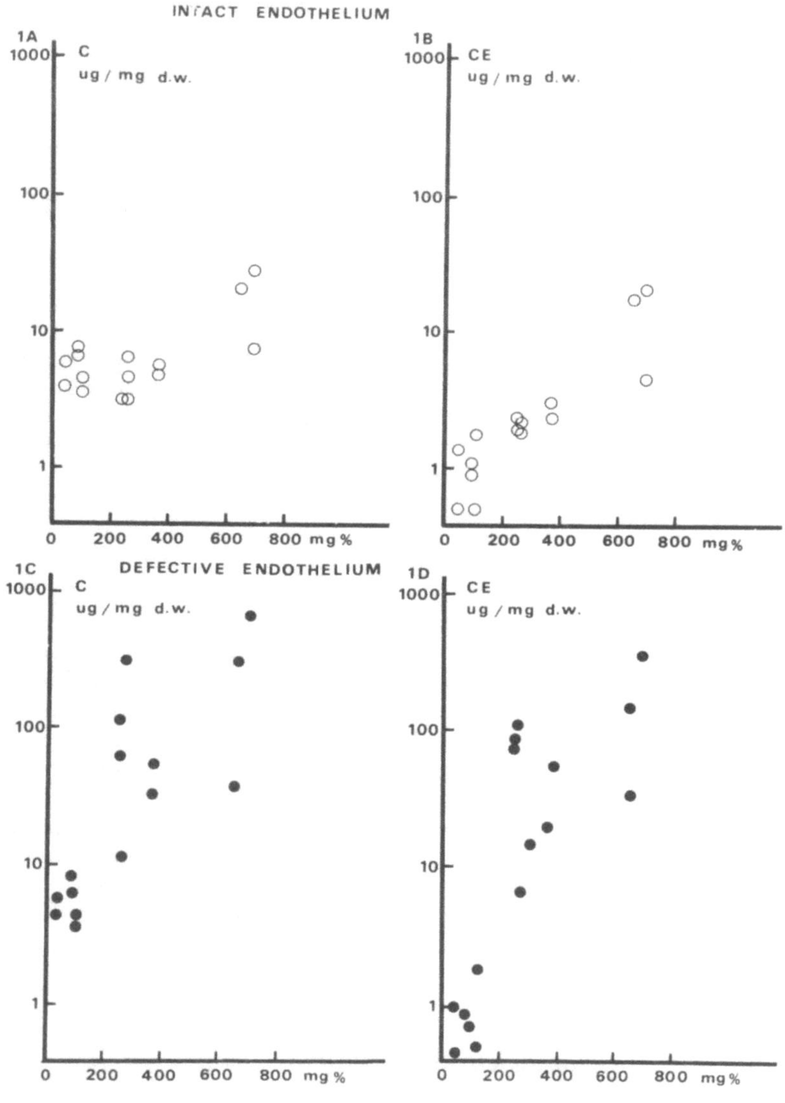

Fig.1. Serum cholesterol (abscissa)vs free (A and C) and esterified (B and D) cholesterol content (ordinate) in samples with intact (A and B) and defective endothelium (C and D).

only up to 400 mg% (2). As there is much evidence indicating that HDL is of critical significance for cholesterol elimination from arterial tissue (3), the decreased proportion of HDL-cholesterol suggests a mechanistic explanation to the net increase of free cholesterol in hypercholesterolemic rabbits with serum cholesterol above 400 mg% through defective elimination of cholesterol.

In contrast to free cholesterol, cholesteryl ester increased in direct proportion to the increasing serum cholesterol levels in aortic tissue with intact endothelium (fig. 1B). Recently, a similar direct relationship to serum cholesterol was reported for the serum lipoprotein concentration in arterial tissue (4). The present results are well compatible with these data, and indicate that cholesteryl ester is present in this tissue largely as a component of serum lipoproteins.

In regions with defective endothelium, the content of both free and esterified cholesterol increased in proportion to the increasing serum cholesterol levels (fig. 1C and D). We have previously observed that the functional cholesterol barrier between the blood and arterial tissue deteriorates when endothelial integrity decreases in normolipidemic rabbits (1). As a consequence of this decay in barrier function, the cholesterol concentration, as well as the influx of cholesterol, was higher in regions with defective endothelium. It was suggested that this difference between tissue with intact and defective endothelium would be exaggerated with increasing serum cholesterol concentrations. The present investigation supports this suggestion (fig. 1A-D). Therefore, it seems probable that the significance of the intact arterial endothelium as a barrier to cholesterol transfer and retention increases with increasing serum cholesterol levels.

REFERENCES

(1) Björkerud,S. and Bondjers,G. Endothelial integrity and viability in the aorta of normal rabbit and rat as evaluated with dye exclusion tests and interference contrast microscopy. Atherosclerosis 15,285-300, 1972.

(2) Bondjers,G., Hansson,G., Brattsand, R. and Björkerud, S. In manuscript.

(3) Bondjers,G., and Björkerud,S. Cholesterol transfer between arterial smooth muscle tissue and serum lipoproteins in vitro. Artery,1, 3-7, 1974.

(4) Smith,E.B., and R.S. Slater. Relationship between low-density lipoproteins in aortic intima and serum lipid levels. The Lancet 1, 463-469, 1972.

(3)

CHOLESTEROL EXCHANGE: EVIDENCE FOR A ROLE IN ARTERIAL CHOLESTEROL ACCUMULATION

Frank P. Bell, Ph.D.

Department of Pathology, McMaster University, Hamilton, Ontario, Canada

Despite the fact that virtually all the cholesterol that accumulates in atherosclerotic arteries has its origin in plasma lipoproteins, the mechanism(s) of net transfer of cholesterol into the arterial wall is unknown. It seems certain that arterial cholesterol accumulation cannot be explained solely on the basis of the simple diffusion of plasma lipoproteins into the artery (1,2). For this reason, other mechanisms such as lipoprotein remnant uptake (3) or cholesterol exchange (4-6) have been proposed. Recent experimental evidence (6) supports the feasibility of the latter mechanism which will be discussed here.

The incubation of aortas with washed erythrocytes labeled *in vivo* with ^{3}H-cholesterol proved to be a simple model system with which to examine the fate of isotopic cholesterol exchanged to the arterial wall (Table I) (6). A portion of the isotopic cholesterol exchanged to the intimal surface of atherosclerotic rabbit aortas was converted to cholesteryl esters indicating that the cholesterol may have further exchanged to the membranes of intracellular organelles in order to reach esterification sites within arterial cells which are, presumably, the endoplasmic reticulum and lysosomes. These organelles are considered since two different cholesterol esterifying systems have been identified in fractionated homogenates of arterial tissue; a microsomal system with a pH optimum of about 7.5 requiring ATP and CoASH (7-9) and a soluble, likely lysosomal system, with a pH optimum of about 5.0 with no requirement for ATP or CoASH (8,9).

The results of experiments with cell-free preparations of atherosclerotic arteries are consistent with the possibility that

TABLE I. Esterification of Erythrocyte ^{3}H-cholesterol Exchanged to Rabbit Aortas in vitro.

AORTAS	n	TOTAL ARTERIAL CHOLESTEROL (mg)	CHOLESTEROL ESTERIFIED (dpm/aorta)
NORMAL	10	0.28 - 0.73	14 ± 3
NORMAL (BOILED)	4	0.35 - 0.44	15 ± 4
ATHEROSCLEROTIC	6	12.22 - 20.10	43 ± 10
ATHEROSCLEROTIC	9	21.00 - 47.20	94 ± 46
ATHEROSCLEROTIC (BOILED)	4	15.18 - 33.20	14 ± 1

Everted aortas were incubated 4 h at 37° in Krebs-Ringer-Bicarbonate buffer, pH 7.4, containing ^{3}H-cholesterol-labeled erythrocytes (S.A. 600 dpm/ug) at a hematocrit of 30%. Values are means ± SEM of the number (n) of aortas used. Aortas boiled for 10 min served as controls.

intracellular cholesterol movement can occur by an exchange process. The addition of ^{3}H-cholesterol-labeled erythrocyte membranes to 1000 x g supernatants from cholesterol-fed rabbit aortas at pH 7.4 and pH 5.0 resulted in the incorporation of ^{3}H-cholesterol into cholesteryl esters (6) thus indicating the suitability of exchangeable membrane-bound cholesterol as a substrate for arterial esterifying enzymes. Microsomes and 165,000 x g supernatant (HSS) were also prepared from cholesterol-fed rabbit aortas at pH 7.4 and pH 5.0, respectively. Incubation of these fractions with labeled erythrocyte membranes resulted in the incorporation of ^{3}H-cholesterol into cholesteryl esters by both fractions (Fig. 1). The sigmoidal curve describing the rate of incorporation of ^{3}H-cholesterol into cholesteryl esters suggests that the ^{3}H-cholesterol was first exchanged to the microsomal membranes before esterification occurred. In contrast, ^{3}H-cholesterol ester formation by the soluble enzyme system at pH 5.0 was essentially linear over the entire incubation period indicating that the enzyme can act directly on the membrane-bound substrate.

The esterification of cholesterol exchanged to the arterial wall is relevant to any mechanism implicating cholesterol exchange in the net movement of cholesterol into arteries. For instance, the exchange of cholesterol between erythrocytes and lipoproteins

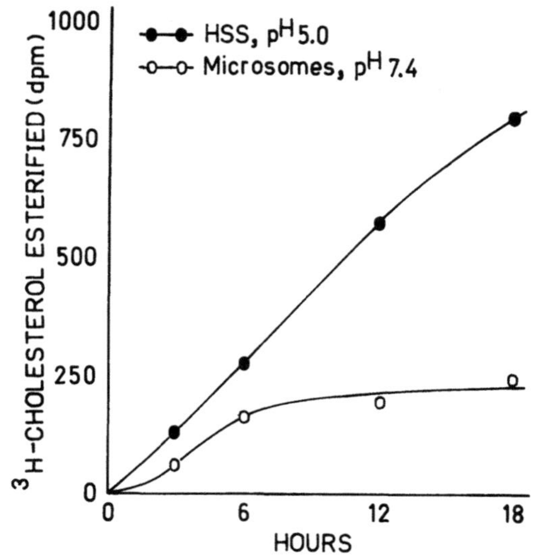

Fig. 1. Incorporation of membrane-bound ^{3}H-cholesterol into cholesteryl esters by cellular fractions from cholesterol-fed rabbit aortas. Aortas were homogenized in 10 vol of McIlvaines citrate-phosphate buffer at either pH 5.0 or pH 7.4. Homogenates were centrifuged 20 min at 10,000 x g and the supernatants centrifuged at 165,000 x g for 45 min to obtain the microsomal pellet and high speed supernatant (HSS). Incubations were performed at 37° in a total vol of 2.45 ml containing 100,000 dpm of ^{3}H-cholesterol-labeled erythrocyte membranes (S.A. 2530 dpm/µg). At pH 7.4, incubations contained 2.38 mg of microsomal protein, 15 µmoles ATP, 1.5 µmoles CoASH, 15 µmoles NaF and 12 µmoles $MgCl_2$. At pH 5.0, incubations contained 4.18 mg of HSS protein without added cofactors.

occurs without a net transfer of sterol (10). However, in the presence of the cholesterol esterifying enzyme LCAT, exchange as well as net transfer of cholesterol to the lipoproteins occurs (11). In effect, the esterification reaction functions as a biochemical trapping mechanism creating a vectoral drain on erythrocyte cholesterol. Thus, the potential for a movement of cholesterol into atherosclerotic arteries by a similar coupling of cholesterol exchange to esterification exists since atherosclerotic tissue has a high enzymic capability to esterify cholesterol and the capability to exchange cholesterol with plasma lipoproteins, particularly in the presence of hypercholesterolemia.

ACKNOWLEDGEMENT

This work was supported by Medical Research Council of Canada (MT 3067), the Canadian Heart Foundation and the Ontario Heart Foundation.

REFERENCES

1. Dayton, S. and Hashimoto, S. Recent advances in molecular pathology: A review. Cholesterol flux and metabolism in arterial tissue and in atheromata. Exp. Mol. Path. 13: 256-268 (1970).
2. Zilversmit, D.B. Mechanisms of cholesterol accumulation in the arterial wall. Amer. J. Cardiol. 35: 559-566 (1975).
3. Zilversmit, D.B. A proposal linking atherogenesis to the interaction of endothelial lipoprotein lipase with triglyceride-rich lipoproteins. Circ. Res. 33: 633-638 (1973).
4. Portman, O.W., Alexander, M. and Maruffo, C.A. Nutritional control of arterial lipid composition in squirrel monkeys: Major ester classes and types of phospholipids. J. Nutr. 91: 35-46 (1967).
5. Geer, J.C., Panganamala, R.V., Newman, H.A.I. and Cornwell, D.G. Arterial wall metabolism. In: The pathogenesis of atherosclerosis, p. 200-213 (The Williams and Wilkins Co., Baltimore, 1972).
6. Bell, F.P. Studies on physico-chemical sterol exchange: Esterification of exchangeable membrane-bound cholesterol by intact aortas and cell-free arterial homogenates from cholesterol-fed rabbits. Artery 1: 86-96 (1974).
7. St. Clair, R.W., Lofland, H.B. and Clarkson, T.B. Influence of duration of cholesterol feeding on esterification of fatty acids by cell-free preparation of pigeon aorta: Studies on the mechanism of cholesterol esterification. Circ. Res. 27: 213-225 (1970).
8. Proudlock, J.W. and Day, A.J. Cholesterol esterifying enzymes of atherosclerotic rabbit intima. Biochim. Biophys. Acta 260: 716-723 (1972).
9. Brecher, P.I. and Chobanian, A.V. Cholesteryl ester synthesis in normal and atherosclerotic aortas of rabbits and rhesus monkeys. Circ. Res. 25: 692-701 (1974).
10. Hagerman, J.S. and Gould, R.G. The in vitro interchange of cholesterol between plasma and red cells. Proc. Soc. Exp. Biol. Med. 78: 329-332 (1951).
11. Murphy, J.R. Erythrocyte metabolism. III. Relationship of energy metabolism and serum factors to the osmotic fragility following incubation. J. Lab. Clin. Med. 60: 86-109 (1962).

(4)

CHOLESTEROL METABOLISM IN HUMAN ENDOTHELIAL CELLS IN CULTURE

S. N. JAGANNATHAN, W. E. CONNOR, L. J. LEWIS

West Virginia University Departments of Pathology and Biochemistry, Morgantown, W. Va. and University of Iowa, Department of Medicine, Iowa City, Ia., U.S.A.

The origin of esterified cholesterol accumulating in cultured human endothelial cells[1] and its influence on cholesterol biosynthesis were investigated in monolayer cultures. Whole plasma (WP) or isolated low density lipoproteins (LDL) from a normolipidemic subject and a hyperlipoproteinemic (Type IIa) patient, were included in McCoy's 5a culture media at 10% level of plasma in the presence of acetate-2-H^3. The free cholesterol of the WP and LDL were previously labeled in vitro with 4-C^{14}-cholesterol. Cultures with plasma-free media served as control. Cell pellets were isolated after incubation at 37°C for 4 hours in an atmosphere of 5% carbon dioxide - 95% air mixture.

In control cells there was no esterified cholesterol. WP elicited some accumulation of esterified cholesterol (5 and 12 μg/mg protein respectively for the normal and Type II samples), whereas LDL provoked an esterified cholesterol response of 18 and 58 μg/mg protein. The uptake of labeled free cholesterol (-4-C^{14}) from LDL was substantially greater than from WP (185 vs 108 dpm/mg cell protein for normal and 925 vs 552 dpm/mg for Type II). The label, however, was found exclusively in the free cholesterol fraction of the cell pellet.

Labeled acetate was incorporated readily into free cholesterol when the media was devoid of cholesterol (1729 dpm/mg protein). Inclusion of Type II plasma elicited a 51% inhibition of cholesterol biosynthesis (849 dpm/mg), whereas isolated LDL almost completely (96%) suppressed biosynthesis (62 dpm/mg). Relative to the respective plasma, inhibition was 93% for Type II LDL (849 vs 62 dpm/mg protein) and 64% for normal LDL (1027 vs 368). In LDL-incubated cells, no significant labeling of the esterified cholesterol fraction occurred either in the cholesterol or fatty acid moiety. With plasma, some minor amounts of labelled cholesterol (0.5 to 10%) were observed in the cholesterol moiety of esterified cholesterol.

It is concluded that the accumulation of esterified cholesterol in cultured endothelial cells is not mediated through uptake of free cholesterol and its esterification, but through uptake of esterified cholesterol as such either from LDL or as LDL. It is further suggested that the accumulation of esterified cholesterol may be the factor responsible for effective inhibition of cholesterol biosynthesis in cultured endothelial cells.

---

[1]S. N. Jagannathan, L. J. Lewis and W. E. Connor (1974): The accumulation of free and esterified cholesterol by human endothelial cells cultured with various plasma lipoproteins. Circulation: 50: III-69

(5)

EFFECT OF LIPOPROTEIN ON IN VITRO SYNTHESIS OF DNA IN AORTIC TISSUE

J. Augustyn, K.E. Fritz, A.S. Daoud, J. Jarmolych

V. A. Hospital and Albany Medical Center Hospital

Albany, New York, U.S.A.

Several factors such as lipoproteins,[1,2] platelets[3] and insulin[4] have been shown to stimulate the proliferation of aortic smooth muscle cells in culture in the presence of serum or serum derivatives. Using an explant system from swine thoracic aorta we have studied the effect of lipoproteins on the synthesis of DNA. Our system, on which we have previously reported in detail,[5] exhibits cell proliferation, cell death and a peripheral growth of smooth muscle cells which secrete collagen, elastic tissue and glycosaminoglycans and is well-suited as a model system for use in the study of the phenomenon characteristic of atherosclerosis. In addition, unlike cultures of smooth muscle cells which are both very time-consuming to obtain and which cannot be easily cultured in large numbers, our system has the advantage of having only a 9-day culture period and of allowing for the assay of large numbers of samples in quadruplicate.

Lipoprotein fractions were obtained by differential flotation.[6] The serum proteins which pelleted at each of the three steps in the fractionation were designated Pellet I, II and III; those which remained in solution at the end of the fractionation procedure were designated as residue. Each fraction was dialyzed extensively against Hanks' salts and sterilized by ultrafiltration. All fractions were monitored by acrylamide electrophoresis[7,8] and by their cholesterol[9]-protein[10] ratio.

Four replicate cultures each consisting of four randomly selected 1.2 mm^2 segments of middle media were incubated for 9 days at 37° in 4 ml of medium (M199) containing either 10% of the serum

TABLE I

Fraction (10%)	Ave Total ug[a] DNA	Re: 10% Serum,%	Ave ^{3}Hdpm[a,b] / ug DNA	Re: Tot dpm Recov.,%	Re: 10% Serum,%
M199	21.3	217	524	--	9
NS	9.8	-	6122	--	-
VLDL	20.1	205	385	2	6
LDL	21.6	220	511	3	8
HDL	24.2	247	544	3	9
Residue	12.9	132	3653	23	60
Pellet I	11.9	121	2537	16	41
Pellet II	16.4	167	2023	16	33
Pellet III	10.0	102	6375	40	104

[a]Average of triplicate cultures

Serum	^{3}H-Tot dpm Recovered[b]	Re: Orig Serum % Recovered	Cholesterol mg/dl
NS	16,028	262	79

TABLE II

Fraction (10%)	Ave Total ug[a] DNA	Re: 10% Serum,%	Ave ^{3}Hdpm[a,b] / ug DNA	Re: Tot dpm Recov.,%	Re: 10% Serum,%
M199	13.7	138	159	--	11
HC	9.9	-	1963	--	-
VLDL	15.3	155	125	5	6
LDL	17.0	172	41	2	2
HDL	13.4	135	93	4	5
Residue	10.7	108	468	19	24
Pellet I	8.5	86	730	30	37
Pellet II	11.2	113	482	20	25
Pellet III	10.2	103	518	21	26

[a]Average of triplicate cultures

Serum	^{3}H-Tot dpm Recovered[b]	Re: Orig Serum % Recovered	Cholesterol mg/dl
HC	2,457	125	402

of origin, 10% of one of the lipoprotein fractions or 10% of one of the serum protein fractions. The effect of each fraction in culture was studied by comparing the incorporation of ^{3}H-thymidine during the last 2 hrs of incubation with that of cultures containing the serum of origin. Tables I and II show data from a representative experiment carried out with both normocholesterolemic (NS) and hypercholesterolemic (HC) porcine serum. Our data show: 1) Neither VLDL, LDL nor HDL account for any appreciable part of the synthetic activity of whole serum. Often they are inhibitory when compared to controls grown in incubation medium alone; 2) There is no difference in activity between lipoprotein fractions derived from either normocholesterolemic or hypercholesterolemic serum; 3) The activity resident in whole serum is recoverable in the pelleted serum protein fractions and in the residue. These data indicate that in the aortic explant model system cell proliferation, as measured by DNA synthesis, cannot be attributed to any one of the lipoprotein fractions but results from the combined activity of a number of factors in serum.

REFERENCES

1. Ross, R. and J.A. Glomset, Science 180, 1332 (1973).

2. Fisher-Dzoga, K., R. Chen and R. W. Wissler in Arterial Mesenchyme and Arteriosclerosis, 1974, p. 299.

3. Ross, R., J.A. Glomset, B. Kariya and L. Harker, Proc. Nat. Acad. Sci. U.S. 71, 1207 (1974).

4. Stout, R. W., E.L. Bierman and R. Ross, Circ. Res. 36, 319 (1975)

5. Daoud, A. S., K.E. Fritz, J. Jarmolych and J.M. Augustyn, Exp. Mol. Path. 18, 177 (1973).

6. Havel, R. J., H.A. Eder and J.H. Bragdon, J. Clin. Invest. 34, 1345 (1955).

7. Davis, B. J., Ann. N.Y. Acad. Sci. 121, 404 (1964).

8. Hall, F.F., C.R. Ratliff, C.L. Westfall and T.W. Culp, Biochem. Med. 6, 464 (1972).

9. Haung, T. C., C.P. Chen, V. Wefler and A. Raftery, Anal. Chem. 33, 1405 (1961).

10. Lowry, O. H., N.J. Rosebrough, A.L. Farr and R.J. Randall, J. Biol. Chem. 193, 265 (1951).

CHAPTER 10
EXPERIMENTAL MODELS OF HYPERLIPIDEMIA

(1)

COMPARISON OF AGE RELATED ALTERATIONS IN ARTERIAL STEROL ACCUMULATION, BLOOD PRESSURE AND CHOLESTEROL BALANCE IN SPONTANEOUSLY ATHEROSCLEROSIS-SUSCEPTIBLE AND ATHEROSCLEROSIS-RESISTANT PIGEONS

M.T.R. Subbiah, Z. Rymaszewski, I.A. Carlo and B.A. Kottke

Mayo Clinic and Founcation
Rochester, Minnesota, U.S.A.

The marked difference in the incidence of spontaneous atherosclerosis between White Carneau and Show Racer pigeons is well documented (1). Although the differences in arterial cholesteryl esters and their metabolism between the two breeds have been studied (2,3), no comparative studies of the age related alteration in blood pressures in these two breeds have been made. Also, it is not known how the pattern of arterial sterol accumulation compares with the changes in blood pressure and cholesterol balance. This communication reports the age related alterations in blood pressure and arterial sterol accumulation in White Carneau and Show Racer breeds of pigeons at 9 months and 17 months of age. Our studies have shown that lipid accumulation in the White Carneau pigeon occurs after 9 months of age (4).

METHODS

White Carneau and Show Racer pigeons were obtained from The Palmetto Pigeon Plant, Sumter, South Carolina. Pigeons were maintained on a cholesterol-free grain diet during the study. All blood pressure measurements were made without anesthesia by inserting a 25-gauge needle into the axillary artery in the wing. For chemical studies aortas from these pigeons were obtained following sacrifice and the content and composition of the sterols and steryl esters were determined as described previously using thin-layer and gas-liquid chromatography (3,5). Cholesterol balance studies in these pigeons were done by placing them individually in metabolic cages as described previously (6).

RESULTS

Table I shows the results of systolic pressures observed in the White Carneau and Show Racer pigeons. As can be seen in the Table the mean systolic pressures of 9-month old White Carneau and Show Racer pigeons were similar. Also, the mean systolic pressure of Show Racers did not change from 9 to 17 months. However, the 17-month old White Carneau showed a higher blood pressure when compared to 9-month old White Carneau ($P < 0.005$). At 17 months of age the blood pressure in White Carneau was significantly higher than that of age matched Show Racer ($P < 0.01$).

Table I. Comparison of Mean Systolic Pressures of White Carneau and Show Racer Pigeons

Breed	Age (Months)	Number of Pigeons	Mean Systolic Blood Pressure ± SEM
Show Racer	9	17	155.0 ± 2.1
White Carneau	9	41	156.9 ± 2.0 ⎤ $P < 0.005$ (vs. White Carneau 17)
Show Racer	17	20	156.2 ± 4.3 ⎤ $P < 0.01$ (vs. White Carneau 17)
White Carneau	17	17	168.8 ± 3.6

The alteration in arterial sterols and steryl esters during these ages in both the breeds is shown in Table II. It is evident that the total sterols in White Carneau increased by 43.6% from 9 to 17 months. When compared to Show Racers the sterol content was higher by 56.2% in the White Carneau ($P < 0.01$). The major increase in the White Carneau occurred in steryl esters (nearly doubled when compared to Show Racers).

Table II. Age Related Changes in Aortic Sterol and Steryl Ester Content[a]

Breed	Age (Months)	Total Sterols (mg/g) Mean ± SD	% Esters Mean ± SD
White Carneau	9	2.91 ± 0.24	12.26 ± 2.66
White Carneau	17	5.16 ± 1.04[b]	24.27 ± 5.98[c]
Show Racer	9	2.67 ± 0.28	12.10 ± 4.99
Show Racer	17	2.26 ± 0.38	12.80 ± 3.12

[a]Values obtained by the analysis of at least 3 pooled samples of 3 birds each.
[b]Values significantly higher than in White Carneau 9 months of age ($P < 0.001$) and in Show Racer 17 months of age ($P < 0.01$).
[c]Values significantly higher than in White Carneau 9 months of age ($P < 0.001$) and in Show Racer 17 months of age ($P < 0.05$).

During this critical period of lipid accumulation there is also a change in the fecal excretion of sterol and bile acids between White Carneau and Show Racer pigeons (Table III). It is

Table III. Fecal Excretion of Neutral Sterols and Bile Acids

Breed	Neutral Sterols	Bile Acids	Total Fecal Steroid Excretion
	(Mean ± SD (mg/kg per day)		
White Carneau(5)	5.83±1.38	10.43±4.60	16.26±3.79
Show Racer (5)	10.09±2.28[a]	18.05±9.52	28.14±10.28[b]

[a]For difference between breeds, $P < 0.01$.
[b]For difference between breeds, $P < 0.05$.

evident that at 1 year of age the fecal excretion of total steroids in the White Carneau is significantly lower than that of Show Racers ($P < 0.05$) with a major difference in the neutral sterol fraction ($P < 0.01$).

In conclusion, this study has demonstrated that during the period of lipid accumulation in the White Carneau pigeon there are also alterations in other metabolic factors (i.e., blood pressure and cholesterol balance) which might contribute to the overall pathogenesis of spontaneous atherosclerosis in this animal model.

REFERENCES

1. Clarkson, T.B., Pritchard, R.W., Netsky, M.G. and Lofland, H.B., Sr.: Arch. Path. 68:193, 1959.

2. Lofland, H.B., Jr., Moory, D.M., Hoffman, C.W. and Clarkson, T.B., J. Lipid Res. 6:112, 1965.

3. Subbiah, M.T.R., Kottke, B.A. and Carlo, I.A.: Inter. J. Biochem. 5:63, 1974.

4. Rymaszewski, Z., Langelier, M., Carlo, I.A., Subbiah, M.T.R. and Kottke, B.A.: Atherosclerosis, in press.

5. Kottke, B.A., Unni, K.K., Carlo, I.A. and Subbiah, M.T.R.: Trans. Assoc. Amer. Phys. 87:263, 1974.

6. Siekert, R.B., Jr., Dicke, B.A., Subbiah, M.T.R. and Kottke, B.A.: Res. Commun. Chem. Path. Pharm. 10:181, 1975.

This study was supported in part by Grant HL 14196 (SCOR) from the National Institutes of Health.

(2)

HEREDITARY HYPERLIPIDEMIA IN CHICKENS - MODEL FOR STUDY OF TOXIC OXIDATION PRODUCTS FOUND IN SIGNIFICANT AMOUNTS IN U.S.P. CHOLESTEROL, POWDERED EGGS AND MILK

C. B. Taylor, S. K. Peng, H. Imai, B. Mikkelson,
K. T. Lee, and N. T. Werthessen
Veterans Administration Hospital and
Albany Medical College, Albany, New York,
and Brown University, Providence, Rhode Island, U.S.A.

In 1948 Chaikoff, et al. (1) induced endogenous hypercholesteremia in chickens by subcutaneous implantation of diethylstilbesterol; in another group of chickens comparable levels of hypercholesterolemia were induced by feeding a 2% cholesterol diet. After 6.5 months on these two regimes these 2 groups of animals and a group of controls were killed and studied. The animals fed cholesterol had numerous, grossly visible atheromata in the thoracic aorta whereas those given endogenous hypercholesteremia by diethylstilbesterol and the controls had only a meager amount of spontaneous atherosclerosis.

For over twenty years sterol chemists have been aware of autoxidation of cholesterol, stored at room temperature and exposed to air. Smith et al. (2), employing two dimensional chromatography demonstrated 32 autoxidation products of cholesterol.

Imai and coworkers have observed an increased number of necrotic medial smooth muscle cells in animals ingesting U.S.P. Cholesterol (3). In the current study both light and electron microscopy were employed to evaluate death of medial smooth muscle cells produced by feeding impurities concentrated from U.S.P. Cholesterol; this study has been published in a short paper (4).

The impurities from lots of U.S.P. Cholesterol were concentrated by recrystallizing cholesterol from methanol solutions and retaining the mother liquor, then evaporating the residue in the mother liquor to dryness, under vacuum. The concentrate contained products of spontaneous oxidation of cholesterol and other contaminants from the original sources of dead aortic smooth muscle cells and induced focal areas of intimal edema in rabbits 24 hours after gavage of

250 mg./kg. (Table 1). Both new and old unpurified U.S.P. Cholesterol were angiotoxic, the older being more toxic than the recently purchased sterol (Table 1). None of the animals in the above study showed hypercholesteremia.

Concentrated impurities administered three times per week and for a total dose of 1g./kg. over a period of seven weeks induced focal intimal fibrotic lesions without foam cells or hypercholesteremia. Purified cholesterol at the same dose over a seven week period produced no effect.

TABLE 1. Data obtained from 15 controls and 5 experimental groups. In interest of conserving space only ranges of aggregate debris and degenerated cells as well as average cell count per animal are given for control animals. All animals in experimental groups are listed.

CONTROLS

No. of Animals	Aggregate Debris-Range	Degenerated Cells-Range	Cells Counted per Animal-Average
15	0.0 to 0.2 %	0.0 to 1.4 %	497
Averages	0.3 %	0.61%	

Animal No.	Aggregate Debris %	Degenerated Cells %	Number of Cells Counted
	Old USP Cholesterol, 1g./kg.		
1	0.2	8.3	542
2	3.0	7.4	500
3	0.2	7.5	426
4	0.1	6.9	870
5	0.0	7.9	933
Averages	0.7*	7.6**	
	New USP Cholesterol, 1g./kg.		
1	0.2	3.4	616
2	0.5	5.0	652
3	0.0	6.2	546
4	0.2	3.8	597
5	0.2	3.5	670
Averages	0.2**	4.4**	

(cont.)

TABLE 1 (cont.)

	New USP Cholesterol, 250 mg./kg.		
1	0.0	1.7	477
2	0.2	.3	416
3	0.0	2.9	423
Averages	0.1	1.6*	
	Concentrate, 250 mg./kg.		
1	13.6	23.6	433
2	4.6	2.7	372
3	4.7	7.6	724
4	12.1	4.3	372
5	0.7	3.6	416
6	0.3	7.5	389
7	3.1	1.5	488
Averages	5.6**	7.3**	
	Concentrate, 10 mg./kg.		
1	1.8	0.7	546
2	0.4	3.1	262
3	0.4	2.6	476
4	1.6	0.4	551
Averages	1.1**	1.7**	

* Probability less than .05 but greater than .01 that difference from the controls could be due to chance.

** Probability less than 0.1 that difference from controls could be due to chance.

Compounds that were necrogenic to arterial smooth muscle cells were isolated by similar chemical methods from powdered whole eggs and powdered whole milk.

Our group has a flock of chickens with hereditary, endogenous hypercholesteremia (5). The carrier of the defect is the rooster which transmits the sex-linked defect to half its hen offsprings. When these genetically defective hens are ingesting a cholesterol-free diet and are changed from a photoperiod of 6 to 18 hours their serum cholesterol increases from 100 to 770 mg.%. These hens with hereditary endogenous hypercholesteremia also have an inability to fully develop and lay eggs. We plan on using this animal, which has only endogenously synthesized cholesterol, in the cholesterol oxidation products study outlined above. If there are no autoxidation products in the cholesterol of these hens, they should be useful in this study.

REFERENCES

1. Chaikoff, I.L., Lindsay, S., Lorenz, F.W., and Entenman, C.: J. Exp. Med., 88:373-387, 1948.

2. Smith, L.L., Matthews, W.S., Price, J.C., Bachmann, R.C., and Reynolds, B.: J. Chromatog. 27:187-205, 1967.

3. Imai, H., Lee, S.K., Pastori, S.J., and Thomas, W.A.: Virchows Arch. Path. Anat. 350:183-204, 1970.

4. Lee, K.T., Imai, H., Werthessen, N.T., and Taylor, C.B.: Proc. III International Symposium on Atheroclerosis. Editors: Schettler and Weizel, Springer-Verlag, New York, 1974, pp. 344-347.

5. Ho, K.J., Lawrence, D.T., Lewis, L.A., Liu, L.B., and Taylor, C.B.: Arch. Path. 98:161-172, 1974.

Supported by Veterans Administration, MRIS No. 8332-01, U.S.P. H.S. NIH Grant HL 14177-03 and U.S.N., ONR Grant No. 00014-67-0191-0028.

(3)

A COMPARATIVE STUDY OF THE EFFECT OF DIETARY CHOLESTEROL ON PLASMA LIPOPROTEINS IN NONHUMAN PRIMATES

R. K. Paula, L. L. Rudel, and T. B. Clarkson

Arteriosclerosis Research Center, Bowman Gray School of Medicine of Wake Forest University
Winston-Salem, N. C., U.S.A.

During the past decade there has been considerable emphasis on the use of nonhuman primates as animal models for atherosclerosis research. The increased emphasis has resulted from the belief by many investigators that experimental data obtained on nonhuman primates is more likely to be directly applicable to man than those derived from lower animals. With the increased emphasis on nonhuman primates, many research opportunities utilizing species differences have been elaborated. Among the differences that have been useful in research on atherosclerosis have been those in lesion morphology and in lipoprotein metabolism.

In this communication, we report on the influence of dietary cholesterol on the plasma lipoproteins of two species in the genus Macaca (*Macaca mulatta* and *Macaca nemestrina*) and an African nonhuman primate (*Erythrocebus patas*) of recent interest to atherosclerosis research workers primarily because the lesions induced by diet bear a considerable resemblance to the atherosclerosis of human beings.

All animals were adult males and were fed a semipurified diet containing 45% of calories as lard and containing 0.05 mg cholesterol/Cal (control) or 1 mg cholesterol/Cal (test). At the time of study, the mean plasma cholesterol concentration in control and test animals was 137 and 822 mg/dl in *M. nemestrina*, 191 and 822 mg/dl in *M. mulatta*, and 136 and 416 mg/dl in *E. patas*. Six animals of each species were in each diet group. Animals were fasted for 24 hours, plasma was collected and its density raised to 1.225 g/ml with solid potassium bromide. Lipoproteins were then isolated by ultracentrifugation and separated and purified by agarose gel filtration. The purity of the separation was checked with agarose gel electrophoresis. Four lipoprotein fractions, namely VLDL, ILDL, LDL, and HDL were studied. In all species, the increased plasma cholesterol concentration was due to an elevation in VLDL, ILDL, and LDL, although in the *E. patas*, changes were less pronounced. The separation of lipoproteins by agarose gel filtration is based on size. Typical elution profiles for control and test diet-fed animals are shown in Figure 1.

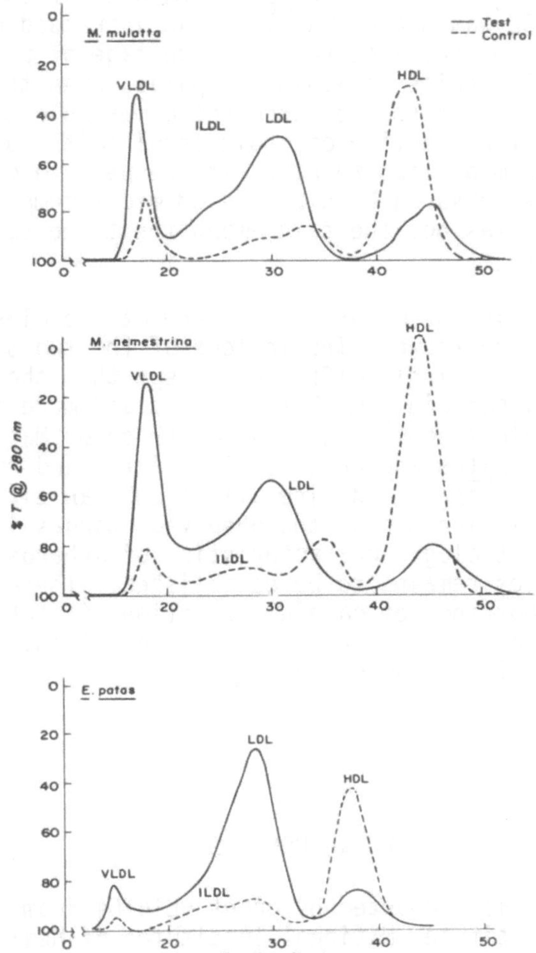

Fig. 1. Agarose gel filtration profiles of plasma lipoproteins of monkeys fed test and control diets.

By using this method, we found that in macaques, the size of VLDL, ILDL, and LDL was increased by dietary cholesterol indicating that a change in lipoprotein structure occurred. No similar size increase was observed among the lipoproteins of E. patas. In test animals of each species, HDL was decreased in concentration but apparently normal in size. The electrophoretic mobility of the VLDL was shifted from pre-β to β in all test animals.

The increased level of dietary cholesterol also induced chemical composition changes in lipoproteins. VLDL of test M. nemestrina and M. mulatta were markedly higher in cholesteryl ester and lower in triglyceride. A similar, but much less marked change was found in VLDL of E. patas. The alteration in the composition of LDL was due primarily to an increased percentage of cholesteryl ester and a decreased percentage of protein, and was found for all species including E. patas, even though size changes for LDL in this species were not comparable to those in macaques. Thus, the addition of cholesterol to the diets altered the entire spectrum of lipoproteins with respect to concentration and structure, as measured by size and chemical composition, although the effect was not the same among the three species of nonhuman primates.

Differences in the morphology of the atherosclerotic lesions of these species are known. The lesions of the two species of macaques are not strikingly different except that the lesions of Macaca nemestrina contain somewhat less fat and more fibrous proteins, particularly collagen, than do those of Macaca mulatta. The lesions of E. patas appear to be less fatty and to have more connective tissue changes and mineralization than either of the macaques. The relationship of the observed changes in the lipoproteins to the pathologic characteristics of atherosclerosis among these species remains to be established. These results emphasize the importance of careful selection of nonhuman primate species for biological similarities to human beings, if they are studied as models for human disease.

ACKNOWLEDGMENTS

This study was supported by grant HL14164 from the National Heart and Lung Institute, National Institutes of Health.

The authors gratefully acknowledge the cooperation of Drs. David Johnson, Donald Fry, and Robert Mahley of the National Heart and Lung Institute in obtaining E. patas plasma.

(4)

LIPOPROTEINS AND THE *IN VITRO* STUDY OF CHOLESTEROL METABOLISM IN GERBILS

R. J. Nicolosi, Y. Kim and K. C. Hayes

Department of Nutrition
Harvard School of Public Health
Boston, Massachusetts, U.S.A.

The Mongolian gerbil has proven a useful model to study diet-induced hyperlipidemia in that it responds to saturated fat and/or cholesterol by raising its serum cholesterol levels 300-400 mg/dl and increasing hepatic lipid synthesis and secretion (*Amer. J. Physiol.* 221: 548, 1971). Despite this degree of hypercholesterolemia, the gerbil aorta remains free of atherosclerotic involvement. In order to determine if this was related to a peculiarity of lipid transport or an obvious difference in cholesterol metabolism by major organs that metabolize cholesterol and its esters, mainly liver and intestine, we examined the gerbil's lipoproteins along with cholesterogenesis by liver and intestine and accumulation of cholesterol in these organs.

Young female gerbils were fed 10% corn oil or butterfat ± 0.1% cholesterol for 4 weeks, after which the animals were fasted for 16 hours and exsanguinated via cardiac puncture. Plasma was prepared and used for determining total, esterified and free cholesterol, and for separation of lipoproteins by agarose gel electrophoresis and density gradient ultracentrifugation. Liver and ileal slices were incubated at 37° for 2 hours in KRB containing sodium octanoate-1-^{14}C, glucose and antibiotics. After incubation, samples were washed, extracted for lipid, and an aliquot fractionated by thin layer chromatography. Silica gel areas containing various lipid classes were scraped and eluted and aliquots taken directly for determining incorporation of radioactive octanoate into lipid, and for chemical determinations of cholesterol and cholesterol ester for calculation of specific activities.

The lipoprotein profile revealed that the LDL:HDL ratio in both butterfat and corn oil-fed gerbils was relatively constant, with the majority of lipid being carried by HDL (Fig. 1), even

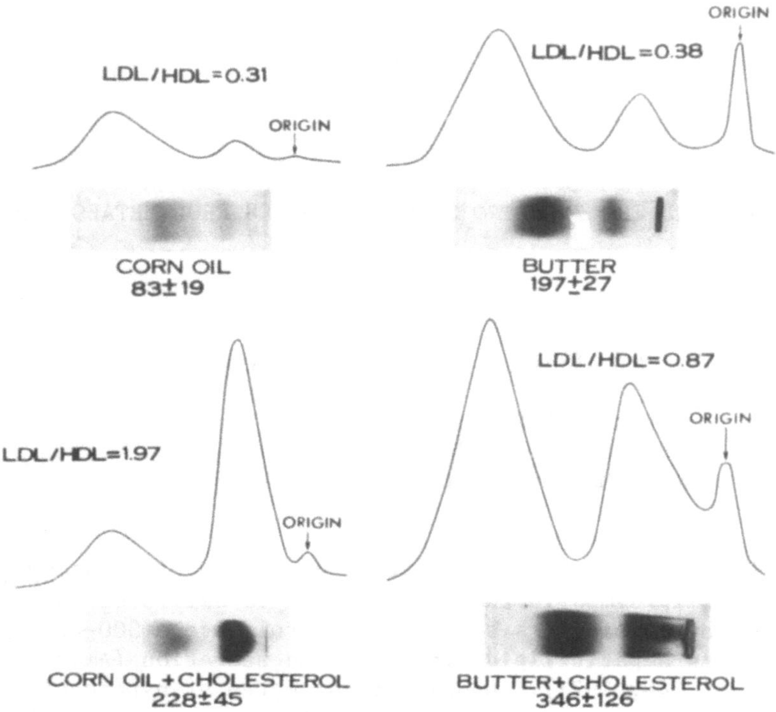

Fig. 1. Agarose gel electrophoresis patterns of gerbil lipoproteins. Plasma cholesterol (mean ± S.D.) beneath diet in mg/dl.

though hypercholesterolemia resulted from butterfat alone. However, when cholesterol was supplemented in the diet, the rise in serum cholesterol was largely accounted for by increased LDL, particularly with corn oil, suggesting separate control mechanism(s) for the elevation of serum cholesterol caused by saturated fat or cholesterol.

While butterfat feeding produced a highly variable increase in hepatic cholesterol ester concentration compared to corn oil-fed gerbils, the addition of cholesterol to both diets caused 10-20 fold increases in hepatic cholesterol esters, whereas the free cholesterol remained stable (Table 1). The lack of inhibition of the gerbil ileum as opposed to the nearly complete inhibition of hepatic cholesterol synthesis due to cholesterol feeding is in keeping with data of other species, suggesting a greater role by the liver than the ileum in regulating the gerbil lipoproteins during cholesterol feeding. The increase in CE:FC ratios in the liver following cholesterol feeding was not seen in the individual gerbil lipoproteins (Table 2) suggesting other homeostatic control mechanisms in the plasma, possibly involving LCAT and LPL enzymes.

The typical response by the gerbil liver and intestine to cholesterol feeding and the lack of effect of high circulating LDL-cholesterol on the arterial wall suggest that the unique resistance of the gerbil to atherosclerosis may reside in the wall itself, independent of the circulating lipid concentration or nature of the lipoprotein carrier.

TABLE 1. DIETARY EFFECT ON HEPATIC AND ILEAL FREE OR ESTERIFIED CHOLESTEROL CONCENTRATION AND SPECIFIC ACTIVITY[1]

Diet	Concentration (μg/100 mg wet wt)			
	Liver			Ileum
	CE	FC	CE:FC	FC
Corn Oil				
No cholesterol	82 ± 47 (302 ± 269)	151 ± 29 (2578 ± 1192)	0.5	208 ± 62 (210 ± 69)
+ cholesterol	1145 ± 310 (1 ± 2)	104 ± 28 (39 ± 24)	11.0	199 ± 57 (173 ± 137)
Butterfat				
No cholesterol	194 ± 183 (329 ± 296)	159 ± 24 (1961 ± 1997)	1.2	151 ± 73 (124 ± 49)
+ cholesterol	1378 ± 597 (21 ± 27)	146 ± 59 (65 ± 44)	9.4	253 ± 115 (112 ± 89)

[1] Mean ± S.D., 4 gerbils/group. Values in parentheses are specific activities (dpm/μg × 10^2).

TABLE 2. DIETARY EFFECT ON THE CE:FC RATIO OF PLASMA LIPOPROTEINS[1]

Diet	CE:FC				
	Chylomicron	VLDL	LDL_1	LDL_2	HDL
Corn Oil					
No cholesterol	7.0	4.6	4.5	10.9	15.1
+ cholesterol	8.1	5.7	5.3	8.1	9.8
Butterfat					
No cholesterol	4.5	3.4	3.6	5.7	9.5
+ cholesterol	8.7	5.9	3.7	6.1	10.3

[1]Plasma samples were pooled from 5 animals for each group.

(5)

A CIRCULATING INHIBITOR OF POST-HEPARIN PLASMA LIPOLYSIS IN THE TYPE IV-V HYPERLIPOPROTEINEMIA INDUCED IN GREEN LYMPHOMA-BEARING HAMSTERS

V. BEAUMONT, M. BERARD and J.L. BEAUMONT

Unité de recherches sur l'Athérosclérose de l'INSERM

Hôpital Henri Mondor, 94010 Créteil, France

Hyperlipidemia, a factor well known to be implicated in atherosclerosis, may be secondary to different physiopathological disorders whose mechanisms are not always clear. For this reason, it is of interest to study the major hypertriglyceridemia following subcutaneous transplantation of Greene lymphoblastic lymphoma in golden hamsters (1,2), because it may be related to the immunological state associated with the tumor growth, and provide an experimental model for those hyperlipoproteinemias in which immunological mechanisms are implicated (3,4,5).

MATERIAL AND METHODS

Greene tumor is maintained by serial transplantations in golden hamsters. For each study, fragments of tumor from a donor are inserted through a large trocar, in the flanks of recipients of the same age and breeding.

Serum cholesterol and triglyceride determinations were made in a group of 100 grafted male hamsters and 50 controls, and electrophoretic patterns were determined according to Noble.

In vivo fat tolerance studies were performed in grafted animals and controls after a I ^{131}-labeled triolein test diet according to Posner. Measures of radioactivity in plasma samples were done 2,3 and 6 hours after the test diet.

Post-heparin lipase activity (PHLA) was studied according to the technic of Schotz et al., in which is measured the power of a post-heparin plasma (PHP) to release labeled fatty acids from a purified lipidic substrate consisting of a mixture of C^{14}-triolein, C^{12} triolein, Tris buffer and normal hamster serum in adequate amounts. The lipase activity is estimated from the measures of radioactivity 10, 20 and 30 minutes after the incubation of PHP and substrate.

The possibility that a serum factor, present in tumor bearing hamsters, may inhibit the lipolysis of the above purified lipidic substrate induced by PHP from normal hamsters was studied in vitro. Serum and several serum fractions : chylomicra, serum without chylomicra, fractions from $SO^4(NH^4)_2$ precipitated serum, were tested. Biochemical and immunochemical methods were applied to isolation, purification and identification of an active fraction present in chylomicra. The same procedures were applied to control and grafted animals, and the results were compared.

RESULTS

The hyperlipidemia is constant.It is related to the tumor growth, begins about 5 to 10 days after transplantation and reaches a maximum at the 15th day. It subsides when the tumor is excised.

It is characterized by serum milkiness, moderate increase of serum cholesterol (177 $\pm$ 55 mg p.100 ml for controls, 226 $\pm$ 97 mg p.100 ml for grafted ; $p < 0.01$), major hypertriglyceridemia (185 $\pm$ 89 mg p.100 ml for controls 1 819 $\pm$ 2 539 mg p.100 ml for grafted ; $p < 0.001$). Chylomicra and VLDL are increased giving a type IV or V pattern.

In vivo fat tolerance studies performed in 5 grafted and 4 controls indicate an impairment of post-prandial triglyceride clearance in tumor-bearing animals, in which peaks of labeled triglyceride are higher and delayed. Mean values of radio-activity are statistically different ($p < 0.001$) 3 and 6 hours after test diet.

Post-heparin lipase activity (PHLA) is greatly decreased (6) in tumor bearing hamsters, as compared to controls. In controls, determination of labeled fatty acids released after 10, 20 and 30mn incubation of lipidic substrate with PHP, was respectively 7, 16 and 33 p. 100. For grafted, it was only 1, 4 and 6 p.100 ($p < 0.001$ for each compared measures).

Determination 5, 10, 15 and 20 days after transplantation indicate that triglyceridemia increases up to the 15th day, while PHLA decreases inversely. There is an inverse correlation between triglyceride level and PHLA ($r = 0.63$; $p < 0.01$)

In vitro, serum from tumor-bearing hamsters, when added to the lipidic labeled substrate,is able to inhibit the lipolysis induced by a PHP from normal hamsters. With 30 µg of protein, the inhibition is 65 p.100.

The inhibiting activity is present in the chylomicra and VLDL (40%) and not in serum without chylomicra (11%), nor in supernatant (4%) or precipitate (0%) from serum treated by 40% $SO^4(NH^4)_2$. An active substance can be extracted from chylomicra of lymphoma-bearing hamsters, to which it is bound, by 2 successive intervent dilution chromatography on DEAE Sephadex A 25 with appropriate fronts.Its inhibiting activity is 54%. There is no activity in the homologous fraction from normal hamsters.

Immunological identification of this substance reveals 2 arcs with hamster gamma-globulin antiserum, instead of one in controls. The possibility of an immunoglobulin with inhibiting lipolytic activity is under study.

REFERENCES

1. ALBRINK,N.S. & ALBRINK M.J. - The hyperlipidemia of Greene lymphoma-bearing hamsters. YALE J. BIOL. MED., 1971,43,288

2. BEAUMONT V. & BEAUMONT J.L. - Hyperlipidemia and tumors : the hyperlipidemia of lymphoma bearing hamsters. BIOMEDICINE,1974,20,68

3. BEAUMONT J.L. - Autoimmune hyperlipidemia : an atherogenic metabolic disease of immune origin. EUROP. J. CLIN. BIOL. RES., 1970, 15,1037

4. BEAUMONT J.L. & LEMORT N. - Les immunoglobulines anti-héparine. Un facteur de thromboses, d'hyperlipidémies et d'athérosclérose. PATH. BIOL., 1974, 22,67

5. GLUECK H.I., MacKENZIE M. & GLUECK C.J. - Crystalline IgG protein in multiple myeloma : identification effects on coagulation and on lipoprotein metabolism. J. LAB. CLIN. MED., 1972,79,731

6. BEAUMONT V., BERARD M,BOISNIER C. & BEAUMONT J.L. - Hyperlipidémie et tumeurs : l'activité lipasique post-héparine du hamster porteur de lymphome malin. C.R. ACAD. SCI. PARIS, D., 280:665, 1975

CHAPTER 11
EXPERIMENTAL HYPERCHOLESTEROLEMIA

(1)

TURNOVER OF CHOLESTEROL IN AORTA OF RABBITS PREVIOUSLY FED A CHOLESTEROL-ENRICHED DIET

Steen Stender

Department of Clinical Chemistry A

Rigshospitalet, University Hospital,
Copenhagen, Denmark

When cholesterol addition to the diet of rabbits is discontinued, there is general agreement about the ability of the rabbits to eliminate cholesterol accumulated in liver and serum. More confusion exists on the fate of cholesterol accumulated in the arteries (1,2).

Fifty-four rabbits of the same strain, sex and age were fed a cholesterol-enriched diet for 8 weeks. At this time the cholesterol-enrichment was discontinued and the rabbits were fed ordinary stock diet for the next 32 weeks. One third of the animals were killed immediately after the 8 weeks of cholesterol-feeding. One third were killed 16 weeks later, when serum cholesterol had normalized. The last third were killed after a further 16 weeks. The content of total cholesterol in serum, liver and inner aorta was determined. The results are shown in Fig. 1. It should be emphasized, that the accumulation of cholesterol in inner aorta continued following discontinuation of cholesterol addition to the diet in spite of a concomitant 20-fold decrease in serum cholesterol concentration. No further increase in concentration of cholesterol in inner aorta was observed during the final 16 weeks when a normal serum cholesterol was maintained.

Whether or not the cholesterol in inner aorta in week 40 was the same as that already present in week 24 was further investigated. The same amount of ^{3}H-cholesterol was injected intravenously to all the rabbits in week 5, thus making it possible to trace at a later time the fate of the cholesterol which had accumulated in the aorta during the hypercholesterolæmia. The average amount of ^{3}H-cholesterol in inner aorta of each of the 3 different groups of rabbits are given in Fig. 2 (open columns). It should be

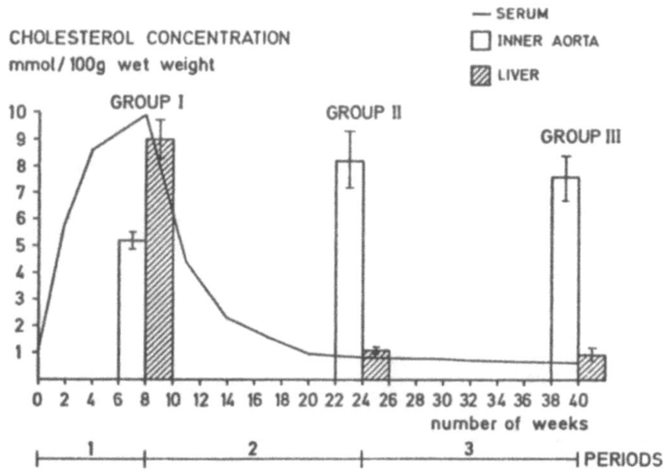

Fig. 1. Concentration of cholesterol in serum, liver and inner aorta of rabbits fed a cholesterol-enriched diet for 8 weeks followed by 32 weeks on a diet without cholesterol addition. The units for serum cholesterol concentration are not indicated. The maximum level obtained in week 8 was 50 mmol/l serum.

noticed how a significant reduction in labeled cholesterol took place at the same time as no net change in cold cholesterol was observed. This suggests that a substantial fraction of cholesterol accumulated by inner aorta during the first 24 hypercholesterolemic weeks exchanged with tritiated serum cholesterol with lower specific activity during the last 16 normocholesterolemic weeks. That the efflux of aortic cholesterol in this period also included some of the cholesterol accumulated in inner aorta from week 19 to week 24 was suggested by the use of ^{14}C-cholesterol intravenously injected at week 19 in 2 subgroups of the animals killed at week 24 and week 40 respectively. Fig. 2 (dotted columns) shows a decrease in the amount of ^{14}C-cholesterol in inner aorta.

Since a measurable efflux of cholesterol from inner aorta has taken place, but no change in amount of aortic cholesterol was observed during the same time, an influx of cholesterol during the normocholesterolemic period has to be postulated.

The entry of ^{14}C-cholesterol from serum into inner aorta during the last 3 days before killing was measured in a subgroup of hypercholesterolemic rabbits at week 8 and in a subgroup of normocholesterolemic rabbits 16 weeks later (3) (Table 1). It is

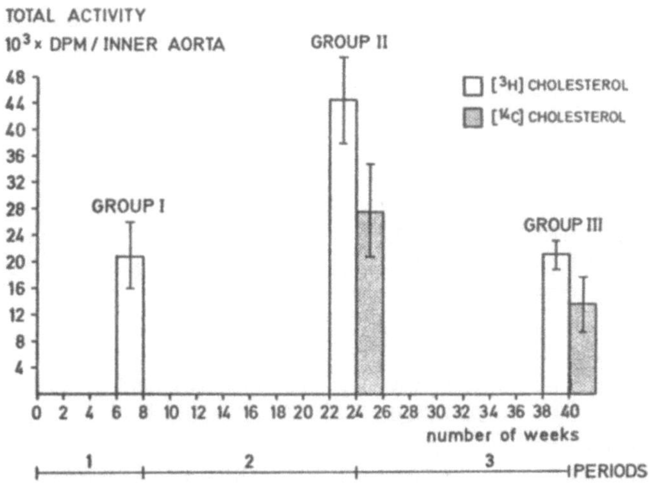

Fig. 2. The total activity in inner aorta of ^{3}H- and ^{14}C-cholesterol intravenously injected in week 5 and week 19 respectively.

	Week 8 n = 10	Week 24 n = 6
Mean serum level during the 3 day period mmol/l	40.4 ± 2.0	2.3 ± 0.3
Calculated influx of serum cholesterol into inner aorta µmol/day	0.83 ± 0.12	0.22 ± 0.05

Table 1. Influx of labeled serum cholesterol into the inner aorta of cholesterol-fed and previously cholesterol-fed rabbits.

observed how the aortic affinity to labeled cholesterol in serum did not decrease in proportion to the level of serum cholesterol.

It is therefore concluded that although a reduction in serum cholesterol caused an efflux of cholesterol previously accumulated in aorta, the effect of this efflux is minimized due to an enhanced entry of serum cholesterol into the inner aorta, which had previously experienced a hypercholesterolæmia.

REFERENCES

1. Adams, C.W.M., Morgan, R.S. & Bayliss, O.B.: Atherosclerosis, 1973, 18, 429.
2. Bortz, W.M.: Circulation Research, 1968, 22, 135.
3. Campbell, D.J., Day, A.J., Skinner, S.L. & Tume, T.K.: Atherosclerosis, 1973, 18, 301.

(2)

TURNOVER AND AORTIC UPTAKE OF VERY LOW DENSITY LIPOPROTEINS (VLDL) FROM HYPERCHOLESTEREMIC RABBITS: EFFECT OF METFORMIN

Cesare R. Sirtori, L. Innocenti, P.G. Grigolato and J. Rodriguez
Center E. Grossi Paloetti for the Study of Metabolic Diseases and Hyperlipidemias, and Institute of Morbid Anatomy
University of Milan, Milan, Italy

Turnover of ^{125}I-labelled very low density lipoproteins (VLDL) from hypercholesteremic (HC) rabbits, is markedly slower than that of VLDL from control rabbits. $T\frac{1}{2}$ of the two lipoproteins, in the log-normal phase, is, respectively, of 22 hours, and of 16 hrs (1). Conversion of VLDL into low density lipoproteins (LDL), and high density lipoproteins (HDL) is very rapid and almost complete in the case of normal VLDL, while HC-VLDL is very slowly converted, and, up to 48 hrs after the injection, over 60% of the radioactivity remains in the VLDL fraction. These findings, i.e. a prolonged log-normal phase, and an inefficient conversion to lipoproteins of the higher density, can be demonstrated also when labelled VLDL from HC rabbits are injected into normal recipients.

These findings are probably related to structural alterations of the HC-VLDL. By examining its lipid and protein composition we noted that HC-VLDL, compared to normal VLDL, has a 12-fold increase of cholesterol esters (63.10 vs 5.14%), with a corresponding decrease of protein (8.10 vs 18.50), and that sphingomyelin concentration is markedly higher (21.58 vs 6.68), phosphatidylcholine/sphingomyelin ratio being 2.89 as compared to 11.14 in control VLDL. Moreover, 18:1 concentration in cholesterol esters is 26.1% in control VLDL, while it rises to 47.5 in HC-VLDL, 18:2 concentration being similar in the two lipoproteins (2). Apoprotein composition shows an increased concentration of R2 and R3 peptides (3), which have been shown to be rich in arginine, and to correspond to the arg-rich peptides in human type III disease and hypothyroidism.

Metformin, a biguanide drug in clinical use for the treatment of maturity onset diabetes, has been shown to markedly reduce atherosclerosis in cholesterol-fed rabbits, while only moderately influencing serum lipid levels (4). We examined the plasma lipoprotein composition and turnover of New Zealand rabbits fed cholesterol (2 g/day), with or without metformin (135 mg/kg/day mixed with the diet and divided into two daily administrations), for a period of 4 weeks.

Lipoproteins from control rabbits, HC, and HC who had received metformin (HC+Met), were also analyzed for their affinity to the aortic lipoprotein complexing factor (ALCF) (5) isolated usually from the thoracic aorta of HC rabbits with initial atheromatosis (in these ALCF, although not structurally different from that of control animals, can be recovered in larger amounts). The different lipoproteins were incubated with the ALCF and cholesterol was determined after a brief ultracentrifugation in the insoluble pellet.

Metformin administration only slightly modified cholesterol induced hyperlipidemia. In the HC group cholesterol was 1403 $\pm$ 148 mg/dl vs 978 $\pm$ 45 in the HC+Met groups. Triglyceride and glucose levels did not differ in the two groups. There was a marked decrease of aortic and liver lipids in the group given metformin, similarly to that reported by Agid (4).

Composition of VLDL differed markedly in the two groups. Protein concentration was increased (HC 8.1%; HC+Met 20.7%), with a decrease of cholesterol esters (HC 63.1%; HC+Met 36.7%). Sphingomyelin content was decreased in the HC+Met group, with a correspondent increase of phosphatidylethanolamine and phosphatidylinositol. Apoprotein analysis demonstrated a marked decrease of the concentration of R2 and R3 peptides (B peptides), with a concomitant increase of C peptides.

Turnover of VLDL of the HC+Met group was markedly accelerated as compared to HC VLDL, and also to control lipoprotein. In the log-normal phase, $t_{\frac{1}{2}}$ of VLDL from the HC+Met group was 11 hrs, both when injected into the same donor animals, and into controls. We also observed that uptake of radioactivity in the aorta, 1 and 2 hours after injection of the labelled lipoproteins, was significantly lower with the HC+Met VLDL than with HC and also with control lipoprotein. In particular, 2 hr after injection into control rabbits, uptake was 4.0 ± 0.2 (% of the injected dose/g) 10^2 with control VLDL, 7.9 ± 0.3 with HC VLDL, and 1.2 ± 0.2 with VLDL from the HC+Met group.

Affinity with ALCF is significantly lower with both VLDL and LDL taken from metformin treated animals. Data are reported in Table 1.

Table 1

Insoluble complexes between aortic complexing factor and different plasma lipoproteins

Lipoproteins	Chol. in complex[+] ($\bar{X}$ ± SEM)	No.of Expt
A) CONTROL		
VLDL	0	(5)
LDL	11.2 ± 4.7	(5)
B) HC GROUP		
VLDL	461 ± 102	(7)
LDL	583 ± 98	(7)
C) HC+MET GROUP		
VLDL	201 ± 25	(7)
LDL	376 ± 31	(7)

[+] µg of cholesterol/mg of aortic protein

These findings point out a dissociation between hyperlipidemia and atherosclerosis in rabbits fed cholesterol and metformin.

References

1) Rodriguez J., Ghiselli G.C., Catapano A. and Sirtori C.R., Atherosclerosis, 1975, in press

2) Rodriguez J., Ghiselli G.C., Torreggiani D. and Sirtori C.R., Atherosclerosis, 1975, in press

3) Shore V.G., Shore B. and Hart R.G., Biochemistry, 13, 1579 (1975)

4) Agid R., Path. Biol. 19, 727 (1971)

5) Camejo G., Lopez A., Vegas A. and Paoli A., Atherosclerosis, 21, 77 (1975)

(3)

INCREASED OXYGEN CONSUMPTION IN CHOLESTEROL-FED RABBITS

Philip D. Henry, M.D.

Cardiovascular Division
Washington University School of Medicine
660 South Euclid Avenue
St. Louis, Missouri, U.S.A.

Aortic walls from animals with diet-induced atherosclerosis have increased oxidative capacities for various substrates (1-3) and mitochondria isolated from atherosclerotic rabbit aortae have increased respiratory rates (4). Atherogenic diets produce multiple systemic disturbances and metabolic changes in the wall of atherosclerotic arteries have been shown to occur in other organs (5-7). As atherosclerosis of the coronary arteries may critically limit the oxygen supply of the heart it would appear important to determine whether oxidative metabolism and oxygen requirements of the myocardium are increased under dietary conditions that promote atherogenesis. To explore whether atherosclerosis induced by a high cholesterol diet is associated with an increase in systemic or myocardial oxidative metabolism, the basal oxygen consumption of cholesterol-fed rabbits and the oxygen uptake of the isolated hearts from these animals were measured.

Male New Zealand rabbits weighing 2.2 to 2.7 kg were fed 2% cholesterol Purina pellets or Standard Purina pellets. After a period of 3 months the diet of the cholesterol-fed animals was changed to Standard pellets. Experiments were started 2 months after removal of the cholesterol from the diet. Body weight, hematocrit, serum cholesterol and serum free fatty acid concentrations in control and cholesterol-fed rabbits immediately after, 2 months after, and 6 months after the period of cholesterol feeding are shown in Table I. After 2 months total body oxygen consumption under basal conditions (VO_2) was significantly increased in cholesterol-fed rabbits, averaging 506 ± 9 ml $(kg \cdot hr)^{-1}$ (mean$\pm$S.E., n=15) compared to 465 ± 3 ml $(kg \cdot hr)^{-1}$ in the control animals (n=15, P<0.001). Serial measurements in cholesterol-fed rabbits revealed a parallel decline in VO_2 and serum cholesterol after the period of cholesterol feeding,

	BODY WEIGHT Grams			HEMATOCRIT per cent			SERUM CHOLESTEROL mg/100 ml			SERUM FREE FATTY ACID mg/100 ml		
	a	b	c	a	b	c	a	b	c	a	b	c
I	3385 ±110 (12)	3711 ±166 (12)	3910 ±180 (12)	41.5±0.6 (20)	42.0±0.5 (12)	41.0±0.5 (12)	48±8 (20)	58± 10 (12)	52±8 (14)	5.5±0.5 (20)	5.9±0.6 (10)	5.6±0.5 (14)
II	2850 ±196 (12)	3594 ±170 (12)	3860 ±178 (12)	30.1±1.0 (12)	39.0±0.9 (12)	40.0±0.8 (12)	1618 ±128 (10)	603 ±83 (10)	63±12 (7)	25±6 (10)	8.9±1.9 (10)	5.8±0.7 (7)
P	<.05	>.05	>.05	<.001	>.05	>.05	<.001	<.001	>.05	<.001	>.05	>.05

I Control Animals

II Cholesterol-fed Animals

Values are mean±S.E.; numbers in parentheses indicate the number of animals studied

a: at the end of cholesterol feeding
b: two months after cholesterol feeding
c: six months after cholesterol feeding

Table I

values returning in each animal concomitantly to control levels within $3\frac{1}{2}$ to 5 months. Difference in VO_2 between the 2 groups could not be attributed to differences in body weight, a determinant of VO_2 in small animals (Table I). Nor could they be ascribed to the cholesterol-induced anemia from which the animals had completely recovered (Table I). Cholesterol-fed and control animals exhibited similar rectal temperatures, heart rates, arterial pressures and PBI values throughout the experimental period. The increased VO_2 did not correlate with increases in the plasma free acid concentrations (Table I).

Isolated hearts from hypercholesterolemic animals 2 months after removal of cholesterol from the diet (n=12) and from normal controls (n=12) were perfused with Krebs buffer containing 5 mM glucose. Myocardial oxygen uptake of the empty beating hearts exhibited similar spontaneous heart rates (183 ± 12 beats/min) and myocardial oxygen consumptions (205 ± 15 μl (g myocardial protein·min)$^{-1}$).

Thus, hypercholesterolemia may be associated with a generalized hypermetabolic state, but does not appear to increase myocardial O_2 uptake under controlled conditions.

REFERENCES

1. Loomeijer, F.J. and Ostendorf, J.P.: Oxygen consumption of the thoracic aorta of normal and hypercholesterolemic rats. Circ. Res., 7:466, 1959.
2. Maier, N. and Haimovici, H.: Oxidative capacity of atherosclerotic tissue of rabbit and dog, with special reference to succinic dehydrogenase and cytochrome oxidase. Circ. Res., 16:65, 1965.
3. Scott, R.F., Morrison, E.S. and Kroms, M.: Aortic respiration and glycolysis in the preproliferative phase of diet-induced atherosclerosis in swine. J. Atheroscler. Res., 9:5, 1969.
4. Whereat, A.F.: Fatty acid synthesis in cell-free system from rabbit aorta. J. Lipid Res., 7:671, 1966.
5. Non-atherosclerotic effects of cholesterol. Nutrition Rev., 20:55, 1962.
6. Hauss, W.H., Junge-Hulsing, G. and Hollander, H.J.: Changes in metabolism of connective tissue associated with aging and arterio- or atherosclerosis. J. Atheroscler. Res., 2:50, 1962.
7. Jacotot, B. and Beaumont, J.L.: Le renouvellement du cholesterol de l'aorte et des granulomes souscutanés chez le rat. Arch. Mal. Coeur., Supple. 1:24, 1969.

(4)

EFFECTS OF DIETARY PROTEINS AND AMINO ACIDS ON THE PLASMA CHOLESTEROL CONCENTRATIONS OF RABBITS FED CHOLESTEROL-FREE DIETS

M. W. Huff, R. M. G. Hamilton and K. K. Carroll[1]

Department of Biochemistry
University of Western Ontario
London, Ontario, Canada

Hypercholesterolemia and atherosclerosis develop in rabbits on cholesterol-free, semisynthetic diets, but not on commercial feed (1). Our studies have shown that dietary protein is important in this response. Proteins from animal sources gave higher plasma cholesterol levels than proteins from vegetable sources (2). The present experiments were designed to investigate reasons for this difference.

Groups of six New Zealand White rabbits of approximately 1 to 1.2 kg in weight were fed experimental diets for 28 days. The composition of the basic low fat diet has been described previously (2). Casein and soy protein isolate were used in these studies because they are readily available in purified form.

Diets containing 27% by weight of casein or soy protein isolate gave cholesterol concentrations of 210 and 70 mg/dl respectively (Fig. 1). Increasing the amount of protein to 54% gave levels of 370 and 60 mg/dl. A diet containing 27% of a 1:1 mixture of casein and soy protein isolate produced a result similar to that obtained with the diet containing soy protein isolate alone.

Average daily weight gains are shown in Fig. 1. Doubling the amount of casein reduced the weight gain relative to other diets. This poor growth performance can be attributed to an excess of certain amino acids compared to estimated requirements. Adamson and Fisher (3) found that a moderate excess of lysine, isoleucine, phenylalanine or threonine depressed food intake and weight gain.

[1] Research Associate of the Medical Research Council of Canada.

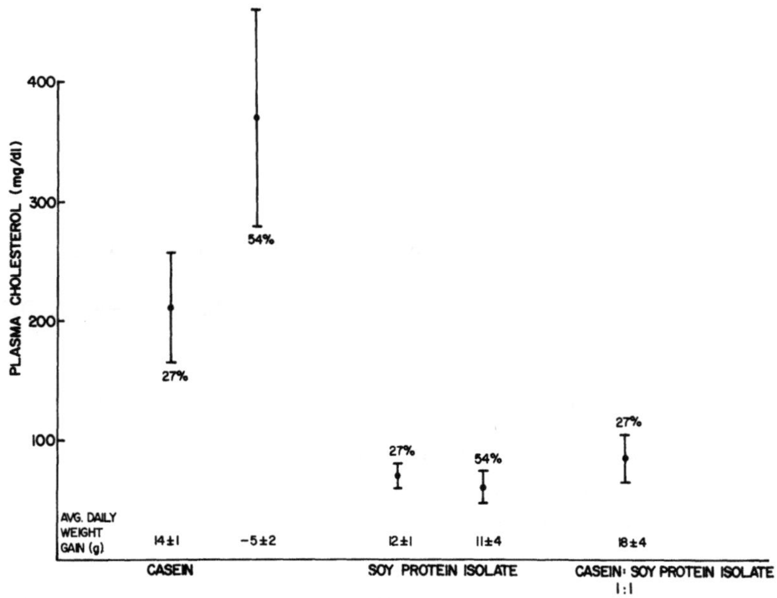

Fig. 1. Plasma cholesterol levels of rabbits fed diets containing different amounts of casein or soy protein isolate. The percentages represent the amount of protein in the basic diet. Proteins fed at the 54% level were added at the expense of carbohydrate. Results expressed as the mean ± S.E.M.

Further experiments were carried out to determine whether the observed differential in plasma cholesterol concentrations was related to amino acid composition (Fig. 2). Mixtures of amino acids corresponding to casein and soy protein isolate gave cholesterol levels of 210 and 125 mg/dl respectively ($P < 0.1$). A greater differential ($P < 0.01$) was observed when the amounts of essential amino acids in these mixtures were reduced by half and non-essential amino acids increased proportionately. The mixture corresponding to soy protein with reduced essential amino acids gave poor growth, probably due to essential amino acid deficiency.

An attempt was made to reverse the observed effects of casein and soy protein isolate by adding amino acids to casein (approx. 1:1) to give a mixture equivalent in amino acid composition to soy protein isolate and by adding amino acids to soy protein isolate to give a mixture corresponding to casein. These two diets gave plasma cholesterol concentrations of 185 and 95 mg/dl respectively (Fig. 2). It appears that the intact protein component of each mixture has an over-riding effect.

These studies suggest that the amino acid composition of the diet influences the plasma cholesterol concentrations of rabbits, but the observed differences in cholesterol levels cannot be explained on the basis of amino acid composition alone. Other factors

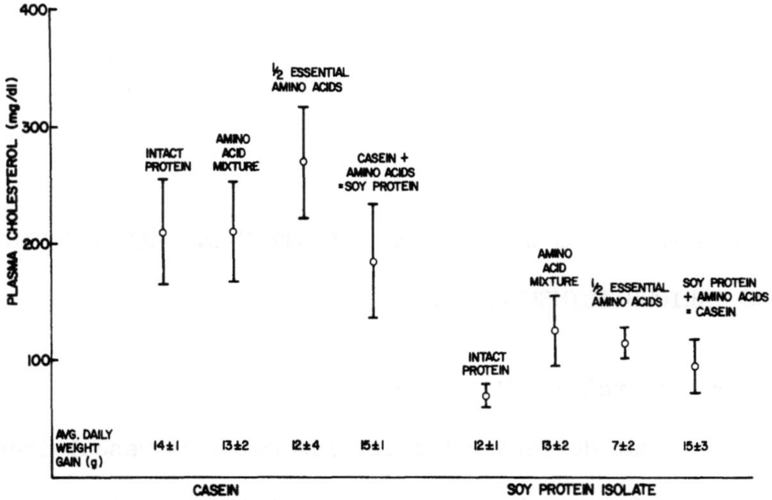

Fig. 2. Plasma cholesterol levels of rabbits fed casein and soy protein isolate or corresponding amino acid mixtures. The intact proteins accounted for 27% of the basic diet and the amino acid mixtures 25%. Results expressed as the mean ± S.E.M.

such as rates of digestion and absorption of the proteins, or the presence of other components in the protein preparations may be involved.

ACKNOWLEDGEMENTS

This work was supported by the Ontario Heart Foundation and the Medical Research Council of Canada. Technical assistance by L. McPhee and R. Rasmussen is gratefully acknowledged. The soy protein isolate (Promine-R) was generously supplied by Dr. E. W. Meyer, Central Soya, Chemurgy Div., Chicago, Ill.

REFERENCES

1. Kritchevsky, D. Experimental atherosclerosis in rabbits fed cholesterol-free diets. J. Atheroscler. Res. 4: 103, 1964.

2. Carroll, K. K., Hamilton, R.M.G. Effects of dietary protein and carbohydrate on plasma cholesterol levels in relation to atherosclerosis. J. Food Sci. 40: 18, 1975.

3. Adamson, I. and Fisher, H. Amino acid requirement of the growing rabbit: An estimate of quantitative needs. J. Nutr. 103: 1306, 1973.

(5)

SERUM AND AORTIC LIPIDS OF RATS FED LONG-TERM EQUILIBRATE DIETS CONTAINING VARIOUS ALIMENTARY FATS

B. Jacotot and M. Claire

Institut de recherches sur les maladies vasculaires

Hopital Henri Mondor, 94010 Creteil, France

In the purpose to study the effect of dietary fats on serum and arterial lipids, male Sprague-Dawley rats are fed during one year with equilibrate diets containing 12 p.100 of one of the following fats: butter, sunflower oil, rapeseed oil, soybean oil, hydrogenated soybean oil, palm oil, canbra oil and arachid oil. Total serum cholesterol is lower in arachid, sunflower and butter groups and higher in palm and hydrogenated soybean groups ($F = 4,41$; $p<0,01$); serum cholesterol esters are lower in arachid, sunflower and soybean groups, but higher in palm and hydrogenated soybean groups ($F = 4,20$; $p<0,01$). Serum triglycerides are lower in sunflower and arachid groups and higher in butter and palm groups ($F = 7,96$; $p<0,01$). There is a positive and significant correlation between serum cholesterol and phospholipids in various groups.

In aortas, free cholesterol levels are the same in different groups, but ester cholesterol levels increase in the following range: canbra, butter, arachid, palm, sunflower, rapeseed, hydrogenated soybean and soybean ($F = 4,73$; $p<0,01$). There is a significant correlation between aorta cholesterol esters and the ratio: $\frac{18:2}{18:0+18:1}$ of the dietary fat ($r = 0,69$; $p<0,001$).

CHAPTER 12

LIPID COMPOSITION AND METABOLISM IN MAN

(1)

THE CHARACTERISTICS OF HUMAN PLASMA LIPOPROTEIN METABOLISM: INFLUENCE OF LOW CALORIC DIET ON HYPERLIPIDEMIA

Seiki Nanbu, Seiichiro Yamasaki, Noboru Kimura, Hiroo Gohda, Masato Ageta, Sumito Kariya, and Takahiko Kamogawa,
The 3rd Department of Internal Medicine, Kurume University School of Medicine,
67 Asahi-machi, Kurume-shi, FUKUOKA, Japan

Diet has a powerful effect on plasma cholesterol concentration; however, cholesterol levels often vary among individual cases on the same diet. Recently we have reported that hypercholesterolemia, which could not be reduced by the low calorie-diet intake, may be related to subclinical hypothyroidism. We found a reciprocal relation between the change of plasma cholesterol and that of very low density lipoprotein (VLDL)-triglyceride in hypercholesterolemia which was reduced by diet (1,2).

In the present study, hyperlipidemia in which the plasma cholesterol was reduced by the diet, has been divided into three groups according to VLDL-triglyceride concentration (for clarifying the characteristics of plasma lipoproteins in hyperlipidemia).

MATERIAL AND METHOD

The fifty-two hospitalized subjects, who suffered from hypertension, ischemic heart disease, and simple obesity, consumed daily a formula diet (1000 calories containing 130-140 gr. of carbohydrate and 80 gr. of protein) for four weeks. Eleven subjects with subclinical hypothyroid function were subsequently treated with 0.6-0.9 gr/day of iodocasein.

Blood samples were drawn (in the morning after an overnight fast) at the beginning of the diet-therapy and during the fourth week of the diet- and iodocasein- therapy. Plasma lipoprotein was determined by preparative ultracentrifugation at densities 1.006, 1.063 and 1.21. The concentrations of total cholesterol (TCh), free cholesterol (FC), triglyceride (TG), and protein were determined in VLDL, the low density lipoprotein (LDL), and the high density lipoprotein (HDL).

The criteria used for classifying hyperlipidemia were plasma

TCh and TG, VLDL-TG, and LDL-TCh above 200, and 100, or 180, and 600 mg/100ml, respectively. The Control group consisted of 19 normolipidemic subjects. The 22 hyperlipidemic subjects, whose plasma TCh concentration was reduced more than 15 mg/100ml by the diet, has been divided into three groups according to the VLDL-TG level during pretreatment period: under 180, between 180 to 260, and over 260 mg/100ml. Plasma TCh of the 11 hyperlipidemic subjects were not reduced by the diet.

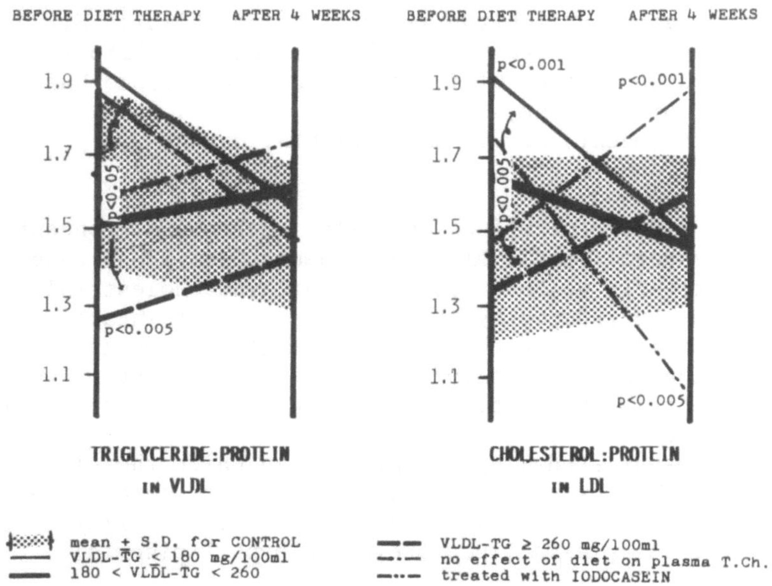

Figure 1. Effect of the Diet on Relative Value of Lipids to Protein in Lipoprotein

RESULTS AND DISCUSSION

The Plasma TCh level before treatment was similar in all five groups and also the mean difference of TCh reduced by the diet was the same level in three groups with different VLDL-TG levels. VLDL-TG in the group with VLDL-TG≤180 mg/100 ml increased with the diet (mean difference + 18 mg/100 ml). On the other hand, VLDL-TG in the two groups with 180<VLDL-TG<260 and VLDL-TG≥260, and in the group with plasma TCh unchanged by the diet were significantly decreased

(45, 161, and 160 mg/100ml of mean difference, respectively), whereas within iodocasein-treated group there was no significant change in VLDL-TG.

These results suggest that calories from dietary carbohydrate are a major determinant of VLDL-TG concentration. Additionally, increased VLDL-TG levels might play a role inhibiting disappearance of plasma cholesterol. This possibility was shown by reciprocal relation between the change of plasma TCh and the change of VLDL-TG as following formulas; $Y=-0.66X-79 (p<0.05)$ for the group with $180<$VLDL-TG<260, $Y=-0.23-99 (p<0.01)$ for the group VLDL-TG≥ 260 and the iodocasein-treated group. Y; decreased level of plasma TCh (Δmg/100ml), X; changed level of VLDL-TG(Δmg/100ml).

To clarify the mechanism of inhibitory effect of VLDL-TG on plasma TCh we determined VLDL-FC. In the group with VLDL-TG$\leq$180 mg/100ml, the percentage of VLDL-FC before treatment was 27.9%, whereas values for the groups with $180<$VLDL-TG<260 and VLDL-TG$\geq$260 mg/100ml were 48.2 and 47.6%, respectively. Additionally, these levels became similar after the diet therapy. As shown in the results, it is suggested that esterification of FC in VLDL was more difficult when VLDL-TG was increased; moreover, the decreased formation of cholesterol-ester might lead to abnormal catabolism of VLDL to LDL.

Table 1. Effects of the Diet and Iodocasein on LDL-Lipids

Group	Total Cholesterol initial level #	Total Cholesterol mean change	Triglyceride initial level#	Triglyceride mean change
VLDL-TG≤180mg/100ml	657(505-782)	-187*	117(89-139)	-6
180<VLDL-TG<260	628(504-730)	-181*	138(101-166)	-39*
VLDL-TG≥260mg/100ml	450(272-684)	-70	128(80-175)	-26
non-effect of the diet	528(382-725)	+359*	143(72-323)	-2
treated with Iodocasein	732(459-942)	-405*	163(113-220)	-58*

mean(range) mg/100ml, * statistically significant.

As shown in Figure 1,TG:protein ratio in VLDL of the group with VLDL-TG$\geq$260 mg/100ml was significantly lower than in the control group or the group with VLDL-TG$\leq$180 mg/100ml, $p<0.005$ or 0.05, respectively. On the other hand, the TCh: protein ratio in LDL of the group with VLDL-TG$\leq$180 mg/100ml was significantly higher(than in the control group or the group with VLDL-TG$\geq$260 mg/100ml) $p<0.001$ or <0.05, respectively. These levels became similar after diet therapy. The TCh: protein ratio in LDL of the group with plasma TCh which was unchanged by the diet rose to the pretreatment level of the group with VLDL-TG$\leq$180 mg/100ml by the diet. This increase in LDL was mainly attributable to elevation of TCh in LDL (see Table).

SUMMARY

We have classified hyperlipidemia into three groups according to different levels of VLDL-TG, and postulated the effect of low calorie-diets on plasma TCh are as follows: 1) Low calorie-diets are effective on VLDL-TG in every type of hyperlipidemia, except hyperlipidemia with VLDL-TG under 180 mg/100ml; 2) There was a reciprocal relation between the decreased amount of plasma TCh and the changed VLDL-TG induced by the diet; 3) Catabolism of VLDL was accelerated by an increased esterification of VLDL-FC; 4) In the group with VLDL-TG≤180 mg/100ml, the LDC showed a high level of TCh: protein ration, and in the group with VLDL-TG≥260 mg/100ml, there was to be low level of TG: protein ratio in VLDL: 5) In hyperlipidemia with plasma TCh unchanged by the diet LDL-TCh increased significantly without any increase in LDL protein and LDL-TG.

REFERENCES

1) S. Nanbu et al.: Significance of Plasma Lipids-From Aspect of Plasma lipoprotein, Jap. J. Clin. Patholgoy, 23:168, 1975.

2) S. Nanbu, H. Gohda, and N. Kimura: The Studies of Cholesterol Metabolism-The Effect of Iodocasein and T3-Analogue on Serum Cholesterol and Thyroid Function, Jap. Circ. J., 37:888, 1973.

(2)

FATTY ACID COMPOSITION OF ADIPOSE TISSUE IN PATIENTS WITH MYOCARDIAL INFARCTION COMPARED WITH SUBJECTS FREE OF CORONARY HEART DISEASE

P.D. Lang, M. Degott, J. Vollmar

Klinisches Institut für Herzinfarktforschung an der Medizinischen Universitäts-Klinik,Heidelberg, Germany

The fatty acid composition of adipose tissue is mainly determined by the kind of dietary fat, but may also be related to the incidence of CHD (Insull et al., 1969). In a previous study, we found a negative association between the degree of pathologically graded coronary arteriosclerosis and the stearic and lauric acid content of depot fat (Insull et al., 1968). The present study attempts to substantiate those findings in a clinical study on patients with a uniform diet.

Thirty-four patients with acute myocardial infarction, confirmed by ECG-changes and enzyme studies, and 33 controls, hospitalized for other diseases but free of CHD by clinical and ECG criteria, were selected. Both groups consisted of males only. Patients with diabetes mellitus, endocrine disorders, liver and kidney diseases and clinical conditions known to be accompanied by alterations in blood lipids, were excluded. Body weight changes were confined to ± 5 kg during the preceding 6 months. Subjects deviating from the "normal" customary diet as evaluated by interview, were omitted. Alcohol consumption was limited to 50 g/day.

Blood for the determination of cholesterol and triglycerides was drawn within 24 hours of admission. Skinfold thickness was measured over the triceps and above the left iliac crest. Subcutaneous fat was obtained by needle biopsy from the abdominal wall and the fatty acid composition analyzed by GLC. Both groups differed significantly in age, relative body weight and abdominal skinfold thickness, but not in triceps skinfold thickness, cholesterol and triglycerides, although cholesterol was higher in CHD patients. The composition of adipose tissue fatty acids is shown in Table 1. A statistically significant difference between the groups was observed only in the proportion of stearic acid.

The results of a multivariate discriminant analysis including

Table 1: Fatty Acid Composition of Adipose Tissue in Patients with and without CHD

Fatty Acids		Relative Proportion (%) (Median, 25th and 75th Percentile)		Statistical Analysis of Differences by Wilcoxon-Test
		Patients without CHD (n = 33)	Patients with acute MI (n = 34)	
Lauric	12:0	0.28 (0.22 - 0.39)	0.27 (0.14 - 0.44)	n.s.
Myristic	14:0	2.54 (2.27 - 3.16)	2.61 (2.09 - 3.02)	n.s.
Palmitic	16:0	25.52 (24.03 - 26.67)	26.30 (24.66 - 27.81)	n.s.
Palmitoleic	16:1	4.40 (3.32 - 4.91)	4.81 (3.69 - 5.90)	n.s.
Stearic	18:0	4.13 (3.71 - 4.66)	3.25 (2.93 - 4.03)	significant
Oleic	18:1	52.48 (50.46 - 54.06)	52.33 (50.23 - 54.07)	n.s.
Linoleic	18:2	10.57 (8.76 - 11.47)	9.44 (7.78 - 11.37)	n.s.

n.s. = not significant

age, relative body weight, skinfold measurements and the fatty acid proportions are shown in Table 2. Other than age and the proportion of stearic acid no other parameters contributed significantly to discrimination between the two groups. Age did not correlate with the proportion of stearic acid in either group or in the combined groups.

Table 2: Rank Order of significant Parameters discriminating between Patients with and without CHD

Parameter	Age	>	Stearic Acid (18 : 0)
Sign	positive		negative

Three to seven months after the acute event it was possible to restudy the lipids in 17 patients of the infarction group. Fifteen of these patients had changed to a diet known to lower blood lipids and 3 were additionally on hypolipidaemic drugs. Although there was a statistically significant median weight-lose of 7%, the cholesterol and triglyceride levels had risen considerably (+ 11% and + 42% respectively; not statistically significant). This indicates that the lipid values determined within 24 hours after admission did not reflect the actual values and were therefore not included in the multivariate discriminant analysis.

The results of this investigation are in close accordance with our previous study (Insull et al., 1968). The metabolic basis of the relationship between CHD and the stearic acid content of adipose tissue is not clear at present. In a single subject, the stearic acid proportion does not predict with certainty the presence or absence of CHD. Since in the present study occult CHD in the control group cannot be ruled out, additional studies to investigate the importance of the fatty acid composition of adipose tissue for the detection of CHD are under way.

REFERENCES

Insull, Wm., Jr., P.D. Lang, and B. Hsi: Adipose tissue fatty acids and extent of coronary atherosclerosis, Circulation 38, Suppl. VI (1968), 11.

Insull, Wm., Jr., P.D. Lang, B. P. Hsi, and S. Yoshimura: Studies of arteriosclerosis in Japanese and American men, I. Comparison of fatty acid composition of adipose tissue, J. Clin. Invest. 48 (1969), 1313.

(3)

CHOLESTEROL SYNTHESIS AND UPTAKE BY FAT CELLS IN FAMILIAL HYPERCHOLESTEROLEMIA

Petri T. Kovanen and Esko A. Nikkilä

Third Department of Medicine, University of Helsinki,

Helsinki, Finland

Clinical studies have shown that in patients heterozygous for familial hypercholesterolemia (FH) the absolute rates of turnover of body cholesterol and of plasma LDL are in the normal range, whereas in FH homozygotes they are often enhanced (Lewis and Myant, 1967; Goodman and Noble, 1968; Grundy and Ahrens, 1969; Langer et al., 1972; Simons et al., 1975). Recent studies with human fibroblasts in vitro have demonstrated that cholesterol synthesis in these cells is regulated by the concentration of LDL in the medium, and that the feedback inhibition is insufficient in heterozygotes and defective in homozygotes with FH (Goldstein and Brown, 1974). Accordingly, high levels of LDL in the medium suppress the rate of cholesterol synthesis to normal in heterozygote, but not in homozygote fibroblasts. In the present study we determined the rates of cholesterol synthesis in adipose tissue and the uptake of LDL-cholesterol by fat cells of patients with FH to examine whether the plasma LDL might regulate cholesterogenesis also in vivo.

PATIENT MATERIAL

The study was made in seven FH patients, one of which was homozygous for the abnormal gene. The control group consisted of 25 normocholesterolemic patients undergoing laparotomy for diverse non-malignant abdominal disorders. Clinical data of the patients are given in Table I.

Table 1. Clinical data of controls and patients with FH

Subjects	Age	RBW	Plasma	
			Cholesterol	Triglyceride
		%	mg/100 ml	
Controls	45 ± 13	116 ± 18	228 ± 38	114 ± 45
FH heterozygotes	44 ± 9	124 ± 22	453 ± 36	128 ± 28
FH homozygote	11	90	1100	220

The values are mean ± s.d.

METHODS

Subcutaneous adipose tissue from abdominal wall was removed under local anesthesia (FH patients and one control patient), or under general anesthesia (controls), and the rate of cholesterol synthesis was determined in pieces of adipose tissue (Kovanen et al., 1975). From another specimen of the tissue the fat cells were separated by collagenase treatment. The cells were incubated with rat LDL labeled with ^{14}C-cholesterol according to Goodman and Noble (1968). The rate of cholesterol exchange was calculated from the cellular uptake of labeled cholesterol.

RESULTS

In normocholesterolemic patients the rate of cholesterol synthesis in adipose tissue was inversely correlated with plasma cholesterol level ($r = -0.51$, $p < 0.01$). The rate of cholesterol synthesis in the adipose tissue of heterozygote FH patients did not differ from corresponding value of control subjects (Table II). On the other hand, the cholesterol synthesis in the adipose tissue of the homozygote FH patient was about 15 times higher than in control subjects.

The rate of cholesterol exchange in vitro between heterozygote fat cells and LDL was significantly less ($p < 0.01$) than the exchange between normal cells and LDL. The rate of cholesterol exchange between homozygote fat cells and LDL was even lower being only one-fifth of the corresponding control value.

Table II. Cholesterol synthesis by adipose tissue and cholesterol exchange between LDL and fat cells of normocholesterolemic subjects and of patients with FH

Subjects	N	Cholesterol		
		Synthesis	Exchange	
		ng/g TG/h	μg/g TG/h	(%)
Controls	6	0.74 ± 0.30	50.0 ± 8.5	(100)
FH heterozygotes	6	0.60 ± 0.03	34.2 ± 6.0	(68)
FH homozygote	1	9.24	10.3	(21)

The values are mean ± s.d.

DISCUSSION

The negative correlation between the rate of cholesterol synthesis in adipose tissue and the level of plasma cholesterol suggests that the synthesis is controlled by plasma cholesterol or LDL levels. In patients heterozygous for FH the rate of cholesterol synthesis was in the normal range showing that the hypercholesterolemia was not caused by enhanced synthesis of cholesterol in the adipose tissue. On the other hand, in spite of elevated levels of plasma cholesterol (and LDL) the cholesterol synthesis in heterozygous fat cells was not suppressed to subnormal values. Hence, the feedback control of cholesterol synthesis by plasma LDL was evidently defective as is the case in cultured skin fibroblasts of patients heterozygous for FH.

In the homozygote patient the rate of cholesterol synthesis was much elevated in spite of extremely high levels of plasma cholesterol and LDL. She had previously undergone ileal bypass operation, but her plasma cholesterol level was uninfluenced by this procedure. Thus the excessive production of cholesterol in the adipose tissue was evidently not caused by the operation but was rather due to a complete absence of feedback control of cholesterol synthesis by plasma LDL.

The decreased incorporation of cholesterol from LDL into fat cells of patients with FH indicates that the defect of LDL receptors is present also in at least this type of native cells. However, the possibility cannot be ruled out that the increased amount of plasma LDL present in the patients' plasma had occupied relatively more receptor sites in vivo, and thus less labeled LDL was bound to the cells in vitro.

REFERENCES

Brown, M.S., and Goldstein, J.L., Science 185: 61 (1974)
Goodman, D.S., and Noble, R.P., J.Clin.Invest. 47: 231 (1968)
Grundy, S.M., and Ahrens, E.H.,Jr., J.Lipid Res. 10: 91 (1969)
Kovanen, P.T., Nikkilä, E.A., and Miettinen, T.A., J.Lipid Res. 16: 211 (1975)
Langer, T., Strober, W., and Levy, R.I., J.Clin.Invest. 51: 1528 (1972)
Lewis, B., and Myant, N.B., Clin.Sci. 32: 201 (1967)
Simons, L.A., Reichl, D., Myant, N.B., and Mancini, M., Atherosclerosis 21: 283 (1975)

(4)

EFFECTS OF CALORIC RESTRICTION ON CHOLESTEROL METABOLISM IN HYPERLIPEMIC OBESE SUBJECTS

H.S. Sodhi and B.J. Kudchodkar

Department of Medicine, University of Saskatchewan,

Saskatoon, Saskatchewan, Canada

It has been known for some time that cholesterol synthesis is decreased on caloric restriction and is increased in obesity[1,2]. It was suggested that the extra body fat may be the actual site for additional synthesis of cholesterol in obesity[2], but studies with human adipose tissue indicated that it was not capable of enough cholesterogenesis to account for this observation[3]. Our studies show that cholesterol synthesis is decreased immediately on caloric restriction and much before there is any significant change in the adipose tissue mass suggesting that, as in normal subjects, most of their cholesterol is also synthesized in the liver.

Six obese and hyperlipemic subjects were investigated by cholesterol balance and kinetics of plasma cholesterol. One of the subjects had Type V hyperlipoproteinemia, and the lipoprotein patterns of the others were of Types IIb or IV. During the first 6 to 15 days of control period the diets were designed to maintain body weight, and then the caloric as well as cholesterol intake was reduced by reducing all foods proportionately. Therefore, the percentages of calories derived from proteins, fats and carbohydrates were constant during both the control and experimental periods.

During the first 9 to 12 days of reducing diet, the mean percentage decrease in their body weight was 3.5±1.6%. In the five subjects without hyperchylomicronemia, the associated decrease in plasma triglycerides was 31-52% and in plasma cholesterol it was 9-24%. In the one subject who had Type V hyperlipoproteinemia, the decreases in triglycerides (77%) and in cholesterol (56%) were much greater than in others without hyperchylomicronemia.

The percentage absorption of dietary cholesterol did not change

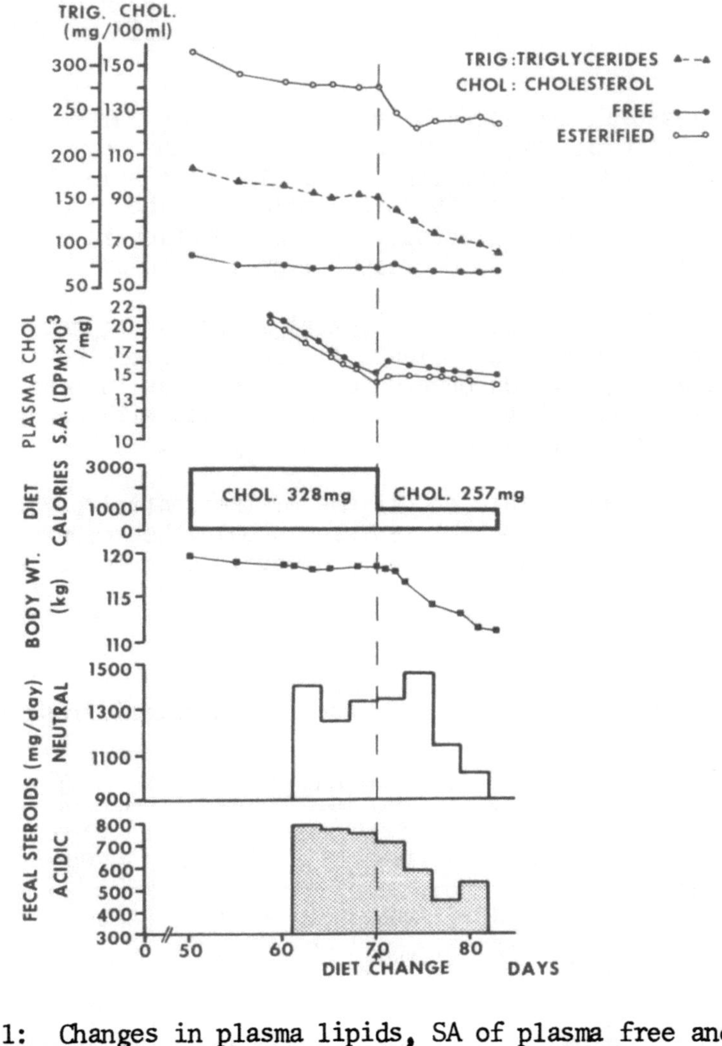

Figure 1: Changes in plasma lipids, SA of plasma free and esterified cholesterol, body weight, and fecal metabolites of endogenous cholesterol on caloric restriction.

on caloric reduction (40.1±2.9% and 42.6±3.2%). However, the actual amounts absorbed per day were reduced from 157-358 mg/day to 110-197 mg/day due to decreased intake.

The fecal excretion of cholesterol and its (intestinal) metabolites showed variable, but modest changes (mean of -11.4%) during the period of caloric restriction (fig. 1). The range of values during control and treatment periods were 520 to 1313 vs 522 to 1240 mg/day.

The decrease in the fecal bile acids was more marked and unlike the fecal cholesterol, the decrease was seen in the very first sample after the change to a reducing diet. The bile acids decreased by 26 to 53% (587 to 938 vs 369 to 566 mg/day). The reduction in deoxycholic acid was much greater than the reduction in lithocholic acid so that their ratio was decreased from 1.62 to 1.17.

Since the fecal excretion of neutral steroids did not decrease as much as that of bile acids (Table 1), the ratio of the neutral to acidic metabolites of endogenous cholesterol was increased on caloric restriction. This may well be associated with changes in the composition of bile making it more lithogenic.

During the steady-state conditions of the control period, the negative balance of cholesterol represents only the amounts of cholesterol synthesized in the body. However, on caloric restric-

Table 1: Changes in cholesterol metabolism on caloric restriction

Subjects	Losses From Plasma Pool (mg/day)	Synthesis + Absorption (mg/day)	Fecal Excretion of Endogenous Cholesterol (mg/day)	Mobilized* From Tissues (mg/day)	Changes in Fecal	
					Neutral Steroids (mg/day)	Bile Acids (mg/day)
1	382	658†	1325	285	-188	-288
2	266	689	1102	147	-176	-191
3	170	726	1209	313	-197	-405
4	275	447	732	10	+2	-201
5	114	731	1696	831	-73	-189
6	94	293	846	459	+106	-74

* Fecal excretion-(synthesis + absorption + losses from plasma pool)

† Calculated using mean % inhibition of the group

tion, losses from tissue and plasma cholesterol pools also enter into this equation. Such data (Table 1) suggested that when the patients were put on reducing diets, approximately 300 mg of tissue cholesterol was mobilized per day. As explained previously[4], the upswing in plasma cholesterol SA seen immediately after the start of caloric restriction also indicated that higher SA tissue cholesterol was acutely mobilized.

The rate of exponential decay in the plasma cholesterol SA was reduced on the reducing diet (Fig. 1). This was primarily due to a decrease in the entry of unlabelled cholesterol (from absorption and synthesis) into the readily miscible pool. Although the amount of dietary cholesterol absorbed was reduced by 38%, the normal negative feedback mechanism on isocaloric diet should have increased synthesis of cholesterol to make up for the reduction in the absorbed cholesterol[5]. Therefore, the SA curve should not change significantly due to reduced cholesterol absorption. The observed significant decrease in the rate of fall therefore reflected a decrease in the synthesis of cholesterol.

REFERENCES

1. Tomkins, G.M., and Chaikoff, I.L., J. Biol. Chem., 196 (1952) 569.
2. Nestel, P.J., Whyte, H.M., and Goodman, D.S., J. Clin. Invest., 48 (1969) 982.
3. Schreibman, P., and Dell, R.B., J. Clin. Invest., 55 (1975) 986.
4. Sodhi, H.S., Kudchodkar, B.J., and Horlick, L., Atherosclerosis, 17 (1973) 1.
5. Sodhi, H.S., Perspect. Biol. Med., 18 (1975) 477.

(5)

RELATIONSHIPS BETWEEN PLASMA LIPOPROTEIN CHOLESTEROL CONCENTRATIONS AND THE POOL SIZE AND METABOLISM OF CHOLESTEROL IN MAN

N.E.Miller, P.J.Nestel and P.Clifton-Bligh

Department of Clinical Science, Australian National University, Canberra, Australia

The plasma concentrations of unesterified and esterified cholesterol within very low density (VLDL), low density (LDL) and high density (HDL) lipoproteins have been examined in relation to cholesterol pool size and metabolism in 5 normal and 10 hyperlipidaemic subjects. Cholesterol metabolism was assessed as faecal endogenous neutral and acidic steroid excretion (14 subjects), a 2-pool model of cholesterol turnover (8 subjects), and in vitro plasma cholesterol esterifying activity (9 subjects).

VLDL total cholesterol (TC) concentration was positively correlated with cholesterol turnover, endogenous neutral steroid excretion, bile acid excretion and the absolute rate of plasma cholesterol esterification. The correlations with cholesterol turnover and neutral steroid excretion, but not that with bile acid excretion, remained significant when these were corrected for their relationships to body weight. LDL TC was negatively correlated with the fractional rate of plasma cholesterol esterification and, in subjects with primary type IIa hyperlipoproteinaemia, also with the rate constant for cholesterol elimination from the rapidly exchanging cholesterol pool. No correlation was found between LDL TC concentration and faecal neutral or acidic steroid excretion. HDL TC concentration was negatively correlated with both the rapidly and slowly exchanging pools of tissue cholesterol, after correction for their relationships to body weight and adiposity (Figure 1). In contrast, cholesterol pool sizes were not correlated with the concentration of VLDL or LDL TC; nor was there any relationship to plasma cholesterol esterifying activity. No correlation was found between the relative proportions of unesterified and esterified cholesterol within any lipoprotein fraction and either the pool size or metabolism of cholesterol.

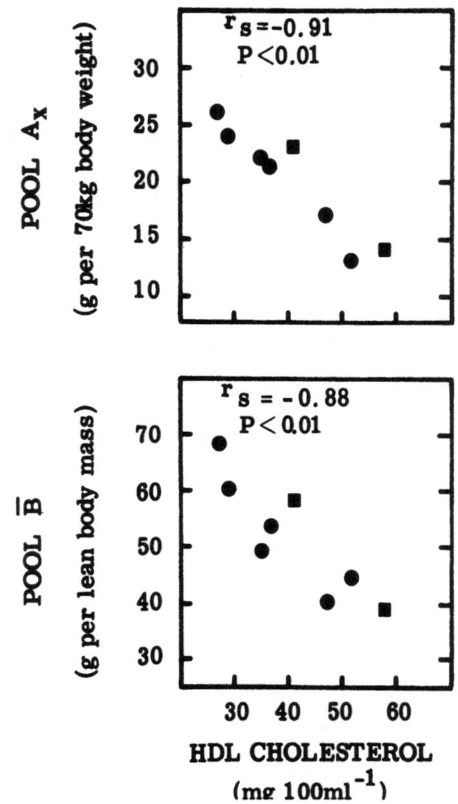

Figure 1 Relationships between HDL cholesterol concentration and body cholesterol pool sizes in eight subjects. Pool A_X, rapidly exchanging cholesterol pool, excluding plasma component; Pool $\bar{B}$, mean of minimum and maximum estimates of slowly exchanging pool; ● , males; ■ , females; r_s = Spearman rank correlation coefficient.

These findings accord with previous reports of enhanced cholesterol metabolism in subjects with elevated VLDL concentrations[1,2] and of impaired plasma LDL[3] and cholesterol[4] clearance in patients with primary type IIa hyperlipoproteinaemia. The demonstration that HDL TC concentration is negatively correlated with body cholesterol pool size supports in vitro evidence for a role of HDL in tissue cholesterol clearance[5], and suggests that the plasma concentration of HDL may be an important determinant of atherogenesis.

References

1. Sodhi, H.S., Kudchodkar, B.J. Lancet, 1 (1973) 513.

2. Nestel, P.J. Clin. Sci., 38 (1970) 593.

3. Langar, T., Strober, W., Levy, R.I. J.Clin.Invest., 51 (1972) 1528.

4. Nestel, P.J., Whyte, H.M., Goodman, DeW.S. J.Clin.Invest., 48 (1969) 982.

5. Glomset, J.A. Amer. J. Clin. Nutr., 23 (1970) 1129.

CHAPTER 13

METABOLIC CONTROL IN ANIMAL TISSUES

(1)

INJECTED 7-OXO CHOLESTEROL AND PLANT STEROL DERIVATIVES AND HEPATIC CHOLESTEROGENESIS

G. Kakis, A. Kuksis and J.J. Myher

Banting and Best Department of Medical Research

University of Toronto, Toronto, Canada

We have demonstrated that intravenously administered cholesterol is an effective inhibitor of hepatic cholesterogenesis, while comparable treatments with plant sterols are ineffective (1). A possible explanation for the divergence in the metabolic effects of the two sterol types exists in the observation (2,3) that rat liver enzymes are incapable of converting plant sterols to the 7α-hydroxy derivatives, which may be the active feed-back regulators of cholesterogenesis. Work with primary liver cell cultures and fibroblasts has shown that the 7-oxo derivatives of cholesterol are much more powerful inhibitors of cholesterol biosynthesis than is cholesterol itself (4). Furthermore, 7α-hydroxylation is known to be the rate limiting step in bile acid formation (5), and both 7α and 7β-hydroxy cholesterols are inhibitors of bile acid biosynthesis (6).

In this study we have examined the effect of synthetic 7-oxo derivatives of cholesterol and β-sitosterol upon the hepatic biogenesis of cholesterol. This work was intended to confirm in vivo, the in vitro effects of 7-oxo cholesterols, as well as to probe for the possible existence of other steroid transformations which are blocked or impaired by the presence of an alkyl group in the side chain of the plant sterols.

For our purpose male Wistar rats (250 g) were injected intravenously with synthetic 7-keto (7) and 7-hydroxy (8) cholesterol and β-sitosterol derivatives, as well as the original sterols (10 mg each sterol in 2 ml of Intralipid) and hepatic cholesterogenesis was monitored by incorporation of 1-^{14}C-acetate by liver slices (9) prepared from these animals 5 hours later. The intravenous administration of the 7-oxo cholesterol derivatives had only marginal effects (20-30% inhibition), while the 7-oxo plant sterol derivatives had no effect on cholesterogenesis. These *in vivo* results with the oxo cholesterols are at variance with the findings *in vitro*, although primary liver cell cultures had shown lower sensitivity toward these inhibitors than the fibroblasts (4). It is also possible that the injected oxo sterols failed to come into contact with the feed-back control system of cholesterol biosynthesis. In any event, the present study shows that the lack of direct effect of injected plant sterols upon cholesterogenesis cannot be attributed to their inefficient oxygenation at C_7.

While the injected 7-oxo-sterols may not have reached the sites of feedback regulation of cholesterogenesis, they were readily cleared from plasma, and entered the liver where they gave rise to both acidic and neutral products. About 80% of the injected 7-hydroxycholesterol-4-^{14}C was cleared in the bile as a 90:10 mixture of acidic and neutral steroids in 29 hours. This is comparable to a 90% conversion of 7α-hydroxycholesterol-4-^{14}C to bile acids in man following parenteral injection (10). Likewise, β-hydroxycholesterol administered to bile fistula rats had been shown (11) to be excreted in bile as 90% acidic fraction. Since our 7-hydroxycholesterol preparation contained 25% α- and 75% β-hydroxy-epimers, it presumably yielded both normal bile acids (10) and their epimers (11), although this was not specifically confirmed. In contrast, only 8% of the 7-hydroxy-β-sitosterol-22,23-^{3}H was cleared into bile in 29 hours, and the proportion of acidic to neutral steroids was 40:60. This indicates a relative inability of the rat liver enzymes to oxidize the 7-hydroxy β-sitosterol to acidic products. Both the acidic and neutral products of the further oxidation of 7-hydroxy-β-sitosterol were made up of several components which require further identification.

Hepatic concentrations of all oxo-sterols were very low 5 hours after injection even though the products of their further oxidation continued to be secreted into the bile, confirming a similar observation by Norii et al (11). It would be expected that intermediates of normal bile acid synthesis other than cholesterol would be very quickly processed to bile acids and secreted, if the rate limiting step in this process is indeed the 7-α-hydroxylation (4). The apparent absence from liver of the bulk of 7-hydroxy-β-sitosterol or its oxidation products, which cannot be converted to normal bile acids, however, is surprising and requires further investigation in view of their limited excretion in bile.

Thus it is obvious that the alkyl group in the side chain of β-sitosterol also interferes with the subsequent metabolic utilization of its 7-hydroxy derivative. It is therefore possible that other enzymes involved in the metabolism of cholesterol also have specific apolar binding sites for the side chain of cholesterol as suggested by Boyd et al (3) for the 7α-hydroxylase.

REFERENCES

1. Kuksis, A. and G. Kakis. Federation Proc. 32, 238A (1973).
2. Aringer, L. and P. Eneroth. J. Lipid Res. 14, 563 (1973).
3. Boyd, G.S., M.J.G. Brown, N.G. Hattersley and K.E. Suckling. Biochim. Biophys. Acta 337, 132 (1975).
4. Kandutsch, A.A. and H.W. Chen. J. Biol. Chem. 248, 8408 (1973).
5. Shefer, S., S. Hauser, I. Bekersky and E.H. Mosbach. J. Lipid Res. 11, 404 (1970).
6. Katayama, K. Yonago Acta Med. 12, 93 (1968).
7. Fieser, L.F., J. Am. Chem. Soc. 75, 4386 (1953).
8. Bjorkem, I. and H. Danielsson. Anal. Biochem. 59, 508 (1974).
9. Dietschy, J. and M.D. Siperstein. J. Lipid Res. 8, 97 (1967).
10. Anderson, K.E., E. Kok and N.B. Javitt. J. Clin. Invest. 51, 112 (1972).
11. Norii, T., N. Yamaga and K. Yamasaki. Steroids 15, 303 (1970).

(2)

THE EFFECTS OF FASTING AND REFEEDING ON IN VITRO LIPOGENESIS AND GLYCOGEN SYNTHESIS FROM U-^{14}C-GLUCOSE IN THE RAT AORTA

Kerin O'Dea

Research Division
Cleveland Clinic Foundation
Cleveland, Ohio, U.S.A.

Tissues of animals fasted for two to three days and subsequently refed a high carbohydrate diet exhibit an extremely high capacity for lipogenesis from non-fat precursors. This adaptive hyperlipogenesis of refeeding has been studied extensively in adipose tissue and liver and is associated with a number of striking changes in enzyme profiles. Increased circulating levels of insulin are considered to play a major role in this phenomenon.

In the present study the in vitro incorporation of U-^{14}C-glucose into lipids and glycogen of rat aortic intima-media was measured in the following groups of animals: ad libitum fed, three day fasted, and three day fasted followed by refeeding for one, three and five days. The aortas were split longitudinally, one half being incubated for two hours in the presence of insulin (lmU/ml) and the other half in its absence and serving as a control. The glucose concentration was 5mM throughout. Male Wistar rats weighing 190-210 gm and fed Purina chow were used in the study. The results are summarized in the accompanying table.

Measurable amounts of radioactivity were found only in the triglyceride and phospholipid components of the aortic lipids. The level of incorporation of ^{14}C-label into triglycerides was found to be extremely sensitive to the nutritional state of the animal : falling to low values after a three day fast and rising dramatically to levels two- to four-fold higher than controls after three to five days refeeding. A significant stimulation by insulin was seen after three days refeeding. This effect was no longer significant, although still evident, after five days refeeding. However, the incorporation of ^{14}C-label into triglycerides was not stimulated by insulin in the control group, the three day fasted or one day refed rats.

Table 1

The effect of fasting and refeeding on the *in vitro* aortic lipogenesis and glycogen synthesis from U-^{14}C-glucose in the rat in the presence and absence of insulin.

	Ad libitum fed		3 days fasted							
			0 days refed		1 day refed		3 days refed		5 days refed	
	n=5		n=6		n=6		n=7		n=8	
	Control no Ins.	Change + Ins.	Cont. no Ins.	Change + Ins.	Cont. no Ins.	Change + Ins.	Cont. no Ins.	Change + Ins.	Cont. no Ins.	Change + Ins.
Triglycerides	31.2 ±8.7	-5.0 ±8.4	11.0 ±1.9	-1.5 ±1.4	33.0 ±7.0	-1.5 ±7.9	47.7 ±5.3	+20.3 ±7.6	79.3 ±15.7	+23.0 ±27.0
Phospholipids	22.6 ±3.0	+0.1 ±3.8	11.6 ±1.4	+2.8 ±3.5	23.9 ±1.2	+0.9 ±0.9	25.3 ±1.8	+3.2 ±1.8	31.8 ±2.0	+1.1 ±2.6
Glycogen	22.8 ±4.5	+1.5 ±3.4	31.7 ±5.6	+2.6 ±2.4	46.4 ±6.3	+10.0 ±5.4	78.0 ±16.4	+30.1 ±7.5	95.9 ±16.8	+2.7 ±16.5

Control values represent nanomoles glucose converted in the absence of insulin, per 100 mg aorta dry wt, per 2 hour incubation ± S.E.M.

Change represents the difference between the control value in the absence of insulin and the value in the presence of insulin ± S.E.M.

In contrast, the incorporation of ^{14}C-label into phospholipids was less affected than the triglycerides by refeeding after a fast. It fell to low levels after the three day fast, returned to control values after one day refeeding and rose slowly to levels 50% greater than controls after refeeding for five days. Aortic glycogen synthesis was found to be very sensitive to refeeding after a fast : being significantly higher than control values at all stages of the refeeding process. Glycogen synthesis was significantly stimulated by insulin after three days of refeeding. Insulin had no effect after five days refeeding. Glycogen synthesis appears to increase and to become sensitive to insulin earlier in the refeeding process than does the lipogenic system.

These results indicate that aortic intima-media reacts in a manner similar to adipose tissue and liver to refeeding after a fast. Metabolic changes occur whereby the tissue becomes sensitized to insulin during refeeding. This could be related to the increased levels of insulin circulating in the animal during this period. Insulin stimulated the incorporation of U-^{14}C-glucose into aortic triglycerides and glycogen in the fasted refed rat, and yet had no effect on the incorporation into phospholipids. Phospholipids are primarily structural lipids in arterial tissue and it is conceivable that their rate of synthesis is tightly controlled by cell membrane turnover rates. On the other hand, triglycerides, if they do have a function at all in the artery wall, can only be an energy store. The rate of triglyceride synthesis may have no such limitations on it as was postulated for phospholipids. During refeeding after a fast the large amounts of glucose and insulin would collaborate to present increasing amounts of glucose to the interior of lipogenic cells. This condition results in a progressive increase in the lipogenic capacity of the cell. From our results this seems to be preceded by an increase in glycogen synthesizing capacity to cope with the increased glucose and insulin in the short-term. Since relatively low concentrations of insulin inhibit a hormone-sensitive lipase in the arterial wall[2], the higher rates of triglyceride synthesis in the fasted refed rat probably do represent a net increase in arterial triglyceride content. Indeed, Howard[3] observed an increased triglyceride and phospholipid synthesis from glucose in atherosclerotic rabbit aortas. Stout[4] has proposed that insulin may play a role in the pathogenesis of atheromatous vascular disease. The present findings suggest that the adaptive hyperlipogenesis associated with refeeding after a fast may exacerbate this role.

References

1. Tepperman, H.M. and Tepperman, J., Fed. Proc. (1964) 23, 73.
2. Mahler, R.F. and Parker, A.B., Europ. J. Clin. Invest. (1970) 1, 137.
3. Howard, C.F., J. Lipid Res. (1971) 12, 725.
4. Stout, R.W., Horm. Metab. Res. (1975) 7, 31.

(3)

CHOLESTEROL ESTER : LYSOLECITHIN ACYLTRANSFERASE ACTIVITY OF THE AORTA

J. Patelski and M. Pioruńska

Lipid Metabolism Laboratory, Department of Biochemistry

Medical Academy, Poznań, Poland

INTRODUCTION

Enzyme-catalyzed transfer from lecithin on cholesterol to form cholesterol ester and lysolecithin (LCAT+) 1/ in the arterial wall has been found (1) but not much is known about the reaction in reverse direction. It seemed to be of interest, therefore, to investigate the cholesterol ester : lysolecithin acyl transfer activity (LCAT-) of the aortic wall, as compared with LCAT+ and cholesterol esterase activities.

MATERIAL AND METHODS

Protein extracts of acetone-butanol powders from thoracic aortas from pigs and substrate hydrosols were prepared and the enzyme activities assayed using sample-type methods based on measuring changes in concentration of reaction products extracted from reaction mixtures, as described elsewhere (2,3). The reaction mixtures contained the enzyme extract, substrates (lysolecithin and/or cholesterol ester at optimum concentration (2), lecithin + cholesterol, and lecithin, and cofactors (reduced glutathione, and EDTA for LCAT or $CaCl_2$ for cholesterol esterase). Substrate and enzyme controls were taken into account.

Results are expressed in nmoles of free (LCAT-) and esterified cholesterol (LCAT+) and free fatty acids (cholesterol esterase) per min per mg of protein of the enzyme preparation (mU/mg).

1/ LCAT = lecithin : cholesterol acyltransferase (EC 2.3.1.43), cholesterol esterase = sterol ester hydrolase (EC 3.1.1.13).

RESULTS AND DISCUSSION

Following reaction products were found: lecithin, lysolecithin, glycerylphosphoryl choline, free and esterified cholesterol and free fatty acids. The reversible reaction lecithin: cholesterol ⇄ lysolecithin: cholesterol ester has thus been proved to be present, along with other enzyme-catalyzed reactions (4), in the experimental systems used.

Optimum experimental conditions for the phospholipid-dependent reaction have been established (substrates: lysolecithin + cholesteryl oleate or lecithin + cholesterol = 3 + 1 mmol/1 respectively, enzyme preparation: 1.16 $\pm$ 0.10 mg of protein/4 ml of the reaction mixture, incubation time: 60 min at 30°C, pH optimum).

Two pH optima, 7.0 and 8.0, for synthesis of cholesterol esters in the presence of lecithin, and only one optimum pH 8.0 for the lysolecithin-dependent decomposition of cholesteryl oleate, were found (figure 1).

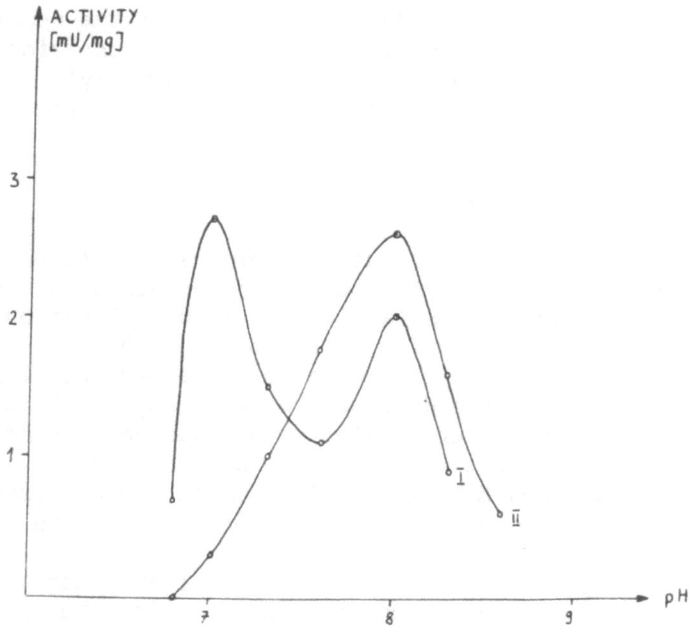

Figure 1. Effect of pH of the reaction mixtures on (I) lecithin: cholesterol and (II) cholesteryl oleate : lysolecithin acyltransferase activities.

This may be due to different affinity of the enzyme to substrates with fatty acids of different chain length and saturation, as demonstrated by the results listed in Table I.

The results seem to indicate the relative importance of these two reactions. The acyl transfer from cholesterol esters on lysolecithin may aid to decomposition of the esters, particularly oleate, by hydrolysis and thus promote their removal from the artery.

Table I. Enzyme activities of the aorta

Substrate fatty acid	LCAT-	Cholesterel esterase
	mU/mg	
$C_{16:0}$	1.1 ± 0.56 1/	8.3 ± 1.01
$C_{18:0}$	0.8 ± 0.22	7.8 ± 1.06
$C_{18:1}$	2.6 ± 0.43	6.6 ± 1.04
$C_{18:2}$	1.3 ± 0.33	11.5 ± 1.42
$C_{18:3}$	1.6 ± 0.67	9.5 ± 1.19

1/ Mean $\pm$ standard deviation from N=4 series of estimates. The means were compared by Analysis of Variance for each enzyme separately ($P \leq 0.01$).

LCAT+ = 2.7 ± 0.69 mU/mg (N=4) at pH 7.0 and 2.0 ± 0.51 mU/mg (N=6) at pH 8.0.

REFERENCES

1. Abdulla, Y.H., Orton, C.C. and Adams, C.W.M., Cholesterol esterification by transacylation in human and experimental atheromatous lesions, J. Atheroscler. Res., 8(1968)967.

2. Patelski, J., Pniewska, B., Pioruńska, M. and Obrębska,M., The arterial acyl-CoA: cholesterol acyltransferase and cholesterol ester hydrolase activities. In vitro effect of substrates with fatty acid of different chain length and saturation, Atherosclerosis, 22(1975) 287-291.

3. Patelski, J. and Pioruńska, M., Cholesterol ester:lysolecithin transacylation in the aorta, to be published.

4. Patelski, J., Participation of phospholipids in arterial metabolism of cholesterol esters, in this book.

(4)

SIGNIFICANCE OF LIPOPROTEIN LIPASE IN RAT SKELETAL MUSCLE

Meng H. Tan, Tsunako Sata and Richard J. Havel

Cardiovascular Research Institute

San Francisco, California, U.S.A.

Lipoprotein lipase (LPL) mediates the removal of plasma triglycerides in extrahepatic tissues. Utilization of plasma triglycerides by adipose tissue is related to its LPL activity. LPL activities in adipose tissue and heart have been extensively studied but that in skeletal muscles has not.

Activity in skeletal muscle was measured by a modification (Diabetes 24 (Suppl 2):417, 1975) of the assay described by Nilsson-Ehle and associates (Clin. Chim. Acta 42:383, 1972) with triolein - ^{3}H, emulsified in 10% lecithin, as substrate. We found that the enzyme activity was reduced by about 90% when serum was absent in the assay medium. Activity was inhibited by about 90% by 1M NaCl and 85% by protamine (1 mg/ml). The pH optimum for the enzyme was between 8.0 and 8.5.

Though most skeletal muscles are heterogeneous in their fibre content, the soleus of the rat consists primarily of red fibres whilst the posterior band of the semitendinosus consists primarily of white fibres. The LPL activity was considerably higher in the soleus (36.8 ± 2.7 μmoles/gm/hour — Mean $\pm$ SEM) than in the semitendinosus (1.08 ± 0.17). The lateral head (mainly red fibres) of the gastrocnemius contained more LPL activity (6.06 ± 1.4) than the body (mainly white fibres) of the muscle (0.46 ± 0.04).

To estimate the total LPL activity in adipose tissue and skeletal muscle of the rat, the enzyme activities of adipose tissue from 4 different sites and those of 11 different muscles were measured. Based upon the average value for each tissue and assuming that adipose tissue and skeletal muscle comprised about 5% and 45%

of body weight respectively, the following values were calculated. In the fed state skeletal muscles contained 691 units and adipose tissue 759 units. In the 24 hour fasted state skeletal muscles contained 635 units and adipose tissue 230 units.

These results suggest that skeletal muscles, and particularly their red fibres, which like heart muscle depend on aerobic metabolism and readily oxidize fatty acids, are an active site of catabolism of plasma triglycerides. This is especially so in the fasted state when the total LPL activity in skeletal muscles is considerably higher than that in adipose tissue.

(5)

DECREASED CARDIAC GLYCOGEN FOLLOWING PHENFORMIN INJECTION IN HYPERGLYCEMIC, HYPERINSULINEMIC ANAESTHETIZED RATS

N. W. Rodger and S. P. Sangal

Departments of Medicine and Epidemiology

University of Western Ontario, London, Canada

The incidence of death due to heart disease in diabetics treated with phenformin was double that of other groups in the University Group Diabetes Program of the U.S.A.[1] Despite some insights into the actions of oral hypoglycemic agents this observation has not been explained. The human diabetic myocardium contains large amounts of glycogen,[2] consumes glucose at rates comparable to those of normal hearts, may experience high serum insulin levels, and is subject to ischemic disease. We have compared the effects of phenformin with insulin on tissue glycogen levels in a model of co-existing hyperinsulinemia and hyperglycemia in which glucose was infused at a rate 6 times greater than that needed to satisfy energy needs.

Methods. Normal male rats (n = 90, BW 270-395 gm;0.37-0.49 $kg^{0.75}$) were injected (i.p.) with pentobarbital (50 mg/kg) and with phenformin at doses (n = 30) of 0, 0.2 mg/$kg^{0.75}$ (similar to that used therapeutically) or 80 mg/$kg^{0.75}$. Insulin infused in albumin: phosphate buffer was started 10 minutes later (subclavian vein) at rates of 0, 3, 30, 300, 3000, 30,000 mU/$kg^{0.75}$/67 min. (n = 15) so that the 3 doses of phenformin applied at each insulin infusion rate. Glucose (32 mmol/$kg^{0.75}$/60 min.) was started after a further 7 minutes. Blood glucose (carotid artery) was sampled at intervals. In some experiments arterial pO_2 was measured. After 60 minutes of glucose infusion heart, liver and skeletal muscle were frozen and glycogen content was measured in aqueous extracts using an enzymatic method. Computer assisted analysis was performed following logarithmic transformation of the data.

Results. Blood glucose rose to hyperglycemic levels in all

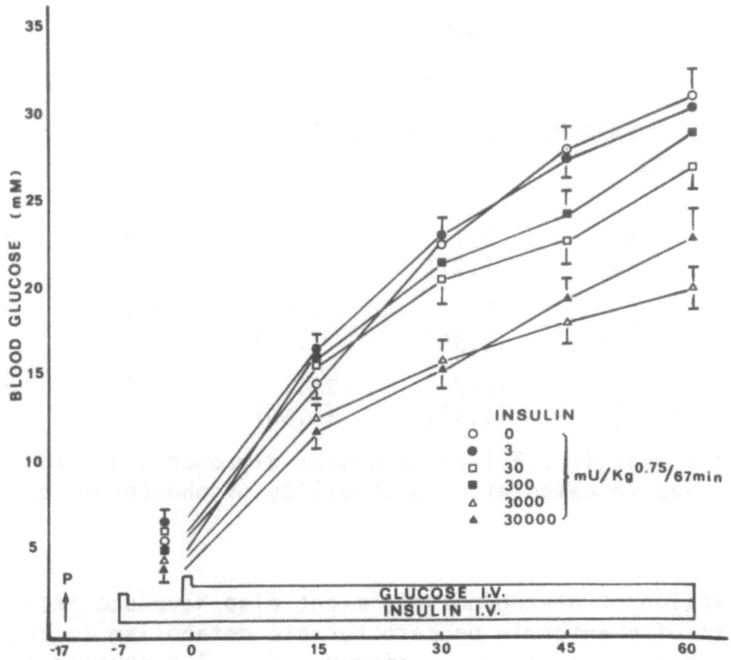

Figure 1. The effect of elapsed time and of insulin dose on arterial blood glucose concentration (mean ± S.E.) following phenformin ingestion at - 17 minutes (P).

treatment groups. A decrease of blood glucose was related to the insulin infusion rate ($p < 0.01$, Figure 1), but phenformin had no such effect. A decrease following phenformin injection of mean cardiac glycogen concentration was seen at the high dose only ($p < 0.01$, Table 1); insulin had no effect. Phenformin did not change skeletal muscle or liver glycogen levels. Arterial O_2 tension rose during infusions when performed.

Discussion. An experimental model of maturity onset diabetes mellitus based on glucose-induced hyperglycemia may be justified on the basis of evidence suggesting an increased glucose turnover rate and the clearly defined role of glucagon (acting to increase hepatic glucose output) in diabetic patients[3]. Analogous to the known increased glycogen content of the human diabetic heart independent of ante-mortem insulin therapy,[2] cardiac glycogen levels in our study exceeded reported values for fed normal rats and were unaffected by added insulin. The stimulus to cardiac glycogenesis reported to occur with exposure of the perfused rat heart to large amounts of glucose (40mM) was reproduced in our study and was blocked by a high dose of phenformin. Although glycogen synthesis may have been inhib-

Table 1

GLYCOGEN CONCENTRATION

(mg/gm wet wt[1])

TISSUE	PHENFORMIN DOSE ($mg/kg^{0.75}$) 0	0.2	80	F^2	p
Heart	8.5* (.36)	8.7 (.21)	6.0 (.28)	25.67	< 0.01
Skeletal Muscle	6.9 (.32)	6.3 (.34)	6.6 (.33)	1.13	> 0.05
Liver	19.6 (1.39)	21.7 (1.31)	21.1 (1.50)	0.71	> 0.05

1. Arithmetic mean (+ S.E.) using oyster glycogen standard.
2. F ratio used in calculating probability of phenformin effect (p).
* n = 30.

ited, activation of glycogenolysis might also have occurred as certain effects of phenformin on carbohydrate metabolism in rats may be reversed by beta-adrenergic blocking agents. A hypoxemic stimulus to catecholamine secretion was unlikely. These data disagree with findings obtained using the perfused rat heart in which insulin increased cardiac glycogen content to levels which were unaffected by concurrent phenformin administration.[4] If stored glycogen is available to the diabetic myocardium, our study suggests that in the presence of high tissue levels of phenformin, as might occur with renal impairment, patients treated with this drug might be denied a source of substrate during ischemic episodes, increasing the chance of cardiac dysfunction at that time.[5] The increased mortality observed might thus be explained.

References

1. The University Group Diabetes Program: V. Evaluation of phenformin therapy. Diabetes 24 (Supp 1):65-184, 1975
2. Mowry RW: Histochemically demonstrable glycogen in the human heart with special reference to glycogen storage disease and diabetes mellitus. Am J Path 27:611-623, 1951
3. Gerich JE, Lorenzi M, Bier DM, et al: Prevention of human diabetic ketoacidosis by somatostatin. N Engl J Med 292:985-989, 1975
4. Williamson JR, Walker RS, Renold AE: Metabolic effects of phenethylbiguanide on the isolated perfused rat heart. Metabolism 12: 1141-1152, 1963
5. Scheuer J, Stezooki SW: Protective role of increased myocardial glycogen stores in cardiac anoxia in the rat. Circ Res 27:835-849, 1970

CHAPTER 14
EXPERIMENTAL LESIONS - MORPHOLOGY

(1)

COMPARATIVE ULTRASTRUCTURE OF PRIMATE FATTY STREAKS

K. C. Hayes and N. P. Westmoreland

Department of Nutrition, Harvard School of Public Health
Boston, Massachusetts, U.S.A.

Extensive investigation of primates as models of human atherosclerosis has called attention to their varied susceptibility to this disease process associated with differences in lipid metabolism (*Atherosclerosis* 20: 405, 1974). This report describes basic differences in the ultrastructure of aortic fatty streaks in five primate species.

Young adult or adult squirrel (34), cebus (25), spider (14), rhesus (3) and cynamolgus (12) monkeys were studied following three to thirty-six months of commercial chow (spontaneous lesions) or semi-purified diets containing 10% butter, coconut oil, safflower oil or corn oil with or without 0.1% cholesterol (30 mg/100 kcal of the diet). Although diet and time influenced the degree of change, species differences provided the overriding characteristics that are described.

The most extensive atherosclerotic change was observed as raised sudanophilic lesions in the aortic arch of squirrel monkeys (20-80% sudan), in association with a typical hypercholesterolemia of 250-300 mg/dl. These lesions included proliferation of intimal smooth muscle cells, intra- and extracellular lipid, extensive interstitial glycosaminoglycans and basement membrane-like material, and moderate collagen and elastin formation. A marked intimal cellularity was largely accounted for by smooth muscle cells and numerous less well-differentiated sub-endothelial cells (Fig. 1). Degenerating cells and extensive extracellular debris were characteristic. Cholesterol feeding increased the hypercholesterolemia slightly and resulted in a striking increase in the intra- and extracellular lipid accumulation of the intima.

By contrast, the fatty streak was a misnomer in cebus which were refractory to sudanophilic lesions (0%) despite a comparable hypercholesterolemia. Intimal changes were characterized by a

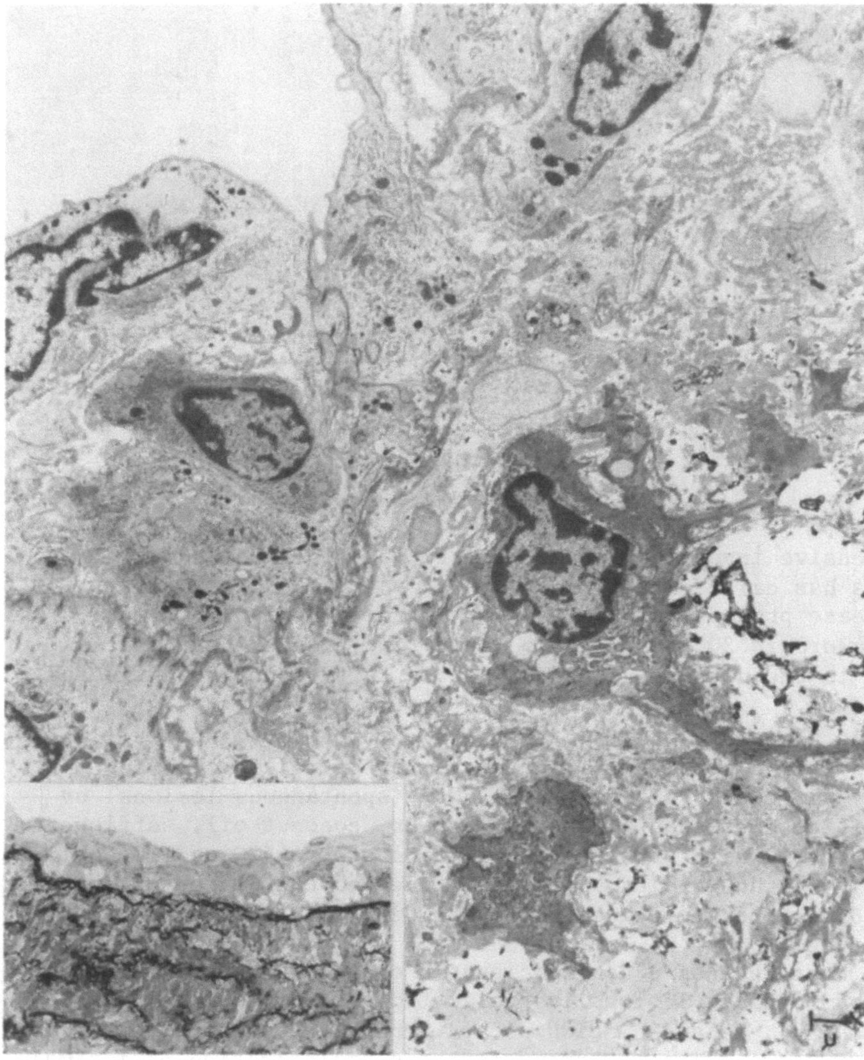

Fig. 1. Squirrel monkey aortic arch. Coconut oil + cholesterol, 9 months. Note extensive cellularity, intra- and extracellular lipid, and connective tissue proliferation. Insert shows reaction and lipid in media.

moderate smooth muscle cell proliferation and extensive collagen and elastin synthesis with essentially no intra- or extracellular lipid. The intimal response was less cellular than that of the squirrel monkey, but the number of degenerating smooth muscle cells and associated extracellular debris was as extensive (Fig. 2). In-

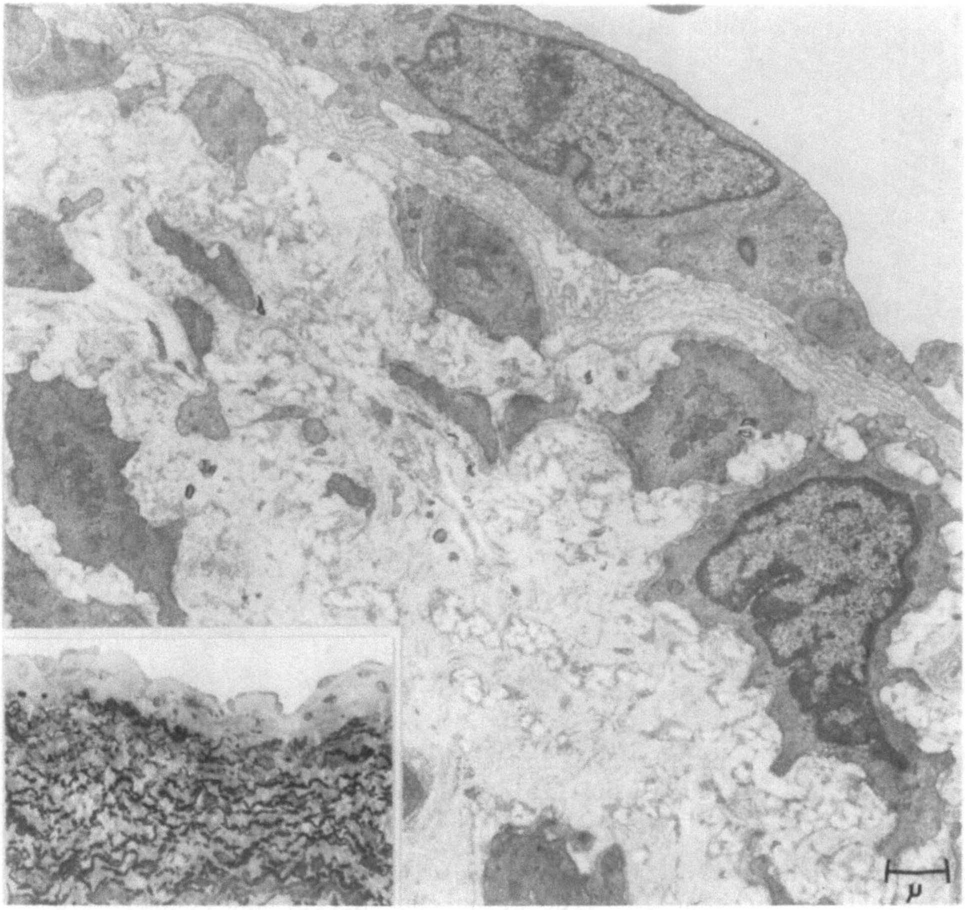

Fig. 2. Cebus aortic arch. Coconut oil + cholesterol, 9 months. Note reactive smooth muscles and proliferation of collagen, elastin and basement membrane.

timal collagen synthesis predominated in the proximal aorta, whereas elastin synthesis was the predominant connective tissue response in the distal aorta in both species. Cholesterol feeding in the cebus monkey had a minimal effect on the hypercholesterolemia and the intima. The spider monkey appeared to be as resistant to atherosclerotic change ($< 2\%$) as the cebus and responded with a similar intimal reaction.

Fatty streaks in Old World macaques (rhesus and cynamolgus) were characterized by marked intracellular lipid resulting in foam cells ($< 10\%$ sudan) and many extracellular dense bodies with moderate glycosaminoglycans and fibrous connective tissue proliferation. The principal intimal cell was the smooth muscle cell, but monocytic

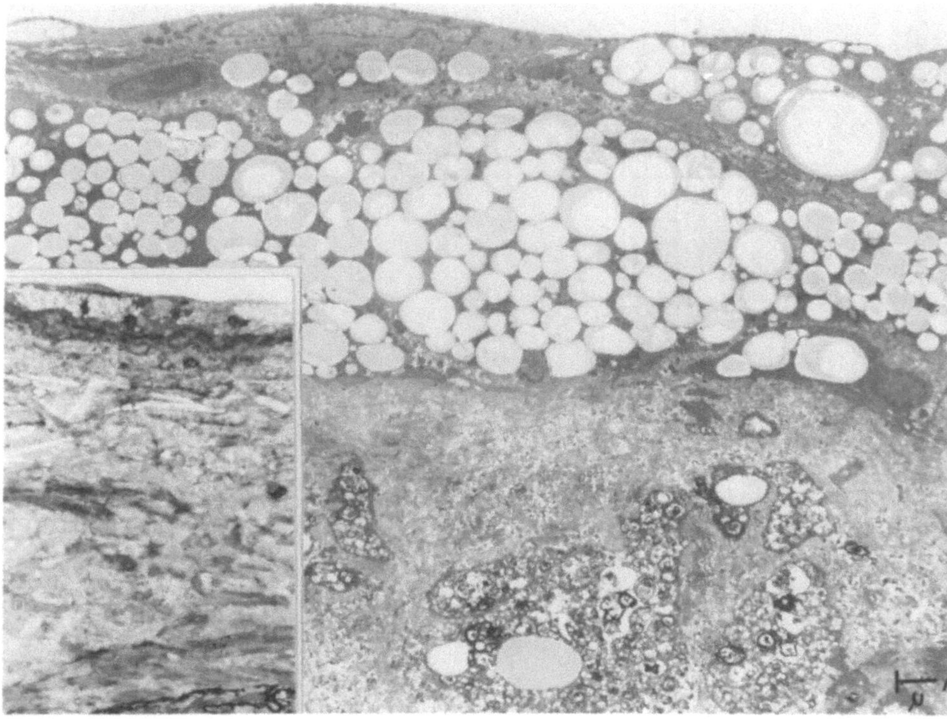

Fig. 3. Rhesus aortic arch. Spontaneous streak-23 year old female. Foam cells and extracellular lipid predominate.

cells were observed. Cholesterol feeding of macaques resulted in the greatest increase in circulating cholesterol and accumulation of foam cells (Fig. 3).

The notable difference between species was the remarkable susceptibility of the squirrel monkey and the relative resistance of the other species to atherosclerotic change under similar dietary treatment. A second difference was the connective tissue proliferation noted in the intima of the cebus and spider monkeys contrasted with the foam cell accumulation in Old World species, with the squirrel monkey representing an intermediate between these two extremes. These data serve to demonstrate the fact that processes of lipid deposition and fibromuscular thickening can occur independently as a function of species.

It will be of interest to determine whether these differences in reactivity represent the nature of the lipid insult associated with transport and metabolism of the lipid by particular lipoproteins, differences in endothelial or intimal permeability, or intrinsic factors related to the metabolism of smooth muscle cells or connective tissue in the wall itself.

(2)

SPONTANEOUS ARTERIAL LESIONS IN NORMAL PIGS AND PIGS WITH VON WILLEBRAND'S DISEASE

V. Fuster, E. J. W. Bowie, and A. L. Brown

Mayo Clinic and Mayo Foundation

Rochester, MN., U.S.A.

To evaluate how significant is the role played by platelets in the initiation of atherosclerosis we thought that a good deal of information might be obtained by investigating whether experimental animals known to have an impairment in platelet function are less prone to the development of atherosclerosis than normal control animals.

For several years a breeding colony of pigs with all the characteristics of human von Willebrand's disease have been maintained in Rochester at Mayo Institute Hills farm. In order to evaluate whether such von Willebrand pigs with impaired platelet adhesiveness are less prone to the development of atherosclerosis than normal control pigs, we initiated a detailed pathological study of the aortas from the pigs with von Willebrand's disease who died in the last 3 years. The study included 11 von Willebrand pigs, 7 male and 4 female and 11 male normal control pigs from the same breed. Both groups of pigs were 1 to 3 years of age and they were all rigidly matched by heart weight. Of the 11 normal pigs, 6 showed multiple arteriosclerotic plaques which microscopically consisted of intimal proliferation, and one pig showed a single plaque of more than 2 mm in diameter. In contrast none of the von Willebrand pigs had multiple plaques and only one showed a single lesion of more than 2 mm in diameter. Three of the von Willebrand pigs showed a single very small lesion of less than 2 mm in diameter (Table 1).

During the course of this study we made a most interesting observation. In over half of the pigs with von Willebrand's disease the macroscopically normal aortas completely free of

TABLE 1

LESIONS	MULTIPLE (4-10)	SINGLE	
DIAMETER	1-10 MM	> 2 MM	≤ 2 MM
CONTROL (11)	6	1	0
VWD (11)	0	1	3

AORTIC PLAQUES

arteriosclerotic plaques showed evidence after staining with Sudan IV of extensive fat deposition infiltrating about 5 to 30% of the aortic surface. Microscopically these non-arteriosclerotic lesions consisted of extensive subendothelial infiltration of fat without significant intimal proliferation. Only one of the control pigs showed an area of infiltration and this was a small area occupying less than 5% of the aortic surface (Table 2).

TABLE 2

AORTIC SURFACE AREA	5-30%	< 5%
CONTROL (11)	0	1
VWD (11)	7	0

AORTIC FAT INFILTRATION

In conclusion, it would appear that the pigs with von Willebrand's disease are resistant to the development of early arteriosclerotic plaques, but are prone to develop extensive intimal fat infiltration. These observations are preliminary and we are reluctant to draw any definite conclusion because of information about the normal animals is inadequate as they were obtained from a slaughter house. We can, however, offer a speculative explanation for our findings. In normal pigs, endothelial injury presumably due to hemodynamic and rheological factors might attract platelets to adhere to the arterial surface and as suggested by the work of L. A. Harker and R. Ross (1), the platelets may promote the development of the intimal hyperplasia seen in the early arteriosclerotic plaques. This would not occur in the von Willebrand aorta because the platelet does not adhere. In addition, as shown by several investigators (2,3,4), the adherence of the platelet to the arterial surface in the normal animal may help to repair the endothelium and reduce its permeability so that very little fat would pass through the endothelium. In the von Willebrand pig, on the other hand, because the platelet does not adhere, endothelial integrity is not restored and permeability is increased allowing the fat to accumulate in the intima.

REFERENCES

1. L. A. Harker, R. Ross and S. J. Slichter: Chronic endothelial cell injury and platelet-factor induced arteriosclerosis. Proceedings Vth Congress of the International Society on Thrombosis and Haemostasis. Paris, 1975, p.56.

2. M. A. Gimbrone, R. H. Aster, R. S. Cotran, J. Corkey, J. H. Jondal, and J. Folkman: Preservation of vascular integrity in organ perfused in vitro with a platelet-rich medium. Nature 222:33, 1969.

3. J. D. Wojcik, D. L. Von Horn, A. J. Webber and S. A. Johnson: Mechanism whereby platelets support the endothelium. Transfusion 9:324, 1969.

4. J. Roskam: Du role de la paroi vasculaire daus l'hemostase spontanee et la pathogenie des etats hemorrhagigues. Thromb. Diath. Haemorrh. (Stuttg) 12:338, 1964.

(3)

INJURY INDUCED ATHEROSCLEROSIS; IS INJURY OR THROMBOSIS RESPONSIBLE FOR PROGRESSION OF LESIONS?

Sean Moore and Robert J. Friedman

Department of Pathology, McMaster University

1200 Main St. W. Hamilton, Ontario, Canada

We have previously shown that repeated or continuous intimal injury caused by mechanical (1) or immunological (2) means causes a variety of lesions in rabbits maintained on a diet unsupplemented by lipid. These include fatty streaks and edematous plaques, lipid free fibro-muscular plaques, and lipid-rich raised thromboatherosclerotic lesions. Regression of lipid rich raised atherosclerotic lesions (3,4) was associated with acquisition of an intact covering layer of endothelial-like cells and the disappearance of thrombus. Fibro-muscular plaques showing no stainable lipid, were seen at 5 weeks following removal of the injury stimulus. These findings suggest that the development of a covering layer of cells and disappearance of thrombus are associated with regression of raised lipid-rich lesions.

Whether lipid-rich raised lesions are a result of injury or coexisting thrombosis or both is not clear. The present experiment was designed to answer this question.

Anti-platelet serum (APS) to washed, sonicated rabbit platelets was raised in sheep. PE 60 polyethylene catheters were placed in the aortas of 35 rabbits by way of a femoral artery. The animals were divided into 2 groups, an experimental and control group. The experimental group (17 rabbits) received an intravascular injection of 1.0 ml. of APS followed 8 hours later by a subcutaneous injection of 0.5 ml. Thereafter, 0.5 ml. APS was given subcutaneously each day for 13 additional days. The control group received no APS. Platelet counts were done prior to surgery, at 5 minutes following injury, at 4 days, 8 days and just prior to killing. Extent of lesions was estimated by photographing the opened aortas, projecting the photographs on cardboard, cutting out the areas occupied by the different lesions and weighing the cardboard.

In a second experiment, the effect of diluted APS was compared with normal sheep serum (NSS). Twenty-one rabbits of either sex paired for weight, age and sex were divided into 2 groups. Subgroup I consisted of 10 rabbits which had indwelling aortic catheters placed and received APS diluted sixteen fold in 0.9% NaCl. Subgroup II comprised 11 rabbits which had catheters placed and received undiluted normal sheep serum (NSS).

Type of Lesions

The morphological characteristics of the resultant lesions have been previously described (1,2,3).

Experiment I

The surface area involved by raised lipid-rich lesions was between 6 and 7 fold less in the group of rabbits receiving APS as compared to the control group. Statistical analysis of this difference employing Welsh's "t" test for unequal variances was highly significant ($P<0.001$). There were no significant differences in fatty streaks between the APS and no-APS groups, however the extent of fibrous lesions was significantly higher ($P<0.05$) in the no-APS group. Platelet counts in the APS group varied from 0 - 20,000/cu mm. at the time of killing. The extent of raised lesions was greater at higher platelet counts. In animals with platelet counts $<$ 1,000/cu mm. raised lesions were completely absent.

Experiment II

The results of experiment II were entirely consistent with those of the first experiment. Raised lesions and fibrous plaques were more extensive in the NSS group, with significance levels of $P<0.001$ and $P<0.05$ respectively as assessed by a Welsh's "t" test. Since experiment II was performed because of doubt about the adequacy of the no-APS control, it is interesting to examine the intergroup comparison. There was no significant difference in comparing the control groups in experiments I and II. Similarly, in the experimental groups (APS and APS 1:16) there was no significant difference in raised or fatty streak lesions. While they differ at the 5% level ($P<0.05$) in the fibrous lesions the difference is so small that it is probably not meaningful.

These findings indicate that raised, lipid-rich thromboatherosclerotic lesions, which are caused by continuous or repeated intimal injury in rabbits, can be significantly inhibited by inducing severe thrombocytopenia. Since the injury stimulus is identical in animals exposed to APS as in those not so treated, these results indicate that thrombosis, rather than injury, is the determining factor in the production of lesions. It is known that a single injury to the arterial wall results in the development of a lipid-free fibro-muscular plaque composed of smooth muscle cells (5,6). Continuous or repeated intimal injury results in lipid-rich thromboatherosclerotic lesions (1,2). These findings suggest that the absence of endothelium may play a permissive role in facilitating continuing or repeated deposition of thrombus material. The results are compatible with the observation of Ross (7) indicating a factor in platelets causing stimulation of smooth muscle cell proliferation. They also suggest that there may be some substance in the repeated or continuing thrombotic process, associated with repeated or continuing intimal injury, which may induce lipid synthesis by the smooth muscle cells of the developing plaque. Thus, the evidence presented in this study indicates that platelets and thrombosis are more important than injury in the genesis of raised lipid-rich thromboatherosclerotic lesions. Supported by a grant from the Medical Research Council of Canada MA-2168.

REFERENCES

1. Moore, S. Thromboatherosclerosis in normolipemic rabbits. A result of continued endothelial damage. Laboratory Investigation 29, 478, 1973.

2. Friedman, R.J., Moore, S. and Singal, D.P. Repeated endothelial injury and induction of atherosclerosis in normolipemic rabbits by human serum. Laboratory Investigation 30, 404, 1975.

3. Friedman, R.J., Moore, S., Singal, D.P. and Gent, M. Regression of injury induced atheromatous lesions in rabbits. Archives of Pathology. In press.

4. Moore, S., Friedman, R.J. and Gent, M. Evolution of fatty streak to fibrous plaque in injury induced atherosclerosis. Federation Proceedings 34, 875, (Abst) 1975.

5. Stemerman, M.B. and Spaet, T.H. The subendothelium and thrombogenesis. Bulletin of the New York Academy of Medicine 48, 289, 1972.

6. Stemerman, M.B. and Ross, R. Experimental atherosclerosis. Fibrous plaque formation in primates, an electron microscopic study. Journal of Experimental Medicine 136, 769, 1972.

7. Ross, R., Glomset, J., Kariya, B. and Harker, L. A platelet dependent serum factor that stimulates the proliferation of arterial smooth muscle cells in vitro. In: Proceedings of the National Academy of Science U.S.A. 71, 1207, 1974.

(4)

THE EFFECT OF HYPERCHOLESTEROLEMIA ON THE RESPONSE PATTERNS AFTER DIFFERENT TYPES OF DEFINED MECHANICAL INJURY

S. Björkerud[x] and G. Bondjers

[x]Astra Läkemedel AB, University of Göteborg, Sweden

[x]S-151 85 Södertälje, Sweden

Dept. of Internal Medicine I, S-413 45 Göteborg, Sweden

Different types of specific mechanical injury to the arterial wall elicit three characteristic and reproducible types of tissue responses. The morphology of these has many similarities with the three major changes in human arteries, i.e. progressive intimal thickening, medial sclerosis, and atherosclerosis. Hyperlipidemia is closely epidemiologically related to early human atherosclerotic disease. To test whether this relationship could be mediated by a modifying effect of hypercholesterolemia on the different arterial tissue responses, the three different types of specific injuries were induced in rabbits, which were kept on cholesterol-supplemented diet for different time periods.

MATERIAL AND METHODS: In each of 16 male albino rabbits the following three types of lesions were induced mechanically with a microsurgical instrument (1, 4): a. superficial injury with small area (regularly developing to a non-atherosclerotic intimal thickening with rapid reendothelialization and consecutive regression and healing in the normolipidemic rabbit), b. deep total local necrosis (regularly undergoing rapid calcification, capillarization, and encapsulation in normolipidemic rabbits, ref. 3) and, c. superficial injury with large area (in the normolipidemic rabbit regularly leading to development of different types of lesions in three sequential phases: the <u>early phase</u> with intimal thickening --- <u>phase of defective reendothelialization</u> with excessive intimal thickening, accumulation of extracellular lipids, formation of mural thrombi --- <u>phase of late reendothelialization</u> with tissue injury manifested as necrosis, demasking of masked lipids, formation of foam cells in combination with invasion by macrophages and the appearance of foreign body giant cells followed by rapid elimination of lipids and regression of the intimal thickening in the normolipidemic rabbit to a condition similar to that following the induction of a total necrosis).

The animals were divided into five groups. Two of the groups C_1 and T_1) were killed after four weeks and three groups (C_2, T_2, T_3) after ten weeks. A supplement to the diet of one percent of cholesterol was given to groups T_1 and T_2 during the period 10 to 25 days after the induction of the lesions and to T_3 during days 20 to 40. The serum cholesterol concentration varied from 14 to 50 mg% in the control groups (C_1, C_2). Mean maximal serum cholesterol values were 662 mg% and 372 mg% for groups T_1+T_2 and T_3, respectively. Evans blue was given intravenously two days before killing as an indicator for areas with increased permeability for albumin-Evans blue complex. The morphology of the lesions was studied light microscopically in sections and block preparations after selective staining of major arterial tissue components (2).

RESULT AND DISCUSSION: Following a superficial injury with small area in the normolipidemic rabbit is a non-atherosclerotic lesion which rapidly undergoes reendothelialization and subsequent regression and healing. The same mechanical type of injury in the hypercholesterolemic rabbit was followed by a clearly atherosclerotic type of response. In the normolipidemic animal corresponding lesions can only be elicited by the infliction of a very large endothelial defect. Thus, hypercholesterolemia transforms a reaction normally leading to complete healing of an arterial injury to a defective healing response with the characteristics of the early human atherosclerotic lesion, i.e. the "gelatinous lesion" or "early fibrous lesion". Lipid-loaded lining cells (endothelium?) and mural thrombi were found on these lesions. One possible factor for the transformation of the tissue response in hypercholesterolemia may, therefore, be interference with endothelial regeneration during the reendothelialization of the lesions, leading to a "phase of defective reendothelialization" encountered after extensive endothelial desquamation (4). Another factor may be overloading of the tissue with serum constituents beyond its capacity for elimination.

After a period of 4 weeks on cholesterol-supplemented diet a further interval of 6 weeks with regular diet did not reconvert the lesions towards complete healing. On the contrary, necrotic regions, foam cells, calcification, and capillarization indicate defective repair. Such changes are also found during regression of lesions induced by <u>large</u> endothelial desquamation and developed under normolipidemic conditions (see above and ref. 4).

Reendothelialization and subsequent regression and healing of the non-atherosclerotic type of lesion induced by a small endothelial desquamation and developed during normolipidemic conditions is usually complete 3-8 weeks after the induction of the injury (1). With dietary supplement of cholesterol during this period (20th-40th day; T_3) and after a month without cholesterol supplement the lesions were <u>incompletely</u> covered with endothelium. As reendothelialization of this type of lesion under normolipidemic conditions is regularly complete within 3 weeks after injury, breakdown of the regenerated endothelium had taken place during the period with dietary cholesterol supplement. The lesions were similar to those following a large desquamation of endothelium developed under normolipidemic conditions with the presence of extracellular lipid in uncovered and intracellular lipid and degenerative and regressive changes in endothelium-covered regions of the plaques.

No effect of cholesterol-feeding was observed on the response pattern following the induction of a total local necrosis. The lesion following this type of injury is characterized by the direct appearance of degenerative changes such as calcification, encapsulation, and aneurysm formation and are rapidly reendothelialized (3). It is possible that the independence of this type of lesion to hypercholesterolemia might be due to the low cellular content and rapid reconstitution of the endothelial permeability barrier.

SUMMARY: The induction of a period of hypercholesterolemia had the following major effects: 1. lesions with regularly heal completely, i.e. lead to complete restitution of the arterial wall structure in the normolipidemic animal, were converted to a more "malign" type which also in the normolipidemic animal leads to defective repair, 2. reinstitution of normolipidemia did not reconvert the lesions to the more "benign" variety but transferred them to the next phase along the regular line of development for the more "malign" variety of lesions, which includes rapid elimination of lipids from the tissue, 3. original lesions of the more "malign" variety were not affected qualitatively; mural thrombi and lipid accumulations were more abundant as was the tendency for necrosis, capillarization, and aneurysm formation, and 4. regions initially rendered necrotic were little affected, possibly due to low cellularity and rapid covering with endothelium. The results support the concept that atherosclerosis is not irreversible. However, the efficiency for reconstitution of the arterial wall varies between the different types of repair processes, and is impaired by increased serum cholesterol levels.

REFERENCES

1. Björkerud, S.: Reaction of the aortic wall of the rabbit after superficial, longitudinal, mechanical trauma. Virchows Arch. Abt. A Path. Anat. 347: 197, 1969.
2. Björkerud, S.: Preparative, staining, and microscopic techniques for the study of whole artery segment. Atherosclerosis 15: 147, 1972.
3. Björkerud, S. and Bondjers. G.: Arterial repair and atherosclerosis after mechanical injury. Part 2. Tissue response after induction of a total local necrosis (deep longitudinal injury). Atherosclerosis 14: 259, 1971.
4. Björkerud, S. and Bondjers, G.: Arterial repair and atherosclerosis after mechanical injury. Part 5. Tissue response after induction of a large superficial transverse injury. Atherosclerosis 18: 235, 1973.

(5)

ARTERIAL SURFACE CHANGES EXAMINED BY SCANNING (SEM) AND TRANSMISSION (TEM) ELECTRON MICROSCOPY

H. Jellinek

Professor of Pathology

2nd Department of Pathology, Semmelweis Medical University, Budapest, Hungary

The problem of hypoxia has been studied by several authors. Scanning electron microscopic studies have been carried out by Nelson et al. (1975), but they did not examine recirculation following hypoxia.

We studied the transitorily ischemized areas of the rat abdominal aorta, double-ligated for one hour and recirculated for one or two hours, or two or 10 days before sacrifice. The SEM of normal aorta revealed the delicately uneven, undulating structure of the luminal surface. The first changes following hypoxia are the crater-like bulgings and processes of the endothelial cells (Fig. 1). In some areas the undulating structure disappeared, depending on the degree of damage rather than on its duration. At such border areas the endothelial cells began to migrate over the damaged areas already after one hour (Fig. 2). The severely damaged areas are easily recognizable by the absence of the regular undulant structure. In this condition we observed at the borders of the damaged areas the appearance of different numbers of thrombocytes and leukocytes. SEM revealed uneven surface of the damaged areas corresponding to the ground substance of the subendothelium. In these areas thrombocytes were found by TEM and also endothelial cell processes were visible.

In areas with totally destroyed intimal surface, the denuded ground substance and the bridge-like or process-like residues of the collagen fibres could be recognized. Occasionally the completely denuded elastic fibres and traces of their stomata were seen as deep craters or holes. In such areas small groups of thrombocytes were anchored. Occasional appearance of leukocytes

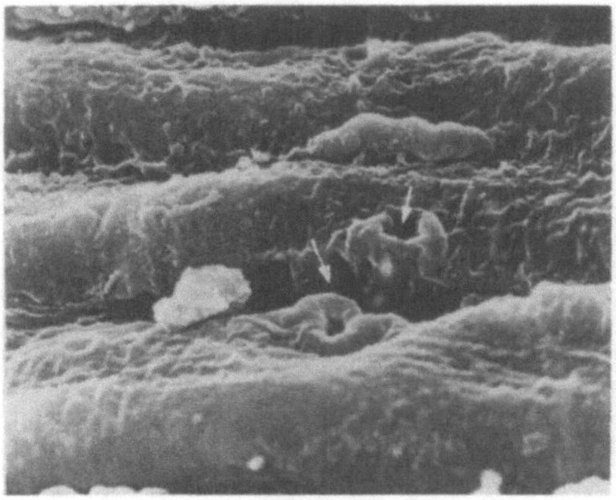

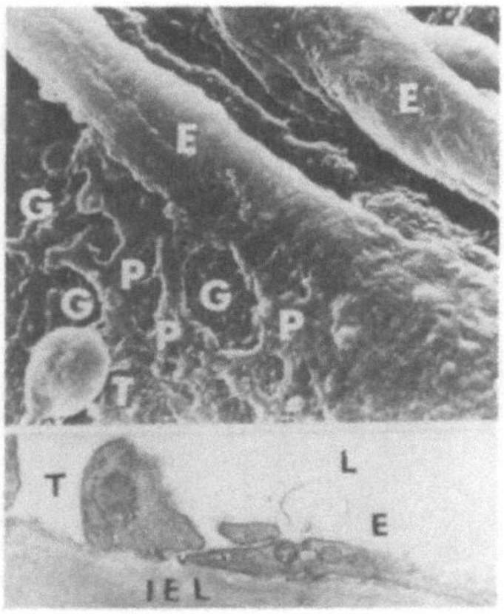

Fig. 1. Scanning electron micrograph. Note bulgings and process formation on the endothelial surface (arrows) x 3000

Fig. 2. Free subendothelial ground substance (G), with a thrombocyte (T) in one field, is well visible in the scanning electron micrograph between the processes of the endothelial cell (PE). Same in transmission electron micrograph: at left the thrombocyte (T), at right the endothelial cell process (E) are well visible. IEL=internal elastic lamina; L=lumen x 10.000; x 24.000

and macrophages was seen. In the same areas also debris of destroyed cells may appear. Similarly to the SEM pictures, also the TEM pictures may show leukocyte just passing across the stoma of an elastic fibre. In the TEM-micrograph a histiocyte-like cell is seen above the newly regenerated endothelial cell (Fig. 3). The early regenerative changes seen already after two hours are demonstrable in SEM pictures by the appearance of swollen endothelial cells having numerous spike-like processes on their surfaces. These cells are bulging deeply into the lumen. The same cells - when viewed by TEM - occasionally exhibit the morphology of mitosis.

The leukocytes and other phagocytic cells become subendothelial as a result of superposition of migrating endothelial cells, as shown by SEM. At some places the localization of a phagocytic cell in a ditch-like cavity, partly covered by an endothelial cell, was visible. In TEM one could clearly trace the formation of new endothelial coat with typical intercellular junctions overlaying the phagocytic cell.

In a later stage of the process the regenerating endothelial cells cover most of the destroyed and denuded areas. The deep

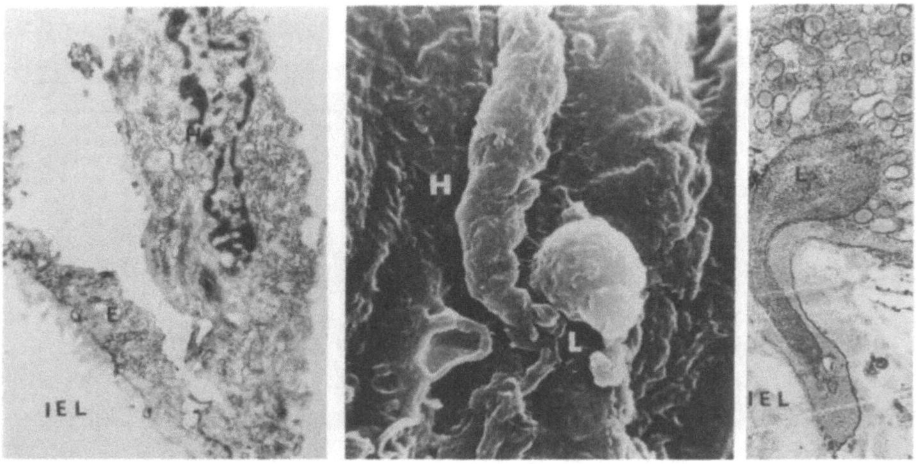

Fig. 3. Leukocytes (L) and histiocytic elements (H) seen in the injured areas can be easily identified also in the transmission electron micrograph (leukocyte at left, histiocyte at right); the leukocyte is just in the process of passing across a stoma of the internal elastic lamina (IEL). E= De novo formed row of endothelial cells. x 12.000; x 6.000; x 18.000

ditches disappear along with the stomata and all subendothelial structures until by the 10th day a "restitutio ad integrum" ensues. The even, undulating structure as seen in the control preparations is missing only in a few areas, in which a minor disturbance of the undulating structure is seen.

Hypertensive vascular lesions produced with noradrenaline showed loss of the regular structure, deterioration of endothelial cells, and appearance of phagocytes and thrombocytes. Similar phenomena are seen when vascular damage is produced at the adventitial side. Alterations of the intimal structure are similar to the above phenomena in scanning electron micrographs.

As in other studies similar changes were observed by SEM, there is reason to postulate that the scanning electron micrographs of intimal lesions developing in response to various injuries are of approximately similar appearance.

REFERENCES

Frost, H. Investigations into the pathogenesis of arteriosclerosis: drug prophylaxis. Atherogenesis II. Ed. T. Shimamoto, 1972, 32-51, Exc. Med.

Nelson, E., Sunaga, T., Shimamoto, T., Kawamura, T., Rennels, M.L., Hebel, R. Ischemic carotid endothelium. Arch. Path. 99, 125-132, 1975.

CHAPTER 15
SURGICAL TECHNIQUES - INVESTIGATION AND TREATMENT

(1)

THE INVESTIGATION OF CEREBRAL PERFUSION USING INTRA-ARTERIAL INJECTION OF ISOTOPICALLY LABELLED ALBUMIN MACRO-AGGREGATES

Allcock, J.M. and Chamberlain, M.

Department of Radiology

University Hospital, London, Ontario, Canada

We have to accept that even with the refinements of magnification and subtraction and selective injection the delineation of the small vessels of the brain leaves much to be desired and we really have no way at all of showing in any kind of detail the arterioles and capillaries.

The information gained from angiography is to a certain extent complemented by that supplied by routine scanning with isotopes. However, this method really gives more of a measure of tissue perfusion. Cerebral blood flow studies by methods such as the injection of xenon gives some information but unfortunately, it is not easily related to cerebral topography except in a gross manner.

In order to try to fill in some of these gaps, we have been using macro-aggregates of albumin. These at present have a mean size of 20 mμ. Approximately 80% of them lie within a 10% variation from this but they do range up to 60 mμ. At present, these aggregates are being labelled with iodine 131 or technetium 99. 150 microcuries of iodine or 300 microcuries of technetium are used, one being injected into one vessel and the other into a second. 10 - 20,000 particles of each are used, and because of their size, they are held up mainly in the distal arterioles. Their biological life is approximately 5 hours so that the patient can be scanned in a routine manner within 3-4 hours of injection. The scan obtained represents a visual freeze of the distribution of these particles in the territory of the vessel injected at the time of injection even though the imaging may be several hours later. There may have been a change in the circulation prior to the time of scanning but this does not affect the situation because there was no reservoir of particles in large vessels to pass on into smaller vessels and change the situation if for instance, dilatation of the smaller vessels does occur after the time of injection.

I would like to show you some representative slides of various studies that we have done. I am not going to show the xrays and will just describe them briefly to save time. The first one is a young man with a normal arteriogram and the anterior cerebral arteries each fill from their own side. The scan shows that there is a very slight crossflow from left to right of blood and no crossflow from right to left. The colour coding represents the distribution of activity analogous to a relief map, but the scale varies with different patients.

The next one shows a man, in whom both the anterior cerebral arteries filled from the left side and you can see isotopes pulling over to the right.

In this next patient, one isotope was injected into the right common carotid and one into the right vertebral and you can see the distribution of blood from these two vessels.

In the next patient, one isotope was injected into the external carotid and one into the internal on the same side and again you can see the distribution.

This next patient had a subarachnoid hemorrhage and had moderate arterial spasm on the right side and very severe spasm on the left and you can see the difference in the perfusion on the two sides.

These two cases show examinations of patients with tumors. In one there was a large left occipital tumor which was very vascular and presumably all the aggregates passed through shunts. The other one was on angiography an avascular frontal tumor but again no isotope is seen within the tumor.

This next one was a lady with a small meningeoma and you can see a concentration of isotope in the external carotid injection in the region of the tumor in the parietal region but not in the internal carotid.

In this next couple, in one there is an old left frontal area of infarction on the angiogram and no isotope was seen within that area. The other lady has had a recent infarct in the posterior frontal region. Angiography showed increased vascularity and this shows on this study also.

The next patient had bilateral carotid stenoses which appeared on angiography to be roughly equal in degree. However, you can see there is good crossflow from right to left, and no crossflow from left to right suggesting that in fact the stenosis on the left is causing more of a reduction in pressure than that on the right.

This lady had a left internal carotid occlusion. There is very little collateral flow through the ophthalmic or other arteries and one only sees the external circulation filling on the scan. The right common carotid was injected, and you can see good crossflow to the left side.

In this next patient, there was a left internal carotid occlusion before operation, with no collateral flow to the head from the external carotid. Anastomosis was performed between the superficial temporal and middle cerebral branch and angiography in this study shows some perfusion to the parietal region. There was good crossflow from right to left.

The next patient had bilateral internal carotid occlusions with very little collateral circulation from the anterior circulation. He had a left superficial temporal-middle cerebral shunt performed, and you can see that there is now excellent crossflow blood to the right supplying both the left and right hemispheres. On the right side the injection shows the external circulation only.

This next man had an occlusion of the left internal carotid artery. The only collateral circulation to this side with this injection that could be seen on the arteriogram was some filling of middle cerebral branches in the posterior parietal region via anastomosis passing through the bone from the superficial temporal artery. This can also be seen and its extent on the scan.

This last patient had a left internal carotid occlusion. Right injection shows good crossflow to the left. On the left, there was no obvious supply from the external carotid to the brain on the angiogram. The scan shows a patchy distribution which appears to be going within the brain and this may also represent leptomeningeal anastomosis.

You may ask whether all this is safe. We have done approximately 50 patients now without any obvious ill-effects. Prior to doing this, we have injected relatively very large quantities of isotope - labelled aggregrates into the cerebral circulation of dogs and killed them at various periods afterwards and no evidence of infarction could be found.

This method has also been used to a large extent in the investigation of renal and cardiac lesions without any ill-effects and its use in the cerebral circulation was in fact described from Montreal about 9 years ago.

I have shown the possible uses of the method at present. It is still fairly experimental and I think its main purpose will probably be to delineate the territory of supply of various vessels particularly in cases of occlusion or stenosis and the affects of operation such as anastomosis and endarterectomies.

I hope to develop it further using especially made microspheres, which could be made to a definite size plus or minus 0.5 mµ. If for instance, we assume that the size of a capillary is 10 mµ. then all spheres of say 15 mu. should be held up in the brain temporarily. If they are not held up in a certain area, the implication would seem to be that there is shunting taking place between the arterial venous systems and bypassing capillaries. We hope by such tests to try and show more clearly for instance, to what level the effects of arterial spasm in subarachnoid hemorrhage extend. I think that other applications will turn up as we pursue the matter further.

(2)

EXTRACRANIAL TO INTRACRANIAL MICROVASCULAR ANASTOMOSIS: A NEW APPROACH TO THE TREATMENT OF CEREBROVASCULAR DISEASE

Gary G. Ferguson

Division of Neurosurgery, Department of Clinical Neurological Sciences, The University of Western Ontario, University Hospital, London, Ontario, Canada.

It is estimated that in the United States alone, 200,000 new strokes occur annually, of which, at least 10% are the result of multiple extracranial or surgically inaccessible intracranial lesions, considered "inoperable" by conventional techniques (1). Recent advances in microsurgery allow revascularization to be undertaken in such patients. The most widely used procedure, first performed by Yasargil in 1967, is an end-to-side anastomosis between the superficial temporal artery and a cortical branch of the middle cerebral artery, vessels only slightly greater than 1 mm in diameter (4). Experience to date indicates that operative mortality and morbidity is less than 5% and that long term anastomosis patency rates approaching 100% are possible (2, 3). The principal difficulty with the procedure has been accurate delineation of the indications for its use in view of the broad clinical spectrum of cerebrovascular disease and the wide variety of lesions which may result in threatened or actual stroke.

The most comprehensive study to date is that of 65 cases from Munich (2). The authors divided their patients into four clinical categories. Ten patients with transient focal cerebral ischemic attacks (TIA's) were assymptomatic post-operatively. Post-operative regional cerebral blood flow studies (rCBF) confirmed improved regional circulation in this group. Prolonged but reversible focal ischemic neurological deficits of greater than 24 hours duration (RIND's) were present in 19 cases. Fifteen of these patients became assymptomatic post-operatively, the remaining four were improved. Stroke-in-evolution was present in seven cases. Surgical intervention proved disastrous in this group. Three patients died within a week of surgery, two more died within a month, and the two survivors were worse. Of 29 patients with a completed stroke, 20 were unchanged at late follow-up, eight had improved, and one had died.

The author has performed 11 anastomoses in 10 patients since September, 1974. The results are in general agreement with the Munich series. One patient with TIA's is now assymptomatic. Of two patients with RIND's, one is assymptomatic, the other is improved. One patient with a stroke-in-evolution remains severely disabled. Of six patients with completed strokes, three with lesser pre-operative deficits are improved, while three with major infarctions are unimproved. There have been no deaths. Angiography at six months in the first five cases has shown a 100% patency rate. In two cases, there were temporarily increased post-operative deficits. One of these cases was of particular interest.

Case Report. This 59 year old man presented with a progressive dementia of three years duration together with frequent TIA's implicating the left carotid territory for three months. There was a history of a major right carotid territory stroke eight years earlier from which he had recovered. Cerebral angiography revealed a right carotid occlusion in the neck, a severe left carotid siphon stenosis, and bilateral vertebral stenosis. A left STA-cortical anastomosis was done. He was well until 72 hours post-operatively when a severe pseudobulbar palsy and dysphasia developed. Angiography at that time revealed a widely patent anastomosis but complete occlusion of the siphon stenosis. The pseudobulbar palsy and dysphasia cleared within a week. When seen at three months, the patient reported a complete cessation of TIA's from the time of surgery, and the family reported that he was more active and mentally alert than in the past three years.

The encouraging initial results suggest that revascularization procedures may have a place in the treatment of threatened strokes, minor strokes, and even dementia, where the cause can be shown to be a conventionally "inoperable" lesion or combination of lesions. The same cannot be said for completed major infarctions, as the results in such cases to date are discouraging. Because of its apparent appropriateness and low morbidity, the procedure is gaining increasing popularity. To prevent its indiscriminate use, however, there is a need to demonstrate that surgical results better those of nature. To this end, plans for a co-operative study have been developed by Reichman (3).

References

1. Chater, N., Mani, J., Tonnemacher, K.: Superficial temporal artery bypass in occlusive cerebral vascular disease. Calif. Med. 119: 9-13, 1973.

2. Gratzl, O., Schmiedek, P., Spetzler, R., Steinhoff, H., Marguth, F.: Clinical experience with extra-intracranial anastomosis in 65 cases. J. Neurosurg. (in press)

3. Reichman, O.H.: Extracranial-intracranial arterial anastomosis. In: Whisnant, J.P., Sandok, B.A. (eds.): Cerebral Vascular Diseases, Ninth Conference. New York, Grune and Stratton, 1975, pp. 175-186.

4. Yasargil, M.G.: Microsurgery Applied to Neurosurgery. New York, Academic Press, 1969, pp. 105-115.

(3)

THE SURGICAL REPAIR OF ACUTE VENTRICULAR SEPTAL DEFECT AS A COMPLICATION OF MYOCARDIAL INFARCTION

John C. Coles

M.Sc., F.R.C.S.(C), Clinical Professor, Chairman, Division Cardiovascular & Thoracic Surgery, U.W.O. London. 111 Waterloo Street, Suite 208, London, Ontario, Canada

Septal perforation is a rare but sinister complication of acute myocardial infarction. It is thought to account for 1 to 2% of all fatal cases.

The purpose of this paper is to present our experience in the surgical repair of such patients, to document a hitherto unrecognized type of septal perforation, and to propose a classification of ventricular septal defect following myocardial infarction. The differentiation of the two types is important because of the different surgical approach.

Material

In a 13 year period at Victoria Hospital, London, 7 patients with septal perforation have been subjected to operation. Preoperative hemodynamic studies confirmed a large left to right shunt at the ventricular level and all showed pulmonary hypertension (pulmonary artery mean $>$ 30 mm of mercury.) Patients varied in ages from 48 to 79, there were five males and two females. Closure of the septal perforation was performed from 4 to 89 days following the myocardial infarction and 2 to 78 days following the onset of the septal perforation. Concomitant surgery included aorto-coronary bypass graft, mitral valve replacement, infarctectomy and left ventricular aneurysm resection.

The high defects (above the papillary muscle) were approached through a high posterior left ventriculotomy. The lower defects were approached through a low antero-apical left ventriculotomy.

The high defect is repaired with a dacron patch of adequate size.

The low defect is handled by amputation of the distal one-third of the heart or a dacron patch closure.

Four of the seven patients gradually improved and were discharged from 25 to 39 days after operation. Three patients died from 24 hours to 10 days postoperatively.

Two of the surviving patients were found to have a residual left to right shunt but with normal right ventricular pressure.

The high defects both developed a persistent left posterior hemiblock postoperatively.

Discussion

Analysis in depth identifies two distinct types of septal perforation following acute myocardial infarction. The high (posterior superior) defect is associated with circumflex and distal right coronary artery occlusion. The left anterior descending artery was not occluded. There was no associated left ventricular aneurysm but akinesis of the posterior superior left ventricular wall was present. The high defects are hidden by the chordae tendenae and mitral leaflets but adequate visualization is accomplished by retraction anteriorly.

The lower defect is associated with occlusion of the distal left anterior descending coronary artery and the posterior descending branch of the right coronary artery. The other vessels are usually the site of atherosclerotic stenotic but not occlusive disease.

Anterior, antero-lateral and/or apical dyskinesis may be present.

Conclusion

We advocate a classification of high and low ventricular septal defects following myocardial infarction. The natural history of the disease and the reasonable surgical results support an aggressive surgical approach in both types of septal perforation.

(4)

THE MEMBRANE LUNG IN ROUTINE BLOODLESS OPEN HEART SURGERY

R. O. Heimbecker, F. N. McKenzie, W. Wall,
K.T.N. Barnicoat and A. Robert
University Hospital, University of Western Ontario,
London, Canada.

INTRODUCTION The principle theoretical attraction claimed for membrane oxygenation is reduction in trauma to blood elements because of the absence of a blood gas interface. Recently, a disposable and inexpensive membrane oxygenator (Travenol "Teflo") has become available. We have used this oxygenator in 40 patients and compared indices of red cell and platelet survival in these patients with 50 patients who underwent open-heart surgery using a conventional bubble diffusion system.

METHODS Relevant data on the patients studied are shown in Table 1. In both groups 2 litres of Ringer's lactate was used to prime the oxygenator and cardiopulmonary by-pass was run at flows greater than 2 L./m^2/min, at 32°C. No arterial line filter was used in either group. Hourly post-operative chest drainage was recorded and platelet count, haemoglobin, haematocrit and plasma haemoglobin were measured before and at intervals after operation.

TABLE 1:

	AGE (Yrs)	PERFUSION TIME (Min)	OPERATIVE PROCEDURE			MORTALITY
			CORONARY BY-PASS	VALVE OPERATIONS	OTHER OPEN HEART	
MEMBRANE (n = 40)	51	61	28	8	4	3
BUBBLER (n = 50)	51	74	33	12	5	3

Supported in part by the Ontario Heart Foundation, the Nelson Hyland Foundation and the Medical Research Council of Canada.

RESULTS:

The mean post-operative chest drainage was approximately halved in the membrane group compared with control (Table 2). This improvement in the haemostatic properties of blood is also reflected in the marked reduction in requirements for blood transfusion in the membrane group. In the bubbler group 38% of patients required no blood during or after surgery, while 75% of patients in the membrane group were managed without blood transfusion. Despite this, the Hb. at the time of hospital discharge in the two groups was comparable. The reduction in the per-operative decrease in platelet count in the membrane compared with the control group provides further evidence of the atraumatic nature of membrane perfusion.

TABLE II:

			BLOOD REQUIREMENTS (units)								
	0 - 12 HR CHEST LOSS ML)	12 HR + CHEST LOSS (ML)	IN O.R.	IN I.C.U.	ON THE WARD	PLATELETS PLASMA (GIVEN)	PLASMA TOTAL HGB (MG%)	% DECREASE PLATELET	HGB (%) ON DISCHARGE	RE-OPERATED FOR BLEEDING	BLOODLESS PUMPS (%)
MEMBRANE	218	242	0	13	16	0	29	19	10.8	0	75
CONTROL	380	290	8	35	47	3	93	30	10.6	1	38

DISCUSSION

Recent improvements in the extracorporeal circulation have emphasized the need to reduce injury to the blood elements. To this end we have eliminated the arterial line filter during bubble oxygenation. (McKenzie et al. 1975). This introduction of membrane perfusion has resulted in further reduction in trauma to circulating blood. There was a modest decrease in plasma haemoglobin, fewer platelets lost and a consequent reduction in chest drainage. These factors combined to markedly reduce blood bank requirements. In addition, we confirmed the excellent gas transfer capabilities of the membrane oxygenator (Powes et al, 1974; Kakvan et al, 1974). In view of its safety and efficiency, membrane oxygenation deserves widespread clinical application.

REFERENCES

1. McKenzie, F.N., Heimbecker, R.O., Barnicoat, K.T.N., Robert, A., Gergely, N.F., DelMaestro, R., and Wall, W: Bloodless open heart surgery with atraumatic extracorporeal circulation. CMAJ 112:1073, 1975.

2. Powes, F.F., Martin, M., Smith, C.P., Beall, A.C., Morris, G.C., and DeBakey, M.E: Clinical experience with the "Teflo" membrane oxygenator. Am.Sect.Proc. 2:80, 1974.

3. Karlson, K.E., Murphy, W.R., Kakvan, M., Anthony, P., Cooper, G.N., Richardson, P.D., Galletti, P.M: Total cardiopulmonary by-pass with a new microporous Teflo membrane oxygenator. Surgery 76:935, 1974.

(5)

NEW SURGICAL APPROACH TO DIFFUSE CORONARY OCCLUSION: SELECTIVE ARTERIALIZATION OF THE CORONARY VEINS

C.J. Chiu, M.D.,Ph.D., & D.S. Mulder, M.D.,F.R.C.S.(C)

McGill University, Montreal, Quebec, Canada

Montreal General Hospital, 1650 Cedar Ave., Montreal, P.Q.

Many patients suffering from coronary heart disease cannot benefit from aorto-coronary bypass (ACB) surgery due to the diffuse coronary arteriosclerosis. The rationale for treating such patients with selective arterialization of the coronary veins include:
1.) Lack of valves in the coronary vein, allowing retrograde blood flow.
2.) The absence of arteriosclerotic changes in the vein even when the accompanying artery is diffusely occluded.
3.) The ability to deliver blood to the specific region of myocardium promptly, in contrast to the myocardial arterial implant procedures.

In 30 sheep (50-60 Kg.), left internal mammary arteries (IMA) were anastamosed to the great cardiac veins (GCV) accompanying the LAD. Proximal ligation of the GCV established prompt retrograde perfusion. LAD was ligated or injected with polyvinyl acetate plastic to produce diffuse occlusion. Flow studies using an electromagnetic flow probe revealed:
1.) Blood flow through IMA-GCV may range from 50 to 200 ml/min. The vein turns pink immediately but branches near the apex may remain relatively blue.
2.) The pulsatile flow pattern is predominantly diastolic, as in ACB.
3.) No reactive hyperemia through IMA-GCV can be elicited following 10 seconds of occlusion, indicating the bypassing of resistance vessels (arterioles) and/or the presence of significant "shunt" flow in this mode of revascularization.

Follow-up studies of up to 5 months showed that the size of infarcts were significantly reduced, but the protection appeared to be partial, as focal or small transmural infarcts were noted near the apecis. The myocardium in the non-infarcted area appeared normal without edema or hemorrhage, and corrosion casts made from such hearts demonstrated the patency of the arterialized vascular tree and the veno-venous runoff channels.

In order to further estimate the extent of the "shunt" blood flow in this preparation, CR-51 tagged microspheres (diameter 15 ± 5 u) suspended in blood were infused into the coronary vessels, and the fraction of the microspheres trapped by the myocardial microcirculation was used as an index of "capillary" or "nutritional" blood flow. When microspheres were injected into the canine LAD, approximately 80% were trapped, in contrast to the less than 5% trapping when they were injected retrograde into canine GCV. Furthermore, the trapping decreased when the accompanying LAD remained patent. In excised sheep heart, 10% trapping occurred with retrograde GCV infusion. It appears that significant veno-venous shunt channels large enough to allow the passage of such microspheres do exist in the myocardium, and thus may divert nutritional blood flow away from the most distant area of the myocardium near the apex.

Although a number of clinical cases of selective coronary vein arterialization have been reported, the experimental studies to date by several investigators have yielded results which ranged from enthusiasm to pessimism. This study indicates both the potential and the possible limitations of this procedure. The long term values of this approach, however, require further elucidation.

REFERENCES

1.) Chiu CJ, Mulder DS: Selective arterialization of coronary veins for diffuse coronary occlusion - An experimental evaluation. J. Thor. Cardiovasc. Surg. 70: 177, 1975.

2.) Park SB, Magovern GJ, Liebler GA, Dixon CM, Begg FR, Fisher DL, Dosios TJ, Gardner RS: Direct selective myocardial revascularization by internal mammary artery-coronary vein anastamosis. J. Thor. Cardiovasc. Surg. 69: 63, 1975.

Section III
Workshop Sessions

SECTION II - (WORKSHOPS)

SUMMARY TABLE

DAY I September 1 P.M.	CHAPTER 1 (WI-1) Lipid Clinic I Objectives, Organization, Biochemical and Dietary Methods Dr. J.A. Little, Canada Dr. H. Peeters, Belgium	CHAPTER 2 (WI-2) New Therapeutic Approaches to Acute Myocardial Infarction (Ml) and its size Dr. R.W. Gunton, Canada Dr. D.B. Hackel, U.S.A.	CHAPTER 3 (WI-3) Fate of Lipoproteins Dr. R.J. Havel, U.S.A. Dr. E.A. Nikkilä, Finland	CHAPTER 4 (WI-4) Regression of Lesions Dr. R.W. Wissler, U.S.A. Dr. M.L. Armstrong, U.S.A.
DAY II September 2 A.M.	CHAPTER 5 (WII-1) Lipid Clinic II Drugs, Genetics and Lipoprotein Dynamics Dr. R. Paoletti, Italy Dr. D. Kritchevsky, U.S.A.	CHAPTER 6 (WII-2) Atherosclerosis and Childhood Dr. Shiela Mitchell, U.S.A. Dr. B.S.L. Kidd, Canada	CHAPTER 7 (WII-3) Plasma Lipids and Thrombosis Dr. A.G. Shaper, England Dr. S. Renaud, France	CHAPTER 8 (WII-4) Animal Models in the Study of Atherosclerosis Dr. T.B. Clarkson, U.S.A. Dr. R. Pick, U.S.A.
DAY II September 2 P.M.	CHAPTER 9 (WII-5) Lipid Clinic III Effects of Nutrition and Treatment on Lipid Metabolism Dr. L.A. Carlson, Sweden Dr. K.K. Carroll, Canada	CHAPTER 10 (WII-6) Current Investigations in Myocardial Perfusion Dr. M. McGregor, Canada Dr. J.B. Armstrong, Canada	CHAPTER 11 (WII-7) Tissue Culture I Dr. G.H. Rothblat, U.S.A. Dr. O.J. Pollak, U.S.A.	CHAPTER 12 (WII-8) Connective Tissues in Atherosclerotic Lesions Dr. R.H. More, Canada Dr. W. Hollander, U.S.A.
DAY III September 3 A.M.	CHAPTER 13 (WIII-1) Recommendations to the Public for Prevention of Atherosclerosis Dr. S. Wolf, U.S.A. Dr. J.F. Mustard, Canada	CHAPTER 14 (WIII-2) Biochemistry of Arterial Wall; Factors in Mural Lipid Accumulation Dr. G.S. Boyd, Scotland Dr. D. Zilversmit, U.S.A.	CHAPTER 15 (WIII-3) Tissue Culture II Dr. A.L. Robertson, Jr., U.S.A. Dr. S. Björkerud, Sweden	CHAPTER 16 (WIII-4) Endothelium and Permeability Dr. J.C.F. Poole, England Dr. E.P. Benditt, U.S.A.

CHAPTER 1

LIPIC CLINIC I

(Objectives, Organization, Biochemical and Dietary Methods)

(1)

INTRODUCTION TO LIPID CLINIC I

Dr. Alick Little

St. Michael's Hospital & University of Toronto

30 Bond Street, Toronto, Ontario, Canada

The development of lipid clinics was necessitated by the increasing recognition of patients with disorders of lipid metabolism. It is interesting to compare Diabetic and Lipid Clinics. After the discovery of insulin in 1921, Diabetic Clinics sprang up quickly. In contrast, Lipid Clinics have evolved slowly over the last 25 years following the realization that there was a strong relationship between the level of plasma lipids and the future risk of atherosclerotic disease, and that this was the major cause of death in our population. Insulin demonstrated life saving properties within a few hours of it's use in ketoacidotic diabetics. For a few non-diabetic severly lipemic patients, lowering plasma lipids can quickly relieve acute pancreatitis or melt away eruptive skin xanthomata. However, the lowering of plasma lipids by diet and/or drugs, while theoretically desirable, has yet to be of proven benefit for the average patient with only moderate elevation of plasma cholesterol and/or triglyceride. But the relatively large number of such persons in the population (approximately 10%) and the high death rate from atherosclerotic disease, make the potential benefits of an effective program very considerable.

Because of this potential for preventing ischemic vascular disease it is important that Lipid Clinics be organized by competent investigators who will collect data in such a way as to be able to tell in future whether the treatment program has any net benefit on health. Indeed I am suggesting that Lipid Clinics around the world should collaborate to help answer the question, "Does lowering plasma cholesterol and triglyceride delay or prevent ischemic vascular disease and improve survival?". There should be an International Registry for all patients in collaborating clinics and a very simple protocol for follow-up with data on plasma cholesterol, triglyceride, smoking, blood pressure, body weight, diet, drugs and clinical events including death, heart attack, stroke and obstruction of a major peripheral artery. This implies some standardization of laboratory techniques and diagnostic reporting. Data analysis would consist of comparing clinical events in patients grouped according to their baseline indices and response to therapy. What the participants of this and other Workshops on Lipid Clinics say may indicate whether this lofty objective is practical. It may be relevant that 50 years after the discovery of insulin, Diabetic Clinics are still struggling with the question, "Does careful chemical control of diabetes prevent the late vascular complications?".

(2)

OBJECTIVES

Alick Little, M.D.

Project Director, University of Toronto-McMaster,
Lipid Research Clinic
St. Michael's Hospital, 30 Bond Street, Toronto, Canada

The prime objectives are to investigate and treat patients with disorders of lipid metabolism. Although there may be a few patients with rare disorders such as abeta lipoproteinemia, the majority of cases have hyperlipoproteinemia (HLP). Although every disease presents a challenge for us to understand the basic mechanisms and the etiology, HLP is a monumental challenge since it is a major risk factor for atherosclerosis. Therefore Lipid Clinics are in the front line trenches for the army of health scientists who are battling to reduce the very high morbidity and mortality from ischemic vascular disease.

Lipid Clinics should not take the myopic view that prevention of atherosclerosis begins and ends with lowering plasma lipid levels. All of the recognized risk factors should be considered in each patient, including hypertension, smoking, diabetes and obesity. Of course complete investigation leads to a consideration of causes of secondary HLP, especially hypothyroidism, oestrogen therapy and abuse of alcohol. Dealing with this array of problems requires collaboration with practically all the other health delivery teams in a large hospital.

Patients with HLP, especially the so-called primary type, require screening of their close relatives for elevation of plasma lipids. In our experience from 25-50% of first degree relatives also have HLP, the percentage depending in part on where the upper limits of normal for cholesterol and triglyceride are placed. This is a very high yield and shows the practical value of family screening. Besides providing important information concerning the modes of genetic transmission of the disorders, the affected relatives are good candidates for programs to study the prevention of complications of HLP.

Although there has been a considerable increase in the understanding of lipid chemistry and metabolism recently there is much more to learn. Thus every patient with a lipid disorder should be studied for variations from the known chemical, metabolic and genetic patterns. Again collaboration between the physician, biochemist, dietitian and geneticist, etc. is indicated. Lipid clinics should be a focal point for teaching and research by several disciplines.

Perhaps the most important issue for Lipid Clinics is to test the hypothesis that lowering plasma lipids will delay or prevent ischemic vascular disease and prolong life. Evidence from previous studies of this problem are suggestive but not conclusive. In some collaborating clinics, projects such as the Lipid Research Clinic(LRC) program and the Multiple Risk Factor Intervention Trial(MRFIT) are evaluating the effect of reducing risk factors like hypercholesterolemia, hypertension and smoking on survival and ischemic heart disease. In the introduction to this Workshop I suggested that there may be other less sophisticated ways of studying this most important public health problem. I would like to emphasize that there is much work to be done and more hands are needed to organize and work in Lipid Clinic programs.

(3)

ORGANIZATION OF LIPID CLINICS

Dr. Bernard M. Wolfe

Chief, Endocrinology & Metabolism, Dept. of Medicine

University Hospital, London, Ontario, Canada

Lipid clinics may be expected to provide facilities for accurate diagnosis and optimal management of hyperlipidemias. By bringing together patients with similar problems, lipid clinics afford the opportunity for more efficient use of time by dietitians who counsel the patients (possibly counselling them in groups) and laboratory technicians who analyze the lipid content of blood samples. The clinics also provide an opportunity for discussion of diagnostic and therapeutic problems by staff physicians, house staff and students of medicine, dietetics and nursing. Such conferences provide an opportunity for members of the medical community to continuously improve their knowledge and may serve as an incentive for physicians to participate in such clinics.

The essential personnel commonly involved in the lipid clinic are the medical secretary, receptionist, physicians (assistants and supervisor), nurse(s), biochemistry technician(s) and dietitian(s). The medical secretary and receptionist are mainly concerned with the administration of the clinic and ensuring that the patient reaches the appropriate personnel or service within the hospital. The physicians, nurses and dietitians are intimately involved with interviewing and counselling the patient while the biochemistry technician may or may not come to the clinic to obtain the blood samples.

The secretary is often the first person the patient contacts. She should inform the patient at that time to abstain from alcohol and to fast for at least twelve hours the night before coming to the lipid clinic so that a specimen of blood can be obtained immediately for determination of fasting lipids. She can assist the physician greatly by obtaining copies of the patient's previous medical records. In co-operation with the receptionist, she schedules the patient's visits to the clinic. She may note the names of patients who did not attend the clinic and, in accord with clinic policy, may send out clinic reminders. She may also keep the accounts.

As in any clinic, the receptionist obtains the names of patients attending the clinic, puts them at ease and ensures that they receive their turn to see their doctor. The receptionist may save the physician a great deal of time by completing requisitions, directing the patient to other hospital services such as the dietary department and the blood-taking station, and by arranging follow-up.

The physician is responsible for obtaining and recording the clinical data base. The data base need not differ from that required for any other new medical patient, although it might be expected to emphasize the detection of early signs of disease. Some clinicians may find a clinical check-list useful (1); however, the present limitations of time do not permit further discussion of this. Base-line investigations such as fasting levels of lipids and glucose are essential. Because of the day-to-day variation in the levels of fasting lipids (2) and the difficulty in ascertaining whether a particular therapeutic regime has been effective, it is advisable that at least two or three base-line measurements of fasting lipids be obtained in general before dietary and/or pharmacologic intervention is undertaken. Urinalysis, electrocardiogram and chest x-ray are mandatory in all adult patients attending a lipid clinic. Patients will comply better and be more successful if the physician explains the rationale of proposed dietary therapy and indicates the results that might be anticipated. Whenever drugs are used, the physician should alert the patient to possible side-effects and what to do about them. Obese patients may need special attention including behavioural counselling. The inactive patient might be persuaded to undertake exercise. The supervising physician should see every patient under his charge with his assistants on completion of each interview, and should ensure that the referring physician receives a prompt report of every clinic visit.

The role of the nurse is summarized as follows. She usually manages the facilities, maintaining the examining tables and chaperoning the female patients. Nurses may obtain the blood samples for measurement of the lipids as well as other specimens. The nurse may play a special role in educating patients, particularly those with diabetes.

The dietitian plays a key role in the therapy of hyperlipidemias. She should always obtain a careful dietary history to assess caloric requirements as well as the kind of food the patient can afford. The dietitian should give a clear explanation of the diet to the patient, and if he is a man, also to the patient's wife. Greater compliance with the diets can be obtained if the patient is informed of all acceptable alternatives with respect to choice of foods. The patient should have a continuing access to the dietitian by telephone.

The essential facilities for a lipid clinic include adequate space for about 10 or 20 patients and the receptionist's desk. Each physician should have an examining room which is provided with the usual equipment required by an internist. Of particular value is the large size blood pressure cuff for the obese patient. Facilities should be available for obtaining an electrocardiogram. If there is a question of quantifying basal energy requirements, measurement of oxygen consumption under basal conditions may be indicated.

With respect to selection of patients, it is seldom easy for a specialist to determine the nature of the medical problems that are referred to him. However, physicians who have a special interest in hyperlipidemia tend to find that patients with all types of hyperlipidemia (3) and those with a family history of premature atherosclerosis are referred to their clinic.

Patients often prefer to come to the clinic early in the morning on their way to work, for example at 8:00 a.m. Usually about 40 to 60 minutes are needed to see a new patient; subsequent visits may require 10 to 20 minutes. Usually patients need to be seen at two or three monthly intervals until control of the hyperlipidemia is achieved. Thereafter, the patient may need to attend at 6 to 12 monthly intervals to ensure maintenance of therapeutic effect and to assess developments.

The lipid clinic naturally has a close relationship with cardiovascular, neurological and renal clinics because of the frequency of cerebrovascular and cardiovascular disease of patients attending those clinics. Patients often pass both ways between these clinics. In summary, it is a particular role of the lipid clinic to provide efficient means for the management of hyperlipidemia and other problems predisposing to atherosclerosis, while maintaining a balanced perspective on the total health profile of the patient.

REFERENCES

1. The problem-oriented system. 1972. J.W. Hurst and H.K. Walker, editors. Medcom Press, New York.

2. Allard, C., P. Jolicoeur and G. Goulet, 1970. Cholesterol determinations: How many? Can. Med. Assoc. J. 102:1398-1399.

3. Beaumont, J.L., L. A. Carlson, G.R. Cooper, Z. Fejfar, D.S. Frederickson and T. Strasser. Classification of hyperlipidaemias and hyperlipoproteinaemias. Memoranda. Bull. World Health Organization 43 and Suppl. 891-908, 1970.

(4)

STANDARDIZATION OF CURRENTLY EMPLOYED BIOCHEMICAL PROCEDURES (CHOLESTEROL, TRIGLYCERIDES, LIPOPROTEIN ELECTROPHORESIS, AND TYPING)

Gerald R. Cooper, Ph.D., M.D.

Center for Disease Control

Atlanta, Georgia, U.S.A.

The most common biochemical procedures employed in studies on atherosclerosis are those that measure lipids, lipoproteins, and associated metabolic products (1). At present, determinations of cholesterol and triglyceride levels appear to be more useful in the clinical classification of hyperlipidemia and hyperlipoproteinemia and in characterizing the patient with a risk factor. Determination of the lipoprotein concentration and the level of lipoprotein apoproteins and enzymes, however, provides a clearer and more definite picture of the patient's lipid metabolic state. Other biochemical procedures for plasma constituents, such as hormones, coagulation factors, and constituents associated with other risk factors, are measured to detect or follow suspected risk factors and complications or sequelae of atherosclerosis. Standardization of all of these tests is essential if results obtained by laboratories participating in clinical and epidemiological studies are to be comparable.

Calibration and standardization of any clinical biochemical test involve use of reference materials, a reference method, and a properly designed quality control system. Procedures used in calibrating and standardizing the various lipid and lipoprotein tests vary because different methods are often used to determine these constituents, and the available standardization materials are not always applicable to all methods.

CHOLESTEROL

Cholesterol does not exist in a free state in the plasma but resides in lipoproteins, with about two-thirds being esterified with fatty acids. This makes accuracy in performing the cholesterol determination more difficult to achieve since all of the color-developing reagents do not react with cholesterol esters to the same extent or rate that they react with cholesterol. In colorimetric methods, sources of error can exist in any of the multiple analytical steps of sampling, hydrolysis, extraction, evaporation, redissolving in a solvent suitable for color production, and color production and measurement. Quality control, calibration, and standardization should cover all steps, particularly those in which errors are usually more significant. In some procedures for determining serum cholesterol, some of these basic steps are omitted. For instance, direct methods omit extraction and hydrolysis and are subject to sources of error from nonspecific reactions with interfering substances, differences in rate and degree of reaction of the reagent with free and esterified cholesterol, and effects of heat convection on the chemical reaction. The degree of heat production varies with small changes in the water content of the sample and in technique. The order and speed of adding reagents is considered the major factor in the uncontrollability of the temperature of the chemical reaction being measured. Various substances can interfere in the various color reactions for cholesterol, such as bilirubin and hemoglobin in the Liebermann reaction and salicylates and protein in iron salt-sulfuric acid reactions. Standardization must, therefore, include not only a comparison of the method with the selected reference or referee procedure on samples from serum pools, but also a comparison of the methods by using results obtained on fresh samples with values in both normal and abnormal ranges.

After enzymatic methods have been examined for completeness of hydrolysis and stability of measurement of the enzymatic process, they must also be standardized against pure standards and serum pools of known values, and their values must be compared with those obtained on fresh normal and abnormal serums determined with a reference method.

The type of sample must be considered in standardizing the cholesterol determination. Results obtained with plasma and serum can differ, depending on the type of anticoagulant used to form the plasma. For instance, at levels near the middle of normal range, little difference in plasma and serum values is noted when heparin is used as the anticoagulant, but plasma values are about 3% lower when disodium ethylenediamine tetra-acetate (EDTA) is used, about 8% lower when oxalate is used, 12% lower when citrate is used, and about 18% lower when fluoride is used (2). Now either plasma prepared with EDTA or serum is used in most studies.

Reference materials needed for calibrating the cholesterol determination are pure standards and serum pools with a labeled value established by the reference procedure. A primary standard of defined purity is distributed by the National Bureau of Standards for evaluating primary standards acquired from commercial sources. Cholesterol preparations of at least 99% purity are available from commercial sources for use as primary standards (3). These pure cholesterol preparations should be stored dry, cool, and in the dark.

Serum reference pool materials are available commercially; some are unlabeled and are for use as a daily bench control, and some have a labeled value established with a selected method that may or may not be an accurate value. Arrangements should be made to acquire at least one serum reference pool material labeled by the current reference method of Abell et al.

A reference method is needed to label reference materials with an accurate value and to study the effects of sampling and conditions on a method under investigation. The CDC Lipids Section uses a modified, manual Abell, Levy, Brodie, and Kendall cholesterol method (4) as its reference method for labeling materials for its WHO-CDC and NHLI lipid standardization programs.

TRIGLYCERIDE

Colorimetric, fluorometric, and enzymatic methods capable of meeting the performance requirements of various proficiency testing and standardization programs are available for use in clinical and research laboratories (5). Use of specific and reproducible analytical procedures and careful collection, transport, and storage of samples are essential to standardization of the method. Serum collected from persons in the fasting state is preferred for measurement of triglycerides. Since most triglyceride exists in lipoproteins, plasma values will be lower than serum values according to the anticoagulant used. Samples stored for analysis must be kept in a frozen, sterile state. Turbidity, hemolysis, and elevated bilirubin necessitates use of blanks or other corrections for some methods. The colorimetric and fluorometric methods acquire specificity by steps that extract the lipids from serum, separate phospholipids and glucose, and hydrolyze the isolated triglycerides before the glycerol content is determined.

Purified preparations of either triolein or tripalmitin are usually employed as primary standards in standardizing the triglyceride determination. If results are expressed in mg/dl, the primary standard used in the analysis should be stated, since its molecular weight must be considered in calculating results. Failure to indicate which primary standard is used can cause confusion in interpreting and comparing reported values. This source of error can be avoided if millimolar concentration is adopted for reporting triglyceride values.

Stable, clear serum reference materials for standardization of the triglyceride determination can be prepared by adding egg yolk extract to animal or human serum (6). Lyophilized pooled serum preparations are available from a few commercial suppliers, but these are often turbid, and many have been assigned labeled values that do not agree with those obtained with reference procedures. A semiautomated colorimetric chromotropic acid method that gives values comparable to those of the manual Carlson method (7) is used in the CDC Lipid Standardization Laboratory for reference purposes. A description of this method is available from the Lipids Section.

LIPOPROTEIN ELECTROPHORESIS

Free migration and size-sensitive types of electrophoresis are used to detect intermediate density lipoproteins (type III) and to confirm obvious lipoprotein pattern types. The test is qualitative, since staining varies with type and subgroups of lipoprotein. Quality control involves a check on the distance of migration and a comparison of the appearance of the stain on fresh specimens and on a frozen serum pool of low triglyceride content. Standardization among collaborators at the present time is attempted by choosing the same method and the same quality control system.

ULTRACENTRIFUGATION

Instability of the lipoproteins causes major problems in standardization of the ultracentrifugal analysis. Standardization consists primarily of three requirements: 1) samples shall be collected under conditions that maintain integrity, 2) both preparatory and analytical ultracentrifugation shall be performed under standard conditions, and 3) the chemical and physical measurements made on lipoprotein fractions shall be made under strict quality control to cover both reproducibility with time and comparability with other laboratories.

POST-HEPARIN LIPOLYTIC ACTIVITY (PHLA) AND LECITHIN CHOLESTEROL ACYLTRANSFERASE ACTIVITY (LCAT)

A gross estimate of PHLA is usually made by comparing the electrophoretic pattern of plasma before and after *in vivo* injection of heparin (8). Standardization of PHLA involves use of an effective quality control system for electrophoresis and use of a heparin preparation proven to be effective in a normal person. LCAT activity is determined by measuring the formation of cholesterol esters after incubation of plasma with radioactive unesterified cholesterol at 37° for several hours (8). Standardization of LCAT involves standardizing the radioassay procedure and the method used to determine free and esterified cholesterol.

PHENOTYPING SYSTEM

Interpretation is the major problem encountered in standardizing a lipoprotein phenotyping system. Lipoprotein patterns are influenced by both genetic and secondary factors. In fact, major components contributing to abnormalities of lipoprotein patterns are environmental. Standardization for genetic studies requires selection and adhering to guidelines for conditions of sample collecting, analysis, calculation, and interpretation (9).

Most samples collected for the clinical laboratory reflect the physiological state of lipoproteins in patients at the time of sample collection and thus cover both genetic and environmental factors (10). The clinical laboratory reports the type of lipoprotein pattern, and the clinician interprets its meaning with respect to genetic, environmental, and disease states. Standardization of the measurement of cholesterol and triglyceride, the procedure for collecting fresh samples, and the technique of the electrophoretic procedure are the basis for standardizing the determination of lipoprotein patterns for clinical studies.

REFERENCES

1. Beaumont, J. L., Carlson, L. A., Cooper, G. R., Fejfar, Z., Fredrickson, D. S., and Strasser, T., Classification of hyperlipidemias and hyperlipoproteinemias. Bull. Wld. Hlth. Org. 43, 891-915 (1970).

2. Cooper, G. R. and Eavenson, E., Unpublished Results (1963).

3. Williams, J. H., Kuchmak, M., and Witter, R. F., Evaluation of the purity of cholesterol primary standards. Clin. Chem. 16, 423-426 (1970).

4. Abell, L. L., Levy, B. B., Brodie, B. B., and Kendall, F. E., A simplified method for the estimation of total cholesterol in serum and demonstration of its specificity. J. Biol. Chem. 195, 357-366 (1952).

5. Cooper, G. R., The World Health Organization-Center for Disease Control lipid standardization program. In Transactions of the VI International Symposium on Quality Control, Geneva, H. Huber, Bern, in press.

6. Williams, J. H., Taylor, L., Kuchmak, M., and Witter, R. F., Preparation of hypercholesterolemic and/or hypertriglyceridemic sera for lipid determinations. Clin. Chim. Acta 28, 247-253 (1970).

7. Carlson, L. A., Determination of serum triglycerides, J. Atheroscler. Res. 3, 334-336 (1963).

8. Fredrickson, D. S., Gotto, A. M., and Levy, R. I., Familial lipoprotein deficiency. In The Metabolic Basis of Inherited Disease, 3rd ed. J. B. Stanbury, J. B. Wyngaarden, and D. S. Fredrickson, Eds. McGraw-Hill, New York, N. Y., 1972.

9. Lipid Research Clinics Program, Manual of Laboratory Operations, Volume 1, Lipid and Lipoprotein Analysis, NHLI, Bethesda, Maryland. DHEW Publication No. (NIH) 75-628, May 1974.

10. Friedewald, W. T., Levy, R. I., and Fredrickson, D. S., Estimation of the concentration of low-density lipoprotein cholesterol in plasma, without the use of the preparative ultracentrifuge. Clin. Chem. 18, 499-502 (1972).

From the Clinical Chemistry Division, Bureau of Laboratories, Center for Disease Control, Public Health Service, U.S. Department of Health, Education, and Welfare, Atlanta, Georgia 30333

(5)

THE DIETARY MANAGEMENT OF HYPERLIPOPROTEINEMIA

Miss Valerie McGuire

Nutrition Coordinator, Toronto-McMaster Lipid Research Clinic, St. Michael's Hospital, 30 Bond Street
Toronto, Ontario, Canada

The patients who attend the Lipid Clinic at St. Michael's Hospital are referred to us by their physician or cardiologist. Some may already have ischemic vascular disease but more and more subjects are only referred because of hyperlipoproteinemia discovered during a routine health examination.

The dietitian interviews the patient on the first visit to the clinic in order to obtain a history of previous dietary habits. This serves two purposes:

1. It helps determine the etiology of the hyperlipoproteinemia. There may be excessive ingestion of calories, sugar, alcohol and foods rich in cholesterol and saturated fat.

2. The patient's eating pattern assists in planning the therapeutic diet that will meet the special nutrient requirements and life-style of that person, such as, restaurant meals and lunches at work.

The interview form consists of 4 pages:

1. Questions regarding occupation, physical activity, number of meals eaten out, former use of a special diet, etc.

2. An activity associated meal pattern. When do you arise? What is the first thing you eat or drink? What do you eat at lunch? Do you snack between meals?

3. Questions about specific fat containing foods: use of butter or margarine, brand of shortening, number of eggs per week.

4. Food frequency: how often the patient eats other foods which might be excluded later in the controlled fat diet, such as: ice cream, desserts, candy, snack items.

The dietitian summarizes this information and does a crude analysis of the composition of the diet in terms of calories, carbohydrate, protein, fat, alcohol, cholesterol, ratio of complex to simple carbohydrate and ratio of polyunsaturated to saturated fatty acids. This report is given to the doctor to help in the assessment of the causes of hyperlipoproteinemia and other conditions.

At the first visit, the patient is also asked to follow a Typical Canadian Diet for two weeks prior to the ultimate blood tests for plasma lipids and lipoprotein fractionation. This diet includes plentiful amounts of meat, eggs, cheese, butter, sugar. This standardizes the diet and makes interpretation of the laboratory tests more reliable. This is necessary because some patients may be following some kind of diet prior to coming to the Lipid Clinic which distorts the lipoprotein pattern.

At Visit I, patients are also asked to keep a 3 day diet record (2 work days and 1 day off). This is returned to the dietitian at Visit 2 and she compares it with, and adds it to her initial information.

THERAPEUTIC DIETS

The most commonly prescribed diets for hyperlipoproteinemia are Type II and Type IV. Types I, III and V are much less common and will not be discussed here.

1. Obese patients are given limited calories for weight reduction.

2. Type II:
   (i) Saturated fat is reduced by limiting meat intake to 4-8oz per day depending on calorie level, using only skim milk products and eliminating all visible animal fats; butter, lard, meat fat.
   (ii) At least half of the fat calories are supplied by fats and oils rich in polyunsaturated fatty acids. This means consuming 6-10 teaspoons (depending on caloric allowance) of liquid vegetable oil (corn, safflower, and sunflower seed oils) per day. Walnuts or sunflower seeds may be substituted for part of this. In addition soft polyunsaturated margarines, other nuts and peanut butter are allowed within certain limits.
   (iii) All foods rich in cholesterol are eliminated including egg yolks, organ meats and shrimp.

3. Type IV: In addition to the above limitations:

   (i) simple sugars are restricted such as: sugar, jam, jelly, honey, soft drinks.

   (ii) alcohol is eliminated.

Most Type IV's are obese and need to achieve ideal weight in order to lower plasma lipids.

TABLE I CHARACTERISTICS OF DIET FOR TYPE II AND TYPE IV HYPERLIPOPROTEINEMIA

DIET	% CALORIES		CHOL mg	P/S	C/S	ALCOHOL
	CARB*	FAT				
Type II	40-50	30-40	< 200	⩾1.8	⩾1.4	in moderation
Type IV	30-40	40-50	< 200	⩾1.5	⩾2.0	none
For Comparison:						
Typical Can. Diet	45-50	30-40	300-800	<0.3	1.0	average: 6% of total cals

* Carbohydrate:
1. Type II - sucrose allowed but should not exceed 20 - 25% of total calories.
2. Type IV - sucrose not allowed. Emphasis on complex carbohydrate.

Chol - cholesterol
P/S - ratio of polyunsaturated to saturated fatty acids
C/S - ratio of complex to simple carbohydrate

All of the diets are based on the exchange system comparable to the diabetic exchange system. This allows the patient variation in food choice within the prescribed nutrient levels and permits the patient to lose weight without counting calories. Patients are encouraged to be conscious of portion sizes but need not weigh and measure all foods.

Once the physician has the results of all the investigation, he makes the diagnosis and prescribes treatment. Diet is the foundation of the treatment program and is always used first. Medication is never used unless the diet is unsuccessful in reducing lipids satisfactorily. Diet instruction is given to patients in groups. Most patients are better motivated by group counselling. They benefit from other patients questions and enthusiasm. Group counselling also results in a more efficient use of dietitians time. Individual instruction is available and may be more suitable for the exceptional case.

The patients are given material to take home and read before the instruction. This includes the booklet "Questions and Answers About Your Controlled Fat Diet". (1)

Group instruction for 4 - 6 patients and their spouses takes place in the evening. The sessions are approximately two hours long.

1. During the first hour the basic principles of the diet and the metabolic effect of various nutrients on plasma lipid levels are discussed. The terms cholesterol, saturated fats, polyunsaturated fats and atherosclerosis are explained. We review foods allowed, foods to avoid, restaurant eating, travel, shopping and cooking hints.

2. During the second hour the patients are given their individual diets with the daily food allowances and are asked to write a sample meal for the day using the food exchanges. Two dietitians are available so that each patient receives some individual help.

3. Displays are used as teaching aids. There are food models to show portion sizes; product information; recipe booklets from the hospital and other sources; and slides to illustrate the presentation. At the coffee/tea break controlled fat snacks are served.

FOLLOW-UP, COMPLIANCE, REINFORCEMENT

Once patients are taught the diet they are given return appointments for plasma lipid estimation and discussion with the dietitian at two week intervals for six weeks.

At the 2-week visit the patient's blood is taken and he is weighed. The 3-day food record is discussed. This serves as a means of checking how well the diet is being followed and if the poly-unsaturated fats are being incorporated into the diet. The patient can ask other questions.

At the 4-week visit the patient's blood is taken, he is weighed and the 3-day food record is reviewed. He is given the results of the first blood tests and although they are not always an accurate evaluation of dietary adherence they may encourage the patient. The dietitian reports the patient's weight, diet adherence and general attitude to the doctor.

At the 6-week visit the doctor assesses the patient's progress. Furture visits are booked at increasing intervals of 1, 3 or 6 months depending on the results. If a patient has a great deal more weight to lose, the dietitian may see him every two weeks until he reaches ideal weight.

The patients are given our telephone number and are encouraged to call anytime they have a question. We try to keep them up-to-date with the latest food product information. We systematically see all patients annually to review the diet. Old patients who have strayed from the diet are re-instructed in groups.

(1) ___________, "Questions and Answers About Your Controlled Fat Diet". Available from the Ontario Hospital Association, 150 Ferrand Drive, Don Mills, Ontario.

(6)

A POINT OF VIEW ON DIETARY MANAGEMENT OF HYPERLIPIDEMIA

Helen B. Brown, Ph.D.

The Cleveland Clinic Foundation

Cleveland, Ohio, U.S.A.

The description of dietary management for treating hyperlipidemia in the previous paper by Valerie McGuire makes several important points I wish to emphasize. You are aware that conditions at Saint Michaels Hospital are close to ideal. Both the facilities and the time available are adequate for the necessary activities.

The physician-dietitian team has a good working relationship; the physician recognizes the importance of nutrition in the overall care of the patient. He also recognizes and depends on the professional knowledge and experience of the dietitian; they communicate easily with each other. The dietitian becomes acquainted with the patient. Information is obtained about the patient's life style, eating habits, likes and dislikes and food practices. The dietitian needs to understand the patient's attitudes toward his medical problem and the relationship of his eating habits to them. The patient should be aware that the dietitian is not a disciplinarian or a judge, but she is there to help him and is fully supported by his physician.

The three day food record that is taken periodically during instruction and the intensive follow-up period is excellent for two reasons: (1) it provides the dietitian with continuing information about food habits and food selection, and (2) it enables the patient to become aware of what food he eats, how much, when he eats it, and maybe, even why. It is an excellent teaching tool.

The dietitian has ample time and information to adapt the prescribed diet to the individual needs of the patient - the packed lunch, the restaurant meals, the late evening snack, and the proper foods management when business and recreation interfere with his necessarily altered daily routine.

The preliminary period of two weeks, before the patient commences the therapeutic diet, is an excellent way to obtain a good baseline of blood lipid values from which to measure the effectiveness of diet therapy. This prior period is often difficult to achieve since some patients are overanxious to adopt some of the dietary changes they have heard about.

During instruction it is most important that the patient help in planning his diet; and his wife or other person buying the food and preparing the meals should be present. Group instruction is often better than individual instruction because of interaction among members of the group. Opportunity for personal discussion with the individual is also necessary during this time.

In the follow-up period, visits at two, four and six weeks after the two hour instruction are certainly adequate. The program, as set up at Saint Michaels Hospital, should be very effective. The physician continues to support the dietary management program during the follow-up period, and interprets the results of treatment to the patient. After the six week intensive follow-up, less frequent visits are required for adherence to the diet pattern. Continued objective measurements of adherence: body weight, blood pressure and lipid levels, encourage the patient to stay on his diet. The National Diet-Heart Study (1) demonstrated that serum cholesterol reduction was less in free-living persons than in those in institutions. Reduction was also less in those eating 4 to 6 meals a week at restaurants, than in those eating 1 to 2 such meals.

The metabolic background for these diets is discussed in other sessions of this Workshop. Basically there is one diet pattern, low in saturated fat and cholesterol, with a sliding scale of total fat, the amount depending on the amount of carbohydrate required. This fact becomes very apparent when food products are selected for implementing the food pattern (2). The only difference between the diets used at Saint Michaels for type II and type IV is the kind of carbohydrate. The total fat is the same for both and depends on the caloric requirement of the individual.

Greater emphasis on a different diet for each type of hyperlipidemia causes needless confusion. Originally the Cleveland Clinic studies used what were called two different diets (3). One was low in fat, with 15% of total calories as fat, and the other, a "vegetable oil" diet, with 38%. Serum lipids were equally reduced with either diet in hypercholesterolemic patients (type IIa) (4). In hyperglyceridemic patients (types VI or IIb and IV) serum lipids were reduced somewhat lower with the 38% fat diet than with the low-fat.

Diets with 15% to 38% total calories as fat are practical for home use. A moderate diet is widely recommended and used (5). It has 30 to 35% total calories as fat, less than 10% saturated fat and 10% or more polyunsaturated. Cholesterol is kept below 300 mg per day. This diet accomplishes many goals: body weight reduction, blood pressure reduction, serum triglyceride and cholesterol reduction (1). It may be taken as a basic guide and the fat content varied up and down a sliding scale.

Table I

MASTER FOOD PATTERNS

Food Pattern	Fat % Cal	Carb % Cal	Sat F.A. % Cal	Poly F.A. % Cal	P/S
Basic low-fat*	12	73	5	<1	-
Moderate low-fat*	20	65	5	8	1.6
Moderate fat*	33	52	7	12	1.7
Customary fat*	38	47	10	15	1.5

*Protein 15% calories (15-20%)
Cholesterol <300 mg (75-300 mg)

It is important to understand the interdependence of nutrients that are manipulated in fat-controlled diets (2). None of these factors--saturated fat and cholesterol, polyunsaturated fat, total fat and total carbohydrate--can be thought of alone. Selection of food follows a simple formula: Lean meat well trimmed of visible fat, low-fat or skimmed milk products, polyunsaturated oil and margarine, with a limited amount of refined sugar. Details may become complicated and confused unless the principles determining food choices are well understood.

The type of hyperlipidemia may not be clearly defined by the fasting lipoprotein pattern. In that case, the lipoprotein fraction that is abnormal is the key to an individual's treatment. Regardless of what other lipoprotein fraction is elevated, the persistent presence of chylomicrons or exogenous triglycerides requires a diet very low in total fat. Here, at first, a diet with only the fat contained in the day's meat supply, 10 to 15 grams, is suitable. When the chylomicrons disappear, oil and margarine may be added, one to two teaspoons at a time. The effect on lipid levels of this additional fat is monitored. If endogenous triglyceride (VLDL) increases during this treatment, it is first controlled by reduction in refined sugar, then with added clofibrate.

When cholesterol in the form of beta lipoprotein (LDL) is high, the basic diet, low in saturated fat and in cholesterol, with additional polyunsaturated oil, will reduce it. When endogenous triglyceride is high, the polyunsaturated fat level is adjusted to provide less than 50% of total calories as carbohydrate.

Diets may be highly structured or low in structure. A high-structured diet is required for use in hospital research and in a metabolic ward. It can be adjusted to treat obesity, diabetes, and blood lipid levels of highly resistant hyperlipidemic individuals. For the out-patient, weighing his food at home teaches portion size and insures that the right amount is eaten. This approach to diet therapy is very helpful to patients who feel threatened by their disease.

Many people needing dietary treatment are active, free-living individuals with many concerns other than food. A less structured diet is required to fit into their living pattern. The food pattern must be suitable to family and friends, and needs to withstand prevailing environmental pressures. Hyperlipemic outpatients (6) have followed a relatively unstructured food pattern for up to ten years and were able to maintain reduced blood lipid levels.

Table 2

Degree of serum cholesterol reduction maintained with diet in hyperlipidemic patients for up to ten years (adapted from ref. 4, figure 3)

Serum Cholesterol Reduction percent	Normal Subjects* n = 98**	Type IIa n = 38**	Type VI(IIb) n = 24**	Type IV n = 19**
0 - 9	11§	35§	0§	0§
10 - 19	53	40	57	0
20 - 29	33	23	43	12
>30	3	2	0	88

* 18 day quantitative diet test
** Number of persons in group
§ percent of persons in group

A change in eating behavior is emphasized in several experimental studies in nutrition education which are nearing completion. Preliminary results were reported at a meeting held by the National Heart and Lung Institute in April of this year, 1975 (7). There were several approaches. One was to change environmental pressures through messages in the public media, reading matter, radio, TV, along with intensive dietary instruction. Another study (8) stressed a low structured diet. It taught the use of foods and food groups within the framework of an overall nutritious food pattern. The use of lean meats, low-fat dairy products and polyunsaturated oils was emphasized. Synchronized slide-tapes were developed to teach the principles of the diet plan, adaptable to group or individual teaching, as well as self instruction.

Another study adapted several established educational methods to the teaching of diets to patients (9). People learn in different ways (10): Some by ideas and symbols (the symbolic mode), some by pictures and images (the ikonic mode), others by actual performance (the enactive mode). In addition to different learning modes, some persons require material that is highly structured, exact and detailed, others do better with much less organized material. Simple ideas, simply explained are necessary for those with few words at their command. Generalities and relationships alone may be suitable for learners with language ability. Such distinctions between individuals is an interesting view point that help the dietitian find new ways to help the patient (11). In this study, new teaching devices were developed, especially for the person who learns by doing (enactive mode).

Complete results are not yet available. However, the teaching method used with one group was reported at the April meeting (7). This group was taught by the best behavioral methods the nutritionists were able to devise. The focus was on the patient and his goals. The diet plan was developed by the participant himself, with guidance from the dietition. The patient contracted with the dietitian concerning the food habits he was willing to change before the next visit. He also agreed to keep a food record. Food servings were stressed with food models of proper size, cartons from a mock grocery store were shown and actual foods were served during the interview. The patient's meal pattern and his snacks were planned. On follow-up visits, only the present situation was dealt with. Value judgements were established and focus kept on the patient's own goals. Flexibility in the teaching approach was found to be important. Over the year, blood cholesterol and triglycerides were significantly reduced, body weight and blood pressure declined.

Another way to change a person's food pattern is to provide him with foods in which the fat composition has been modified by the processor. In an early study (12) a group of medical students and their wives were provided fat-controlled foods through a special commissary. They followed no diet pattern, choosing foods as they wished. Serum cholesterol levels were reduced by 14%. A few groups in the Diet-Heart Study (1) controlled only their meat intake, the remaining special Diet-Heart foods were eaten as desired. This freer regimen gave a serum cholesterol reduction equal to that obtained by the stricter diets.

In summary, fat-modified food patterns have been successfully administered in several different ways and varied according to the individual, his special medical and personal needs and his living situation. Dietary management, under all conditions, requires an on-going physician-dietitian-patient team. The diet itself is a lifetime food pattern, based on principles of good nutrition. Emphasis is placed on the changing of food habits, eating behavior and proper choice of foods.

REFERENCES

1. National Diet-Heart Study Research Group: The National Diet-Heart Study Final Report. Circulation 37: Suppl. I, 1968.

2. Brown, H.B.: Food patterns that lower blood lipids in man. J. Amer. Diet Assn. 58: 303, 1971.

3. Brown, H.B. and Page, I.H.: Lowering blood lipid levels by changing food patterns. JAMA 168: 1989, 1958.

4. Brown, H.B., Lewis, L.A. and Page, I.H.: Mixed hyperlipemia, a sixth type of hyperlipoproteinemia. Atherosclerosis 17: 181, 1973.

5. Inter-Society Commission for Heart Disease Resources, Athero-sclerosis and Epidemiology Study Groups. Primary prevention of the atherosclerotic diseases. Circulation 42: A-55, 1970.

6. Lewis, L.A., Brown, H.B. and Page, I.H.: Ten years' dietary treatment of primary hyperlipidemia. Geriatrics 25: 64, 1970.

7. Nutritional Behavior Research Conference, National Heart and Lung Institute, Bethesda, Maryland. April 29-30, 1975. In press.

8. Mojonnier, L., Hall, Y., Shekelle, R., Pardo, E., Davis, S. and Berkson, D.M.: A study of effective methods of changing eating habits in hypercholesteremic men and women. Chicago Heart Assoc-iation Nutrition Education Project. July 1972 to 1974. Reported at the Nutritional Behavior Research Conferences, NHLI, 1975. In press.

9. Jones, R., Turner, D., Slowie, L.A., Brandt, B., Ginther, J.R.: Reported at the Nutritional Behavior Research Conferences, NHLI, 1975. In press.

10. Ginther, J.R.: Educational diagnosis of patients. J. Amer. Diet Assoc. 59: 560, 1971.

11. Slowie, L.A.: Patient learning - segments from case histories. J. Amer. Diet Assoc. 59: 563, 1971.

12. Green, J.G., Brown, H.B., Meredith, A.P., Page, I.H.: Use of fat-modified foods for serum cholesterol reduction. JAMA 183:5, 1963.

(7)

DISCUSSION (LIPID CLINIC I)

Dr. Jean Palmer, Australia

The multivariate analysis of factors associated with the dietary lowering of serum cholesterol in a group of patients with type II hyperlipoproteiemia and obesity, averaging 112% of ideal weight, suggested that weight loss was the most important factor, having three times the effect of reduced dietary saturated fat.

Dr. Alick Little

Other investigators also have shown that a negative energy balance lowers serum cholesterol. However, there are patients with hypercholesterolemia who are not obese and weight reduction is not practical for them. Furthermore, studies where weight was held constant have shown a positive effect of dietary saturated fat and cholesterol and a negative effect of polyunsaturated fatty acids on serum cholesterol concentration.

Dr. Jean Palmer

Should one consider the kind of protein in diets for patients with hyperlipoproteinemia?

Dr. Bernard Wolfe

We do not yet know the answer to this question. In rabbits substitution of animal for vegetable protein raised serum cholesterol. Studies of this type are just now being undertaken in humans.

Dr. Gerald Berensen, New Orleans

Studies in primates have shown that lowering total dietary protein from 25% to 8% of calories decreased serum cholesterol. This was prevented by giving sulphur containing amino acids. Lowering dietary protein below 8% resulted in an increase of serum cholesterol.

Dr. Wm. Godolphin, Vancouver

What is the cost of operating a lipid clinic?

Dr. Bernard Wolfe

The major costs are for salaries for the secretary, dietitian, nurse and technician which is about $100 per half day. In addition there is the professional component for the physician and biochemist. Laboratory reagents are not expensive and the equipment is fairly standard for a clinical biochemistry lab.

Dr. Alick Little

Aside from the biochemical laboratory costs, a lipid clinic is equivalent to the cost of operating a diabetic clinic. Indeed it may be cost-effective to combine diabetic and hyperlipoproteinemic patients in the same clinic, especially in smaller centres.

Dr. Hubert Peeters

In some European countries the government sponsored health programs will only pay for lab tests which are abnormal while in the United States laboratory tests may be charged directly to private patients. Under these circumstances laboratory investigation must be kept within practical limits.

Dr. Alick Little

We must be careful to distinguish between what is necessary for a strictly consultative service clinic as compared to a research clinic like Dr. Gotto's Lipid Research Clinic at Houston or Dr. Ahren's Specialized Centre of Research(SCOR) at Rockefeller University in New York. Service clinics only need to coordinate the efforts of the physician, biochemist and dietitian which can be done in any large hospital. Every Lipid Clinic does not need to have an ultracentrifuge. Serum samples from problem cases can be sent to the nearest research lipid laboratory or the patient could be referred there instead. In the case where healthy people are being screened for hyperlipoproteinemia, this is a research function and needs to be financed as such.

Question from unidentified person

Who interprets the lab data, the biochemist or the doctor?

Dr. Gerald Cooper

The lab reports the data and the lipoprotein pattern. The biochemist is responsible for the reliability of the data. It is up to the physician to interpret it along with the clinical findings.

Dr. Helen Brown

Many physicians cannot interpret the lab data logically and are confused by the typing system.

Dr. Gerald Cooper

With simple guide lines which have been published (Bull. Wld. Hlth. Org. 1970, 43, 891-915) and using a few basic assumptions concerning the ratio of cholesterol to triglyceride in the VLDL fraction and the amount of cholesterol in the HDL fraction, it is possible to type every patient with reasonable accuracy.

Dr. Hubert Peeters

I would like to comment on lipoprotein typing. One can be biased in the interpretation of the lipoprotein electropherograms by knowing the cholesterol and triglyceride values. Perhaps typing should be done first without knowing the lipid levels. However, the lipoprotein pattern is only useful where serum cholesterol and triglyceride are elevated. Although I was formerly against typing, I am a convert to the use of lipoprotein electrophoresis, especially if it is done carefully such that it can almost be scanned quantitatively. Unfortunately, quantitative scanning is made difficult because of disproportionate losses of lipids from the lipoprotein fractions during processing and staining.

Dr. Gerald Cooper

I agree that the lipoprotein pherograms are not quantitative. You need cholesterol and triglyceride for quantitative data. Electrophoresis detects gross abnormalities in distribution of lipoproteins.

Dr. Alick Little

In our clinic we see the chemical data and lipoprotein pherograms together with the patient and the other clinical and laboratory findings. If the results do not agree with each other, then they are reviewed with the biochemist and dietitian after the clinic and further studies are planned to clarify the diagnosis.

Dr. David Bassett, Michigan, U.S.A.

Because of the cost and confusion in some centres there is pressure to discontinue lipoprotein electrophoresis and use only total serum cholesterol and triglyceride values. What do others think about this?

Dr. Alick Little

Because we are still in a relatively early stage of investigating diseases of lipid metabolism we should not try to do without all the necessary information.

Dr. Gerald Cooper

I like to have measurement of total serum cholesterol and triglyceride and the cholesterol in the alpha (HDL) lipoprotein. From these I calculate the amount of cholesterol in the beta (LDL) lipoprotein. The lipoprotein pherograms are visually examined to confirm the impression from the chemical data. If all the data do not agree, one should suspect the presence of sinking pre-beta lipoprotein, floating beta lipoprotein, or other usugual conditions. However, for screening purposes in healthy populations one requires less data such as total serum cholesterol plus the appearance of the fasting serum after standing 16 hours at 4°C or the total serum triglyceride.

Dr. Harold Taylor, Indianpolis

I would like to ask Dr. Helen Brown and Miss Valerie McGuire how much do diets lower serum lipids from base-line measurements and do you have trouble getting patients already on a therapeutic diet to go back on a typical North American diet?

Dr. Helen Brown

It is important to obtain several estimations of serum cholesterol and triglycerides while the patient is on his customary diet. Some patients claim they have already adopted a diet to lower serum cholesterol but questioning reveals that they really have not changed their diet to an important extent. After starting the patient on his prescribed diet one sees significant lowering of serum lipids within a few weeks.*

Dr. D. Shapcott, Sherbrooke, Quebec

Do you distinguish between types of carbohydrates, especially between sugar and starch?

Miss Valerie McGuire

Yes, in my presentation I mentioned that for type IV (and other triglyceridemic types) we limit sugar and replace it with starch.

---

*Chairmens' footnote: Under ideal, metabolic ward conditions the maximum effect of a controlled fat diet on lowering serum lipids is usually seen in three to four weeks. Depending on the type of hyperlipoproteinemia and the diet this varies from 10% to 30% or more. Type II hypercholesterolemia is more resistant to lipid lowering while the hypertriglyceridemias have much more dramatic falls in serum lipids. In outpatients, with less rigorous dietary changes, the decrease in serum lipids may be less marked and more delayed depending in part on patient adherence to the diet.

Dr. Helen Brown

We do this also in Cleveland. We divide foods into five groups: (1) low fat meats (2) dairy products (3) visible fats and oils (4) low fat products such as fruits, cereals and vegetables (5) sugar, sweets and alcohol. In teaching patients about their diet we de-emphasize group 5 by warning them that these are "empty calories" and they should choose from the other four groups.

Miss Betty Chua, Sudbury, Ontario

Do patients have difficulty ingesting the amounts of polyunsaturated fats which are prescribed.

Miss Valerie McGuire

Some patients may have initial problems, but if they use the recipes which are provided during diet counselling there should be no problem.

Dr. Alick Little

I would like to ask Dr. Cooper to comment on the problems experienced by the private physicians served by a variety of laboratories which have varying accuracy and precision and different so called "normal limits" for cholesterol and triglyceride. As a teacher of post-graduate medicine, I find it difficult to help private physicians learn how to diagnose and treat hyperlipoproteinemia. The lab which they use may give 350 mg% as the upper normal limit for cholesterol at all ages, which contradicts my statement that 270 mg%, the 95th percentile in our laboratory, is abnormal in middle aged adults. (indeed a value in excess of 230 mg% is abnormal for persons under age 20) Also, in following patients during treatment the doctor may become discouraged because the treatment appears to have no consistent effect on serum lipid levels, whereas in fact it is the laboratory which may be providing unreliable, variable results.

Dr. Gerald Cooper

We know from the examination of the same serum pool by different laboratories that they report different results. This is because of the use of different methods, standards, reagents and equipment. Therefore each clinical laboratory should determine the "normal limits" for their routine method. This can be done by using accurately labelled reference serum materials and comparing the values obtained by their routine method with those given for the reference method or by comparing values obtained on a series of subjects' serum samples by their routine method with those obtained by a reference method. Finally the clinical laboratory should take age and sex specific "normal limits" from a reputable survey of the local population using a reference method and adjust these for the results which would have been obtained if the routine method had been used. The physician is still left with the problem of interpreting results from laboratories with different normal limits and variances. For this reason we still need to strive to develop stable, accurately labelled reference materials and to improve methodologies for serum lipids around the world.

Summary, Dr. H. Peeters

In Europe there are no lipid clinics similar to those in North America. However, from the experience gained in the study of serum lipids in Belgian Postmen, a visit to the Lipid Research Clinic at Houston, Texas and listening to the presentations at this workshop I have some comments to make. Unfortunately unlike Diabetic Clinics we do not have a magic drug like insulin. Instead, we must emphasize diets to lower serum lipids. In Belgium hyperlipoproteinemia is relatively rare, possibly because of the information in the lay literature about diets to lower blood lipids. I wonder if lipid clinics reach the lower income groups. Perhaps we should use the family doctor more, either by having him work in the clinics or by referring the patients back to him for management. Could we do more screening of healthy populations at an earlier age?

We should not chop off funds for lipid biochemical investigation. A new generation of investigative tests is appearing. These are the immunoassays for apolipoproteins and serum lipid profiles using gas chromatography [(x)] or column chromatography [(xx)]. There is good evidence that the ratio of sphingomyelin to lecithin in plasma and in alpha lipoproteins may be very important indeed.

In Belgium the diets differ from one city to another and possibly this is also true in North America. We need to develop better methods for evaluating what people eat. I have experimented with a method using photographic slides of various foods and a synchronized tape asking the subject questions about the pictures. This helps to eliminate interobservor bias.

I think that it is important for the clinician to examine the laboratory data and to interpret it in the light of the clinical findings. If we in Europe are going to develop lipid clinics, perhaps we should not make them a carbon copy of the ones in North America. Instead we should develop second generation lipid clinics which will look at diseases of lipid metabolism from a different view point.

[(x)] Determination of Plasma Lipid Profiles by Automated Gas Chromatography and Computerized Data Analysis. Kuksis, A., Majher, J.J., Marai, L., Geher, K., J. Chromatogr. Sc. 13: 423-430, 1975.

[(xx)] A universal gradient apparatus for multiple organic solvents. II. Fractionation and elution of serum lipids. D. Vandamme, B. Declercq, A. Denoo, V. Blaton, H. Peeters, Anal. Biochem., in press.

CHAPTER 2
NEW THERAPEUTIC APPROACHES TO ACUTE MYOCARDIAL INFARCTION (MI) AND ITS SIZE

(1)

LESSONS FROM THE MYOCARDIAL INFARCTION RESEARCH UNITS

H.J.C. SWAN, M.D., Ph.D.

CEDARS-SINAI MEDICAL CENTER

LOS ANGELES, CALIFORNIA, U.S.A.

The broad areas of concern of the Myocardial Infarction Research Unit Program have been: The biology of ischemic myocardium; the recognition of its clinical presentation as acute myocardial infarction; and the management of patients with established infarction. Significant progress has been made in an understanding of the pathophysiology of severe power failure of the heart (1), and hence the development of more optimal form of therapy. It has been recognized that in certain hearts the magnitude of myocardial necrosis, usually combined with pre-existing myocardial destruction, precludes survival (2). In a number of instances, however, important changes have been made both short-term and long-term relative to the attainment of a more favorable outcome.

1. Development of subsets relative to prognosis (3): It is clear that the taxonomic descriptor--acute myocardial infarction--is inappropriate to effectively and meaningfully encompass illnesses with such widely differing therapeutic needs and outcomes as acute myocardial infarction. Four major subsets based on presenting hemodynamics have been identified:

    a. Hyperdynamic

    b. Normal

    c. Moderate depression

    d. Severe depression (pre-shock and shock)

The first subset is characterized by an exaggerated catecholamine response and accounts for approximately 10% of patients with acute myocardial infarction. The second, with minor or moderate myocardial damage, has relatively normal dynamics and an equally good prognosis. The third is frequently characterized by moderate or even severe degrees of pulmonary congestion and the fourth by varying degrees of pulmonary congestion but also severely depressed cardiac pump performance. The mortality prognosis in each of these subsets should approximate 0, 5, 15 and 60 percent.

2. Techniques for safe and effective bedside catheterization of the right heart have been developed (4). They depend principally on the introduction of the balloon flotation catheter systems which allow for the measurement of right atrial, right ventricular, pulmonary artery and pulmonary capillary wedge pressures. In addition, the development of the thermodilution technique utilizing a single catheter for both injection and detection of thermal changes and computation of the resulting values now makes practical the measurement of cardiac output at the bedside with an error of 5%. In addition, the development of electrodes for sensing of endocardial potentials and pacing of the atrium or ventricle has facilitated the accurate hemodynamic evaluation of such influences.

3. In the management of severe power failure, the first objective is to obtain a sinus rhythm with an optimal heart rate. Probably the optimal rate varies from patient to patient and is within the range of 90 to 110 beats per minute.

4. It is now possible to identify the optimal level of left ventricular filling pressure (5) by use of the flotation catheter and the measurement of the pulmonary wedge pressure. Pulmonary wedge pressures of between 14 and 18 mm Hg are optimal. Increases in filling pressures beyond approximately 16 mm Hg do not result in any substantive increase in cardiac output. Reductions in filling pressure from values in excess of 30 mm Hg into the range of 14 to 18 mm Hg are not associated with a reduction in cardiac output. Pulmonary congestion commences at filling pressures in excess of 20 mm Hg, and pulmonary edema in the presence of filling pressures in excess of 26 mm Hg. Hence, it is now possible by use of fluid loading or diuretic therapy to optimize filling pressures at between 14 and 18 mm Hg.

5. Hemodynamic measurements have indicated the limitations of benefit of inotropic intervention (6). In patients with severe power failure and major depression of cardiac performance the effects of inotropic agents on hemodynamics is usually small. This is particularly true in the more seriously ill patients.

Application of inotropic agents causes an obligatory increase in cardiac metabolism. It is possible that in certain patients the use of inotropic agents has caused an increase in the severity of ischemia and in the magnitude of ultimate cell death.

6. Impedance reduction by use of vasodilator drugs (7) or intra-aortic balloon counterpulsation (8) has been shown to have a profound and beneficial effect on cardiac performance. Increases of approximately 30% in cardiac output with optimization of left ventricular filling pressure can be achieved with sodium nitroprusside in the majority of patients seriously ill with power failure of the heart. Similar hemodynamic alterations have been reported in patients in which aortic impedance is reduced by intra-aortic balloon counterpulsation.

The therapy of power failure of the heart has been substantively changed. It is now recognized that destruction of the myocardium is not necessarily complete at the time that the patient enters the medical care system; necrosis may be a continuing function and must be minimized (9). Maximization of the output of the heart by sequential application of the above factors appears to result in a substantive reduction in hospital mortality. Such hemodynamic improvement is at least a first step to a further increases in survival in patients with myocardial infarction.

REFERENCES

1. Swan HJC, Forrester JS, Diamond G, et al: Hemodynamic spectrum of myocardial infarction and cardiogenic shock: A conceptual model. Circulation 45: 1097, 1972

2. Page DL, Couldfield JB, Kastor JA, et al: Myocardial changes associated with cardiogenic shock. New Eng J Med 285: 133, 1971

3. Forrester JS, Diamond G, Swan HJC: Functional subsets of myocardial infarction: A basis for acute coronary triage. Submitted for publication, Circulation, 1975.

4. Swan HJC, Ganz W, Forrester JS, et al: Catheterization of the heart in man with the use of a flow-directed balloon-tipped catheter. New Eng J Med 283: 447, 1970

5. Crexells C, Chatterjee K, Forrester JS, et al: Optimal level of filling pressure in the left side of the heart in acute myocardial infarction. New Eng J Med 289: 1263, 1973

6. Abrams E, Forrester JS, Chatterjee K, et al: Variability in response to norepinephrine in acute myocardial infarction. Am J Cardiol 32: 919, 1973

7. Chatterjee K, Parmley WW, Ganz W, et al: Hemodynamic and metabolic responses to vasodilator therapy in acute myocardial infarction. Circulation 48: 1183, 1973

8. Dunkman WB, Linebach RC, Buckley MJ, et al: Clinical and hemodynamic results of intraaortic balloon pumping and surgery for cardiogenic shock. Circulation 46: 465, 1972

9. Braunwald E, Maroko PR: The reduction of infarct size--an idea whose time (for testing) has come. Circulation 50: 206, 1974

(2)

THE EFFECT OF LOCAL VASODILATING AGENTS

DAVID R. REDWOOD, M.D.

Cardiology Branch, National Heart and Lung Institute
Bethesda, Maryland, U.S.A.

Contrary to the previously widely held concept that nitroglycerin is contraindicated in acute myocardial infarction, it has recently been shown that the administration of nitroglycerin to patients with acute myocardial infarction and elevated left ventricular filling pressures results in a reduction in filling pressure and in an increase in cardiac output, while in those patients with normal filling pressures, cardiac output is unchanged or may decrease. Similarly, it has been demonstrated that another potent vasodilator, nitroprusside, is also capable of inducing similar beneficial hemodynamic changes resulting in improved pump performance in patients with acute myocardial infarction and left ventricular failure. However, improvement in pump performance in patients with acute myocardial infarction does not necessarily mean improvement in the degree of ischemia, since therapy might result in enhancement of function of non-ischemic portions of the ventricle while the ischemic areas remain unchanged or even extend. Nitroglycerin, however, has been shown experimentally to result in substantial reduction in ischemic damage to the myocardium following acute coronary occlusion in the dog. Moreover, this effect is potentiated when the nitroglycerin-induced hypotension and reflex tachycardia are eliminated by the simultaneous administration of methoxamine or phenylephrine, both alpha adrenergic agonists. We have also shown that in the experimental animal, nitroglycerin and the combination of nitroglycerin and an alpha adrenergic agonist has beneficial effects on the electrical stability of the heart following coronary occlusion. Thus, both the ease with which ventricular fibrillation can be induced electrically (ventricular fibrillation threshold) and the incidence of ventricular fibrillation that occurs spontaneously during experimental myocardial infarction, are reduced. These observations have recently been extended to the study of the effects of nitroglycerin on the degree of myocardial ischemia during acute myocardial infarction in man. The results suggest that the responsiveness to nitroglycerin in terms of reduction in ischemia, as estimated by precordial ST segment mapping, depends on whether or not the patient manifests left ventricular failure. Thus in patients without left ventricular failure, the administration of nitroglycerin alone often reduces but occasionally can increase the degree of ischemic injury. However, ischemic injury is always reduced in such patients when phenylephrine is infused in a dose sufficient to reverse the fall in arterial pressure and the reflex tachycardia induced by nitroglycerin. In contrast, in patients with left ventricular failure, nitroglycerin alone consistently reduces ischemic injury. In these patients it appears that the addition of phenylephrine to abolish the nitroglycerin-induced fall in arterial pressure, usually partially reverses the beneficial effects observed with nitroglycerin alone.

The results in the patients without left ventricular failure are entirely consistent with the experimental studies performed in our laboratories. Thus, in dogs with acute single vessel occlusion and otherwise normal coronary arteries, administration of nitroglycerin alone reduces the degree of ST elevation recorded from intramyocardial electrodes. Further significant reduction in the degree of ST segment elevation occurs when the nitroglycerin-induced fall in arterial pressure and reflex increase in heart rate are abolished by the administration of the alpha adrenergic agonist, methoxamine. Moreover, using a similar model, improvement in intramyocardial ST segment abnormalities during therapy with nitroglycerin and phenylephrine was found to correlate with reduction in gross morphologic and biochemical evidence of infarction. When nitroglycerin was administered alone and in combination with phenylephrine during acute myocardial infarction with chronic multivessel occlusions, nitroglycerin alone caused diminution in the degree of myocardial ischemic injury only in those dogs developing a reflex tachycardia in response to nitroglycerin which was less than 50% above control heart rate. In contrast, ischemic injury increased in those dogs developing a more marked tachycardia (in excess of 50% above control heart rate). When the nitroglycerin-induced hypotension and reflex tachycardia were abolished with phenylephrine, ischemic injury consistently decreased in all animals. A similar increase in the degree of ischemia has been observed by us in a patient during acute myocardial infarction when sublingual nitroglycerin resulted in a marked reflex tachycardia, an effect which was reversed when phenylephrine was given in doses sufficient to return arterial pressure to control levels and hence abolish the tachycardia. It has recently been suggested that a more gradual onset of action of nitroglycerin and thus possibly a greater degree of control of the hemodynamic response can be achieved by using the intravenous rather than sublingual route of administration. However, further studies would be necessary in order to compare the relative degree of reflex tachycardia obtained when the drug is given either by the sublingual or by intravenous route. In contrast to the reflex tachycardia induced by nitroglycerin when administered to patients without left ventricular failure, the reflex responses are blunted in patients with left ventricular failure. Thus, in acute myocardial infarction accompanied by failure, nitroglycerin would probably cause tachycardia only rarely.

The possible mechanisms by which the pharmacologic agents reduce the degree of ischemia are complex. Nitroglycerin is a potent dilator of both arteries and veins. This action leads to a reduction in myocardial preload and afterload, both of which effects would result in a reduction in wall tension, a reduction in oxygen consumption, and thereby a reduction in myocardial ischemia. Nitroglycerin also has been shown to dilate coronary arteries, reduce the resistance to coronary collateral flow, and to increase myocardial flow to ischemic areas. Infusion of phenylephrine (a relatively pure alpha agonist) causes arteriolar constriction and thus reverses the reduction in arterial pressure induced by nitroglycerin, a change accompanied by abolition of nitroglycerin-induced reflex tachycardia. These two effects contribute to a reduction in ischemia by increasing coronary perfusion pressure (secondary to increased arterial pressure) and decreasing myocardial oxygen consumption (by decreasing heart rate).

In conclusion, the use of vasodilators and in particular nitroglycerin provides an exciting new therapeutic approach to the treatment of acute myocardial infarction in man. Not only has it proved possible acutely to improve left ventricular performance, but it also appears possible to salvage ischemic myocardium. Thus it is to be hoped that these innovative approaches to therapy may lead to an improvement in both the acute and the long term survival of patients with acute myocardial infarction.

(3)

INFARCT SIZE: ITS ESTIMATION AND MODIFICATION.

Robert Roberts, M.D.,FRCP(C) and Burton E. Sobel, M.D.,FACC

Department of Medicine, Washington University

St. Louis, Missouri, U.S.A.

Clinical assessment of patients with acute myocardial infarction and evaluation of factors which may affect the prognosis have been hampered in the past by lack of adequate objective methods for estimating infarct size in vivo. Accordingly, stimulated by interest in protection of ischemic myocardium, several investigators have explored approaches to quantify the extent of myocardial injury. We have attempted to estimate infarct size (IS) in conscious dogs and in patients based on analysis of serial changes in plasma creatine phosphokinase (CPK) activity. In initial studies, we assumed that the rate of change of plasma CPK activity after myocardial infarction reflected; 1) release of CPK from the heart, and 2) disappearance from the circulation according to first order kinetics with a constant fractional disappearance rate (k_d). (1)

In conscious dogs, CPK released from the heart estimated from serial plasma CPK changes correlated closely with CPK depleted from the myocardium measured directly. In other studies, myocardial CPK depletion was found to correlate with independent indices of infarct size. Subsequently, we estimated infarct size in patients from changes in plasma CPK activity and demonstrated that infarct size was an important determinant of early mortality. Patients with infarct size of less than 65 CPK-gram-equivalents had an early mortality of 5% within six months. In contrast, early mortality was 65% in patients with infarct size exceeding 65 CPK-gram-equivalents. (2)

Recently, we and others have shown estimates of infarct size based on plasma CPK changes correlate closely with impairment of left ventricular function, the frequency of early ventricular dysrhythmia, the severity of

TABLE I

CPK DISAPPEARANCE (k_d) IN 30 CONSCIOUS DOGS

Experiment Number	Half-life $t_{\frac{1}{2}}$	k_d (min^{-1})	SD of slope	Correlation Coefficient r	Distribution Volume (% body wgt.)
1	150	.0046	9.2%	-.97	5.3
2	178	.0039	7.5%	-.96	5.8
3	119	.0058	6.0%	-.92	5.9
4	144	.0048	11.2%	-.95	5.4
5	161	.0043	16.4%	-.99	5.0
6	131	.0053	9.3%	-.93	6.2
7	187	.0037	8.7%	-.96	4.9
8	100	.0069	6.9%	-.92	5.9
9	150	.0046	10.5%	-.95	5.5
10	178	.0039	9.6%	-.96	4.9
11	112	.0062	6.2%	-.94	5.2
12	161	.0043	13.2%	-.97	5.6
13	115	.0060	14.3%	-.95	5.2
14	154	.0045	11.2%	-.93	5.6
15	173	.0040	9.1%	-.95	5.4
16	88	.0078	8.2%	-.97	4.8
17	144	.0048	7.5%	-.96	5.2
18	100	.0054	9.6%	-.96	5.2
19	165	.0042	10.2%	-.98	5.7
20	105	.0066	7.2%	-.95	5.0
21	161	.0043	6.2%	-.95	5.2
22	133	.0052	5.2%	-.94	4.6
23	173	.0040	7.5%	-.96	5.7
24	131	.0053	8.6%	-.97	5.4
25	128	.0054	10.9%	-.93	5.2
26	157	.0044	9.5%	-.92	5.2
27	150	.0046	7.8%	-.99	4.9
28	178	.0039	11.2%	-.96	5.7
29	173	.0040	9.6%	-.95	5.2
30	110	.0063	9.0%	-.95	5.6
mean	144.0	.0048	9.2%	-.95	5.4

clinical manifestations as well as mortality and morbidity during the first six months after infarction. Furthermore, Bleifeld et al., have shown that infarct size estimated from serial CPK changes correlates closely with morphological estimates of infarct size in patients who succumb.

Despite the clinical utility of our initial formulation, refinements and modifications of the method have been pursued vigorously. Since marked hemodynamic alterations may occur in association with myocardial infarction, CPK disappearance from the circulation may be altered, thereby spuriously affecting estimates of infarct size. To evaluate this possibility and to characterize further the kinetics of CPK disappearance, we determined k_d in conscious dogs (n=30) after the intravenous injection of radioactively labelled, partially purified dog heart CPK. Results showed that k_d varied markedly between animals (range of 3.7 to 7.8 x $10^{-3}min^{-1}$), but that CPK disappearance conformed closely to first order kinetics (r=-.95)(Table I). In addition, k_d determined repetitively in the same animal (n=5) on three consecutive days remained virtually constant (<10% variation). To determine whether hemodynamic perturbations alter k_d, 30 conscious dogs were subjected to thoracotomy or laparotomy, and instrumented for subsequent studies performed when the animals had recovered completely. CPK was injected intravenously and the k_d determined before and during selected hemodynamic interventions. Reduction of cardiac output by 67%, monitored by an aortic electromagnetic flow probe and induced by constriction of the inferior vena cava (n=5), did not affect k_d. When both renal arteries were completely occluded (n=5), celiac flow reduced by 70% (n=5), or hepatic arterial flow completely interrupted (n=5), no significant alteration of k_d occurred. Thus, the difference between control k_d and k_d during the intervention was <10% in all cases.

To determine the effect of myocardial infarction per se on k_d, ^{14}C-CPK was injected intravenously and used to determine k_d before, during and after infarction in conscious dogs produced by occlusion of the left anterior descending coronary artery. Under those conditions, tracer disappearance is independent of release of endogenous enzyme. The k_d before, during and after infarction in the same animal was virtually identical (n=5).

In early studies, we utilized a log normal curve fitting technique based on least squares approximation to project the entire CPK curve from early plasma CPK values. The projected values were used to predict infarct size (ISP). Comparison of ISP with infarct size obtained (ISO) from actual CPK values provided an index to evaluate the effect of selected interventions on jeopardized ischemic myocardium. In 14 patients with acute myocardial infarction and hypertension, ISP was obtained from curves derived from plasma

CPK changes during the first seven hours of increased plasma CPK activity. Subsequently, blood pressure was decreased by continuous infusion of trimethaphan to reduce myocardial oxygen requirements. Mean arterial pressure was reduced from an average of 114 ± 4 (S.E.) to 88 ± 2 mmHg and pulmonary artery wedge pressure decreased from 18 ± 2 (S.E.) to 13 ± 2 mmHg. There was no significant change in heart rate or cardiac index. Results of this intervention on the evolution of infarction was evaluated as indicated in the following table by comparing ISO and ISP in treated vs. control patients with comparable hypertension. (3)

	Number of Patients	ISP CPK-g-eq.	ISO CPK-g-eq.
Treated	14	105 ± 21	80 ± 20
Control	14	94 ± 20	94 ± 20

As can be seen in the treated group, observed infarct size (ISO) was 24% less than predicted (ISP)($p<0.01$).

External counterpulsation was assessed in a similar manner by comparing ISP with ISO in 12 patients with myocardial infarction. After prediction of infarct size, patients were treated with counterpulsation for 18 hours with a schedule of 45 minutes of support alternating with 15 minute rest periods. The results are shown below.

	Number of Patients	ISP CPK-g-eq.	ISO CPK-g-eq.
Treated	12	89.1	90.2
Control	12	94.2	92.1

Thus, circulatory assist by external counterpulsation initiated seven hours after the initial plasma CPK elevation did not reduce infarct size. (4)

Thus, infarct size can be estimated from serial plasma changes and estimates correlate with independent parameters including clinical sequelae, acute prognosis, impaired ventricular function, and morphological criteria of necrosis. k_d can be individualized by analysis of the descending portion of each patient's CPK curve (Norris, et al.). Our results suggest that hemodynamic alterations do not significantly affect k_d, and thus, calculations of infarct size need not be modified because of variance in this parameter.

Comparison of infarct size predicted to that observed (estimated from actual CPK changes) has shown that ischemic myocardium can be protected by decreased afterload and reduction of myocardial oxygen requirements. The same methodology has been useful in evaluating other interventions as well. Recent studies indicate that estimates and predictions of infarct size based on quantitative analysis of MB CPK isoenzyme activity is a more specific marker of myocardial injury than total CPK. This allows one to estimate infarct size in patients with complications such as cardiogenic shock or intramuscular injections since release of MB CPK from noncardiac tissues is insignificant. (5)

REFERENCES

1. Shell, W.E., Kjekshus, J.K. and Sobel, B.E.: Quantitative assessment of the extent of myocardial infarction in the conscious dog by means of analysis of serial changes in serum creatine phosphokinase (CPK) activity. J. Clin. Invest. 50: 2614, 1971.

2. Roberts, R., and Sobel, B.E.: Disappearance of creatine phosphokinase (CPK) from the circulation. Annals of the Royal College of Physicians. 8: 1: 16, 1975.

3. Shell, W.E., and Sobel, B.E.: Protection of jeopardiazed ischemic myocardium by reduction of ventricular afterload. New England J. Medicine. 291: 481, 1974.

4. Gowda, K.S., Roberts, R., Ambos, H.D., and Sobel, B.E.: Salutary effects of external counterpulsation in patients with acute myocardial infarction. Amer. J. Cardiol. 35: 140, 1975.

5. Roberts, R., Gowda, K.S., Ludbrook, P.A., and Sobel, B.E.: The specificity of elevated serum MB CPK activity in the diagnosis of acute myocardial infarction. Amer. J. Cardiol., In press.

(4)

MECHANICAL ASSIST IN THE TREATMENT OF IMPENDING OR ESTABLISHED MYOCARDIAL INFARCTION AND CARDIOGENIC SHOCK

DR. R. O. HEIMBECKER

University Hospital, University of Western Ontario, London, Canada

In recent years many methods of circulatory assistance, ranging from the mechanical heart, to transplantation, have been proposed for the acute cardiac problems. Of these, intra-aortic balloon assist and pump oxygenator support are the two methods which have best survived the test of time.

(A) AORTIC BALLOON PUMPING (IABP)

Intra-aortic phase-shift balloon pumping is a bedside technique of mechanical circulatory assistance that is becoming increasingly relevant to the clinician. The procedure is applied easily and rapidly in patients with early,acute ischaemia or shock secondary to acute myocardial infarction. In general, adjunctive clinical management is directed toward improving cardiac function and careful, sequential correction of systemic abnormalities. The cumulative experience of a number of groups indicates that the risk of complications is slight.

Several groups of investigators have reported [1,3,4,5] evidence that phase-shift pumping improves physiologically important haemodynamic and other variables, both in patients with severely impaired left ventricular function and in various experimental models. In particular, evidence has been obtained that myocardial oxygenation and cardiac output are enhanced, while oxygen needs are reduced. Studies in our laboratory have indicated that a left ventricular afterload phase angle of approximately 180° is one of the necessary conditions for maximal effectiveness.

The principles of aortic balloon implementation are well described elsewhere.[2]

The following groups of patients are most amenable to aortic coronary balloon pumping, to be followed by coronary angiography and surgery, when feasible:

A. Unstable Angina Syndromes

Def: 1) New angina 2) Angina at rest 3) Prolonged chest pain	Bal.Crit: 1) Pain after 12 hrs of bed rest 2) Transient EKG changes. Normal enzymes 3) Failure of medical R_x

B. Acute Inf. - Recurrent Pain

	Bal.Crit: 1) Continuous isch. pain over 12 hrs 2) Completed inf.,

C. Acute Inf. Haemodynamically Unstable, No Shock

Def: 1) S_3 gallop 2) Sinus tach. or A.F. 3) PCW above 18 mm.Hg. 4) C.I. $<$ 2.5 but $>$ 1.9 5) Syst.BP $>$ 100 mm.Hg.	Bal.Crit: 1) Fresh ant. MI. 2) Any combination of old and new inf.

D. Acute Inf. with Mech.Defect

VSD MR	Bal.Crit: All patients

E. Acute Inf. - Cardio. Shock

Def: 1) Syst. BP $<$ 100 mm.Hg. 2) PCW $>$ 18 mm.Hg. 3) C.I. below 1.9 4) Oliguria, anuria 5) Change in mental state	Bal.Crit: Only for younger patients seen early - if coronary anatomy optimal

RESULTS:

Results in the unstable angina (Group A) are most encouraging with an overall mortality rate of less than 5% reported in most centres.(4,6,9)

By contrast, in Groups B to D the risks are higher with mortality rates up to 25%.

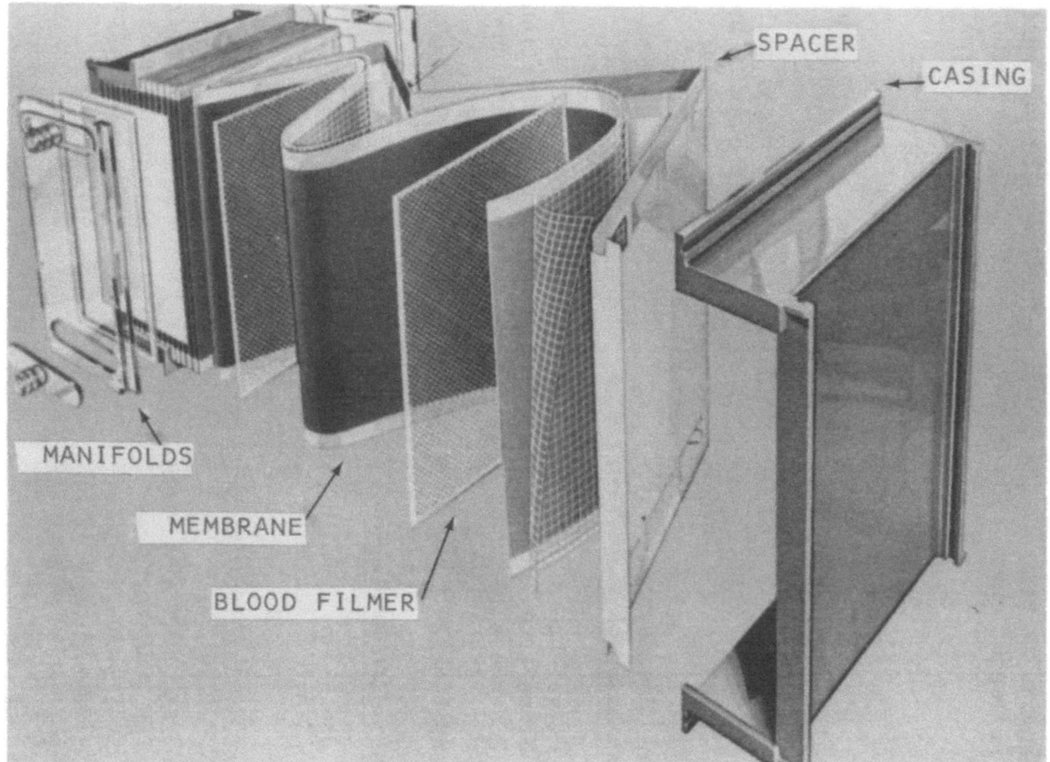

FIGURE 1
Exploded view of disposable membrane oxygenator which appears so effective for post-operative mechanical assist, with flow rates of 6L./min for 12-18 hours, to be followed by simple replacement for a further period of support.

Group E is a high risk group with an almost hopeless prognosis without help (90% mortality), and a survival of some 30% with surgery (5,9).

All centres would stress the importance of initiating mechanical cardiac assistance early after the onset of circulatory decompensation.

Due to its simplicity and low risk, performance of phase-shift pumping in patients with uncomplicated myocardial infarction is well established as a method of reducing the frequency of such sequelae as arrhythmias, congestive failure, shock; to prepare patients for coronary angiography, and to prepare the patient for possible cardiac surgery.

(B) MEMBRANE OXYGENATOR SUPPORT

Early success in the use of pump-oxygenator for support was recorded by R. Baird, J. Kennedy, and many others, but the techniques were limited to an hour or two because of inevitable blood trauma, most of which occurred in the early oxygenators.

The recent advent of a simple, efficient, atraumatic membrane lung has reopened this approach with support of 12-24 hours being quite feasible. Especially in post-operative mechanical support this is preferred(7) to the aortic balloon, for the patient is already fully cannulated for continuation of the same membrane perfusion into the post-operative period.

We have successfully applied this post-operative membrane support in five patients for periods ranging from half an hour to 3 hours, with very gratifying results(8) as shown in the following table:

TABLE I

POST-OPERATIVE MEMBRANE SUPPORT

# of patients		
3	Coronary by-pass	2 survivors
2	Aortic valve replacement	2 survivors
5		4 survivors

In contrast to aortic balloon assist:

1. Fully oxygenated blood is constantly reaching the capillary bed - especially the myocardium.

2. Perfusion is still effective when the patient's heart is generating no output.

3. Cardiac arrhythmias do not interfere.

Further experience is necessary to assess the true value of this approach, but the early results are most encouraging with excellent resuscitation and minimal blood trauma after hours of perfusion support with the membrane unit.

SUMMARY:

In summary IABP is now a simple, well established technique which effectively supports patients undergoing acute myocardial ischaemia, to prepare them for coronary angiography and possible, subsequent surgery.

Post-operative mechanical assist is also very satisfactory with IABP., but the membrane lung with its many advantages may prove to be much more effective.

REFERENCES

1. Kantrowitz, A., Akutsu, T., Chaptal, P.-A., Krakauer, J., Kantrowitz., Arthur and Jones, R.T. (1966): A clinical experience with an implanted mechanical auxiliary ventricle. JAMA., 197, 525.

2. Kantrowitz, A., Tjønneland, S., Krakauer, J.S., Butner,A.N., Phillips, S.J., Yahr, W.Z., Shapiro, M., Jaron, D and Sherman Jr., J.L. (1968c): Clinical experience with cardiac assistance by means of intraortic phase-shift balloon pumping. Trans Amer. Soc. artif.intern. Org., 14, 344.

3. Tyberg, J.V., Keon, W.J., Sonnenblick, E.H., and Urschel,C.W. (1970): Effectiveness of intra-aortic balloon counterpulsation in the experimental low output state. Amer. Heart J. 80, 89.

4. Urschel, C.W., Eber, L., Forrester, J., Matloff, J., Carpenter, R. and Sonnenblick, E.H. (1970): Alteration of mechanical performance of the ventricle by intraortic balloon counterpulsation. Amer. J. Cardiol. 75, 546.

5. Dunkman W., Leinback, R.C., Buckley, M.J., Mundth, E.D., Kantrowitz, A.R., Austen, W.G., and Sanders, C.A. (1972): Clinical and hemodynamic results of intraortic balloon pumping and surgery for cardiogenic shock. Circ. XLVI, 465.

6. Gold, H.K., Leinback, R.C., Sanders, C.A., Buckley, M.J., Mundth, E.D., and Austen, W.G. (1973): Intraortic Balloon Pumping for Control of Recurrent Myocardial Ischemia. Cir. XLVII, 1197.

7. Beall, A. Personal communication.

8. Heimbecker, R., et al. (1975): The membrane lung in routine cardiac surgery - Annual Meeting, American Heart Association, Anaheim, California. 17 Nov. 1975.

9. Gunstensen, J., et al - personal communication.

(5)

NEW THERAPEUTIC APPROACHES TO ACUTE MYOCARDIAL INFARCTION (MI) AND ITS SIZE: THE SURGICAL APPROACH

W.J. Keon, M.D.

University of Ottawa Cardiac Unit, Ottawa Civic Hospital

1053 Carling Avenue, Ottawa, Ontario, Canada

We have been performing aorto-coronary venous bypass graft surgery on patients with acute myocardial infarction and in cardiogenic shock following infarction since 1970. We have also performed surgery on an emergency basis on patients with pre-infarctional angina or an angiographic emergency.

Our general objectives in emergency surgery are to prevent the loss of myocardial tissue due to ischemia, to minimize the size of a myocardial infarct, to alleviate the complications of acute myocardial infarction by correcting arrhythmias and closing perforations, and to restore cardiac pump function to a point where the heart can sustain the circulation.

We define cardiogenic shock as a blood pressure below 80 mm Hg, a venous pressure of 15 mm Hg or higher, signs of peripheral vascular insufficiency, a clouded sensorium, and a urine output of less than 20 cc per hour. In addition, in patients classified as being in cardiogenic shock, we have demonstrated at catheterization a left ventricular end-diastolic pressure of 30 mm Hg or above, a systolic pressure of 80 or below, and a cardiac index of less than two litres per meter squared.

As of December 31, 1974, 21 of our emergency patients were classified as being in cardiogenic shock. (Table I) Fourteen (66.6%) of the patients died at operation while 2 died later for a total mortality of 16 or 76%. One of the late deaths was due to a cerebrovascular accident occurring during catheter study at 3 months following operation. The other patient died 4 years after operation due to congestive heart failure and an arrhythmia.

Table 1: MORTALITY

		Deaths		
	#	Operative	Late	Total
CARDIOGENIC SHOCK	21	14 (66.6%)	2 (9.5%)	16 (76%)
ACUTE INFARCTION	39	0	4 (11 %)	4 (11%)

The patient entering hospital is evaluated at once, and if he meets the cardiogenic shock criteria, we proceed immediately with angiography. Then the patient is quickly evaluated by the surgical team, and if surgical relief of ischemia is deemed feasible, the patient is placed on cardiopulmonary bypass. Bypass grafts are performed only on major lesions and surgery is accomplished without cardiac arrest and without cardiac hypoxia. If the patient is in cardio-respiratory failure when he is removed from bypass, we put him on the intra-aortic balloon assist. Although some surgeons also use the balloon during angiography, we have not found this to be necessary.

The time factor in cardiogenic shock is of importance. Of the 5 patients who now survive, none had been in shock for more than 9 hours with the average being 6.1 hours. However, some of those who did not survive had been in shock as long as 36 hours with the average being 8.4 hours. (Table 2) We have also noted that the average time between myocardial infarction and the onset of shock has been shorter in those who died than in those who survived. The number of previous infarcts in cardiogenic shock patients was calculated and found to be slightly although not significantly lower in surviving patients. (Table 3) The 21 cardiogenic shock patients received 31 grafts and had an average myocardial blood flow of 89.7 cc/min. (Table 4)

Table 2: TIME FACTOR IN CARDIOGENIC SHOCK

		Shock to Surgery		
	#	Max.	Min.	Aver.
SURVIVING PATIENTS	5	9.66 hrs	1 hr	6.1 hrs
NON-SURVIVING PATIENTS	16	36 hrs	1 hr	8.4 hrs

Table 3: CARDIOGENIC SHOCK PREVIOUS INFARCTS

	#	# of Previous Infarcts	Average
SURVIVING PATIENTS	5	4	.80
NON-SURVIVING PATIENTS	16	14	.87

Emergency bypass grafts are performed by us on patients with acute unstable infarction in four situations: if the infarction occurs during cardiac catheterization, in extending infarction (that is, ECG changes, recurrent chest pain, or recurrent enzyme changes following acute infarction), in the case of uncontrollable arrhythmias such as recurrent ventricular fibrillation or ventricular tachycardia, or when infarction is accompanied by low cardiac output and hypotension.

There are 39 acute unstable infarction patients in our series. Twenty-five fell into the extending infarction category, 11 had progressive hypotension, 2 infarcted during catheter study, and 1 had an uncontrollable arrhythmia. We had no deaths at operation. 4 (11%) died later. (Table 1) Two of the late deaths occurred 6 weeks after operation, 1 due to a cardiac arrest and the other a cardiac arrest caused by congestive heart failure. One patient died 2 months post-operatively as a result of an arrhythmia and another at 4 months from congestive heart failure and pulmonary embolism.

The key to successful management of acute unstable infarction patients is rapid angiography, prompt institution of cardiopulmonary bypass, and corrective surgery on an emergency basis. Acute infarction patients are not as seriously ill as those in cardiogenic shock so we perform bypass grafts not only on the occluded vessels but also on other significant lesions. If a vessel is not graftable,

Table 4: INCREASE MYOCARDIAL BLOOD FLOW

	Patients	Grafts	Flow
CARDIOGENIC SHOCK	21	31	89.7 (20-130)
ACUTE INFARCTION	39	85	175.0 (50-385)

we perform an endarterectomy in order to improve myocardial function. The increase in myocardial blood flow for these patients is considerably better than in the cardiogenic shock patients, the average being 175 cc/min. (Table 4)

We feel it is mandatory to improve myocardial blood flow to ischemic areas if myocardial function is to improve. Some patients operated upon in the presence of acute infarction had good left ventricular function at postoperative follow-up, while in others left ventricular function was impaired with the appearance of an aneurysm in two cases. For this reason, we have restricted operation in the presence of acute infarction to the four groups of patients described.

This experience suggests that it may be advantageous to defer myocardial revascularization for about 3 months following an acute myocardial infarction so that the extent of muscle damage can be definitively evaluated and appropriate resection of aneurysmal tissue can be accomplished at the same operation. It should be emphasized that patients who are operated on in the presence of acute complicated myocardial infarction are operated on because of coexistent continuing ischemia to non-infarcted muscle secondary to stenotic lesions which may or may not have been responsible for the actual infarct.

We feel that surgery will salvage some patients in acute myocardial infarction with shock who otherwise would be destined to almost certain death. Angiography should be performed immediately on these patients. We believe that only the major lesions of cardiogenic shock patients should be bypassed. We use normothermic perfusion and avoid ventricular fibrillation and severe hemodilution. In patients with complicated acute myocardial infarction who are not in shock, more extensive operations can be safely performed and short periods of anoxia (15 minutes or less) are well tolerated. The intra-aortic balloon assist is used in patients who have myocardial pump failure post-operatively.

(6)

DISCUSSION (NEW THERAPEUTIC APPROACHES TO ACUTE MYOCARDIAL INFARCTION (MI) AND ITS SIZE)

Discussion following Dr. Swan's presentation

An unidentified Discussor: I would like to ask Dr. Swan what proportion of patients who develop cardiovascular shock after myocardial infarction actually have surgically correctible lesions such as mitral insufficiency, ventricular septal defect, etc.

Dr. Swan, Los Angeles, USA: It is small. It is about 14-15%. We have a retrospective autopsied series of 100 cases, and I think we have about 8 with mitral regurgitation and 5 or 6 perforated ventricular septums. The options to treat these patients surgically at the time of the acute event are really rather restricted. There are some people who have been successful in operating on these patients, but by and large it is a risky matter at best. Of the remaining patients, approximately one-third have got basically terminal heart disease. They do not necessarily come in with a massive acute infarction, they come in with their third infarct or fourth infarct and they now have enough further damage to just totally compromise their circulation. About half or a little more come in really with a first heart attack and I believe they are the spectrum of sudden death that has not died. They have a sufficiently large myocardial involvement that they will ultimately go into myocardial shock and probably die from that. There are a group of these patients that are potentially salvagable if they are reached at a sufficiently rapid period of time and if they have truly bypassable vessels. I think this is an exciting experimental approach to the problem.

Dr. Gunton, London, Canada: Dr. Swan, how would you reduce myocardial metabolism? By avoidance of catecholamines, digoxin, etc?

Dr. Swan: Yes. I think that is the first thing, that the physician do no wrong, and hopefully do some right. Right now we have got to be careful that the treatments that we impose are not deleterious and there is some evidence emerging that most of the things we appear to be doing have a more adverse effect than we would like to admit.

An unidentified Discussor: Can you give us your clinical indication for the use of intra-aortic balloon and vasodilator therapy.

Dr. Swan: Let me take the second one first. Vasodilator therapy is very easy. It is essentially if you have the ability to do haemodynamic monitoring which I believe most Intensive Care Units are becoming able to do. The introduction of graded levels of impedance reduction is very, very simple, and therefore in our particular situation, it is the first line of approach to the patient with severe depression of cardiac performance. Intra-aortic balloon counter pulsation we reserve for the patients who really come to us with failure of other forms of therapy. Our experience with intra-aortic balloon counter-pulsation is somewhat similar to most other people, that is that you can haemodynamically benefit the patient, but in the long run the patient will succumb, with the result that the last five patients that we used the aortic balloon on, we got a very nice result but it did not affect the ultimate outcome. Nor did we believe it would. So our indication for use of the balloon at the present time is failure of other therapy. We would like to be able to feel that we had the ability to get the patient into a surgical possibility. We may be able to hold some ground with the balloon under that circumstance but we are still a long way from that.

Discussion following Dr. Redwood's presentation

Dr. Swan: I would like to ask Dr. Redwood about ST segment mapping and the question of endocardial and epicardial relationships in respect to ischaemia.

Dr. Redwood, Bethesda, USA: While there is experimental evidence to suggest that interventions known to improve epimyocardial ischaemia also favourably influence endocardial ischaemia, it is still possible that some manoeuvres resulting in decrease in precordial or epimyocardial ST segment elevation may not affect endocardial blood flow.

An unidentified Discussor: I do not understand why the administration of phenylephrine together with nitroglycerine improves the effect of the vasodilator.

Dr. Redwood: The relationships are very complex. It is a balance between pre-load, after-load, wall-tension, coronary perfusion pressure, heart rate and a number of other factors and it may also be some local effects of nitroglycerine rather than effects on collateral circulation. So the relationship is extremely complex, but even if one looks at it very simply if one were able to reverse the tachycardia effects of nitroglycerine or given an agent which did not give a tachycardia, one is clearly going to get more benefit than if you are giving the same agent which does give tachycardia. Secondly, it may well be that the coronary perfusion pressure is more critical in the context of patients without failure which is the group we are discussing, than we believe, and it may well be that by increasing after-load to a certain critical level, to control levels, is important, and it may not have to go back to control levels, maybe a small increase in afterload or in coronary perfusion pressure is important.

Discussion following Dr. Heimbecker's presentation

An unidentified Discussor: Dr. Heimbecker, I understand that the membrane oxygenator is used on patients who are on bypass.

Dr. Heimbecker, London, Canada: Yes, that is right. We use it routinely in all our open heart procedures now, but this second application that I am referring to right now is used in our experience only in the post-operative patients who may have to go back on a period of mechanical support. Exposure is very similar to the aortic balloon pumping. Femoral artery exposure, femoral vein exposure, but not necessarily thoracotomy.

Discussion following Dr. Keon's presentation

An unidentified Discussor: Dr. Keon could you use infarctectomy with acute M.I.

Dr. Keon, Ottawa, Canada: We had three patients with cardiac perforations. Two of them died and one survived. You have to do an infarctectomy if there is a cardiac perforation. In the one that survived we put a teflon patch in the wall. In the two that did not survive we also used some teflon and excised the infarct. I think it is more important to try to get some blood supply in early than to concentrate on infarctectomy. It is a very difficult thing to do.

An unidentified Discussor: Do you have a comment to make on the practice that has been advocated by some that in the early phases of acute myocardial infarction, the problem is the obstruction of blood flow to a region of the heart and they should be re-vascularised.

Dr. Keon: I think compromised function is due to two things - to an overall reduction in coronary blood flow, and the second thing is an abnormal distribution of blood. But I think to operate on an acute infarct that is localised to the circumflex system for example is just a mistake at this point in time. We just do not know what is going to happen to the myocardium. There are too many variables.

GENERAL DISCUSSION

Dr. John Parker, Kingston, Canada: I would like to ask Dr. Roberts or Dr. Swan to comment on their experience with infarct extension. We are looking at methods of precordial mapping, CPK curves to assess infarct size, with recent reports that as many as 50% of patients using these two criteria may have infarct extension. Obviously this will have to be settled before we can rule out what the various interventions are doing. I would very much like some comment on this rather controversial question.

Dr. Swan: Dr. Parker is really asking a question which we do not have specific data to answer and that is laboratory evidence to support the context of extension. Clinically extension occurs in something between 5 and 15% of cases of infarction and in properly managed patients, I do not think it should be even that. However, there is a definite group of patients who have a peculiar anatomy in which compromise of different areas of the circulation are occasioned by occlusion of a specific vessel. For example, in the presence of multiple triple vessel disease with involvement of the circumflex and anterior descending systems, occlusion of the right coronary artery will initially produce an inferior infarction. As the patient gets better he may then start to develop the signs of lateral wall ischaemia. The reason he has done that is because he lost his collaterals from right to left and this can present in a very typical manner and Dr. Favaloro has discussed this matter in terms of the anatomical inter-relationships that accompany extension of infarcts. I think that the question that you are really getting at could best be answered by Dr. Roberts if he is familiar or not with the large amount of CPK data, to look at the incidence of deviations outside the projected area, late, that is at 36, 48 or 72 hours. ST segment mapping can be quite tedious and I do not know, and Dr. Redwood may, of groups who have continued ST mapping in large groups of patients on a clinical basis. I do not know of it.

Dr. Redwood: I have nothing to add to what Dr. Swan has said. The longest we have followed patients is up to two hours following infarction with precordial mapping, so we have no evidence to add to Dr. Swan's comments. I do not know of any studies in which precordial mapping has been done for a longer period of time than that.

Dr. Robert Roberts, St. Louis, USA: We have analysed data on about 80 patients and the incidence of extension as defined, as Dr. Swan mentioned, is looking at CPK curves. In other words, at 48 hours we still have continuing release of CPK, or there is actually another peak, and in about 30% of our patients we see a second peak or this continued release of CPK. This includes all the patients in shock as well. It is interesting that we have now analysed the patient in shock and although it is not absolutely firm on a small number of patients, it seems to be one of their characteristics that most of them are releasing CPK well up into 48 to 72 hours, the ones that stay alive that long. So it looks like from our data, it is somewhere around 30%. Some of those extensions may only be in CPK gram equivalents about 3-5, so it is very small, but taking the group as a whole we see 30%. I might say that Pitts' group have followed the ST segments for extension for 72 hours or for two weeks, and they show an incidence of extension based on the ST segments of 70% as reported in the NEJM. I would rather Dr. Redwood comment on what he thinks of that number, I do not know what to make of it, but we have used ST mapping and have not seen that incidence, even with the map.

Dr. Swan: I would like to comment on that very high incidence. I think that this is not clinical extension, it is just a prolonged process of release and I doubt that this can be identified in the manner that they apparently have, as true extension. Would you like to comment, Dr. Roberts, on CPK and the fact that animal experiments are all based upon an instantaneous event, whereas many of us believe that myocardial infarction on a clinical basis is not always an instantaneous event.

Dr. Roberts: I think that is one of the problems with our prediction programme and that is why in most of our studies, as I so well know, at the moment only about 40 or 50% of the patients we get, that would otherwise qualify for an intervention, can be used, because their CPK's dribble on, they go up to our upper limit of normal 50, they probably go to 80, stay there, go up to 95 or so, and then there is another slight rise and that kind of curve of course does not correspond to our equation and we cannot use it. Unfortunately this is fairly frequent.

Dr. Maseri, Pisa, Italy: Dr. Roberts do you have any information on the enzyme release from the dying cells. How much is released in the active form, which is actually what you are measuring as CPK activity and how much is released maybe in the inactive form in different forms of necrosis. Secondly, I would like you to comment on the curves that you show, in predicting vs. actual curves. The most striking deviation from prediction is not in the peak of the curve but is rather on the final slope which becomes much steeper as in one curve you showed today or much slower.

Could you comment on this changing final slope rather than on change in peak activity.

Dr. Roberts: The first question I take is related to the CPK that is released into the blood after a cell dies. Do we know anything about CPK that is released but because it is not active, we cannot measure it? That is the question. I would say that we have a little bit of data on that subject. One, we are now doing experiments where we are looking at CPK incubated in blood versus CPK incubated in lymph. The half-life in blood in a dog is around 2½ hours. In the lymph it is about one-third that. So I suspect that based on that a lot of CPK that is released from a dead cell that we cannot account for in our original model is in fact released into lymph and prior to getting into the venous blood is inactivated and therefore we do not measure it. I am hoping that is the case and it would tie up the story and we would not have one more big mystery about where it is going. The second thing is that I now have an antibody to all three isoenzymes and I can recognise the molecule even without activity. Initial results suggest that there is some floating around. I would not want to put a number on it at this time.

The second question was why do we see most of the difference after the peak. That is an astute observation. Unfortunately our model does not predict infarct size until after about 7 hours of enzyme rise. We are close to the peak before we can intervene and I suspect that is why we do not see dramatic changes we would like to see. We are intervening at a reasonably late time, very close to the peak, and so our results would be after the peak.

Dr. Maseri: You say that disappearance constant is constant in the same patient and yet what we see is change in the disappearance constant produced by the intervention.

Dr. Roberts: We are saying that that change, whether it is a flat high or the slope has altered is because there is continued release of CPK. The curves you saw today are at the end of 48 hours. Our disappearance is not taken until well after that. You do the CPK for the disappearance rate, 96 hours at present. We usually take our disappearance rate between 60 and 80 hours.

Dr. Maseri: This accounts for the slope becoming less steep but I cannot figure out how this occurs when the slope becomes steeper.

Dr. Roberts: You are saying that the actual disappearance rate is faster on some of those.

Dr. Maseri: Yes.

Dr. Roberts: Is faster on the observed than the predicted? I would have to look at those slides. I know that in the case of the counter-pulsation one, at that time we were using the mean k_d, so that means it was deviated from the true k_d.

An unidentified Discussor: In the discussion of the balloon assist, there was no mention made of external counter-pulsation. I wondered if you could consider it of little or no value at the present time. A year or so back it was first advocated that it may be external counter-pulsation might work in a small community hospital where there are not people available to insert intra-aortic balloon assist.

Dr. Heimbecker: We have had no experience ourselves. This of course is a type of pressure costume that is similarly synchronised to an electrocardiogram. Some of the haemodynamic data from other centres has been quite encouraging, even to suggest that it is more effective than the aortic type of counter pulsation but it is certainly a much newer approach. Not enough people have studied it to really come to any proper conclusions. There is a ray of hope.

Dr. Roberts: Our results with the external pulsation showed significant haemodynamic improvement. In fact the mean drop in wedge pressure was from a mean of 17 down to a mean of about 10 on the machine. The patients tolerated it well - 18 hours - with 15 minutes rest per hour. The effect on arrhythmias in the first two hours on the machine was beneficial, there was a significant decrease, although it was transient, and had no lasting effect beyond two hours. Infarct size was unaffected. So we felt from the infarct size point of view, it was not of value intervening at the 7th hour as we did, but certainly it was very simple to operate and the patients tolerated it well. I do not know the results of the co-operative study with external counter- pulsation. Dr. Swan might be able to comment on that.

Dr. Swan: There is a study in which a group of individuals have randomised patients with Class 1 or 2 acute myocardial infarction and intervened immediately on admission with counter-pulsation. As the data was being evaluated it became clearly evident, as Dr. Roberts has indicated, that there was an apparent beneficial effect in that the patients who had been subjected to counter-pulsation did have lower overall mortality. The incidence of cardiac enlargement was less in the group so treated. I believe there were one or two other positive phenomena. The data have been subjected to a certain amount of criticism on the basis of randomisation and how the randomisation was actually conducted. I think there is a small effect, a small positive effect to this device. At the present time that study is still underway and I do not know what the further outcome will be.

Dr. Armstrong, Kingston, Canada: I want to address a comment and a question to Dr. Redwood in relationship to the discussion on vasodilators. Particularly to comment about nitroglycerine, whether to use less, and about the combination of nitroglycerine and phenylephrine. As I understand the data, the wedge pressure in the failure group fell from 25 to 10 and the mean arterial pressure from 110 to 80. There was a substantially greater fall in the mean arterial pressure than wedge pressure, presumably reduction in transmyocardial gradient and propensity to increase flow.. I presume in turn that the major effect, if not the only effect of phenylephrine, would be to restore some sort of increment in coronary perfusion pressure. If one looks at a dose response for nitroglycerine and looks at the fall in wedge pressure that precedes much change in mean arterial pressure , presumably because of its effect on venous pooling before its effect on arteriolar pressure, why would you consider that it might not be reasonable to use less nitroglycerine in relationship to your studies?

Dr. Redwood: That is a good point. One of the problems of course is that with this study through using sub-lingual nitroglycerine, and it is very difficult as you all know, to involve haemodynamic effects of nitroglycerine given in that way, we were judging the dose of nitroglycerine to induce mean arterial pressure drop of the order of 15-20 mmHg., and at the same time, as you saw, there was a fairly substantial fall in wedge pressure. One does not know the results as far as ischaemia is concerned as measured by this precordial mapping technique.

Two things would be an advantage - one is to have a means by which one can control the haemodynamic effects of nitroglycerine at will and hopefully intravenous nitroglycerine might allow this to be achieved, and secondly a means by which one can quantitate precordial ST segment elevation or any other measure of myocardial ischaemia on line so that one can adjust the various haemodynamic influences one wants to achieve at will. It seems intravenous nitroglycerine is going to be more useful than sublingual although there are technical problems with using the drug. It is not as stable in solution. As for "on line" quantitation of ST segment elevation, I understand that Smith and his colleagues in Halifax are doing this and it would add a whole new parameter.

Dr. Armstrong: Does phenylephrine have any other effect that the pure alpha effect of raising coronary perfusion pressure?

Dr. Redwood: As you know it has a minuscule beta effect which is probably of no importance. It reverses the reflex tachycardia effect in the non-failure group - that is it reverses one of the deleterious effects of nitroglycerine.

(1)

THE ORIGIN AND FATE OF CHYLOMICRONS AND VLDL

Richard J. Havel, M.D.

Cardiovascular Research Insitute

University of California, San Francisco, California, U.S.A.

The intracellular processes of the formation of chylomicrons and VLDL are probably quite similar (1). Electron microscopy has provided evidence that precursor-particles are present within the profiles of the smooth endoplasmic reticulum and Golgi apparatus of intestinal mucosal and hepatic parenchymal cells. By use of peroxidase-labeled Fab of gamma globulin directed against the B apoprotein of rat LDL, the B apoprotein has been demonstrated at the electron microscopic level in the rough endoplasmic reticulum of rat liver cells in the absence of a particle. Particles containing the B apoprotein can be seen by this technique within the smooth-surfaced terminal ends of the rough endoplasmic reticulum and in the Golgi apparatus but almost never in association with particles in the smooth endoplasmic reticulum (2). This has led to the hypothesis that triglyceride-rich particles are formed in the smooth endoplasmic reticulum in the absence of the B apoprotein and receive it only after migrating to the junction of the smooth and rough reticulum. The site at which other VLDL apoproteins become part of the nascent VLDL particles has not been determined. These proteins are labeled as rapidly as the component lipids of VLDL secreted from perfused rat liver whereas the B apoprotein becomes labeled later suggesting that a preformed pool of B protein exists in the rough reticulum (3). However, VLDL isolated from the Golgi apparatus contain not only the B apoprotein but also the arginine-rich protein and the several rapidly migrating C apoproteins (1). Certain carbohydrate moieties, including sialic acid, are added to the apoproteins in the Golgi apparatus (4-6) where the nascent VLDL are concentrated in secretory vesicles. The emiocytotic release from the cell of VLDL and other proteins in these vesicles is mediated by the microtubular system (7, 8).

The "core" of nascent VLDL, isolated from a Golgi apparatus-rich fraction of livers from rats on a standard chow diet, closely resembles plasma VLDL: percentage content by weight of triglycerides and cholesteryl esters, as well as their component fatty acids, are almost the same as those of VLDL isolated from blood plasma (9). The surface components of the nascent VLDL differ from their counterparts in blood plasma in having more phospholipids and less of the C apoproteins. These differences disappear when nascent VLDL are mixed with plasma HDL suggesting that phospholipids and proteins transfer reciprocally between these two species without change in particle dimensions (1).

The surface components of newly secreted rat chylomicrons differ from those of VLDL in at least three respects: 1) C apoproteins evidently are not present in the nascent particles but are added entirely after they enter the lymph (10); 2) the proportion of B apoprotein is much smaller than in VLDL (11); 3) the A-1 apoprotein is the major protein of intermediate molecular weight (10-12). Thus in the rat the liver and gut both secrete the B apoprotein (see 10), but only the liver appears to secrete the rapidly migrating C apoproteins. The hepatic parenchymal cell evidently secretes the arginine-rich apoprotein and the intestinal mucosal cell the A-1 apoprotein but the extent to which these proteins are secreted from the alternative cell type remains to be determined. It should be emphasized that these observations may not apply in other species and that, even in the rat, they may not hold under all conditions.

The transfer of C apoproteins to triglyceride-rich lipoproteins renders their component triglycerides a more suitable substrate for the lipoprotein lipase in the capillary beds of extrahepatic tissues. Physiological evidence from several mammalian species (rat, dog and sheep) suggests that the hepatic lipase which, like lipoprotein lipase is rapidly released into the blood when heparin is injected intravenously, does not participate in the removal of chylomicron triglycerides in this initial step, during which 80-90% of the triglyceride is removed from the core of the particles (13-15). The remaining particle, still containing substantial triglyceride, is now commonly called a "remant" (16). From studies in the perfused rat heart, it appears that once most of the triglycerides have been removed from chylomicrons or VLDL, the remaining triglycerides in remnant particles do not compete effectively with "native" particles for the enzyme (17). The composition and structure of chylomicron and VLDL remnants have been studied in functionally eviscerated ("supradiaphragmatic") rats (11). VLDL remnants, obtained after VLDL are allowed to circulate for one hour in the absence of the liver, retain the "pseudomicellar" structure of their precursors. By electron microscopy, they appear to remain spherical and their content of "surface" and "core" components remains appropriate to their volume-average diameter, but they are more homogeneous in size. Calculations based upon volume and chemical composition of the particles indicate that they have lost most of their core triglycerides; by contrast the content of cholesteryl esters (per particle) increases significantly by about 60%. The particles retain their original complement of B apoprotein and of arginine-rich apoprotein, but most of the C apoproteins have been lost, together with much of the original complement of phospholipids. The content of cholesterol (presumed also to be a surface component) remains constant. To isolate chylomicron remnants, uncontaminated with remnants from plasma VLDL, rats were pretreated with 4-aminopyrazolopyrimidine to prevent secretion of VLDL. Remnants were then obtained by injecting supradiaphragmatic preparations from such animals with "large" (1250 Å diameter) and "small" (550 Å diameter) chylomicrons from thoracic duct lymph. With certain exceptions these particles were altered in a manner similar to that of VLDL. In the case of large chylomicrons, however, the remnants appeared to contain excessive amounts of surface components for their size, as determined both by electron microscopy and by analysis of chemical composition. The drug injected into these animals not only eliminated VLDL and LDL from the blood, but it also depleted the content of HDL by about 75%. Earlier studies in man provided evidence that both phospholipids and C apoproteins may return to HDL from chylomicrons as remnants are formed (18). The chylomicron remnants from rats treated with the pyrimidine derivatives also contained less cholesteryl esters than those prepared from VLDL. The particles that accumulated in these drug-treated rats thus resembled the large, very low density particles that accumulate in plasma of individuals with genetically determined LCAT deficiency (19). These observations suggest that HDL and the action of LCAT upon HDL may be necessary for normal removal of some surface lipids and proteins from triglyceride-rich lipoproteins when remnants are formed, so as to maintain the basic pseudomicellar structure in which a core of polar lipid is surrounded by a monomolecular layer of polar lipids and proteins. Similar formation of remnant particles during the catabolism of triglyceride-rich lipoproteins in humans is suggested by studies with radioiodine-labeled VLDL (20) and from demonstration of particles resembling remnants in individuals with primary dysbetalipoproteinemia (21,22).

Whereas available evidence suggests that the liver does not normally participate in the first phase of the catabolism of triglyceride-rich lipoproteins, it clearly plays a major role subsequently in the metabolism of remnants. In the three species mentioned earlier and also in the rabbit, the liver rapidly removes almost all of the component cholesteryl esters (and most of the cholesterol) from chylomicrons and their remnants (13-16, 23, 24). Our recent studies indicate that this is also the case for these components of VLDL in the rat (25) and guinea pig (26). The cholesterol is first concentrated at the plasma membrane of hepatic parenchymal cells and the esters are then gradually hydrolyzed as they are taken up into the cell (27). The B apoprotein of VLDL is also rapidly and almost completely taken up by the liver in the rat (28-30), suggesting that the remnant particle may be incorporated by a process of adsorptive endocytosis. Like cholesteryl esters, the B apoprotein of rat VLDL is first concentrated at the plasma membrane and gradually taken up into the cell (31). A small fraction (<5%) of the B apoprotein remains in the blood and is recognized as LDL (30). It has not been established that the liver participates in the formation of LDL or, alternatively, that it constitutes a completely separate pathway of VLDL metabolism. Similar studies have not been conducted with chylomicrons and it is not known that they contribute to LDL formation.

To conclude this summary of the processes of formation and catabolism of triglyceride-rich lipoproteins, it is worth emphasizing that many of them have been studied only in a single species, the rat. From what is known about other species, including man, caution in extrapolating these results is in order. Two examples of major species differences may be cited. First, in the rat all VLDL cholesteryl esters appear to be derived from the liver. The acyl-CoA cholesterol acyltransferase of rat liver is highly active (32). In the guinea pig, in which the activity of this enzyme is very low (32), only a minor fraction of the cholesterol of VLDL is esterified (26, 33). In humans, in whom this enzyme is reported to be virtually absent in liver (32), about one-half of the cholesterol is esterified, however the fatty acid composition of these esters suggests that they are derived mainly from the action of LCAT (34). Second, about 90% of the B apoprotein of VLDL appears in LDL in humans (35), indicating that very little is rapidly taken up by the liver from remnant particles. These differences, and perhaps others yet to be defined in the metabolism of lipid and protein components of lipoproteins, may account for the large species differences in concentration and composition of the plasma lipoproteins and also for some of the differences in atherogenic responses to specific stimuli.

REFERENCES

1. Hamilton, R.L. Adv. Exp. Med. Biol. 26:1 (1972)

2. Alexander, C. Doctoral dissertation. University of California at Los Angeles. (1974)

3. Kook, A.I. and D. Rubinstein. Can. J. Biochem. 51:490 (1973)

4. Lo, C. and J.B. Marsh. J. Biol. Chem. 245:5001 (1970)

5. Mookerjea, S. and C. Miller. Can. J. Biochem. 52:767 (1974)

6. Wetmore, S., R.W. Mahley, W.V. Brown and H. Schachter. Can. J. Biochem. 52:655 (1974)

7. Stein, O., L. Sanger and Y. Stein. J. Cell Biol. 62:90 (1974)

8. Le Marchand, Y., C. Patzelt, F. Assimacopoulos-Jeannet, E.G. Loten and B. Jeanrenaud. J. Clin. Invest. 53:1512 (1974)

9. Hamilton, R.L. and R.J. Havel. Unpublished data.

10. Windmueller, H.G., P.N. Herbert and R.I. Levy. J. Lipid Res. 14:215 (1973)

11. Mjøs, O.D., O. Faergeman, R.L. Hamilton and R.J. Havel. J. Clin. Invest. 56:603 (1975)

12. Glickman, R.M. and K. Kirsch. J. Clin. Invest. 52:2910 (1973)

13. Goodman, D.S. J. Clin. Invest. 41:1886 (1962)

14. Nestel, P.J., R.J. Havel and A. Bezman. J. Clin. Invest. 42:1313 (1963)

15. Bergman, E.N., R.J. Havel, B.M. Wolfe and T. Bøhmer. J. Clin. Invest. 50:1831 (1971)

16. Redgrave, T.G. J. Clin. Invest. 49:465 (1970)

17. Higgins, J.M. and C.J. Fielding. Biochemistry 14:2288 (1975)

18. Havel, R.J., J.P. Kane and M.D. Kashyap. J. Clin. Invest. 52:32 (1973)

19. Glomset, J.A. and K.R. Norum. Adv. Lipid Res. 11:1 (1973)

20. Bilheimer, D.W., S. Eisenberg and R.I. Levy. Biochim. Biophys. Acta 260:212 (1972)

21. Havel, R.J. and J.P. Kane. Proc. Natl. Acad. Sci. U.S.A. 70:2015 (1973)

22. Havel, R.J. Adv. Exp. Med. Biol. In press (1975)

23. Redgrave, T.G. Biochem. J. 136:109 (1973)

24. Noel, S.-P., P.J. Dolphin and D. Rubinstein. Biochem. Biophys. Res. Comm. 63:764 (1975)

25. Faergeman, O. and R.J. Havel. J. Clin. Invest. 55:1210 (1975)

26. Barter, P.J., O. Faergeman and R.J. Havel. Unpublished data.

27. Stein, O., Y. Stein, D.W. Goodman and N.H. Fidge. J. Cell Biol. 43:410 (1969)

28. Eisenberg, S. and D. Rachmilewitz. Biochim. Biophys. Acta 260:212 (1973)

29. Roheim, P.S., D.I. Edelstein, G. Vega and H.A. Eder. Fed. Proc. 32:672 (1973)

30. Faergeman, O., J.P. Kane, T. Sata and R.J. Havel. J. Clin. Invest. In press (1975)

31. Stein, O., D. Rachmilewitz, L. Sanger, S. Eisenberg and Y. Stein. Biochim. Biophys. Acta 360:205 (1974)

32. Stokke, K.T. Atherosclerosis 19:393 (1974)

33. Bøhmer, T., R.J. Havel and J.A. Long. J. Lipid Res. 13:371 (1972)

34. Nichols, A.V. Adv. Biol. Med. Physics 11:109 (1967)

35. Sigurdsson, G., A. Nichol and B. Lewis. J. Clin. Invest. In press (1975)

(2)

THE ORIGIN AND FATE OF LDL

Yechezkiel Stein and Olga Stein

Lipid Research Laboratory, Department of Medicine B, Hadassah University Hospital and Department of Experimental Medicine and Cancer Research, Hebrew University-Hadassah Medical School, Jerusalem, Israel

Serum low density lipoprotein (LDL) is derived from serum very low density lipoprotein (VLDL) by a multistep process, during which an intermediate particle is formed. Studies carried out in vitro (1) and in the supradiaphragmatic rat (2) have shown that there is conservation of the B apoprotein and of cholesterol during formation of both the intermediate particle (so-called remnant) and of LDL and it has been postulated that one VLDL produces one remnant and/or one LDL. In the rat, only a small fraction of VLDL derived B protein is transformed into LDL and more than 90% is cleared from the circulation in 60 min, after injection of ^{125}I-labeled VLDL. During that time most of the ^{125}I-apoC remains in the circulation, thus indicating that remnant particles are being cleared. We have followed the fate of the particles cleared from the circulation with the help of radioautography (3). In the rat, the main site responsible for remnant uptake is the liver and up to 30% of the injected radioactivity was recovered in this organ (Table 1). The uptake is a two-stage process consisting of binding to the cell surface, followed by internalization and these stages have been visualized by radioautography at the electron microscope level. In Table 2 a summary of the grain counts is shown and it can be seen that at 5 min after injection there is a concentration of the label at the sinusoidal cell surface, which disappears at 120 min (3). In man, in contradistinction to the rat, about 40% of the label is still in the circulation 24 h after injection of ^{125}I-VLDL and most of the labeled B protein is in LDL (4). The LDL thus formed is the main carrier of esterified cholesterol in the human serum and several studies have dealt with the elucidation of the site of LDL degradation When rats were

Table 1

Effect of Dose on the Uptake of ^{125}I-Labeled Very Low Density Lipoprotein by Rat Liver 5 min after Injection

In the liver 88-95% of the label were trichloroacetic acid precipitable and the ratio of chloroform-extractable counts in the liver to chloroform-extractable counts in the injected material ranged between 1.05 and 1.3. Values are means ±S.E.

No. of rats	Injected very low density lipoprotein (mg)	Percent of injected radioactivity	
		Plasma	Liver
5	0.50	53.6 ± 4.0	28.1 ± 1.9
5	1.05	54.2 ± 6.2	23.8 ± 1.3
4	2.10	63.4 ± 0.9	13.9 ± 0.96
2	3.00	60	8.1

Reproduced from Biochim. Biophys. Acta, 360: 205-216, 1974

injected with ^{125}I-LDL a rather high percent of the injected label was recovered in the liver (5). However, studies in pigs have shown that removal of the liver not only does not result in a longer intravascular survival of injected LDL, but on the contrary is accompanied by a shortening of its half life in the circulation (6, 7). These findings have redirected the attention from the liver to the peripheral tissue as the primary sites of LDL degradation.

LDL has to enter the extravascular space, i. e. to cross the endothelial barrier of capillaries in order to reach the "peripheral" tissues. The mode of transcapillary transport involves most probably the plasmalemmal vesicles. These organelles do transport proteins such as ferritin and peroxidase and have been implicated in transport of LDL in studies with rat aorta (8). The presence of B apolipoprotein has been demonstrated in human interstitial fluid of the foot (9), thus providing evidence that this apoprotein does reach peripheral tissues.

Table 2

Relative Concentration of Label over Rat Liver after Injection of ^{125}I-labeled Very Low Density Lipoprotein

Total number of grains counted 404 and total number of random points recorded 8000 for 5 min; 632 and 14,400 for 30 min and 680 and 10,000 for 120 min, respectively.

Compartment	Silver grains (%)	Grain density*	Silver grains (%)	Grain density*	Silver grains (%)	Grain density*
Time (min):	5	5	30	30	120	120
Hepatocyte cytoplasm	42.8	0.61	51.7	0.71	83,2	1.07
Hepatocyte nucleus	0.9	0.28	0.8	0.42	0.4	0.30
Hepatocyte cell boundary	39.1	3.18	39.0	3.58	8.3	1.15
Sinusoid lumen	6.3	0.77	5.3	0.56	1.9	0.27
Littoral cells**	10.9	1.98	3.2	0.69	6.2	0.88

* Percent of grains assigned to each compartment divided by percent of random point hits over each compartment.

** Includes Kupffer cells and endothelial cells.

Adapted from Biochim. Biophys. Acta, 360: 205–216, 1974.

In order to determine the role of peripheral tissues in LDL catabolism some investigators have used mesenchymal cells in culture (10-19). In most studies the LDL was labeled in its protein moiety with ^{125}I and the rates of uptake and degradation of the labeled particles were determined in smooth muscle cells and in fibroblasts. In analogy to the liver, the process of LDL interiorization by cells in culture is also a two-stage process (13). The first stage is defined as binding of the lipoprotein to the cell surface and some investigators have invoked the presence of specific receptors for such a process (17-19). The binding is rapid, does not require energy and thus occurs also at 0°, and at that time most of the lipoprotein can be removed from its binding site with the help of trypsin (20). When the incubation is carried out at 37° the second stage becomes operative and progressively more labeled protein becomes internalized, i. e. is not accessible to trypsinization (10-13). The two processes of binding and uptake increase with the lipoprotein concentration in the medium (Fig. 1). As shown also in Fig. 1, binding and uptake of LDL by rat smooth muscle cells was higher than that of rat HDL at similar lipoprotein-protein concentration. This difference is very much enhanced when human LDL is compared to human HDL. The latter lipoprotein, although bound to the cell surface is interiorized only very poorly (13). After a lag of 30-60 min a third process can be measured, i. e. the degradation of the labeled protein which manifests itself by the appearance of non-iodide - TCA soluble radioactivity in the medium (10). When the rate of degradation is related to the rate of uptake one can demonstrate differences between cell type and species (Fig. 2). Thus it seems that in rat smooth muscle cells the LDL degradation proceeds at a slower rate than in human skin fibroblasts. The site of degradation of the labeled protein is the secondary lysosome, which forms following the fusion of endocytic vesicles bearing the lipoprotein with the enzyme-carrying primary lysosome. This organelle is active also in the hydrolysis of the esterified cholesterol present in the LDL. The evidence that lysosomal enzymes are indeed involved in these processes is based on several different findings. There is concentration of a radioautographic reaction over secondary lysosomes when rat smooth muscle cells had been incubated with labeled LDL for 24 h (Fig. 3). Additional support for the lysosomal location of catabolism of LDL was obtained in experiments with human skin fibroblasts (20). Pretreatment of the cells with concanavalin A prevents the fusion between endocytic vacuoles and lysosomes (21). When human skin fibroblasts were preincubated for 30 min with concanavalin A and then incubated with ^{125}I-labeled LDL the rate of LDL degradation was reduced by about 40%. Interestingly enough pretreatment with concanavalin A resulted also in a very significant reduction of the feedback inhibition of cholesterol synthesis by human LDL (20).

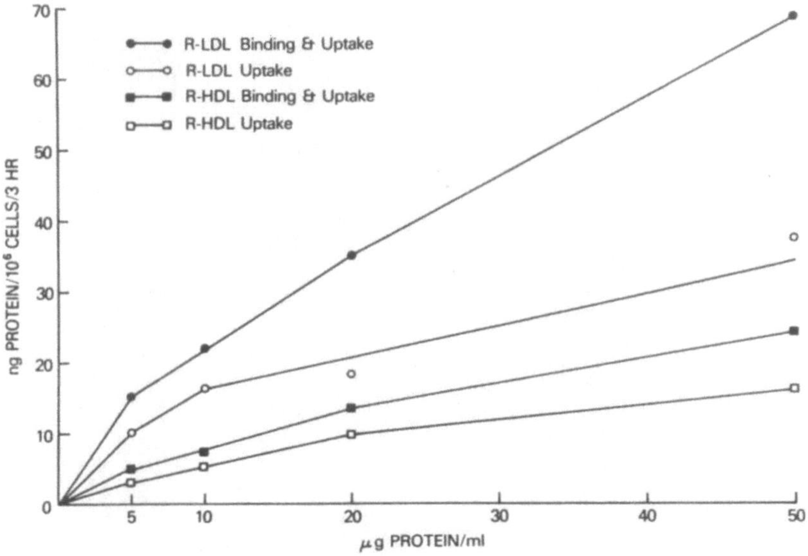

Figure 1. Binding and Uptake of Homologous Lipoproteins by Rat Smooth Muscle Cells.

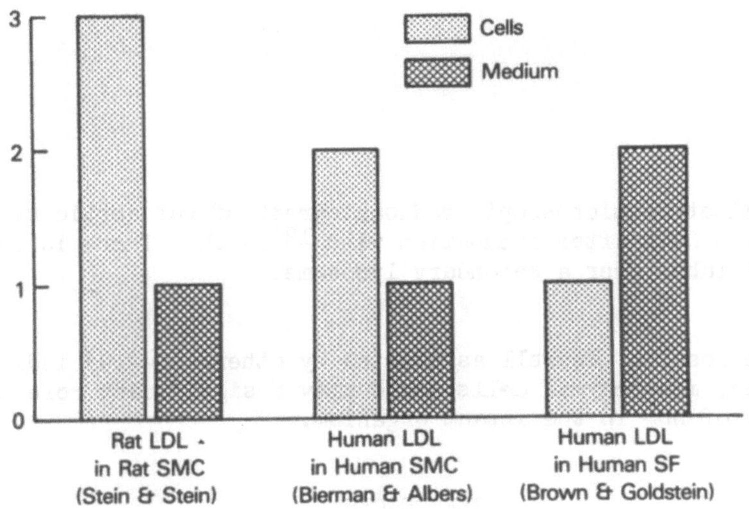

Figure 2. Ratio of Cellular ^{125}I-Protein to ^{125}I-Protein Degradation Products in Medium after 3 Hour Incubation.

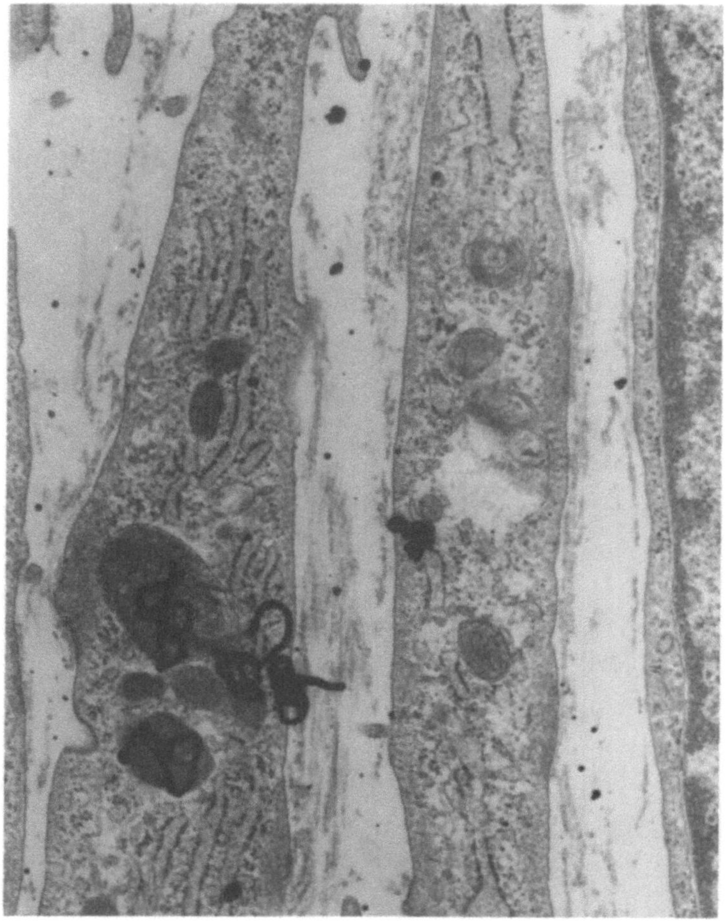

Fig. 3. Electron microscopic radioautograph of rat aortic smooth muscle cells 24 h after incubation with ^{125}I-LDL. There is concentration of label over a secondary lysosome.

These results, as well as studies by others (14-19) indicate that indeed, mesenchymal cells could play a significant role in the catabolism of LDL in the intact organism.

REFERENCES

1. Eisenberg, S. and Rachmilewitz, D.: The interaction of rat plasma very low density lipoprotein with lipoprotein lipase rich (post heparin) plasma. J. Lipid Res. In press, 1975.

2. Mjøs, O.D., Faergeman, O., Hamilton, R.L. and Havel, R.J.: Characterization of remnants of lymph chylomicrons and lymph and plasma very low density lipoproteins in "supra-diaphragmatic" rats. Eur. J. Clin. Invest. 4:382, 1974.
3. Stein, O., Rachmilewitz, D., Sanger, L., Eisenberg, S. and Stein Y.: Metabolism of iodinated very low density lipoprotein in the rat. Autoradiographic localization in the liver. Biochim. Biophys. Acta 360:205, 1974.
4. Eisenberg, S., Bilheimer, D.W., Levy, R.I. and Lindgren, F.T.: On the metabolic conversion of human plasma very low density lipoprotein to low density lipoprotein. Biochim. Biophys. Acta 326:361, 1973.
5. Hay, R.V., Pottenger, L.A., Reingold, A.L., Getz, G.S. and Wissler, R.W.: Degradation of ^{125}I-labelled serum low density lipoprotein in normal and estrogen-treated male rats. Biochim. Biophys. Res. Commun. 44:1471, 1971.
6. Sniderman, A.D., Carew, T.E., Chandler, J.G. and Steinberg, D.: Paradoxical increase in rate of catabolism of low density lipoproteins after hepatectomy. Science, 183:526, 1974.
7. Steinberg, D.E., Carew, T.E., Chandler, J.G. and Sniderman, A.D.: The role of the liver in metabolism of plasma lipoproteins, in: Regulation of Hepatic Metabolism, F. Lundquist, Ed. (Academic Press, 1974), pp. 144-156.
8. Stein, O., Stein, Y. and Eisenberg, S.: A radioautographic study of the transport of ^{125}I-labelled serum lipoproteins in rat aorta. Cell & Tissue Res. 138:223, 1973.
9. Reichl, D., Simons, L.A., Myant, N.B., Pflug, J.J. and Mills, G.L.: The lipids and lipoproteins of human peripheral lymph, with observations on the transport of cholesterol from plasma and tissues into lymph. Clin. Sci. and Mol. Med. 45:313, 1973.
10. Bierman, E.L., Eisenberg, S., Stein, O. and Stein, Y.: Very low density lipoprotein "remnant" particles; uptake by aortic smooth muscle cells in culture. Biochim. Biophys. Acta 329:163, 1973.
11. Bierman, E.L., Stein, O. and Stein, Y.: Lipoprotein uptake and metabolism by rat aortic smooth muscle cells in tissue culture. Circulation Res. 35:136, 1974.
12. Stein, O. and Stein, Y.: Comparative uptake of rat and human serum low density lipoproteins by rat aortic smooth muscle cells in culture. Circulation Res. 36:436, 1975.
13. Stein, O. and Stein, Y.: Surface binding and interiorization of homologous and heterologous serum lipoproteins by rat aortic smooth muscle cells in culture. Biochim. Biophys. Acta, in press.
14. Bierman, E.L. and Albers, J.J.: Lipoprotein uptake by cultured human arterial smooth muscle cells. Biochim. Biophys. Acta 388:198, 1975.

15. Weinstein, D.B., Carew, T.E. and Steinberg, D.: Uptake and degradation of low density lipoprotein by porcine arterial smooth muscle cells with inhibition of cholesterol biosynthesis. Circulation 50:111, 1974.

16. Assman, G., Brown, B.G., and Mahley, R.W.: Regulation of 3-hydroxy-3-methylglutaryl coenzyme A reductase activity in cultured swine aortic smooth muscle cells by plasma lipoproteins. In press, 1975.

17. Brown, M.S. and Goldstein, J.L.: Familial hypercholesterolemia: defective binding of lipoproteins to cultured fibroblasts associated with impaired regulation of 3-hydroxy-3-methylglutaryl coenzyme A reductase activity. Proc. Nat. Acad. Sci. U.S.A. 71:788, 1974.

18. Brown, M.S., Dana, S.E. and Goldstein, J.L.: Regulation of 3-hydroxy-3-methylglutaryl coenzyme A reductase activity in cultured human fibroblasts. Comparison of cells from a normal subject and from a patient with homozygous familial hypercholesterolemia. J. Biol. Chem. 240:789, 1974.

19. Goldstein, J.L. and Brown, M.S.: Binding and degradation of low density lipoproteins by cultured human fibroblasts. Comparison of cells from a normal subject and from a patient with homozygous familial hypercholesterolemia. J. Biol. Chem. 249:5153, 1974.

20. Stein, O., Weinstein, D.B., Stein, Y. and Steinberg, D.: Binding, internalization and degradation of low density lipoprotein by normal human fibroblasts and by fibroblasts from a new case of homozygous familial hypercholesterolemia. In press, 1975.

21. Edelson, P.J. and Cohn, Z.A.: Effects of concanavalin A on mouse peritoneal macrophages. II. Metabolism of endocytized proteins and reversibility of the effects by mannose. J. Exp. Med. 140:1387, 1974.

(3)

THE ORIGIN AND FATE OF HDL

Dr. P.S. Roheim

Albert Einstein College of Medicine of Yeshiva University
Department of Medicine & Physiology
1300 Morris Park Avenue, Bronx, N.Y., U.S.A.

High density lipoproteins (HDL) are one of the major serum lipoprotein fractions. In my presentation I will focus on the metabolism of the protein moiety of HDL. I shall discuss the sites of synthesis and catabolism as well as the rates of removal of HDL and its apoproteins. The interrelationship between the apoproteins of HDL and the apoproteins of very low density lipoproteins (VLDL) will also be discussed.

It has been shown in the past twenty years by several investigators (Marsh and Whereat 1959, Radding and Steinberg 1960, Haft et al 1962), that the liver is the main source of HDL. We have also shown that there is extrahepatic synthesis of lipoproteins in hepatectomized dogs (Roheim et al 1966). Windmueller et al (1973) showed that lipoprotein synthesis takes place in the isolated perfused intestine. They demonstrated that during intestinal perfusion labeled amino acid is incorporated both into plasma (perfusate) and lymph HDL.

It is known that the different lipoprotein classes contain several apoprotein constituents (Shore and Shore 1972), and some of the apoproteins mainly the "C" apoproteins, are present both in HDL and VLDL. The question arises whether the liver and intestine are equally capable of synthesizing all apoproteins. This problem was studied by Windmueller et al (1973) who determined the incorporation of labeled amino acid into the different apoprotein constituents of lipoproteins during liver and intestinal perfusions. Incorporation into all apoproteins was found during liver perfusions however, in the intestinal perfusions no incorporation into the "C" apoprotein could be demonstrated, in either HDL or VLDL. This observation brings up the question of chylomicron formation, i.e. how and where do chylomicrons obtain their "C" apoproteins. Havel et al (1973) showed that during fat absorption HDL serves as a reservoir of chylomicron "C" apoproteins. During fat absorption the plasma "C" apoprotein concentrations do not change but the distribution of "C" apoproteins among VLDL, chylomicrons and HDL is altered.

The rate of removal of HDL was studied in different species by several investigators and the $t_{1/2}$ varied from 10 hours in the rat, to 4.5 days in humans. We have studied the catabolism of HDL in rats. ^{125}I-HDL was injected; the disappearance and uptake by different organs of the labeled HDL was determined (Roheim et al 1971). Fig. 1 shows the turnover curve of ^{125}I-HDL in rats. In these studies the $t_{1/2}$ of HDL was 10.5 hours.

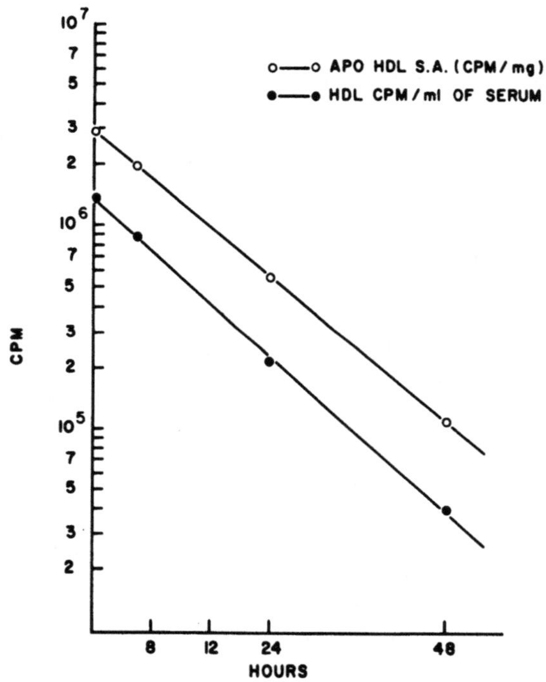

Fig. 1. Radioactivity present in isolated high density lipoprotein and the specific activity (cpm/mg) of the apoproteins of high density lipoprotein after injection of radioiodinated high density lipoprotein.

We also studied the disappearance rate of the different apoproteins of HDL. The distribution of radioactivity in the different apoproteins was determined after subjecting HDL to polyacrylamide gel electrophoresis in 8 M urea (Roheim et al 1972). This is shown in Fig. 2. When the rate of removal of the different bands was determined we found very similar $t_{1/2}$ in all apoproteins. (Fig. 3 and Fig. 4).

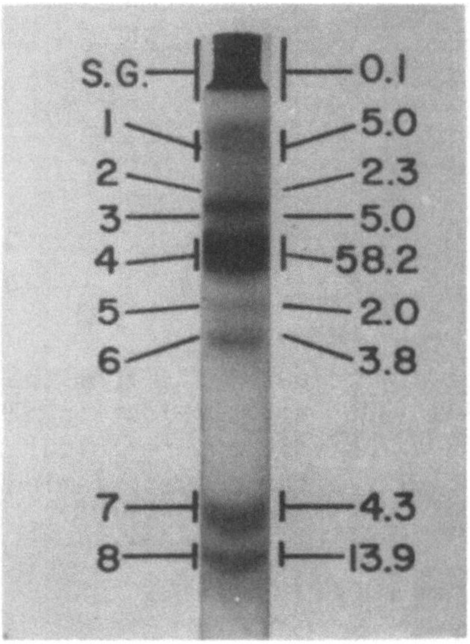

Fig. 2. Distribution of Radioactivity (right) among different apoprotein bands (left) after polyacrylamide gel electrophoresis of ^{125}I-HDL.

Some of the apoproteins present in HDL are also present in VLDL. These apoproteins are the "C" apoproteins and the Arginine rich apoprotein (ARP), (Shore and Shore 1973, Shelbourne and Quarfordt 1974, and Swaney et al 1974). It has been shown that the "C" apoproteins exchange freely between HDL and VLDL (Eisenberg et al 1972). However, we do not have any information on the exchangeability of ARP between HDL and VLDL, therefore we incubated rat ^{125}I-HDL with whole rat serum and reseparated the lipoproteins. After in vitro incubation 5-10% of the original radioactivity present in HDL was found in the VLDL. When the apoproteins of the

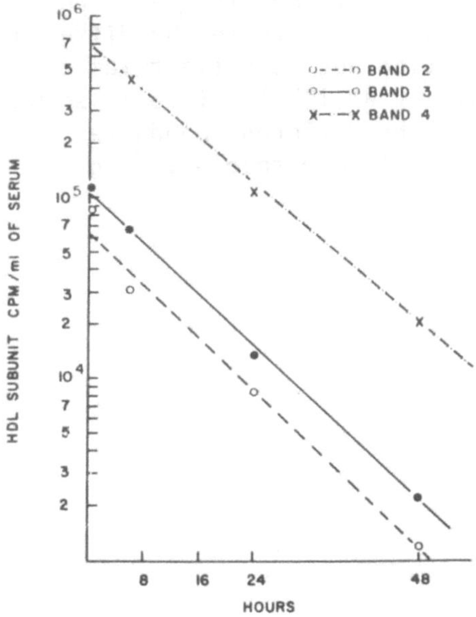

Fig. 3

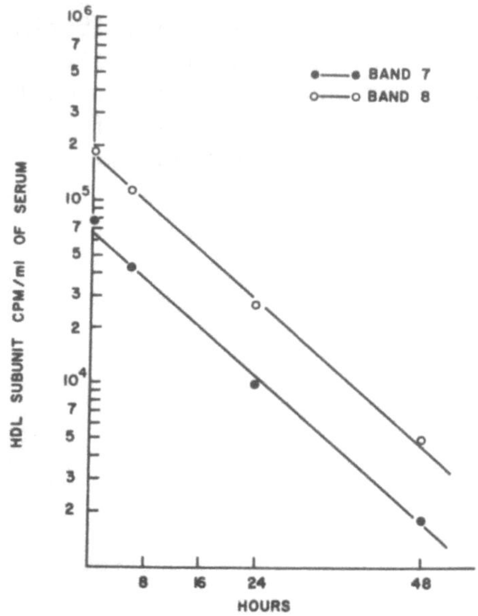

Fig. 4

Fig. 3-4. Disappearance of radioactivity from the subunits of high density lipoproteins (HDL) after injection of radioiodinated high density lipoprotein. The values were calculated from the distribution of radioactivity after polyacrylamide gel electrophoresis and are the mean values of 5-6 gels.

in vitro labeled VLDL were separated, we found radioactivity only in the "C" apoproteins and no radioactivity in ARP. Thus we could conclude that unlike the "C" apoproteins, the ARP does not exchange in vitro when labeled HDL is incubated with unlabeled serum. It is possible that there is no in vitro exchange of ARP but there is an in vivo transfer of ARP between HDL and VLDL. Therefore, we injected rats with ^{125}I-HDL and the appearance of radioactivity in the different lipoprotein fractions was determined. The VLDL contained 5-10% of total radioactivity at all time intervals studied. All the radioactivity found in VLDL was present in the "C" apoproteins, and no radioactivity could be detected in ARP.

The site of removal of labeled HDL in rats has also been studied (Roheim et al 1971, Eisenberg et al 1973). It was found that most of the radioactivity was removed by the liver but significant amounts were also removed by other organs.

We have also studied the intracellular localization of ^{125}I-HDL in the liver (Rachmilewitz et al 1972). When the liver of rats after ^{125}I-HDL injection was subjected to radioautography, we found that most of the radioactivity was localized to the parenchymal cells. By electronmicroscopic radioautography we have shown a concentration of label in the lysosomes which probably participate in the degradation of HDL.

Lastly I will discuss alterations of HDL concentrations and changes in HDL apoprotein composition in different types of experimentally induced hyperlipidemia. We have shown (Lasser et al 1973) that cholesterol feeding of rats results in an increase of the VLDL ($d<1.006$) while HDL decreases and a new intermediate density fraction (IDL) d 1.006-1.030 appears. We compared the apoprotein composition of the different lipoprotein fractions from sera of normal and cholesterol fed rats and we found that HDL from sera of cholesterol fed rats has a remarkable decrease of "C" apoproteins and does not contain detectable amounts of ARP (Kuehl et al 1973). The newly formed intermediate density fraction contains all apoproteins which could be found in HDL in addition to apo-B. Thus the HDL apoprotein composition could be altered by dietary manipulation and HDL apoproteins which are normally present only in HDL can also be found in other lipoprotein fractions. These data suggest that the lipoprotein fractions cannot be rigidly classified according to their density, since in abnormal conditions lipoprotein fractions similar in apoprotein composition to that of HDL (d 1.063-1.21) also appear in the IDL (d 1.006-1.030). It will be of interest to elucidate the mechanism and pathophysiological significance of these changes.

Summary

High density lipoproteins are synthesized both in the liver and intestine. All apoproteins can be synthesized in the liver and intestine except the "C" apoproteins which could not be synthesized by the intestine.

After injection of ^{125}I-HDL its different apoproteins are removed from the circulation at a similar rate. Most of the HDL is removed by the liver and the degradation of the protein moiety of HDL was localized to the lysozomes of the parenchymal cells.

Cholesterol feeding alters the distribution of lipoprotein fractions and results in the appearance of a new intermediate density class, in which all HDL apoproteins are present in addition to apo-B. Cholesterol feeding also results in an alteration of apoprotein composition of HDL.

REFERENCES

Eisenberg, S., D.W. Bilheimer and R.I. Levy, Biochim. Biophys. Acta, 280 (1972) 94.

Eisenberg, S., H.G. Windmueller and R.I. Levy, J. Lipid Res., 14 (1973) 446.

Haft, D.E., P.S. Roheim, A. White and H.A. Eder, J. Clin. Invest., 41 (1962) 842.

Havel, R.J., J.P. Kane and M.L. Kashyap, J. Clin. Invest., 52 (1973) 32.

Kuehl, K., P.S. Roheim and H.A. Eder, Fed. Proc., 33 (1974) 828.

Lasser, N.L., P.S. Roheim, D. Edelstein and H.A. Eder, J. Lipid Res., 14 (1973) 1.

Marsh, J.B. and A.F. Whereat, J. Biol. Chem., 234 (1959) 3196.

Rachmilewitz, D., O. Stein, P.S. Roheim and Y. Stein, Biochim. Biophys. Acta, 270 (1972) 414.

Radding, C.M. and D. Steinberg, J. Clin. Invest., 39 (1960) 1560.

Roheim, P.S., L. J. Gidez and H.A. Eder, J. Clin. Invest., 45 (1966) 297.

Roheim, P.S., D. Rachmilewitz, O. Stein and Y. Stein, Biochim. Biophys. Acta, 248 (1971) 315.

Roheim, P.S., H. Hirsch, D. Edelstein and D. Rachmilewitz, Biochim. Biophys. Acta, 278 (1972) 517.

Shelbourne, F.A. and S. H. Quarfordt, J. Biol. Chem., 249 (1974) 1428.

Shore, V.G. and B. Shore, Blood Lipids and Lipoproteins. Editor: Gary J. Nelson, Wiley - Interscience 1972, p. 789.

Shore, V.G. and B. Shore, Biochem., 12 (1973) 502.

Swaney, J.B., H. Reese and H.A. Eder, Biochem. Biophys. Res. Com., 59 (1974) 513.

Windmueller, H.G., P.N. Herbert and R.I. Levy, J. Lipid Res. 14 (1973) 215.

(4)

THE ROLE OF LCAT IN CHOLESTEROL TRANSPORT

Kaare R. Norum

Institute for Nutrition Research, School of Medicine, University of Oslo, Norway.
P.O. Box 1046, Blindern, Oslo 3, Norway.

The metabolic role of lecithin:cholesterol acyltransferase (LCAT) has recently been subject for review (1). In this short paper I will only draw attention to some aspects concerning the role of LCAT in cholesterol transport.

Isotopic experiments have shown that lipoprotein cholesterol molecules exchange rapidly between the different species of plasma lipoproteins, and with cholesterol in biological membranes. Cholesterol in circulating lipoproteins is therefore in a dynamic equilibrium with cholesterol in cellular plasma membranes. It is reason to believe that intracellular cholesterol is in close equilibrium with that of the cell surface. The cholesterol exchange is non-enzymic, and although it takes place in simple in vitro systems it is probable that the process in vivo is enhanced by sterol carrier proteins (2). This exchange and the dynamic equilibrium form the basis for a net transfer of cholesterol between lipoproteins and plasma membranes.

The dynamic equilibrium of cholesterol between circulating lipoproteins and cells may be affected by both intra- and extracellular processes. Net uptake of cholesterol will take place in cells which convert cholesterol into nonexchangable products (cholesteryl esters, steroid hormones, bile acids) faster than their cholesterol biosynthesis, or if the cholesterol of lipoproteins in plasma or interstitial fluid is increased by a great secretion of cholesterol from liver and/or mucosa cells. Net transport of cholesterol from cells will occur if the rate of cholesterol biosynthesis or hydrolysis of cholesteryl esters exceeds that of cholesterol conversion to nonexchangable products. Important for the transport of cholesterol to and from cells are also enzymic processes taking place in plasma or interstitial fluid.

Lipoprotein lipase catalyzes the removal of the triglyceride core of chylomicrons and very low density lipoproteins (VLDL). This process will lead to a relative excess of lipoprotein surface and to changes in the physico-chemical properties of the lipoprotein remnant. The excess of unesterified cholesterol will most probably be rapidly distributed to other lipoproteins and adjacent plasma membranes. Under normal circumstances, therefore, plasma membranes and circulating lipoproteins may function as cholesterol buffers. The superfluous cholesterol of the buffers will in time be removed due to the continous esterification of cholesterol which takes place in plasma and interstitial fluid and is catalyzed by LCAT.

LCAT catalyzes the transfer of the acyl group from the 2-position of lecithin to cholesterol. Only lipids of high density lipoproteins (HDL) may serve as direct substrates for LCAT (3). The reason for this is probably that the reaction is activated by the main protein of HDL, apolipoprotein A I. Several reports have shown that the activity of LCAT is dependent of both apolipoprotein and lipid ratios in plasma. We know, however, too little about plasma constituents which influence the formation of plasma cholesteryl esters. Conflicting results exist on the consequence of triglyceride-rich lipoproteins for the LCAT reaction, and some find a positive correlation between plasma unesterified cholesterol and LCAT activity (4), while others do not (5). This probably reflects that amounts and lipid load on certain types of lipoproteins have more importance for the LCAT activity than total plasma lipid values. Although LCAT only acts directly on smaller HDL, it indirectly diminishes cholesterol of other plasma lipoproteins because of the rapid equilibration of cholesterol among lipoproteins.

An important feature of the LCAT/HDL cholesterol transport system is the transfer of cholesteryl esters from HDL to VLDL. It has been suggested that this transfer may be associated with a reciprocal transfer of triglycerides from VLDL to HDL (6). Incubation studies with plasma from patients with familial LCAT deficiency have shown that an interchange of triglycerides and cholesteryl esters is not necessary for the transfer of cholesteryl esters from HDL to VLDL (7). It must be stressed, however, that more studies are needed to get more understanding of this important step in the cholesterol metabolism.

LCAT's role in cholesterol transport can be deduced from findings in patients with familial LCAT deficiency (8). These patients have deposits of cholesterol in several organs and tissues. Studies of plasma lipoproteins of the patients have also given valuable information about the role of LCAT in metabolism and interconversion of plasma lipoproteins (1). The VLDL and LDL fractions of the patients contain large particles rich in cholesterol and lecithin. The amounts of these lipoproteins vary in relation to the long-chain triglycerides in the diet (9). The HDL fraction of the patients' plasma is heterogenous and contains at least two populations of particles. Most of the particles are disc-shaped and have larger diameter than normal HDL. They are much like the nascent HDL found in liver perfusion studies (10). Another population of HDL is smaller than normal and of probable intestinal origin (9). Furthermore, most of the arginine-rich apolipoproteins are found in the HDL fraction.

When patient plasma was incubated in presence of LCAT (7), the concentration of the large VLDL and LDL decreased. The concentration of apolipoprotein B in LDL increased concomitantly with an increase in apolipoprotein A I in the HDL. A major component of the HDL fraction became identical in appearance to normal HDL. The concentration of arginine-rich apolipoprotein decreased in HDL and increased in VLDL. Upon incubation of patients' isolated VLDL in the presence of LCAT, lipoproteins with properties similar to normal LDL were formed. Incubation of isolated large HDL and small HDL yielded lipoproteins with the appearance of HDL_2 and HDL_3 respectively. These experiments show that the LCAT reaction can alter the apolipoprotein content and physical properties as well as the lipid content of the patients' lipoproteins, and suggest that the HDL/LCAT system also has an important role in the normal metabolism of lipoproteins. In normal plasma it is, however, difficult to show any dramatic effect of an incubation in the presence of LCAT, because the major effect of the LCAT reaction of the lipoproteins already have occurred. We have in such experiments only found a small loss of the apolipoprotein C from HDL.

Some metabolic studies have indicated the importance of LCAT in cholesterol transport. As most of the unesterified cholesterol entering the plasma compartment is located on the surface of triglyceride-rich lipoproteins, one would expect an increased demand for plasma cholesterol esterification when triglyceride turnover is high. Thus, an increased activity of LCAT has been reported in obesity (4) and in hypertriglyceridemia (11), and turnover of cholesteryl esters was found to be increased in type IV hyperlipoproteinemia, carbohydrate feeding and nephrotic syndrome (12).

The role of LCAT in the normal transport of cholesterol suggests that the activity of the enzyme may have some importance for the development of atherosclerosis. The few studies published till now, however, do not indicate that variations in LCAT activity may be a major risk factor for coronary heart disease, although patients with familial LCAT deficiency develop early atherosclerosis.

Recent research on LCAT covers enzyme purification, studies on LCAT and liver diseases, and the role of the enzyme in lipoprotein metabolism. A lot of valuable information has appeared in the last few years. Much more data, however, are needed before we fully understand the role of the HDL/LCAT system. I feel that we specially need more knowledge on: What regulates production and degradation of LCAT? What roles have apolipoproteins and other lipid carrier proteins in the transfer of cholesterol and cholesteryl esters among the lipoproteins? How is LCAT transported from blood to tissues, and what is the role of the enzyme in normal and pathological arterial intima?

REFERENCES

1. Glomset, J.A. and Norum, K.R.: Adv. Lipid Res. 11:1, 1973.
2. Scallen, T.J., Seetharam, B., Srikantaiah, M.V., Hansbury, E. and Lewis, M.K.: Life Sci. 16:853, 1975.
3. Glomset, J.A.: J. Lipid Res. 9:155, 1968.
4. Akanuma, Y., Kuzuya, T., Hayashi, M., Ide, T. and Kuzuya, N.: Eur. J. Clin. Invest. 3:136, 1973.
5. Barter, P.J.: J. Lipid Res. 15:234, 1974.
6. Nichols, A.V. and Smith, L.: J. Lipid Res. 6:206, 1965.
7. Norum, K.R., Glomset, J.A., Nichols, A.V., Forte, T., Albers, J.J., King, W.C., Mitchell, C.D., Applegate, K.R., Gong, E.L., Cabana, V. and Gjone, E.: Scand. J. Clin. Lab. Invest. 35: Suppl. 142, p. 31, 1975.

8. Norum, K.R., Glomset, J.A. and Gjone, E.: p. 531 in The Metabolic Basis of Inherited Disease (Stanbury, J.R., Wyngaarden, J.H. and Fredrickson, D.S., Eds.), McGraw-Hill, New York, 1972.
9. Glomset, J.A., Norum, K.R., Nichols, A.V., King, W.C., Mitchell, C.D., Applegate, K.R., Gong, E.L. and Gjone, E.: Scand. J. Clin. Lab. Invest. 35: Suppl. 142, p. 3, 1975.
10. Hamilton, R.L. and Kayden, H.J.: p. 531 in The Liver: Normal and Abnormal Functions, Part A. (Becker, F.F., Ed.), Marcel Dekker Inc., New York, 1974.
11. Sodhi, H.S.: Scand. J. Clin. Lab. Invest. 33: Suppl. 137, p. 161, 1974.
12. Nestel, P.J., Miller, N.E. and Clifton-Bligh, P.: Scand. J. Clin. Lab. Invest. 33: Suppl. 137, p. 157, 1974.

CHAPTER 4
REGRESSION OF LESIONS

(1)

INTRODUCTION

Dr. Robert W. Wissler

University of Chicago

Chicago, Illinois, U.S.A.

Dr. Robert W.Wissler of Chicago opened the workshop on regression by stating that a number of recent studies have furnished both indirect and direct evidence that atherosclerotic plaques in man and experimental animals may be substantially reduced in size by the sustained reduction of serum cholesterol to the levels that appear to be usual and normal in each species when it is receiving a low fat and low cholesterol diet throughout life.

The purpose of this workshop is to report some of the recent studies of regression and encourage further discussion and further study of the potential regression of advanced atherosclerotic lesions.

The most promising pioneering work on regression of stenosing coronary atherosclerosis has been reported by the co-chairman of this session, Dr. Mark Armstrong and his coworkers at the University of Iowa who have published data indicating that atheromatous plaques in rhesus monkeys that filled in the lumen by as much as 65% could be opened up so that they only filled in 20 - 30% of the lumen by the simple expedient of lowering the serum cholesterol to 130 - 140 mg%, using a low fat,low cholesterol ration or a polyunsaturated fat, low cholesterol ration. He and his colleagues also reported evidence of a substantial decrease in the collagen content of some of these lesions.

Our own most recent and unpublished studies in this same species have also indicated consistent and significant regression of advanced atherosclerotic lesions in the coronary, carotid and femoral arteries as well as in the aorta when a low fat, low cholesterol ration is fed for 12 - 18 months.

This regression can be increased substantially by use of cholestyramine along with the low fat, low cholesterol ration.

Recent evidence published by Dr. Vesselinovitch of Chicago indicates that severe atherosclerotic lesions in rabbits can also be reduced in size rather remarkably if a therapeutic regimen combining daily increased oxygen administration, a low fat, low cholesterol diet and either estrogen or cholestyramine therapy is maintained. This, too, is encouraging since the resistance of the cholesterol-induced rabbit lesions to regression has been a major cause for pessimism regarding the reversibility of atherosclerosis.

(2)

PROGRESSION AND REGRESSION OF EXPERIMENTAL ATHEROSCLEROTIC LESIONS

J. C. Geer, H. M. Sharma, R. V. Panganamala and D. G. Cornwell

Departments of Pathology and Physiological Chemistry
College of Medicine, The Ohio State University
Columbus, Ohio, U.S.A.

The prerequisite for development of experimental atherosclerosis in the rabbit and all other experimental models is hyperlipemia. Hyperlipemia can be induced in the rabbit by adding cholesterol to the diet or using a diet with a high content of saturated fat. Lipid infiltration into the wall of the proximal aorta begins within hours following the increase in blood cholesterol[1]. The earliest lesion morphologically is granular appearing stainable lipid in the interstitial tissue often associated with elastic fibers. Continued hypercholesterolemia eventuates in a foam cellular infiltrate in the intima and inner media associated with proliferation of smooth muscle cells and appearance of a band of smooth muscle cells beneath the endothelial lining[1,2]. Necrotic cells are found in the lesion usually near the media[2]. The lipid content of this lesion like that of all other experimental models and man is mostly cholesterol as cholesteryl esters[3]. The cholesterol in the lesions is derived from the blood[4].

Factors and mechanisms concerned with induction and progression of the rabbit experimental atheroma are: hyperlipemia; endothelial permeability; lipid transport or entrapment in the artery wall; lipid metabolism in smooth muscle and foam cells; cellular connective tissue synthesis; cell necrosis; movement of foam cells into or out of the artery wall. Each of these factors or mechanisms plays a role in lesion progression; their relative roles as major or minor for lesion progression are not known for certain. In this presentation we are concentrating on possible causes for altered endothelial permeability, cell proliferation, and cell death.

Studies with Trypan blue, Evans blue and labeled albumin have shown variations in endothelial permeability that are local and focal and display the same pattern as induced experimental lesions[1,5-7]. Injured or altered endothelium (hemodynamic, trauma[8], immune complex[9], cholesterol[10], vasoactive substances) shows increased permeability to vital dyes, albumin, lipid, and fibrinogen. The mechanism(s) by which lipid moves from the blood into the artery wall is unknown. When the lipid composition of the artery wall is studied progressing from very early to advanced lesions the composition changes from one of predominantly free cholesterol and sphingomyelin[11] to massive accumulation of cholesteryl esters[3]. The human lesion differs in part from the lesion in the experimental animal. In the human, there is no simple progression in either relative lipid composition or total lipid content from normal intima to fibrous plaques; however, both fatty streaks and fibrous plaques show elevations in free cholesterol[12]. The influx of free cholesterol in early experimental lesions is much greater than that of cholesteryl esters. Plaque lesions show a large influx of cholesteryl esters[13]. These observations on influx and composition in animals suggest that in the early stage of cholesterol accumulation serum lipoprotein is not transported in toto across the endothelium. We have hypothesized that there may be an exchange of free cholesterol between serum lipoproteins and cell membranes which alters the membrane and thus cellular function leading to a movement of cholesterol into the artery wall. There is ample evidence that an excess of free cholesterol modifies membranes and damages cells[14], but whether such plays a role in endothelial permeability and lipid transport remains to be proven. In the following we will expand on this theory and discuss possible mechanisms by which cholesterol may lead to cell proliferation and necrosis.

The fatty streak lesion containing large numbers of foam cells has a lipid content that is primarily cholesteryl esters[3,14]. Metabolic studies have shown cholesterol esterification in the artery wall to occur in situ[14]. The cholesteryl ester fatty acid (CEFA) composition of foam cellular lesions differs from that of blood cholesteryl esters by having a much larger oleic and 8,11,14-eicosatrienoic acid content and lower linoleic acid[3,14]. The composition of CEFA in foam cell lesions suggests limited availability of linoleic acid for esterification. In support of this suggestion is the finding of a small amount of the 5,8,11 isomer of eicosatrienoic acid which characterizes essential fatty acid deficiency[3,14]. The lipid composition of lesions poses the questions of why the massive accumulation of cholesteryl esters rather than free cholesterol, phospholipid, or triglycerides; and why does the lesion CEFA vary from that of blood CEFA? The answer to the first question probably is that phospholipid and triglycerides can be catabolized and cholesterol can not thus leading to cholesterol accumulation. A corollary to this conclusion is that removal of cholesterol from the artery wall must be physical. The variation of CEFA composition between the arterial lesion and blood almost certainly is a reflection of in situ esterification utilizing fatty acids readily available by de novo synthesis such as oleic acid and depletion of available linoleic acid. We propose that cholesterol esterification is a protective or detoxification type reaction in the artery wall. Free cholesterol available for exchange can alter cell membranes and thus alter cell function and lead to cell death. Cholesteryl esters form anisotropic mesophases that appear to be inert to membranes[3,14]. It seems reasonable therefore that conversion of free to esterified cholesterol in the artery wall is serving a protective or detoxifying action changing biologically active free cholesterol to inactive esters.

The CEFA pattern, cholesteryl ester synthetase studies, and saturation of phospholipids suggest another but closely related mechanism for cell injury. The large linoleic and 8,11,14-eicosatrienoic acid requirement for cholesterol esterification depletes the available pool. The principal source for these fatty acids is lecithin which Bottcher[15] has shown becomes more saturated as lesions progress. Lecithins are the source of linoleic acid for esterification by lecithin-cholesterol acyl transferase (LCAT). The increasing saturation of lecithins probably reflects esterification of lysolecithin by endogenously available fatty acids. We propose that the depletion of 8,11,14-eicosatrienoic acid results in decreased prostaglandins E_1 and F_1 (PGE_1 and PGF_1) or their endoperoxide precursors. These prostaglandins inhibit cholesteryl ester synthetase in rat liver[16] and ovarian tissues[17]. Thus an essential fatty acid deficiency has been shown to increase cholesterol esterification in liver and plasma[18]. PGE_1 enhances the activity of cholesteryl ester hydrolase in rat adrenal gland, an action that may be mediated by cyclic adenosine-3',5'-monophosphate (cAMP)[19]. If similar actions for PGE_1 obtain in arteries, the net effect of PGE_1 deficiency would be accelerated cholesteryl ester synthesis.

If cholesteryl ester formation serves as a detoxification type reaction as we propose, accelerated synthesis of esters is a beneficial or desirable effect of PGE_1 deficiency. There are, however, other possible effects of PGE_1 deficiency. PGE_1 stabilizes lysosomes in macrophages and stimulates adenylate cyclase in leukocytes. PGE_1 and cAMP act synergistically to reduce hydrolase release[20,21]. PGE_1 has been shown to increase the cAMP level in cells suggesting that the effect of PGE_1 is mediated through cAMP[22]. Reduced cAMP level in cells is associated with cell proliferation[23]. Thus, it is conceivable that PGE_1 deficiency could result in proliferation of intimal cells due to decreased cAMP and cell death due to lysosomal destabilization. A role for prostaglandins in arterial reactions to injury is at present only hypothetical.

Analytical problems have prevented our being able to directly measure prostaglandins in arterial tissue. Indirectly we have evidence of a role for PGE_2 altering endothelium[24].

An alternative but closely related hypothesis for the mechanism of arterial cell proliferation and necrosis has been proposed by Papahadjopoulos[25]. Increased cholesterol in the cell membrane inhibits Na-K adenosine triphosphatase (ATPase) and adenylate cyclase. cAMP is reduced and cell proliferation and necrosis are promoted. Low density lipoprotein stimulation of smooth muscle cell proliferation in vitro[26] could be mediated by either ATPase inhibition or prostaglandin deficiency. The final pathway, decreased cAMP, is the same for both mechanisms. It remains for future studies to test the validity of these hypotheses and additionally to determine the roles of cyclic guanosine-3',5'-monophosphate as an antagonist for cAMP.

Regression of experimental atherosclerotic lesions follows normalization of blood lipids[2]. Normalization of blood lipids stops or at least markedly reduces the influx of lipid into the artery and permits an unobstructed view of the mechanisms by which lipid is removed from the lesions. The time required for lesion regression are similar in all models: foam cells disappear; an extracellular mass of lipid appears deep in the intima and often extends into the inner media (atheroma); the band of smooth muscle cells adjacent to the endothelium thickens; smooth muscle cells at the margins of the extracellular lipid proliferate; elastic and collagen fibers increase in number in the subendothelial band of smooth muscle cells and about the margins of the extracellular lipid mass; and the extracellular lipid mass (atheroma) slowly disappears[2,27].

Factors and mechanisms operative in regression include normalization of blood lipids, loss of foam cells, cellular necrosis forming the atheroma, smooth muscle cell proliferation, connective tissue synthesis, and removal of extracellular lipid. Although this overall process is widely described as regression, the resultant lesion for a number of months after normalization of blood lipids is from a morphological view point a fibrous plaque. Cell proliferation, connective tissue synthesis, and cell necrosis probably are processes more a part of lesion progression than regression; however, in the rabbit model where influx of lipid is stopped, we are observing a pure reparative process.

The loss of lipid that occurs from the lesions is a truly regressive change. The loss of lipid in the early regression period is due to removal of foam cells from the lesion[2,27,28]. This removal is associated with a marked reduction in cholesteryl ester content[28,29] which almost certainly reflects the ester content of the foam cells. The loss of foam cells can occur by two processes. The cells could undergo necrosis releasing their ester rich content into the extracellular space. Lipid composition studies offer no support for this being the only mechanism for their disappearance. The second mechanism is migration of foam cells from the lesion through the lumen endothelium or through the media to adventitial vessels. Foam cells penetrating the endothelium have been observed in rabbits[30]. Dog experimental lesions appear to regress by transmedial foam cell migration to adventitial vessels[31]. Lipid composition studies are consistent with the cell migration mechanism for foam cell disappearance. The foam cell is thus acting as a mononuclear phagocyte with an action phagocytes are well known to have in other tissues. Most investigators regard the arterial foam cell to be derived from smooth muscle[31]; there is no proof for this. In view of the highly significant role of the foam cell in lesion regression, the origin and factors that promote emigration of these cells are of great importance. Further, since these cells contribute by necrosis lipid to the atheroma and thus progression to more advanced and potentially clinically significant lesions, the factors that cause necrosis of these cells are of similar importance. We previously discussed necrosis and proliferation with regard to cyclic nucleotides and prostaglandins. Other possible factors are cell age, oxygen deficiency, and effects of associated conditions such as diabetes mellitus or hypertension.

There is supporting evidence, morphologic[2,30] and lipid composition[29], that foam cell emigration from lesions is the mechanism for the disappearance of these cells and the reduction of cholesteryl ester content in lesions. Their loss also accounts for the decrease in lesion mass. The mechanism(s) by which the extracellular lipid (atheroma) slowly disappears over a very long period of time relative to the induction time is unknown.

ACKNOWLEDGMENT

These studies were supported in part by grants from the Harkers Fund and U.S. Public Health Service Grant HL-11897.

REFERENCES

1. Duff, G. L., A. M. A. Arch. Pathol. 20:81 (1935).
2. Anitschkow, N., in Arteriosclerosis, ed. by C. V. Cowdry. Macmillan Co., New York (1933) pp. 271-322.
3. Cornwell, D. G., J. C. Geer and R. V. Panganamala, in Pharmacology of Lipid Transport and Atherosclerotic Processes, ed. by E. J. Masoro (1975) Section 24, Vol. 1, pp. 445-483.
4. Dayton, S. and S. Hashimoto, Exper. Mol. Pathol. 13:253 (1970).

5. Bell, R. P., A. J. Day, M. Gent and C. J. Schwartz, Exper. Mol. Pathol. 22:366 (1975).
6. Bell, F. P., I. L. Adamson and C. J. Schwartz, Exper. Mol. Pathol. 20:57 (1974).
7. Bell, F. P., A. Gallus and C. J. Schwartz, Exper. Mol. Pathol. 20:281 (1974).
8. Bondjers, G. and S. Bjorkerud, Atherosclerosis 15:273 (1972).
9. Minick, C. R. and G. E. Murphy, Am. J. Pathol. 73:265 (1973).
10. Shimamoto, T., Jap. Heart J. 16:76 (1975).
11. Portman, O. W., Ann. N. Y. Acad. Sci. 162:120 (1969).
12. Panganamala, R. V., J. C. Geer, H. M. Sharma and D. G. Cornwell, Atherosclerosis 29:93 (1974).
13. Lofland, H. D. and T. B. Clarkson, Proc. Soc. Exper. Biol. and Med. 133:1 (1970).
14. Geer, J. C., R. V. Panganamala, H. A. I. Newman and D. G. Cornwell, in Pathogenesis of Atherosclerosis, ed. by Wissler, R. W. and Geer, J. C., Williams and Wilkins Co., Baltimore (1972) pp. 200-213.
15. Bottcher, C. J. F., Proc. Roy. Soc. Med. 57:34 (1964).
16. Schweppe, J. S. and R. A. Jungmann, Proc. Soc. Exp. Biol. and Med. 133:1307 (1972).
17. Behrman, H. R., G. J. MacDonald and R. O. Greep, Lipids 6: 791 (1971).
18. Sugano, M and O. W. Portman, Arch. Biochem. Biophys. 109:302 (1965).
19. Simpson, E. R., W. H. Trzeciak, J. L. McCarthy, C. R. Jefcoate and G. S. Boyd, Proc. Biochem. Soc 10P (1972).
20. Weissmann, G., P. Dukor and R. E. Zurier, Nature (New Biol.) 231:131 (1971).
21. Zurier, R. E. and G. Weissmann, in Prostaglandin in Cellular Biology, ed. by P. W. Ramwell and B. B. Pharriss, Plenum Press, N. Y. (1972) pp. 151-172.
22. LaRaia, P. J. and W. J. Reddy, Circulation 37, suppl. VI:222 (abstr.), (1968).
23. Pastan, I., Am. J. Clin. Pathol. 63:669 (1975).
24. Sharma, H. M., R. V. Panganamala, J. C. Geer and D. G. Cornwell, unpublished observations.
25. Papahadjopoulos, D., J. Theor. Biol. 43:329 (1974).
26. Ross, R. and J. A. Glomset, Science 180:1332 (1973).
27. Armstrong, M. L., E. D. Warner and W. E. Connor, Circ. Res. 27:59 (1970).
28. Clarkson, T. B., J. S. King, H. B. Lofland and M. A. Feldner, Circulation 44 (suppl. II), II-48 (abstr.) (1971).
29. Armstrong, M. L. and M. B. Megan, Circ. Res. 30:675 (1972).
30. Geer, J. C. and M. D. Haust, in Monographs on Atherosclerosis, ed. by O. J. Pollack, H. S. Simms and J. E. Kirk. S. Karger, Basel (1972) Vol. 2.
31. Bevans, M., J. D. Davidson and F. E. Kendall, Arch. Path. 51: 288 (1951).

(3)

DIETARY RESTRICTION AND PROGRESS OF ATHEROMA

C. W. M. ADAMS

Department of Pathology
Guy's Hospital Medical School
London University, London, Great Britain

1. Dietary Restriction

Sporadic comments in the literature, particularly after the experiences of World War II, suggest that dietary restriction might have some beneficial effect on atherosclerosis. This circumstantial evidence led us to see what effect calorie restriction would have on established atheroma in the rabbit. Thirty four animals were fed 1% cholesterol for 12 weeks and then returned to the stock low-lipid diet for 6 months. Ten animals were baseline controls, while the other 24 were pair matched for cholesterol levels and assigned to ad libitum and restricted dietary groups. The restricted group, after a period of trial-and-error, were fed approximately half of that eaten by the ad libitum group. Both groups received vitamin supplements of brewer's yeast and Vionate (Squibb).

Fig. 1 shows that the restricted group lost weight by about 30% of that of the ad libitum group. Five animals died within a few weeks after stopping the cholesterol-enriched diet: two with otitis media and meningitis, two with biliary cirrhosis and one with undiagnosed jaundice.

Fig. 2 shows the fall in blood cholesterol levels after stopping the cholesterol-enriched diet. From 8 weeks onwards the cholesterol level fell more slowly in the restricted group; breakdown of muscle tissue probably caused this delay in the fall.

At 3 months three restricted animals and six ad libitum animals were killed. The thoracic aorta in the restricted animals showed less atheroma as adjudged chemically (Table 1), by graticule

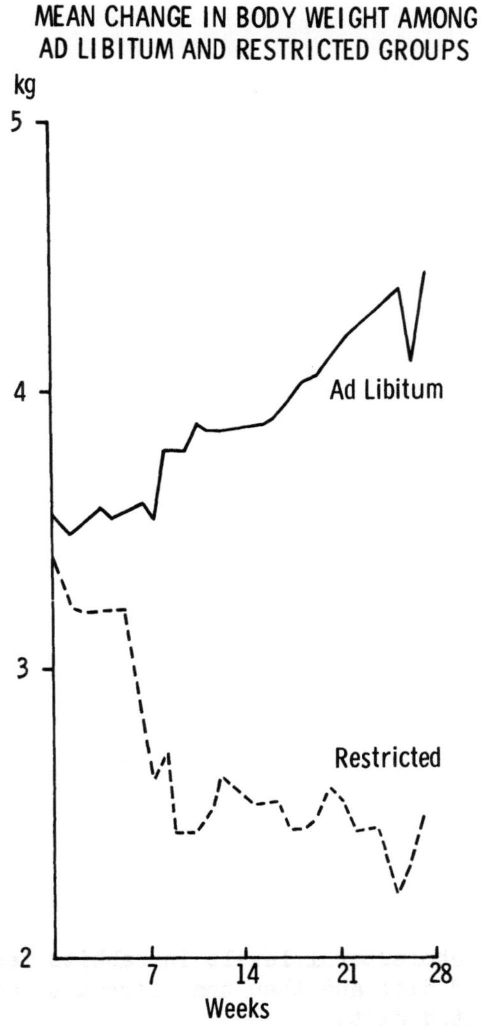

Figure 1. Weight changes in rabbits fed a cholesterol-enriched diet and then transferred to ad libitum or restricted diets.

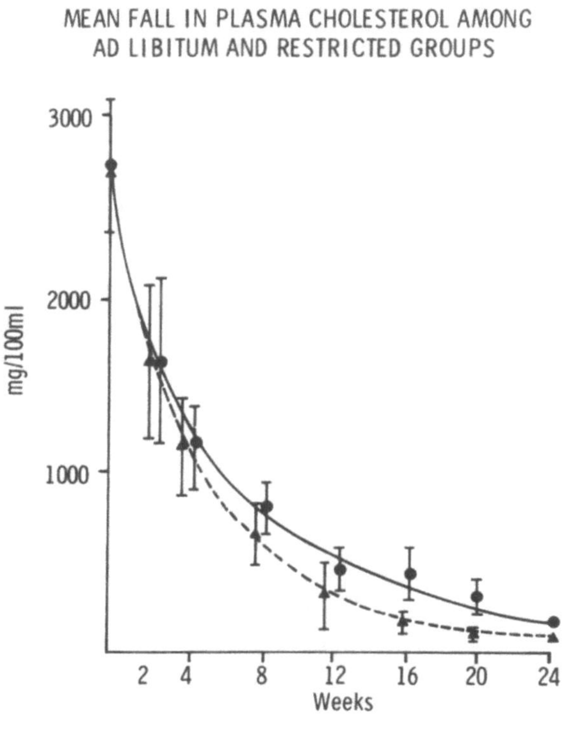

Figure 2. Plasma cholesterol levels in rabbits fed a cholesterol-enriched diet and then transferred to ad libitum or restricted diets.

TABLE 1. TOTAL AORTIC CHOLESTEROL AMONG DIETARY GROUPS

	End of 1% Cholesterol Diet	Ad Libitum		Restricted	
		3 mo.	6 mo.	3 mo.	6 mo.
Thoracic mg/g	52.37	54.59	24.16[a,d]	27.88[g]	32.88[j]
Arch mg/g	43.27	44.81	25.14[b,e]	62.13[h]	41.21[k]
Thoracic mg/5 cm	15.84	25.92	15.71[f]	7.19[i]	19.04[l]
Thoracic and Arch % as ester	64%	54%	38%	53%	40%

Statistical analyses by courtesy of Dr. R.W.R. Baker:-
a-c = 6 mo vs. end of diet; P ≤ 0.002, 0.05, NS.
d-f = 6 mo vs. 3 mo. ad lib; P ≤ 0.001, 0.001, 0.090.
g-i = 3 mo restricted vs. 3 mo ad lib; P ≤ 0.016, 0.0007, 0.26.
j-l = 6 mo restricted vs. 6 mo ad lib; P ≤ 0.10, 0.006, 0.20.

TABLE 2. GRATICULE COUNT (%) OF AORTIC AREA INVOLVED AMONG DIETARY GROUPS

	End of 1% Cholesterol Diet	Ad Libitum		Restricted	
		3 mo.	6 mo.	3 mo.	6 mo.
Mean	91.9	94.7	94.2	65.3[a]	88.2[b]
	10	6	5	3	5
SD	19.91	8.42	4.87	25.32	21.50

a, P = 0.007; b, P = 0.022

count (Table 2) and by histology. The aortic arch, in the restricted animals, showed no improvement at this time and in fact was somewhat worse (Table 1). This improvement in the thoracic aorta only and in such a small group seems unreliable evidence of regressions. Moreover, if the cholesterol contents of arch and thoracic aorta were summated, then there was no improvement at 3 months.

The animals killed at 6 months of restricted diet showed no resorbtion in either arch or thoracic aorta, as adjudged chemically (Table 1), by graticule count (Table 2) and by histology. Atherosclerosis and particularly calcification were, in fact, more severe in the restricted than in the ad libitum group.

This somewhat increased atherosclerosis after 6 months' dietary restriction does not accord with reports from Leningrad, Belsen and Norwegian concentration camps during or after World War II (Helwig-Larsen et al., 1952; Katz and Pick, 1963; De Navasquez, 1964). However, post mortem material obtained from Belsen at the end of the war may have been largely from those younger subjects who managed to survive that length of time. Of five hearts from Belsen prisoners in the museum at the Royal College of Surgeons, London, only one is from a subject older than the 3rd decade.* This subject, a woman of 35, has two small yellow fibrofatty plaques in her ascending aorta. Perhaps more to the point is the report based on 10,000 autopsies at Dachau of severe atherosclerosis in emaciated prisoners (Blaga, 1963). Severe dietary restriction may cause resorption of muscle and other tissue. Cholesterol would then be released from cell-membrane, would accumulate in the blood and would be expected to enhance atherosclerosis.

2. Regression on Ad Libitum Low Lipid Diet

Cholesterol results expressed on a wet weight basis did suggest that atherosclerosis regressed on the ad libitum diet. However, this apparent regression between baseline and 6 months was no longer apparent when results were expressed on a 5 cm-length basis. Possibly the increased connective tissues at 6 months led to a dilution of cholesterol on a weight basis, and hence gave an impression of regression between baseline and 6 months. Nevertheless, leaving aside the baseline-6 months results, aortic cholesterol fell between 3 months and 6 months of ad libitum diet - no matter how results were expressed. This might imply that cholesterol recently added during the "run-down" period of hypercholesterolaemia after the cholesterol-enriched diet had been stopped was labile and susceptible to resorption. A similar lability of recently deposited cholesterol has been reported in

* By courtesy of the curator, Dr. Martin Israel

pigeon by Lofland et al. (1972).

Another confusing feature is that staining of aortas from baseline and 6 month animals with the standard Sudan black procedure showed that sudanophilic lipid apparently decreased during this period. Sudan dyes, however, are unreliable in this context because they only stain droplet esterified cholesterol and not crystalline free cholesterol (i.e. Sudan dyes stain liquid and liquid-crystal, but not solid lipids). During "regression" aortic esterified cholesterol markedly falls and free cholesterol increases. In this instance the mean percentage of cholesterol as ester fell from $\sim$65 to $\sim$38. Hence, it is not surprising that Sudan-staining declined. However, free cholesterol can be converted to liquid sudanophilic droplets with bromine, and the Bromine-Sudan black method (Bayliss and Adams, 1973) revealed as much total staining for lipids in aortic sections at 6 months as at the point of stopping the cholesterol-enriched diet. Thus, the histochemical results agree with the chemical results expressed on a length basis. Apart from the fall between 3 and 6 months, this conclusion accords with a variety of recent studies on attempted regression with low-fat diets in rabbits (e.g. Constantinides, 1965; Adams et al., 1973; Vesselinovitch et al., 1974).

3. Early Versus Established Lesions

Early mild lesions in the cholesterol-fed rabbit - as in certain other species - seem in part to be reversible, particularly where the lipid is mainly intra-endothelial and produced in 2-3 weeks with a blood cholesterol of 900-1000 mg/100 ml (Bortz, 1968; see Adams et al., 1975a). Cholesterol in mature established rabbit atherosclerotic lesions shows little if any metabolic equilibration or physical exchange with plasma cholesterol (Adams, 1973; Adams et al., 1973), whereas the specific activity of cholesterol in the early mild lesion tends to follow that in plasma more closely (Adams et al., 1975a). This points to the greater accessibility of cholesterol in early rabbit lesions and would be consistent with a greater potential for resorption at this early stage.

4. Some Factors Concerned in Slow or Absent Reversibility

A. Physical Accessibility. Atheroma lipid still attached to lipoprotein might be expected to be in metabolic equilibrium with plasma lipoproteins (Adams, 1973), while high-density lipoprotein may provide a shuttle for carrying cholesterol out of the arterial wall and tissue (Bailey, 1973; Stein et al., 1975). Autoradiographic studies show that intracellular lipid and dispersed extracellular lipid rapidly exchange with plasma lipoproteins, but crystalline lipid does not (Adams et al., 1975b). Thus, crystalline cholesterol probably constitutes an inert accessible pool with a sluggish metabolic turnover (Adams, 1973), which is probably - in part - responsible for the slow or absent reversibility of the lipid in atherosclerotic lesions.

B. Phagocytosis. Atheroma lipids and cholesterol-phospholipid mixture injected subcutaneously are resorbed within 6-12 weeks (Admas *et al.*, 1975a). The cells in such lesions are macrophages and can be selectively displayed by catalase and cytochrome oxidase techniques (Adams et al., 1976). Such cells are normally only seen in the subendothelial region of atherosclerotic arteries. However, when organization has occurred after mural thrombosis or intimal haemorrhage, new capillaries enter the lesion and are accompanied by stainable macrophages. The apparent relative absence of actively phagocytic reticuloendothelial cells from uncomplicated atherosclerotic plaques also may partly account for the relative metabolic inertia of the lesions.

REFERENCES

Adams, C.W.M., Morgan, R.S. and Bayliss, O.B. 1973. *Atherosclerosis*, 18, 429.

Adams, C.W.M., Knox, J. and Morgan, R.S. 1975a. *Atherosclerosis*, 22, 79.

Adams, C.W.M., Knox, J. and Morgan, R.S. 1975b. *Atherosclerosis*, 22,

Adams, C.W.M. 1973. In *Atherogenesis: Initiating Factors*, CIBA Foundation Symposium 12 (NS), 5.

Bailey, J.M. 1973. In *Atherogenesis: Initiating Factors*, CIBA Foundation Symposium 12 (NS), 63.

Bayliss, O.B. and Adams, C.W.M. 1973. *Histochem. J.*, 4, 505.

Blaga, F. 1963. Архuф пamoлoгuu (Arkh. Pat.) 25, 13, Transl. in Abst. Wld. Med., 35, 267 (1964).

Bortz, W.M. 1968. *Circulation Research*, 22, 13J.

Constantinides, P. 1965. *Experimental Atherosclerosis*, Elsevier, Amsterdam.

De Navasquez, S.J. 1964. Personal communication.

Helweg-Larsen, P. *et. al*. 1952. *Acta Med. Scand.* 144 Suppl. 274.

Katz, L.N. and Pick, R. 1963. In R.J. Jones (Ed.), *Evolution of the Atherosclerotic Plaque*, Chicago University Press, Chicago, p. 251.

Lofland, H.B. Jr., St. Clair, R.W. and Clarkson, T.B. 1972. *Adv. Exp. Biol. Med.*, 26, 91.

Stein, Y., Glangeaud, M.C., Fainaru, M. and Stein, O. 1975. *Biochim. biophys. Acta*, 380, 106.

Vesselinovitch, D., Wissler, R.W., Fischer-Dzoga, K., Hughes, R. and Dubien, L. 1974. *Atherosclerosis*, 19, 259.

Adams, C.W.M., Bayliss, O.B. and Turner, D.R. *Atherosclerosis*, 1976, in press.

(4)

REGRESSION OF COMPLICATED ATHEROSCLEROTIC LESIONS IN THE ABDOMINAL AORTAS OF SWINE

A. S. Daoud, K. E. Fritz, J. Jarmolych, J. M. Augustyn, K. T. Lee, and W. A. Thomas
From the Departments of Pathology of the Veterans Administration Hospital and Albany Medical College, Albany, New York, U.S.A.

A number of studies have shown that diet-induced proliferative non-complicated atherosclerotic lesions can regress after removal of the dietary stimulus.[1-7] In contrast there is no clear evidence of regression of advanced necrotic lesions with their complications such as calcification, hemorrhage and thrombosis. The reason for this lack of information is the difficulty in producing advanced complicated lesions in experimental animals in a reasonable time.

We have recently devised a method for producing advanced complicated atherosclerotic lesions in swine in a relatively short time. The method involves abrading the intima of an artery with a balloon-catheter followed by a hypercholesterolemic diet. This combination of diet and mechanical injury results in a greatly accelerated atherosclerotic process which produced advanced complicated lesions within a few months.

We have carried out a study involving 40 young male miniature swine weighing from 7-22 kg at the outset. Details of the study are being [8-9]published and only a summary of the results is being presented here.

The intima of the abdominal aortas of all was abraded at the beginning of the experiment with an inflated balloon attached to a catheter. Immediately following ballooning, 30 randomly chosen swine were fed a high-cholesterol (HC) diet for 4 months. Five died shortly before the end of this phase. Of the remaining 25 on an HC diet 11 were sacrificed at the end of the fourth month to serve as a baseline (Group I). The remaining 14 swine were shifted to a commercial mash diet for 14 months and sacrificed at the end of the period (Group III - "regression group"). The 5 animals on HC diet that expired shortly prior to the time for sacrifice were included in the baseline group, but only for morphological studies.

The remaining 10 swine from the original 40 that were ballooned were fed a mash diet throughout the entire experiment. Seven of these survived and were divided into 2 groups. One group of 4 was sacrificed at the end of the 4th month (Group II) to serve as a control for baseline Group I and the other 3 were sacrificed at the end of 18 months (Group IV) as a control for the regression Group III.

The results of the morphologic portion of the study are summarized in Fig. 1 and Tables 1 and 2. It is apparent from these tables that the baseline group had extensive necrotic atheromatous lesions including some with hemorrhage, thrombosis and calcification. Since these were chosen randomly for sacrifice we can assume that the regression group had similar atherosclerotic lesions at this time.

After 14 months on the low fat, cholesterol-free mash diet the necrotic lesions had virtually all healed and been replaced by scars which did not infringe significantly on the lumen. The numbers of calcified areas were similar in the baseline and the regression groups, however, the size of the calcifications was much smaller in the regression group (Fig. 1).

The results of the biochemical portions of the study are shown in Table 3. Biosynthetic processes are elevated in the active lesions of the baseline group as is well known from other studies. In the regression group these activities have returned to near control levels which suggests that the atherosclerotic process has been halted. The expected increase in lipids in the active lesions of the baseline group is seen in the table and it is evident that much of the excess has been removed in the regression group.

These data indicate that in swine advanced atherosclerotic lesions can regress in both structural and biochemical aspects. We do not know whether similar regression can be achieved in man, but these favorable results in an experimental animal do permit at least guarded optimism.

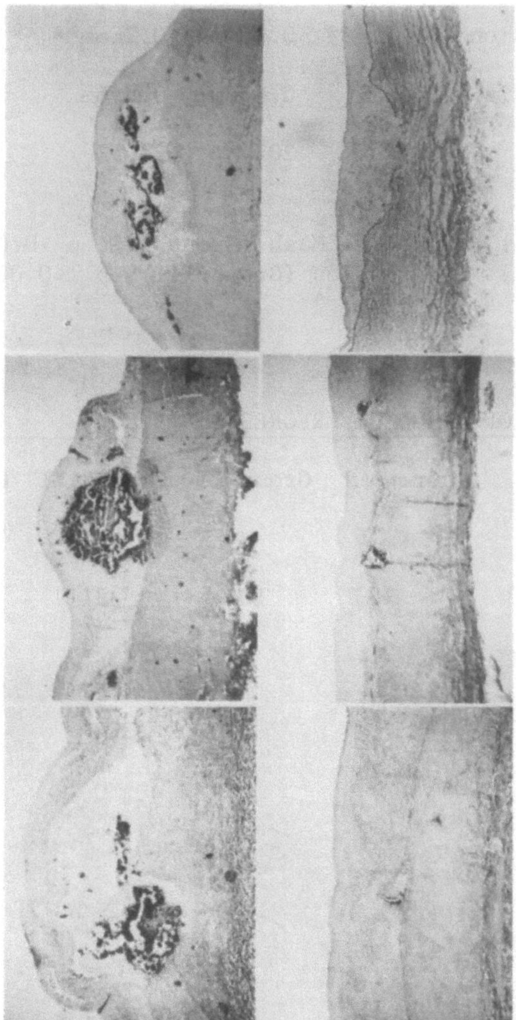

Figure 1 - In the upper half raised complicated atheromata from Group 1 showing "gruel", fibrous cap, calcification and medial involvement. In the lower half are representative lesions from Group III. They are smaller, flat and fibrotic without necrosis and little calcification.

TABLE 1

SUMMARY OF RESULTS: REGRESSION STUDY

	Group I	Group II	Group III	Group IV
Aver. % surface involve.	20.8%	1.0%	3.2%	1.0%
Aver. thickness of lesion	0.41mm**	0.15mm**	0.26mm**	0.26mm
Aver. thickness of media	0.64mm	0.63mm	0.89mm	1.03mm
Ratio lesion media	65%	20%	28.5%	25%

*Baseline HC (Group I) Baseline Mash (Group II), p 0.005
**Baseline HC (Group I) Regression (Group III), p 0.005

TABLE 2

SUMMARY OF RESULTS: REGRESSION STUDY

Number of	Group I	Group II	Group III	Group IV
Animals	16	4	14	3
Segments examined	203	105	391	91
Animals with atheroma**	14	-	1	-
Segments with atheroma	50	-	1	-
No. of atheromata	73	-	1	-
Animals with thrombus	3	-	-	-
Segments with thrombus	4	-	-	-
Segments with hemorrhage	1	-	-	-
Animals with calcification	11	-	13	1
Segments with calcification	28	-	48	5
% of ^{3}HTdR labeled cells	1.36%*	not done	0.07%	not done

*Group I (Baseline) Group III (Regression), p 0.005
**Atheroma indicates the necrotic, grumatous lesion of atherosclerosis

Table 3. Regression Lesions vs Baseline Lesions [(a)]

	DNA, ug	dpm ^{3}H-thy / ug DNA	dpm ^{14}C-Leuc / ug DNA	Cholesterol ug/mg dry wt			Phospholipid umoles Px10^{-9} / mg dry wt	Triglyceride ug/mg dry wt
				Total	Free	Ester.		
Group III	4.2	201	2358	3.8	3.5	0.4	15.0	2.2
Group I	6.6	846	3408	15.0	3.8	11.2	32.0	2.7
Group IV[(b)]	4.4	212	1530	2.0	3.5	0.6	12.5	2.1
Group III-Lesion	Group I ,	Group I ,	NS	Group I ,	NS	Group I ,	Group I ,	
vs								
Group I-Lesion	p 0.005	p 0.01		p 0.005		p 0.005	p 0.005	

(a) Regression (Group III) vs Baseline (Group I)

(b) Group IV = Control Abdominal non-lesion

BIBLIOGRAPHY

1. Armstrong ML, Warner, ED, Connor, WE: Regression of coronary atheromatosis in rhesus monkeys. Circ Res 27: 59-67 1970.

2. Eggen DA, Strong JP, Newman WP III, et al: Regression of diet-induced fatty streaks in rhesus monkeys. Lab Invest 31: 294-301 1974.

3. Vesselinovitch D, Hughes R, Frazier L, et al: Studies of the reversal of advanced atherosclerosis in the rhesus monkey. Am J Pathol 70: 41a, 1973.

4. Clarkson TB, King JS, Lofland HB, et al: Changes in pathologic characteristics and composition of plaques during regression. Circulation 44 (Suppl. II): II-48, 1971.

5. DePalma RG, Insull W Jr, Bellon EM, et al: Animal models for the progression and regression of atherosclerosis. Surgery 72: 268-278, 1972.

6. Pick R, Stamler J, Rodbard S, et al: Estrogen-induced regression of coronary atherosclerosis in cholesterol-fed chicks. Circulation 6: 858-861, 1952.

7. Friedman M, Byers SO: Observations concerning the evolution of atherosclerosis in the rabbit after cessation of cholesterol feeding. Am J Pathol 43: 349-354, 1963.

8. Daoud AS, Jarmolych J, Augustyn JM, Fritz KE, Singh JK, Lee, KT: Regression of advanced swine atherosclerosis (morphological studies) Accepted for publication. Arch Pathol, 1975.

9. Fritz KE, Augustyn JM, Jarmolych J, Daoud AS, and Lee, KT: Regression of advanced atherosclerosis in swine (chemical studies) Accepted for publication. Arch Pathol, 1975.

(5)

STUDIES OF REGRESSION/PROGRESSION OF ATHEROSCLEROSIS IN MAN

David H. Blankenhorn, M.D.

University of Southern California

Los Angeles, California, U.S.A.

Since atherosclerosis in the experimental animal is reversible, it is possible that regression may occur in man. Epidemiologic studies provide evidence of atheroma progression through incidence data on ischemic heart disease and cerebral vascular accidents, but no information about atheroma regression. Atherosclerosis intervention trials, such as the Coronary Drug Project and Multiple Risk Factor Intervention Trial, are based on the premise that atherosclerosis regression can occur and will lead to a lowered incidence of overt ischemic heart disease. It would be useful to have more direct evidence of atherosclerosis regression/progression in man.

This report describes serial assessment of atherosclerosis by angiographic visualization. This has been possible through the efforts of a group of investigators in the USC Specialized Center of Research in Atherosclerosis Program whose contribution I wish to acknowledge. We visualize both coronary and femoral vessels and make serial measurements, usually at an interval approximating one year. We perform coronary angiography for clinical management of patients who require this examination. Our coronary studies have been limited to men with previous myocardial infarction. At the time of coronary arteriography we also visualize one femoral artery. The femoral artery is frequently involved by atherosclerosis and is the safest major vessel to angiogram. In addition, the femoral artery is long, straight, and relatively motionless which make it ideal for high resolution radiography.

METHODS

We evaluate coronary angiograms in two ways: 1) by usual clinical criteria, classifying number of vessels involved and designating degree of coronary obstruction and 2) by simultaneous projection of matched film pairs taken one year apart. A panel of radiologists and cardiologists examines identical views of the coronary tree for change in lesions. Each panelist records a separate opinion without knowledge of which film was taken first. Judgement of lesion change is made without knowing whether the change represents regression or progression. The panel consists of one member from USC and three members from other universities.

We evaluate femoral angiograms in two ways: 1) by panel examination for visual change in matched film pairs, essentially the procedure used for coronary angiograms, but a different panel and 2) by computer controlled densitometer. Development of computer densitometry for atheroma assessment has yielded a great deal of information about angiographic appearance of non-obstructive atherosclerosis. Much of this information is new. Heretofore, radiographers have been principally concerned with obstructive aspects of atherosclerosis and development of collateral circulation. We have just completed a two year study of femoral atherosclerosis in cadavers employing radiographic methods which exactly simulate the appearance of clinical angiograms.

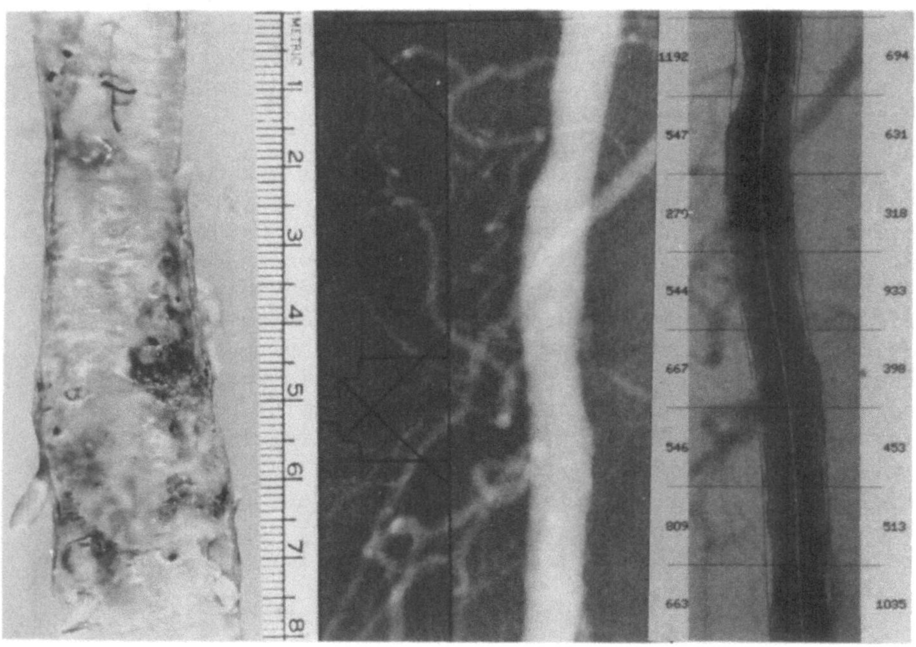

Figure 1

Figure 1 illustrates materials from our postmortem study. Shown on the left is a photograph of an excised femoral artery. The cholesterol content of this vessel was later determined to be 29.6 mg/gram dry weight. Shown in the middle is the postmortem angiogram. Shown on the right is a computer densitometer image of the angiogram with a computer derived measurement (lumen 90 with taper) on each centimeter of vessel. We have completed 64 such comparisons in 21 cadavers (1). The computer measures most highly correlated with visual grade of the excised arterial segment and cholesterol content of the same arterial segment are shown in Table 1. All correlations are significant ($p < .001$).

Table 1

Computer Measure	Type	Correlation With Cholesterol Content	Correlation With Visual Grading
Roughness 1	Edge	0.733	0.788
Lumen 90 with Taper	Edge	0.732	0.756
Outer Density Average N2	Density	0.517	0.728
Outer Density Sum N2	Density	0.577	0.604

We have evaluated one of the computer measures, lumen 90 with taper in a second manner, computer assessment of a clinical film versus human assessment. Human assessment of angiograms is a complex neurovisual process, but one feature appears to be similar to the procedure for "lumen" measures by computer. The "mind's eye" seems to project a nominal vessel edge across large edge indentations and estimate the size of enclosed areas. When we compare clinical evaluation of femoral angiograms with the computer assessment lumen 90 with taper, the correlation is high, $r = .81$ ($p < .001$).

PATIENTS

One hundred men with premature atherosclerosis manifest by myocardial infarction between ages 40 and 49 have been studied by coronary and femoral angiography. On first examination we found single vessel coronary disease in 21, two vessel disease in 19, and three vessel disease in 60. Femoral atherosclerosis was absent or minimal in 8, mild in 50, moderate in 34, and severe in 8. The distribution of risk factors among patients with varying degrees of femoral atherosclerosis is shown in Table 2.

Table 2

	Femoral Atherosclerosis			
	Normal	Mild	Moderate	Severe
Number of Patients	8	50	34	8
% Ideal Weight	108	114	112	128*
Cholesterol mg%	200	235	238	235
Triglyceride mg%	170	206	180	203
Diastolic BP mmHg	82	84	86	96*
Abnormal IVGTT	50%	45%	56%	88%*

The trends indicated by an asterisk are significant ($p < .01$).

Comparison of coronary and femoral atherosclerosis in the same patient indicates a complex relationship. Salient features can be summarized: it is possible to have normal or minimally involved femoral artery and severe coronary artery disease. On the other hand, if femoral atherosclerosis is moderate or severe, the odds are extremely high that three vessel coronary disease will be present.

RESULTS

Panel assessment of change after one year is now available for femoral atherosclerosis in 40 men and coronary atherosclerosis in 15. Coronary assessment is significantly more complex and time consuming. The overall direction of change is shown in Table 3.

Table 3

Artery	Patients	Progression	No Change	Regression
Femoral	40	14	17	9
Coronary	15	7	7	1

We are delaying consideration of coronary change until more film pairs have been evaluated. The remainder of this discussion deals only with femoral artery change. The magnitude of change in those showing progression is on the average very slightly greater than the magnitude of change in those showing regression. Between angiograms these men have been enrolled in a weekly program for exercise and weight loss. They have been assigned at random to one of two groups: a high level group where exercise level is to achieve pulse rates of 130 to 150 and target for weight reduction is 10% below ideal body weight or, a low level group where exercise level is to achieve pulse rates of less than 110 and target for weight reduction is 10% above ideal body weight. On the average, the high level group shows very slightly less progression of atherosclerosis than the low level group. This seems encouraging, but it is important to state that the difference between groups is not statistically significant.

Our data allow a preliminary estimate of how many years we should continue to study the men in our program to ascertain if a significant difference exists between groups. We currently estimate that repeat study after four years could reveal a significant difference between groups if the observed trend in atherosclerosis regression/progression persists. Implicit in this calculation is the possibility of studying more men for a shorter interval. For example, if we had enrolled 133 men in each study group a two year interval between femoral angiograms would be sufficient to test the significance of the trend we have observed.

CONCLUSIONS

1. Visual inspection and computer measurement of angiograms are highly correlated with direct examination of atherosclerosis in a specified vessel segment.

2. Computer assessment of an angiogram is highly correlated with cholesterol content of atherosclerosis in a specified vessel segment.

3. Serial change in human atherosclerosis can be measured by angiography.

4. Approximately 50% of men with premature atherosclerosis manifest by myocardial infarction between ages 40 and 49 will show progression in femoral atherosclerosis in one year. An equal number will have lesions which are apparently stable or show regression.

5. Small scale clinical trials employing atheroma regression/progression assessment by angiography are feasible.

ACKNOWLEDGEMENTS

Members of the USC Specialized Center of Research in Atherosclerosis Program who made a major contribution to this work are: Drs. Robert Barndt, Jr., Edwin S. Beckenbach, Samuel H. Brooks, H.P. Chin, Donald W. Crawford, Paul K. Hanashiro, H. Ralph Haymond, Miguel E. Sanmarco, Ronald H. Selvester, and Mr. Robert H. Selzer.

Members of the coronary review panel from other universities are: Drs. C. Michael Criley, UCLA; Melvin P. Judkins, Loma Linda University; and George G. Rowe, University of Wisconsin.

This work was supported by the USC Specialized Center of Research in Atherosclerosis Program, NHLI Grant HL14138.

REFERENCE

1. Crawford, D.W., Selzer, R.H., Brooks, S.H., Barndt, R., Jr., Beckenbach, E.S., and Blankenhorn, D.H.: Computer densitometry for angiographic assessment of arterial cholesterol content and gross pathology in human atherosclerosis. J. CLIN. INVEST. Submitted for publication.

(6)

APPROACHES TO EVALUATING REGRESSION OF EXPERIMENTAL ATHEROSCLEROSIS

Ralph G. DePalma, Errol M. Bellon, LeRoy Klein,
Simon Koletsky, William Insull, Jr.
Departments of Surgery, Radiology and Pathology
Case Western Reserve University, Cleveland Ohio and
Rockefeller University, New York, New York, U.S.A.

The ability to document changes in atherosclerotic plaques by direct observation _in seriatim_ is important in designing experiments in progression or regression of atherosclerosis. There are variable responses in degree and development among lesions in a single animal and variable occurrence of segmental lesions in groups of animals. The operational goal of experiments is, therefore, to determine the location, state, size and segmental distribution of lesions at preselected times. This can be done by autopsy studies when accomplished by experienced investigators familiar with particular experimental models (1) . However, autopsy observations are limited in that information about plaque dynamics must be inferred from one set of observations in time. Our experience has accordingly emphasized studies of plaque dynamics including detection, serial observation and sampling of individual or paired lesions.

In order to characterize the regressive process, one should, at each stage of the plaque and before intervention: measure its gross size and luminal encroachment; detect its hemodynamic effects; describe its histology; and, establish its chemical composition. By doing this during progression to more advanced or complicated plaques or during regression, the natural history of lesions will be established.

This report details surgical and angiographic approaches for serial evaluation of plaques in the arteries of dogs and subhuman primates. The localization of lesions in characteristic sites of subhuman primates, especially in paired central and peripheral arteries is emphasized, since these provide important opportunities for sampling during lesion development and regression.

EXPERIMENTAL MODELS AND TECHNIQUES

Studies have been made in dogs in which atherosclerosis has been induced by thyroid ablation and cholesterol feeding. In Rhesus and Fascicularis monkeys, atherogenic regimens described by Wissler (2) and Armstrong (3) have been used. Regression of established plaques was accomplished by reduction in serum cholesterol to less than 175 mg./100 ml. by means of diet changes, internal biliary diversion and, sometimes, drug therapy (D-thyroxin or cholestyramine).

Techniques of serial observation of regression of individual plaques visualized at repeated laparotomy and aortotomy were first reported in 1968 (4) and later used to show regression of more advanced disease in dogs (5,6) and to demonstrate regression of experimental lesions in monkeys (7). They were elaborated to permit repeated observation and tissue sampling in selected portions of the arterial tree in atherosclerotic Rhesus monkeys under sequential observation for over six years. More recently, we have studied collagen dynamics (8) in Fascicularis monkeys labeled with ^{3}H-proline by sampling the femoral and carotid arteries.

Sequential angiography combined with surgical sampling of peripheral arteries was used to establish general location, size and distribution of lesions and demonstrate comparable disease in symmetrically paired arteries. Proof of angiographic symmetry guides selection ofone of the pair for biopsy, thus providing a basis for serial morphologic or chemical study of regression in the remaining artery. Finally, techniques at sacrifice were developed to obtain comparable lengths of arteries perfused at arterial pressure.

Sequential angiography combined with surgical sampling of peripheral arteries was used to establish general location, size and distribution of lesions and demonstrate comparable disease in symmetrically paired arteries. Proof of angiographic symmetry guides selection of one of the pair for biopsy, thus providing a basis for serial morphologic or chemical study of regression in the remaining artery. Finally, techniques at sacrifice were developed to obtain comparable lengths of arteries perfused at arterial pressure.

METHODS OF OBSERVATION AND SAMPLING

The ideal data on lesion development or regression should describe quantitatively the major characteristics of lesions and enable their correlations. The characteristics of atherosclerotic lesions important for these studies are summarized in Table I. Apart from the fact that regression of the mass of gross plaques

Table 1. Comprehensive Characterization of Atherosclerotic Lesions

GROSS MORPHOLOGY	MICROSCOPIC and FINE STRUCTURE	CHEMICAL COMPOSITION	FUNCTIONAL CHARACTERISTICS
LOCATION & SIZE Internal area External extent Luminal encroachment CONSISTENCY/ FRIABILITY COMPLICATIONS Hemorrhage Ulceration Dissection Calcification Necrosis	CELL TYPES SMOOTH MUSCLE PROLIFERATION NECROSIS COLLAGEN ELASTIN LIPIDS Physicochemical form Intra/extracellular STRUCTURAL RELATIONSHIPS	LIPID Lipoproteins Cholesterol ester Free cholesterol COLLAGEN ELASTIN OTHER COMPONENTS Glycosaminoglycans Fibrin Muscle proteins	HEMODYNAMICS Local/distal DISTENSIBILITY PERMEABILITY Macromolecules Metabolites INTIMAL ATTACHMENT

does occur (3,4,5) and that this is associated with depletion of plaque lipid, (9) published reports of such comprehensive information about regression is still fragmentary. The techniques described here have been designed to establish a correlative data base in experimental protocols. Serial observations are obtained by a sequence of angiography, operation, and finally, controlled sacrifice.

Physical measurement of lesion size, visual observation and photographic recording are simple and straightforward means of documenting changes in the mass of plaques. This is performed easily by investigators with minimal surgical skills. Laparotomy in dogs, Rhesus or Fascicularis monkeys can reveal characteristic plaques at the origin of the inferior mesenteric artery and diffusely in the paired spermatic vessels. The severity of these plaques is usually an index of lesion development elsewhere, i.e., in the carotids, coronary arteries or aorta (5,6) . In dogs extensive small, yellow beaded plaques of the vasa recta of the mesentery regress within several weeks; the reduction of the number and size of these plaques can be quantitated at surgery (4) .

In order to provide objective quantitative data, the external extent of the plaque can be measured using ophthalmic calipers (Fig. 1). Lesion intrusion into the arterial lumen can also be measured by transillumination of thin-walled vessels but is best evaluated by angiography performed just prior to or after laparotomy. Lesion regression is characterized grossly by diminution of external bulk, lessening of the lumenal intrusion, and a change of external color from yellow to an ivory or whitish hue. The microscopic appearance of regressed plaques in both dogs and monkeys suggest disappearance of lipid and dense residual mass of fibrous tissue (3,5) .

A more precise technique for measuring and sampling plaques involves aortotomy or arteriotomy and a greater sophistication in surgical skill. The infra-renal abdominal aorta is suitable for this intervention since disease frequently occurs in its more severe form there. Extensive dissection or mobilization of the perivascular aortic tissues or the application of clamps should be avoided in order to circumvent provoking or altering lesions as a result of surgical manipulation itself. Hemostasis is obtained with a double loop snare of rubber (Fig. 2). In the peripheral vessels, the brachial or common femoral arteries can be used doubly to obtain access to the aorta for angiography as well as for local biopsy. This is accomplished in subhuman primates under sedation with phencyclidine and 1% local Xylocaine anesthesia. A technique for insertion of a guide wire, 5F Gensini catheter, and excisions of the femoral artery for histologic and chemical analysis is shown in Fig. 3. Posterior "collar button" lesions

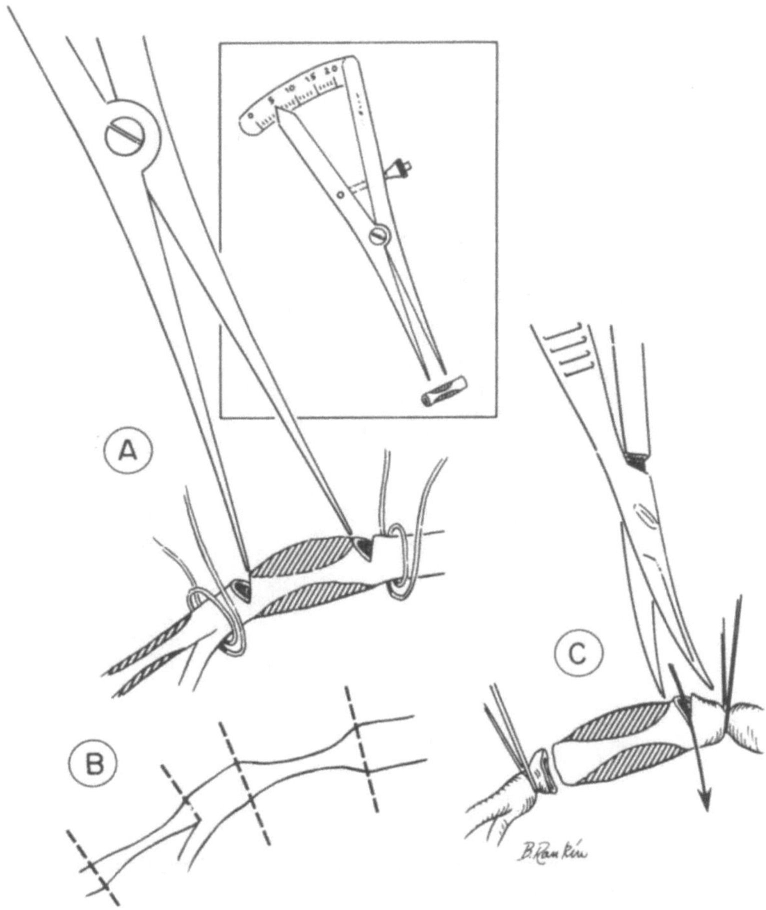

FIG. 1. A, Measurement of external extent of plaque using ophthalmic calipers. B, Angiographic appearance of luminal encroachment. C, Technique of excision of a measured arterial segment.

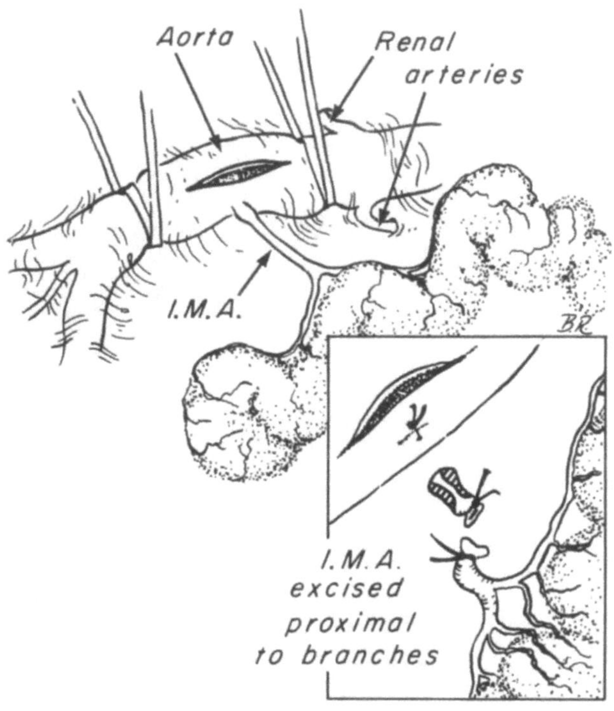

FIG. 2. Technique of aortotomy and excision of plaque at origin of inferior mesenteric artery.

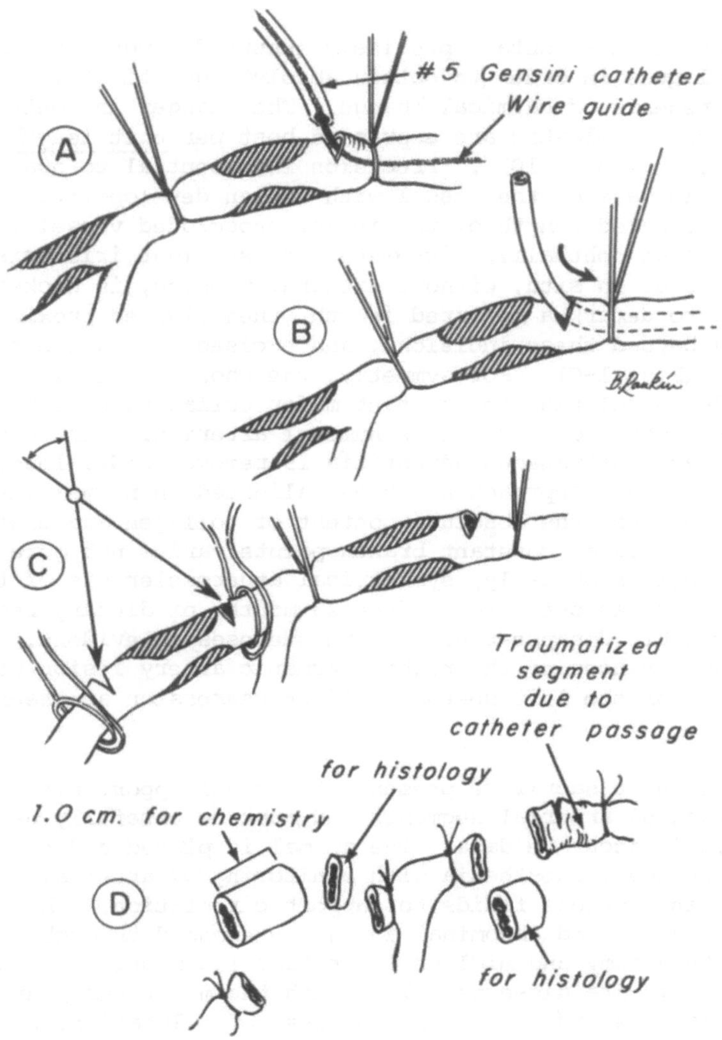

FIG. 3. A & B, Technique of insertion of wire guide and Gensini catheter for arteriography via common femoral artery. C, Measurement and excision of 1 cm. arterial segment of distal adjacent superficial femoral artery containing plaque. D, Distribution of segments obtained for chemistry and histology.

of the lumbar vessels on lateral arteriographic views indicate that elevated fibrous plaques will be encountered on the posterior aortic wall (Fig. 4). These are usually symmetrical and, thus, may be excised for further examination.

It is critical to obtain precisely measured lengths of arteries containing plaques in order to obtain absolute quantitative increments or decrements of chemical change. The changes in content of lipid, collagen or elastin are expressed best per unit length of vessel, e.g., mg./cm. (10) . Precision is essential to quantitate the increase in mass of the vessel with lesion development. At operation a measured length of the intact unoccluded vessel is obtained using an ophthalmic micrometer and straight iris scissors. The intact vessel in situ, without external tension, is nicked at right angles to demark a measured length, then ligated proximally and distally beyond these incisions, and excised by transsection at the nicks (Fig. 1-C). For symmetry, the choice of excision sites is made in relation to constant major collaterals such as the profunda femoris or circumflex humoral arteries. For subsequent chemical analyses extraneous adventitia is removed under loupe magnification. This approach has been validated in normal vessels of dogs and monkeys; the absolute content of collagen and elastin from paired vessels at constant branch points varies not more than 5% to 12%. Angiographically, symmetrical atherosclerosis of the spermatic artery was obtained. After 23 months of dietary regression, angiographic disappearance of the stenoses is evident. The histologic appearances of the right spermatic artery lesion before regression and of the left spermatic after regression are seen in Fig. 5.

Examination at sacrifice presents the final opportunity for obtaining measured arterial segments and must be carefully performed to obtain accurate data. The animal is placed under light general endotracheal anesthesia with monitoring of arterial pressure and intravenous fluids to support circulation. The heart, mediastinal vessels and abdominal aorta are exposed through a continuous sternotomy and midline laparotomy incision. The neck and great vessels are dissected along with the major peripheral vessels of the upper and lower extremities. The location, distribution and size of lesions is then recorded. Beginning peripherally, measured paired segments of arteries containing lesions are obtained for histologic and chemical examination at constant predetermined branch points. The plaques at the origins of the internal carotid arteries are excised last, and then the animal is sacrificed by removal of the heart. This pre-autopsy technique is also useful for insertion of a left ventricular cannula and fixation of the arterial tree by perfusion with glutaraldehyde at arterial pressure.

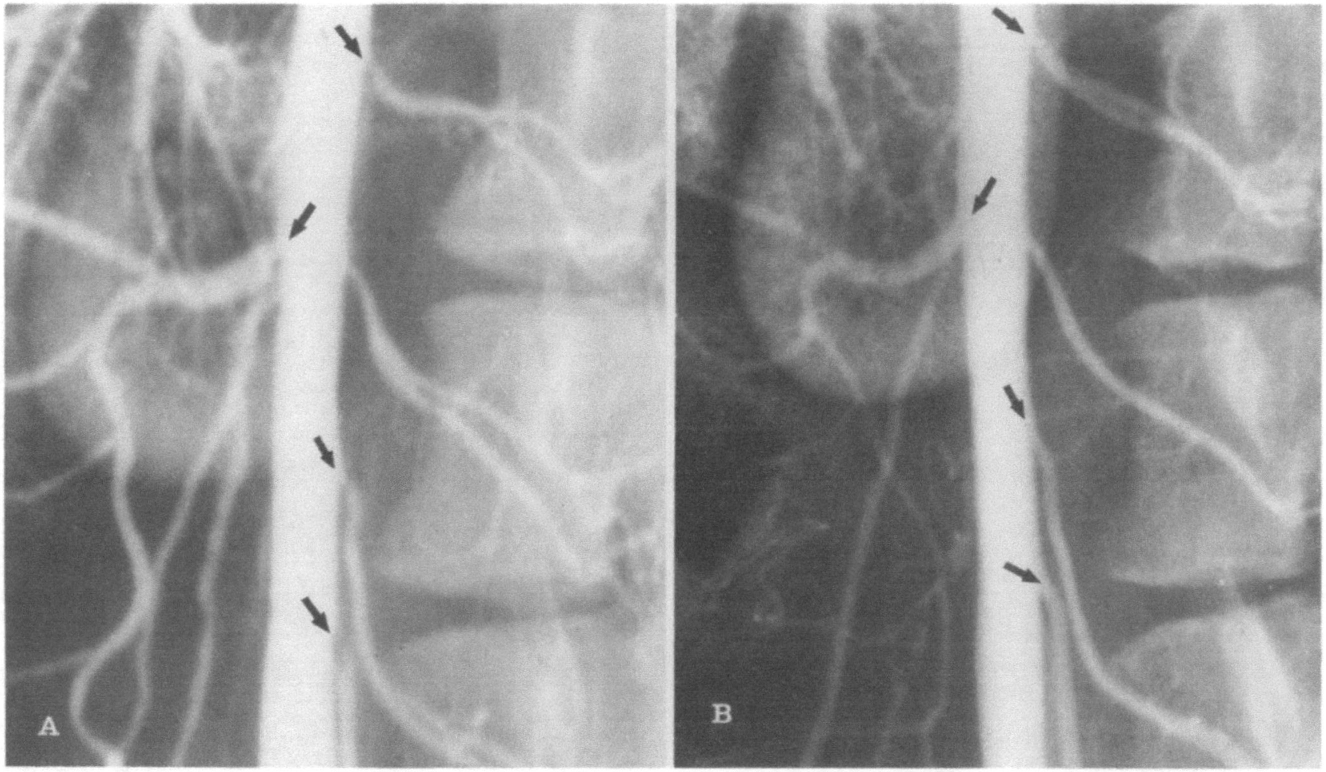

FIG. 4. Angiographic demonstration of regression of atherosclerotic stenoses in Rhesus monkey. A, Lesions after 48 months of cholesterol feeding: serum cholesterol average, 520 mg./100 ml. B, Lesion regression after 23 months control diet: serum cholesterol average, 152 mg./100 ml. Similar changes seen in spermatics on original film (Ref. #5, Monkey D3).

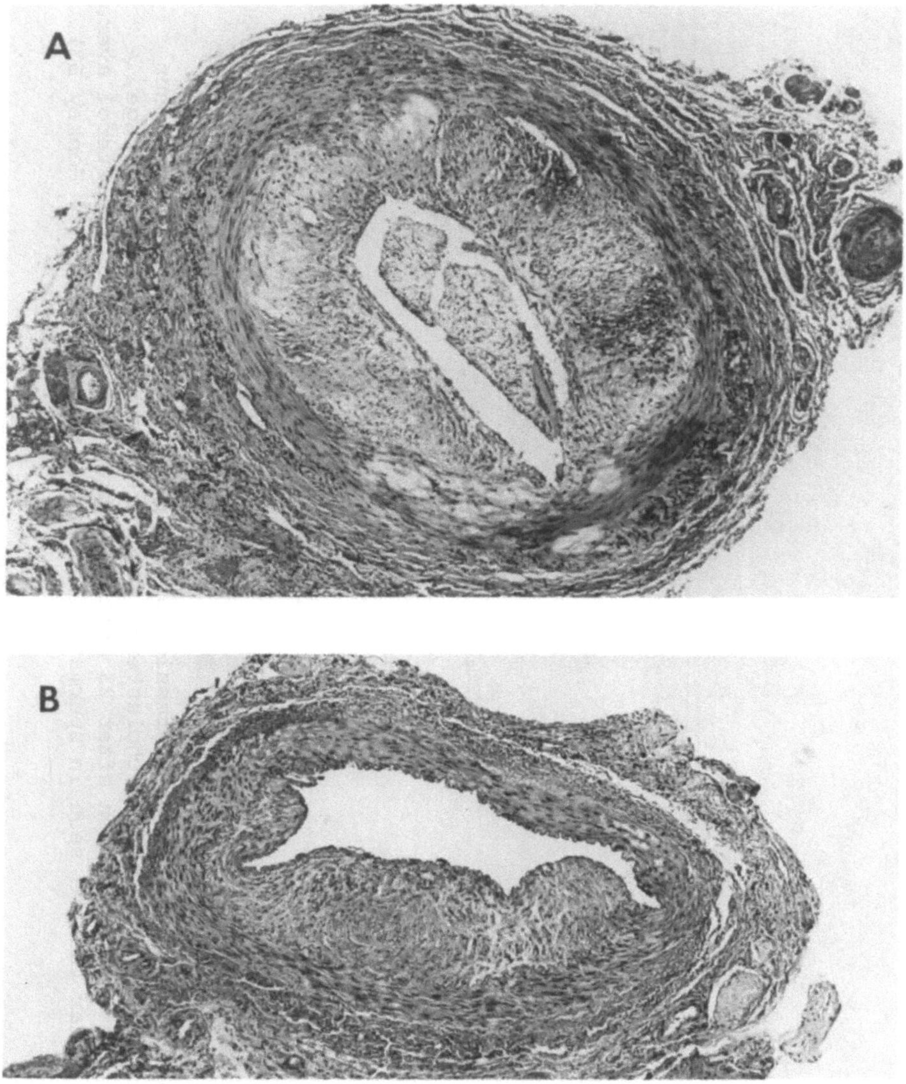

FIG. 5. A, Right spermatic artery before regression (H&E x 25) Intima shows marked deposit of lipid extending focally into media and smooth muscle cell proliferation. B, Left spermatic artery after regression (H&E x 25). Intima shows a compact fibrous plaque with only slight lipid content and condensation of collagen.

IMPLICATIONS

The information gained from serial observation promises a more complete knowledge of lesion development and regression. To date, unequivocal evidence of gross regression with lessening of angiographic stenoses in non-complicated intermediate fibrofatty plaques has been obtained in subhuman primates (6,7). In these animals, hemodynamic effects and clinical complications have not yet been seen. In dogs, instances of ulcerated carotid plaques with stroke and functional hemodynamic deficits in the form of gangrene of the tail occurred. Because of these responses the canine model offers a means of studying plaques with complications.

Thus far, it has been possible to: obtain a rigorous measure of lesion size; correlate gross appearance with angiographic and histologic findings; and, measure the content of cholesterol, cholesterol ester, collagen, and elastin in individual segmental plaques. Direct serial observation offers documentation of changes in experimental plaques providing unequivocal evidence that regression has occurred as a result of experimental interventions. This promises a better comprehension of atherosclerosis by enabling characterization of those lesions capable of regression or arrest as well as plaques which might progress inexorably.

REFERENCES

1. Vesselinovitch, D., Wissler, R.W., Hughes, R., and Borensztajn, J.: Reversal of advanced atherosclerosis in Rhesus monkeys, Part I: Light Microscopic Studies, Atherosclerosis 21: in press, 1975.

2. Wissler, R.W.: Recent Progress in Studies of Experimental Primate Atherosclerosis, In Progress in Biochemical Pharmacology, Vol. IV, Recent Advances in Atherosclerosis, pp. 378-392. Karger, Basel, 1968. Editors: Miras, C.J., Howard, A.N. and Paoletti, R.

3. Armstrong, M.L., Warner, E.D., and Connor, W.E.: Regression of coronary atheromatosis in rhesus monkeys. Circ. Res. 27: 59-67, 1970.

4. DePalma, R.G., Hubay, C.A., Vogt, C., Insull, W.Jr., Hartman, P. and Robinson, A.V.: Regression and prevention of experimental atherosclerosis: effects of diet and bile diversion in the dog. Surg. Forum 19: 308-310, 1968.

5. DePalma, R.G., Hubay, C.A., Insull, W.Jr., Robinson, A.V., Hartman, P.H.: Progression and regression of experimental atherosclerosis. Surg. Gynec. & Obst. 131: 633-647, 1970.

6. DePalma, R.G., Insull, W.Jr., Bellon, E.M., Roth, W.T., and Robinson, A.V.: Animal models for study of progression and regression of atherosclerosis. Surgery 72: 268-278, 1972.

7. DePalma, R.G., Bellon, E.M., Insull, W.Jr., Roth, W.T. and Robinson, A.V.: Studies on progression and regression of experimental atherosclerosis: techniques and application to the rhesus monkey. Medical Primatology 1972, Proc. 3rd Conf. Exp. Med. Surg. Primates, Lyon, 1972, Part III, pp. 313-323 (Karger, Basel, 1972), editors: Edward J. Goldsmith and J. Moor-Jankowski.

8. Klein, L. and Lewis, J.A.: Simultaneous quantification of ^{3}H-collagen loss and ^{1}H-collagen replacement during healing of rat tendon grafts. J. Bone and Joint Surg. 54-A: 137-146, 1972.

9. Armstrong, M.L., and Megan, M.B.: Lipid depletion in atheromatous coronary arteries in rhesus monkeys after regression diets. Circ. Res. 30: 675-680, 1972.

10. Wolinsky, H.: Response of the rat aortic wall to hypertension: importance of comparing absolute amounts of wall components. Atherosclerosis 11: 251-255, 1970.

(7)

DISCUSSION (REGRESSION OF LESIONS)

Discussion Following Dr. Geer's paper

Dr. Werner Hauss of Munster, W. Germany, asked a question about the origin of the cells in the atherosclerotic plaque and during the healing phases of arterial injury to which Dr. Geer responded that in his opinion both during progression and regression of the rabbit lesions there were foam cells moving in and out of the lesion and possibly in and out of the artery wall. He raised the question of whether they migrate into the necrotic lesions that are filled with lipid. He emphasized that it is often difficult to categorize these cells and that it is very important to develop ways to determine the origin of these cells.

Dr. Günter Schlierf of Heidelberg, W. Germany, then asked whether free cholesterol can be catabolized by the arterial wall to which Dr. Geer responded that he thought that the evidence for breakdown of cholesterol in the artery wall was not at hand and that this was particularly true in terms of the cholesterol fed rabbit with diet induced atheromatous lesions where the cholesterol appears to be unusually aloof.

Dr. Dieter Kramsch from Boston, Mass., briefly described some regression experiments that he had conducted with rabbits in which most of the foam cells and other lipid-containing cells disappeared, leaving only the connective tissue components, especially collagen and elastin. The fibrous plaques in the rabbits he studied were mostly associated with and contained abnormal lipoproteins. Dr. Wissler indicated that he, too, had found that most of the remaining lipid was associated with elastin in regression lesions, although he admitted the possibility that some of it could be associated with glycosaminoglycans. He also asked Dr. Geer whether he thought that one could improve the regression of atheromatous lesions by making better use of known relationships between the prostaglandins and lipid metabolism.

Dr. Geer stated that he felt that this would be a fruitful area for more study.

Dr. William Hollander of Boston, Mass., then commented that while the artery makes several of the prostaglandins the main effect of these substances may be on vascular permeability. They also have vasoactive effects with particular potency for influencing contractility of the endothelial cell. He described some work in which angiotensin II had been shown to stimulate cultures of smooth muscle cells to increase the release of prostaglandins from these cells. Dr. Geer responded that there may be a problem in interpretation and that may depend partly on the choice of the artery to be studied as well as the species. He also indicated that the amount of conversion of arachidonate to prostaglandins might be important. He pointed out that in the paper that Dr. Hollander had cited there was only a 1 - 2% conversion of arachidonate to prostaglandins, but that in small muscular arteries from bovine material there was often a 10 - 30% conversion.

Dr. Mark Armstrong of Iowa City then asked whether Dr. Geer was making a distinction between the smooth muscle cells seen in the arterial media and the types of cells seen in atheromatous lesions. Dr. Geer responded that he really could not be absolutely certain about the type of cells that occurred in the lesions and that more sophisticated methods were needed in order to answer this type of question.

Discussion Following C. Adams' paper

Dr. Paris Constantinides of Vancouver led off the discussion by stating that there may be a very special cell type that operates in the atherosclerotic rabbit and he referred to Professor Earl Benditt's observation which may indicate that atherosclerotic plaque cells are a mutant from normal cells and may equate the atheromatous disease with a storage disease. Both Dr. Wissler and Dr. Wilbur Thomas of Albany, New York, commented on the unusual situation in the rabbit where many characterisitcs of a storage disease are present, not only in arteries but also in many other parts of the body. Dr. Thomas in particular noted how sluggish the reticuloendothelial system must be in handling cholesterol. Dr. Zilversmit of Ithica, New York, stated that he had done comparative studies of the rat and the rabbit, and that the rat could release isotopic cholesterol from its reticulo-endothelial system in six or seven hours following loading, but that in the rabbit the same degree of release took four to five days. He indicated that this is related to differences in metabolic pattern that may apply to the arterial wall as well.

Dr. John Poole of Oxford, England, then asked whether there was any evidence of a catalase negative material or of other markers in the cells of the rabbit atheroma to which Dr. Adams responded that he felt there was an acid esterase deficiency at least deep in the lesion. Dr. Lindner from Hamburg, Germany, indicated that additional study of the enzyme activities during the regression phase of athero-sclerosis in humans as well as animals might be helpful in obtaining a better understanding of the differences that we see from species to species. Dr. Adams responded by saying that he thought that the work by R. N. Wollmann indicated that acid esterase was deficient in species that developed atheroma. He cited the work of his colleague, Dr. Alvin Bayliss, who is finding rabbit plaque cells which he has been able to identify histochemically as monocytes or macrophages, to be strongly positive for acid esterase, whereas the smooth muscle cells deeper in the lesion are deficient in acid esterase. He pointed out that if one relates this to the work done by Peeters and the group from Albert Einstein, it would appear that acid esterase is probably arterial cholesterol esterase. He continued that one of the main problems with the smooth muscle cell is that it apparently is deficient in lysosomal acid esterase so that it accumulates cholesterol ester.

The final comment was made by Dr. S. Stender from Denmark. He indicated that when cholesterol-fed rabbits were fasted they had the same concentration of serum cholesterol after 12 weeks even though their body weight was markedly reduced, so that the cholesterol coming into the blood from the stores in the tissues probably helped to maintain the serum cholesterol during a regression phase.

Discussion Following Dr. Thomas' paper

Dr. Geer opened the discussion by making some comments about the amount of free cholesterol in the atheromatous lesions. Both Dr. Thomas and Dr. Armstrong indicated that both free and ester cholesterol were removed from the lesions and that both lipid-laden cells and the extracellular deposits of lipid in the atheromatous plaque were sites of cholesterol depletion in regression. Dr. Adams indicated that in his rabbit studies it appeared that larger deposits of crystalline cholesterol remained in the aortic lesions following the period of treatment than there was in the original reference lesions. There was also discussion of the reason that the tritium labeled proline had failed to give helpful information on collagen kinetics in the studies that Dr. Thomas reported. He indicated that he thought that this was a matter of inadequate radioactive proline leading to inadequate numbers of counts in the hydroxyproline to give a reasonable assessment of whether the collagen was being mobilized or not.

Dr. Sean Moore of McMaster University asked whether all of the animals that were treated with the low fat, low cholesterol diet showed regression to which Dr. Thomas responded affirmatively. There was also considerable discussion, led by Dr. Colin Adams as well as Dr. Geer, as to whether the crystalline cholesterol could be removed from the lesions during the regression process. Dr. Thomas indicated that it was not evaluated in the particular study that he was reporting but that in other studies using both a regression diet and clofibrate, Dr. Ted Daoud had indeed observed an apparent loss of crystalline cholesterol from the atheromatous lesions during regression. Dr. Constantinides questioned whether there were many smooth muscle cells remaining in the lesions of the animals that had been treated with a regression regimen and both Dr. Thomas and Dr. Daoud indicated that the numbers of cells and the rate of cell division seemed to decrease rather remarkably during the process of regression.

Dr. Constantinides made the suggestion that the average thickness of the lesion should have been used as the main measure for both the reference group and the regression group and Dr. Daoud indicated that this had been done and while there was some increase per unit weight of collagen in the lesion, the actual lesion mass was decreased by about half no matter how one evaluated the lesions.

Dr. Armstrong noted that one of the most interesting facets of the study reported by Dr. Thomas was the change in wall thickness. Dr. Daoud indicated that this increase in wall thickness in the animals in which the intimal lesions are undergoing regression is not caused by an increase in fibrous tissue. He indicated that additional study was necessary in order to understand this paradoxical result. He added that calcium is best judged by chemical analysis since it is almost impossible to make any quantitative assessment of calcium in tissues using ordinary light microscopy.

Discussion Following Dr. David Blankenhorn's paper

In answer to a question regarding the type of exercise in which the subjects were participating, Dr. Blankenhorn said that the high level group was supervised in exercises to achieve a pulse rate of between 130 and 150. They are asked to exercise at least once a week and they are supposed to do it at home. They are also encouraged to exercise similarly at least two more times during each week. The low level exercise group has a record of much less vigorous activity, but did engage in a rather regular exercise regimen. There appeared to be general agreement that exercise probably was not the major factor in the results as they have been analyzed thus far. Dr. Blankenhorn also indicated that they are in the process of trying to find out whether the levels of serum cholesterol during the period of therapy were correlated with whether or not the lesions underwent regression. Dr. Blankenhorn's response to questions about the effect of pulse rate and/or smoking on regression indicated that these parameters are still at the stage of being evaluated. Dr. Wissler indicated that these studies in human subjects should offer a remarkable opportunity to find out whether the very low levels of serum cholesterol that seem to be effective in producing definite and substantial regression of atherosclerosis in the nonhuman primates as well as in the swine and in the dog would be effective in man. Dr. Blankenhorn agreed and said that now that they have perfected the measurement technique they should be able to undertake studies in which much more rigorous conditions of serum cholesterol lowering would be tested in relation to the degree of regression. Dr. Constantinides indicated that we should concentrate on advanced disease with severe atherosclerosis and calcification. He also emphasized that one has to be very careful about how one evaluates the size of the lesions both in these studies in living human subjects and in those that are being done which rely on histological approaches as applied to experimental animals. Dr. Blankenhorn indicated his complete agreement and pointed out that his group is now engaged in rather careful correlations between the arteriographic evaluation of the size of lesions and the results of careful histological quantitation of the lesions, using morphometry of the post-morten specimens. Dr. Colin Adams suggested that blood pressure levels might be quite important in these subjects and that one ought to also correlate the responsiveness or the unresponsiveness of the individual subjects to various kinds of therapy. Dr. Blankenhorn also indicated that his group is exploring a number of procedures and proposed improvements in clinical arteriography which may help in the quantitation of coronary artery disease. He also described studies that are being initiated to develop more standard radiographic techniques and to utilize electronic evaluation of the data so that one should be able to quantitate the coronary artery sclerosis and stenosis more adequately.

Discussion Following Dr. DePalma's paper

The remaining general discussion took place following the presentation by Dr. Ralph DePalma of Case Western Reserve University in Cleveland, Ohio. Following this presentation, Dr. DePalma was questioned as to whether the types of surgical procedures that he is utilizing in his studies might have some effect on the results of progression or regression. Dr. A. G. Shaper of London, England and Dr. Wissler both indicated that factors in the arterial adventitia might be more important than they are usually considered to be in relation to either progression or regression of lesions in the atherosclerotic artery. Dr. Shaper also pointed out that it was interesting that very little mention had been made during this workshop about the role of thrombosis in the development of the atheromatous lesion. He indicated that more work probably should be done on the role of thrombosis in the types of arterial lesions showing regression in Dr. Blankenhorn's studies. The question of thrombosis on severely atherosclerotic and carotid arteries and the role of embolism from these kinds of plaques in producing cerebral ischemia were also discussed. The obvious implication is that carotid plaques should be subjected to the same kind of close scrutiny as femoral artery plaques and coronary plaques. Dr. Gotthard Schettler of Heidelberg, Germany, indicated that much of what is being found now in experimental animals and in human atherosclerotic lesions was forecast by the experience of clinicians during and shortly after World War II, when heart attacks due to coronary disease were sharply decreased. He indicated that during this period in some instances serum cholesterol levels decreased from something over 200 mg% to about 110 mg%. He also pointed out that during this same period from about 1945 to 1948, there was a decreased incidence of cerebrovascular accidents and that pulmonary infarcts and pulmonary embolism also appeared to decrease. This suggests that whatever was causing regression of atherosclerotic lesions was also producing a marked decrease in the incidence of thrombosis of arteries as well as veins.

Dr. Jeremiah Stamler of Chicago said that he would like to bring up three points that had been raised over the years in relation to atherosclerosis. He stated that in general there was agreement that without severe atherosclerosis there was little or no coronary heart disease or cerebral ischemia. Therefore if one prevents or reverses severe atherosclerosis, one should then prevent thrombosis and ischemic disease. He also indicated that in his opinion one can really get valid data from the type of experimental studies now being used by Dr. Thomas, Dr. Armstrong, the group at the University of Chicago, and others. In other words, it is not necessary to use the same animal as his control. If one uses well defined models then this kind of study is very useful and can be done without huge numbers of animals. He also commented on Dr. Schettler's point and made a plea that serum lipid data be assessed in conjunction with other factors such as cigarette smoking or high blood pressure when one is trying to evaluate environmental influences on the clinical attack rate resulting from atherosclerosis. In other words, the success or failure of attaining regression may ultimately be a function of not only the height of serum cholesterol but also on whether or not cigarette smoking and elevated blood pressure were controlled.

Dr. Shimamoto of Tokyo then reported some of his work with pyridinolcarbamate in which he has found both in experimental animals and in patients that the use of this therapeutic agent will stop progression and perhaps induce regression of atherosclerosis. Dr. Thomas said in response to Dr. Stamler's comments that in his opinion we should continue our studies on the regression of the severe advanced lesions produced by hypercholesterolemia and that the more complex studies can be done as time goes on. He pointed out that true atherosclerosis could not be produced in the experimental animal without hypercholesterolemia. Dr. Constantinides indicated that he believes that a great deal of progress has been made in the development of an approach to learning more about the potential for regression of advanced atherosclerotic lesions. Dr. S. Björkerud of Södertälje, Sweden, also responded to Dr. Thomas' and Dr. Constantinides' comments by indicating that he believes that true atherosclerotic lesions can be produced in normocholesterolemic animals. He noted that recent studies indicate that if one produces endothelial desquamation sufficiently and for a sustained interval, a lesion that is very similar to the advanced atherosclerotic plaque will develop. Examples are chronic injury from prolonged catheter trauma, which produce progressive lesions in the absence of hypercholesterolemia. The implanted nylon suture or the implanted catheter such as the approach that Dr. Sean Moore has utilized will result in typical atherosclerotic lesions in normocholesterolemic animals.

In lieu of a more lengthy summation, Dr. Mark Armstrong closed the session with two short passages from the King James version of the Bible. The first states: "We are saved by hope." and the second one states : "We are perplexed, but not unto despair."

CHAPTER 5
LIPID CLINIC II
(Drugs, Genetics and Lipoprotein Dynamics)

(1)

EXPERIMENTAL INVESTIGATION OF HYPOLIPIDEMIC AND ANTI-ATHEROSCLEROTIC DRUGS WITH DIFFERENT MECHANISM OF ACTION

A. N. Klimov, V. E. Ryzhenkov, L. A. Petrova,
E. D. Polyakova.
Institute for Experimental Medicine of the USSR
Leningrad, USSR.

In the Soviet Union the following drugs are used to reduce the plasma level of cholesterol and triglycerides in patients with hyperlipidemias: miscleron (clofibrate), nicotinic acid, β-sitosterol and the preparations containing unsaturated fatty acids. Amongst them there are arachiden and conlitol. Arachiden is a mixture of ethyl esters of arachidonic, linoleic, linolenic, pentaene and hexaene acids. It is prepared from the lipid fraction of cattle pancreas. Conlitol is a mixture of ethyl esters of unsaturated fatty acids isolated from linseed oil. Both preparations are used orally.

At the N.N. Anitchkov Department of Atherosclerosis of the Institute for Experimental Medicine (Leningrad) the action of 3 groups of drugs on lipid metabolism and the development of experimental atherosclerosis was studied.

CHOLESTEROL BIOSYNTHESIS INHIBITORS STRUCTURALLY SIMILAR TO 5-DEOXY-MEVALONIC ACID

Sodium salts of some 3-hydroxypentanoic acid derivatives demonstrate an inhibitory action on the biosynthesis of cholesterol from 2-^{14}C-acetate and 2-^{14}C-mevalonate in rat liver extracts (Klimov et al., 1971).

The administration of sodium salts of 2,3-diphenyl-3-hydroxypentanoic and 2-phenyl-3-hydroxy-3-methylpentanoic acids to different species of animals lead to a hypolipidemic effect (Table 1). Both compounds decrease the concentration of cholesterol and triglycerides in serum. A slight hypolipidemic effect was observed also

Table 1 Effect of Hydroxypentanoic Acid Derivatives on Serum Lipids (per cent decrease)

Preparations	Animals	Number of animals, control/experimental	Daily dose, mg/100 g	Time of drug's introduction, days	Cholesterol	Triglycerides
2-phenyl-3-methyl-3-hydroxypentanoic acid (sodium salt)	Rats	20/20	20	7, s.c.	16*	37*
	Mice	22/17	20	7, s.c.	25**	21
	Hamsters	19/15	20	7, s.c.	20**	25
	Guinea pigs	10/11	57	45, p.o.	20	14
	Rabbits	6/12	19	90, p.o.	16**	57*
2,3-diphenyl-3-hydroxypentanoic acid (sodium salt)	Rats	20/24	12	7, s.c.	15*	26**
	Mice	22/15	12	7, s.c.	30**	28
	Hamsters	19/14	12	7, s.c.	12	31**
	Guinea pigs	10/10	19	45, p.o.	18	28
	Rabbits	6/12	6.3	90, p.o.	24**	60*

* $p < 0.001$; ** $p < 0.05$

Table 2

Effect of Parmidin and Aethirazol on Cholesterol and Total Lipids in the Rabbit Liver and Aorta (mg/g)

Group of animals	Aorta cholesterol	Liver cholesterol	Liver total lipids
		Parmidin	
1	3.43 ±0.5 (6)	4.2+0.67 (6)	39.5+4.3 (6)
2	38.8 + 5.9 (6)	58.3+6.3 (9)	167.5±22.3 (6)
3	16.7 ± 1.8 (6)	32.0+4.5 (9)	83.7±11.2 (9)
		Aethirazol	
4	2.9±o.6 (5)	4.5±0.9 (5)	22.1±3.5 (5)
5	33.9±6.0 (6)	80.5±4.8 (6)	110.9±8.4 (6)
6	16.3±3.3 (7)	64.7±4.4 (7)	88.8±6.7 (7)

1,4 - animals of the control groups; 2 - animals on atherogenic diet (0.25 g/kg cholesterol for 16 weeks); 3 - animals on atherogenic diet (0.25 g/kg cholesterol) receiving 10 mg/kg parmidin for 16 weeks; 5 - animals on atherogenic diet (0.3 g/kg cholesterol during 12 weeks); 6 - animals on atherogenic diet (0.3 g/kg cholesterol) receiving 30 mg/kg aethirazol for 12 weeks.
In parentheses - number of animals.

Table 3

Effect of Chondroitin Sulfate A on Serum Lipids and Aorta Cholesterol in Rabbits

Group	No. of animals	Serum cholesterol mg%		Serum triglycerides mg%		Serum phospholipids mg%		Aorta cholesterol (mg/g)
		Before treatment	After 12 weeks of treatment	Before treatment	After 12 weeks of treatment	Before treatment	After 12 weeks of treatment	
1	6	61.7±8	70.0±10	11.8±17	106±10	165±10	160± 10	2.99± 0.6
2	6	58.6±5.6	2246±364	80.8±19	335±48	119±9.4	585±88	33.9±6
3	7	63.5±7.2	724±90	92.7±14	140±51	102±12.6	224±42	12.4±4.9

1 - animals of control group; 2 - animals on atherogenic diet (o.3 g/kg cholesterol for 12 weeks); 3 - animals on atherogenic diet (0.3 g/kg cholesterol) receiving subcutaneously 40 mg/kg chondroitin sulfate A for 12 weeks.

in dogs after oral administration of 2-phenyl-3-hydroxy-3-methyl-pentanoic acid in dose 25 mg/kg for 75 days. Both compounds protected the development of hyperlipidemia in rats provoked by a single intravenous administration of Triton 1339.

AETHIRAZOL AND PARMIDIN

In the experiments on rabbits with experimental cholesterol atherosclerosis we investigated aethirazol (bis-methylamide-1-ethyl-pyrazol-3,4-dicarbonic acid) synthesized at the Institute for Experimental Medicine as well as parmidin (pyridinolcarbamate) synthesized at the Chemical Pharmaceutical Institute (Moscow).

The results obtained in this study show that both drugs have an antiatherosclerotic action. The degree of visible atherosclerotic lesions in experiments with aethirazol was $19.7 \pm 7.1\%$ against 52.3 ± 8.9 in the animals who received only cholesterol. In experiments with parmidin the results were correspondingly 19.2 ± 4.6 and $40.0 \pm 5.2\%$.

Table 2 shows that the investigated compounds decreased the content of cholesterol in aorta and liver of rabbits. At the same time, serum cholesterol and triglyceride content was not markedly changed by these drugs. It should be noted that the structural similarities of aethirazol and parmidin and the data obtained by Shimamoto et al. (1965, 1975) on the ability of pyridinolcarbamate to decrease the permeability of arterial wall enabled us to propose that aethirazol has the same properties as parmidin. The Pharmacological Committee of the USSR authorized the clinical application of parmidin.

CHONDROITIN SULFATE A

The hypolipidemic and antiatherosclerotic action of this drug (provided for our investigation by Professor L. M. Morrison, USA) was studied in experiments on rabbits fed cholesterol for three months (Table 3). The administration of chondroitin sulfate A to rabbits inhibited the development of atheroma in the aorta. The degree of atherosclerotic lesions in the aorta of rabbits receiving chondroitin sulfate A was 11.4 ± 5.1 against 52.3 ± 8.9 in the control group of animals who received cholesterol only. The results obtained in this study are in good agreement with data reported by Morrison et al. (1971, 1972) and recently by Day et al. (1975).

According to the above authors, a number of factors are involved in the mechanism of action of sulfated polysaccharides (stimulation of cellular metabolism, prevention of the proliferation of smooth muscle cells, activation of clearing factor, inhibition of the fibrotic component of atherogenesis, anti-inflammatory effect, etc.). In spite of this uncertainty on the mechanism of action of sulfated polysaccharides we agree with Day et al. that there is clearly enough evidence to warrant more intensive clinical evaluation of these important compounds.

REFERENCES

1. Day, C.E., Powell, J.R., Levy, R.S.: Sulfated polysaccharide inhibition of aortic uptake of low density lipoproteins. Artery 1:126-137, 1975.
2. Klimov, A.N., Poliakova, E.D., Remizov, A.L., Petrova, L.A.: The study of the effect of some possible antimetabolites of mevalonic acid on the biosynthesis of cholesterol in rat liver. Biochimia 32:88-92, 1967. In Russian.
3. Morrison, L.M.: Reduction of ischemic coronary heart disease by chondroitin sulfate A. Angiology 22:165-174, 1971.
4. Morrison, L.M., Bajwa, G.S., Alein-Slater, R.B., Ershoff, B.H.: Prevention of vascular lesions by chondroitin sulfate A in the coronary artery and aorta of rats induced by a hypervitaminosis D, cholesterol-containing diet. Atherosclerosis 16:105-118, 1972.
5. Shimamoto, T., Numano, F., Fujita, T.: Atherosclerosis-inhibiting effect of an antibradykinin agent, pyridinolcarbamate. Am. Heart J. 71:216-227, 1966.
6. Shimamoto, T.: New concept on atherogenesis and treatment of atherosclerotic diseases with endothelial cell relaxant. Jap. Heart J. 13:537-562, 1972.

(2)

TREATMENT OF HYPERLIPOPROTEINEMIAS WITH NEOMYCIN, PROBUCOL AND TIBRIC ACID

Tatu A. Miettinen

Second Department of Medicine, University of Helsinki

00290 Helsinki 29, Finland

Neomycin was introduced for the treatment of hypercholesterolemia more than 15 years ago (1) and has been used successfully for the long-term reduction of serum cholesterol without harmful side effects (2). Its use has been fairly limited, however, though it is effective even in severe forms of familial hypercholesterolemia with tendon xanthomata in which the normalization of serum cholesterol is usually unsuccessful with dietary and drug measures and is achieved only in a part of the patients even with the ileal by-pass operation (3).

Frequently occurring gastrointestinal side effects and reports of ototoxicity are the major reasons for the limited use of neomycin as a hypercholesterolemic agent. Though neomycin is considered a nonabsorbable drug, a few percent is absorbed even after rectal administration (4). Renal dysfunction may potentiate the risk of ototoxicity because absorbed neomycin is eliminated mostly by the renal route. Most of the ototoxic complications have been reported in patients with renal failure, inflammatory bowel disease, intestinal fistulas or hepatic encephalopathy, the total administration of antibiotic ranging from 500 to 2500 g (5). For unknown reasons no ototoxic side effects have been reported in patients treated for hypercholesterolemia with neomycin, though apparently a sizeable number of patients have been treated and though the total amount of the drug, owing to long-term therapy, increase to several kilograms in each patient. Thus, in our lipid clinic material several of the patients have been on neomycin (1.5-2 g/day) up to five years and have each used 2.5-3.5 kg of the drug.

Earlier clinical studies indicated that neomycin when used in fairly large doses (6-12 g/day) caused diarrhea and a malabsorption syndrome which concerned, in addition to lipids, a great variety of different substances (cf. 6); serum cholesterol reduction was associated with an increase of both acidic and neutral steroids into the stools (7,8). More recent investigations have indicated, however, that smaller doses, 1-2 g/day, used currently for the treatment of hypercholesterolemia, decrease serum cholesterol in short-term experiments by enhancing cholesterol elimination as fecal neutral sterols, not as bile acids, and interfere fairly little with fat absorption (9,10). This is illustrated also by the long-term study in Table I, which shows that after about 15 months on neomycin the serum cholesterol is still decreased by 23%, fecal steroids are elevated as neutral sterols and fecal fat is inconsistently increased. It thus seems apparent that though neomycin precipitates micellar sterols, bile acids, phospholipids and fatty acids from the bile and particularly from intestinal contents obtained during fat digestion (11,12), fatty acids and bile acids are still mostly reabsorbed when passing down in the small intestine while the reabsorption of sterols is impaired, resulting in an increased fecal output and proportionate decrease in serum cholesterol (9). Since the disruption of the micellar phase by neomycin is dose-dependent in vitro, larger neomycin doses can be expected to interfere with bile acid and fatty acid absorption also in vivo (12). That this apparently is the case is illustrated in Table I, in which the increase of neomycin to 2-6 g/day resulted actually in a small increase of fecal bile acids and fat. As compared to the serum cholesterol decrease effected by the small dose, the further serum cholesterol reduction by the larger doses was fairly small (9%) despite a 20% further increase in fecal steroid elimination. The decrease in serum cholesterol correlated positively with the increase in fecal steroid output in acute experiments ($n = 0.736$; $P<0.05$), and still tended to do so in the long-term study of Table I ($r = 0.480$) and also after the large doses ($r = 0.430$). Thus, the larger the increase of fecal cholesterol elimination the greater the decrease of serum cholesterol.

TABLE I. Effects of neomycin on serum and fecal lipids in long-term study. Mean ± SE of five subjects.

Dose g/day	Serum lipids		Fecal lipids			
	Cholesterol mg%	Triglyc. mmol/l	Steroids, mg/day Acidic	Neutral	Total	Fat g/day
0	381±30	2.0±0.2	211±24	635±73	846±95	2.9±0.3
1.5	293±24[1]	1.6±0.2	277±39	731±84	1008±106[1]	4.9±1.4
2-6	268±20[1,2]	1.7±0.2	386±99[1]	817±89[1,2]	1203±121[1] [2]	8.7±2.4[1,2]

After recording the zero-values the patients were put on neomycin (1.5 g/day) for 56-94 weeks when they were restudied; third studies were performed after the 2-6 g doses had been on for additional 10-12 days. Statistically significant ($P<0.05$) change from initial[1] or small dose[2] values.

The increase in cholesterol elimination in the long-term study in Table I ranged from 20 to 180 g. This amount is hardly balanced solely by the mobilization of tissue cholesterol but is apparently associated with an increased synthesis, too. A reduction of the rapidly miscible tissue pool has actually been demonstrated by measurement of cholesterol kinetics (13) and an increase of synthesis with radioactive precursors (14). That the increased synthesis is not seen as an increased slope of the serum cholesterol specific activity-time curve during the neomycin-induced decrease of serum cholesterol is apparently due to a simultaneous decrease in absorption and mobilization of tissue cholesterol with a high specific activity (10).

Serum cholesterol reduction by 1.5-2 g/day of neomycin is on an average about 20% in those who tolerate the drug. In our experience 10-20% of the patients discontinue to use neomycin because of diarrhea, nausea and abdominal cramps. Since a satisfactory reduction in the serum cholesterol was obtained in 80% of those who tolerate the drug it can be concluded that neomycin can be used successfully for the treatment of hypercholesterolemia in 60-70% of patients.

Probucol [4,4'-(Isopropylidenenedithio) bis-(2,6-di-t-butylphenol)] is a new hypolipidemic agent which reduces primarily serum cholesterol and has practically no effect on triglycerides (cf. 15), though occasionally a significant decrease has been recorded (16). The drug is primarily indicated for the treatment of type II hyperlipoproteinemia, type II A in particular. Probucol has very few side effects even during long-term treatment. Minor drug-related symptoms arise from the gastrointestinal site, consisting mainly of flatulence and diarrhea. A sizeable proportion of patients may exhibit eosinophilia of unknown significance.

The mechanism of the hypercholesterolemic action of probucol is not known. Animal experiments have indicated that cholesterol synthesis is not inhibited from acetate and mevalonate (17). Metabolic studies in man have shown that the drug transiently enhances fecal bile acid excretion, inhibits cholesterol and fat absorption and decreases fecal output of endogenous cholesterol (18). A marked reduction of plasma methyl sterols (18) may be a sign of decreased cholesterol synthesis (19). Thus the latter associated with a transient malabsorption state may be the primary reason for the probucol-induced decrease of serum cholesterol. The decreased slope of the serum cholesterol specific activity-time curve during the probucol-induced decrease of serum cholesterol may be a sign of tissue cholesterol mobilization (18), though the decreased cholesterol absorption and reduced removal of endogenous cholesterol have a similar effect on the curve. Anyhow, recent studies have indicated that during long-term treatment the tissue deposits of cholesterol are slowly reduced in size or disappear with probucol (cf. 15,16): a phenomenon apparently associated with any decrease in serum cholesterol.

TABLE II. Effect of probucol (1 g/day) on serum cholesterol in different groups of hypercholesterolemia. Mean ± SE.

Series	Number of cases	Serum cholesterol, mg/100 ml				
		Initial	Diet	Months of probucol 3-4	6-8	9-12
I	23	472±12	-	398±18[x]	417±18[x]	420±20[x]
II	15	345±9	-	263±9[x]	293±10[x]	-
III B	6	337±23	-	262±17[x]	267±11[x]	-
III P	8	311±12	-	305±13	286±17	-
IV B	25	321±7	317±7	259±6[x]	263±7[x]	263±5[x]
IV D	10	294±10	255±7[x]	244±6[x]	259±12[x]	255±8[x]

I Patients with tendon xanthomata and familial type II hypercholesterolemia, some of the patients had been for years on a cholesterol-lowering diet; II Patients with type II A hypercholesterolemia, no tendon xanthomata, family history less clear, no special dietary arrangements; III Double blind trial on volunteers of series II, P = placebo, B = probucol; IV Subjects as in series II, after recording initial values the patients were put on a cholesterol-lowering weigh reducing diet for four months after which the diet resistant cases (B) were put on probucol while the others (D) continued on the diet only. Serum triglycerides were not changed significantly in any group by probucol; [x]Statistically significant ($P<0.05$) from initial or diet values.

The mean cholesterol decrease induced by probucol ranges from 9 to 27%, a significant loss of the effect being seen in some series (cf. 15), while an increasing effect up to one year has also been reported (20). A more than 10% reduction is seen in 55-80% of the patients, those with a severe form of familial hypercholesterolemia (15) or diet-resistant subjects responding less favorably (21). An increase of the dose from the usual 1 g/day to 2 g/day further decrease serum cholesterol (15). Our results in Table II show, however, that serum cholesterol was decreased by about 16% even in the diet-resistant subjects with mild type II A hyperlipoproteinemia. Serum triglycerides were not changed significantly in any of the series in Table II.

Tibric acid is one of the newest hypolipidemic agents which appears to be free of major side effects and is useful for the treatment of pre-β-hyperlipoproteinemia; its effect seems to be dose-dependent when the serum triglyceride level on 1.25 g/day is reduced by 30% in patients with type IV hyperlipoproteinemia, a small decrease being detectable in serum cholesterol, too (22). Our results (Table III) on six patients with type IV and one with type II B hyperlipoproteinemia showed that tibric acid significantly decreased (35%) serum total triglycerides, while total and free cholesterol and methyl sterols (cholesterol precursors) were decreased only

TABLE III. Effects of tibric acid on serum and fecal lipids in short-term study. Mean ± SE of seven subjects.

Frac-tion	Plasma lipids			Fecal steroids, mg/day		
	Chol., mg%	Trigl., mmol/l	DMS, μg%	Acidic	Neutral	Total
			Control			
Total	270±55	6.98±1.91	27.3±3.6	606.4±102.9	1015.0±95.8	1620.9±99.5
VLDL	105±27	6.23±1.89	18.9±5.2			
LDL	131±47	0.57±0.16	6.9±2.9			
HDL	34±5	0.18±0.03	1.8±0.4			
			Tibric acid, 1.5 g/day			
Total	205±20	3.55±0.53	17.4±2.8	648.4±169.2	1017.4±85.4	1666.7±144.0
VLDL	48±11	3.01±0.55	8.1±1.8			
LDL	115±17	0.44±0.04	8.1±3.1			
HDL	41±7	0.10±0.03	1.4±0.4			

Tibric acid (1.5 g/day as a single dose) for 2 weeks. DMS = dimethyl sterol from serum methyl sterol (cholesterol precursors) mixture used as an index of possible changes in cholesterol synthesis (19). Statistically significant ($P<0.05$) reductions were seen in serum total (35%) and VLDL (37%) triglycerides. Initial LDL cholesterol concentration and tibric acid-induced change (range from -195 mg% to +45 mg%) in it were negatively correlated with each other ($r = -0.988$). For HDL the corresponding r-value was 0.542, and for VLDL cholesterol and triglycerides -0.905 and -0.963, respectively.

inconsistently. Ultracentrifuge analysis of lipoprotein fractions revealed that VLDL was significantly decreased (37%), while the response of LDL varied according to its initial level and was significantly ($r = -0.988$ for cholesterol) correlated with the initial LDL concentration. Thus, as is the case with many other VLDL-reducing agents (cf. 23), tibric acid increased the low and reduced the high LDL levels, HDL being frequently increased. In contrast to the effect of clofibrate (24, 25), fecal cholesterol elimination as neutral sterols was not increased significantly by tibric acid (Table III), nor was the bile rendered more supersaturated for cholesterol by the drug; the percent molar concentration of cholesterol was 11.5% off and 10.5% on tibric acid in patients of Table III.

REFERENCES

1. P.Samuel and A.Steiner, *Proc. Soc. Exp. Biol. Med.* 100,193(1959).
2. P.Samuel, C.M.Holtzman, and J.Goldstein, *Circulation* 35,938 (1967).
3. H.Buchwald, R.B.Moore, and R.L.Varco, *Circulation* 49,Suppl. 1 (1974).

4. K.J.Breen, R.E.Bryant, J.D.Levinson, and S.Schenker, *Ann. Int. Med.* 76,211(1972).
5. D.P.Berk and T.Chalmers, *Ann. Int. Med.* 73,393(1970).
6. W.W.Faloon, *Am. J. clin. Nutr.* 23,645(1970).
7. G.A.Goldsmith, J.G.Hamilton, and O.N.Miller, *Arch. Int. Med.* 105,512(1960).
8. R.C.Powell, W.T.Nunes, R.S.Harding, and J.B.Vacca, *Am. J. clin. Nutrition* 11,156(1962).
9. T.A.Miettinen, Exerpta Med., 1973 Int. Congr. Ser. No. 283,77.
10. A.Sedeghat, P.Samuel, J.R.Crouse, and E.H.Ahrens,Jr., *J. clin. Invest.* 55,12(1975).
11. G.R.Thompson, J.Barrowman, L.Gutierrez, and R.H.Dowling, *J. clin. Invest.* 50,319(1971).
12. T.A.Miettinen, *in* Proceedings of 6th Int. Congr. Pharmacol. 1974 in press.
13. P.Samuel, C.M.Holtzman, E.Meilman, and W.Perl, *J. clin. Invest.* 47,1806(1968).
14. T.A.Miettinen, *Eur. J. clin. Invest.* 3,256(1973).
15. T.A.Miettinen, *Postgrad. J. Med.* 51,71(1975).
16. R.S.Harris, H.R.Gilmore, L.A.Bricker, I.M.Kiern, and E.Rubin, *J.Am. Ger. Soc.* 22,167(1974).
17. J.W.Barnhart, J.A.Sefranka, and D.D.McIntosh, *Am. J. clin. Nutr.* 23,1229(1970).
18. T.A.Miettinen, *Atheroscler.* 15,163(1972).
19. T.A.Miettinen, *Ann. Clin. Res.* 2,300(1970).
20. A.A.Polachek, H.M.Katz, J.Sack, J.Selig, and M.L.Littman, *Current Med. Res. Opinion* 1,323(1973).
21. H.Brown, and V.G.deWolfe, *Clin. Pharmacol. Ther.* 16,44(1974).
22. P.Bielmann, D.Brun, S.Moorjani, C.Gagné, P.Lupien, and Tētreault, *Clin. Pharmacol. Ther.* 17,606(1975).
23. L.A.Carlson, A.G.Olsson, L.Orö, S.Rössner, and G.Walldius, *in* Atherosclerosis III, Schettler,G. and Weizel,A.(eds.), Springer-Verlag, Berlin-Heidelberg-New York 1974, p.768.
24. S.M.Grundy, E.H.Ahrens,Jr., G.Salen, P.H.Schreibman, and P.J.Nestel, *J. Lipid Res.* 13,531(1972).
25. D.Pertsemlidis, D.Panveliswalla, and E.H.Ahrens,Jr., *Gastroenterology* 66,565(1974).

(3)

CHOLESTEROL TURNOVER AND METABOLISM IN NORMAL AND HYPERLIPIDEMIC PATIENTS

F.R. Smith, R.B. Dell, R.P. Noble and DeW.S. Goodman

Columbia University College of Physicians and Surgeons

New York, New York, U.S.A.

The turnover of plasma cholesterol has been studied in recent years in order to provide information about the metabolism of cholesterol in humans. Initial studies of the plasma cholesterol specific radioactivity-time curves in subjects studied as outpatients during a 10 week interval indicated that the turnover curves conformed to a simple two-pool model (1,2). In 1970 Samuel and Perl (3) reported that in some patients the slow slope of the plasma decay curve deviated from monoexponential behavior. Subsequent studies with six subjects for periods of 32-41 weeks indicated that the best description of long-term data was provided by a three-pool rather than a two-pool model (4). These studies have now been extended to include 24 subjects in whom plasma cholesterol turnover has been examined for intervals of 32-49 weeks. In an additional 5 normal subjects a greatly simplified sampling strategy has been tested in a preliminary fashion.

In the 24 long-term studies, 8 subjects were normolipidemic, 6 had hypercholesterolemia alone, 8 had hypercholesterolemia and hypertriglyceridemia (mixed hyperlipidemia) and 2 had hypertriglyceridemia alone. In each of the groups studied the mean value for percent of ideal body weight did not differ significantly from 100% nor were there significant differences in the mean percent of ideal body weight values between groups. In each of the subjects the previously described three-pool model gave the best fit for the data using a weighted, least squares non-linear regression technique. The three-pool mammillary model is illustrated in Fig. 1. The pools are denoted by Arabic numbers (pools 1, 2, and 3); rate constants are noted by k; the rate of transfer of cholesterol mass (in g/day) into or out of a pool is denoted by R; cholesterol production rate (PR) is given by R_{01}; pool sizes are designated M_1, M_2, and M_3. For this model, the equation for the specific activity of pool 1 is:

$$\text{specific activity} = A_1 e^{-\alpha_1 t} + A_2 e^{-\alpha_2 t} + A_3 e^{-\alpha_3 t}$$

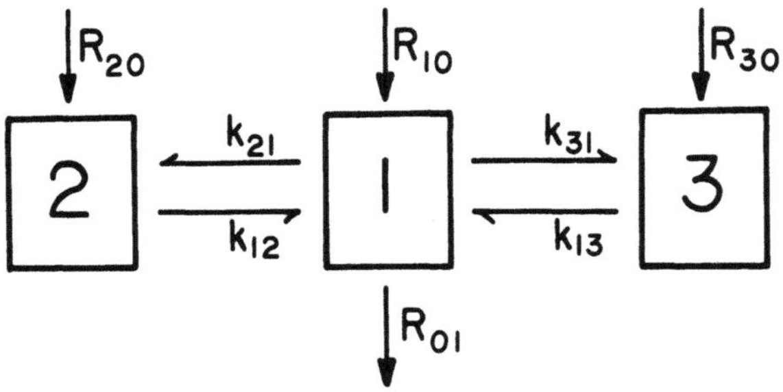

Figure 1. Model of cholesterol turnover in man.

Analysis of the turnover data in terms of this three-pool model provides unique values for each of the rate constants for transfer between pools (k_{21}, k_{12}, k_{31}, and k_{13}); for PR; and for M_1 (the size of the rapidly turning over pool). Although unique values cannot be obtained for the sizes of the more slowly turning over pools 2 and 3, upper and lower limiting values for M_2 and M_3 can be calculated, as described previously (4).

For this study population, the parameters of the three-pool model observed in the normal subjects were compared with the model parameters found in the patients with the different kinds of hyperlipidemia. In addition, single and multiple regression analyses were conducted in order to explore the relationships between the model parameters and various physiological variables including age, body size, and serum lipid concentrations. Using this approach, significant differences between groups, or correlations with serum lipid levels were seen for several parameters of the three-pool model: the PR; the size of pool 1 (M_1); all estimates of the size of pool 3 (M_3); and the rate constant k_{21}.

The PR in normal subjects (1.14 $\pm$ 0.19 g/day, mean $\pm$ SD) was not significantly different from that found in patients with hypercholesterolemia alone ((0.98 $\pm$ 0.25 g/day) or with mixed hyperlipidemia (1.19 $\pm$ 0.28 g/day). The major determinant of cholesterol PR was overall body size, expressed either as total body weight or as surface area (correlation coefficients 0.80). The correlations between PR and indices of adiposity (percent ideal weight and excess weight), although statistically significant, were much weaker in this nonobese population. In these subjects approximately 64% of the observed differences in PR, in the range of 0.71 to 1.47 g/day, could be accounted for by differences in total body size.

Total weight and excess weight have been reported previously to influence cholesterol PR (2,5,6). In the morbidly obese patients (mean percent ideal body weight 257) studied by Nestel, Schreibman and Ahrens (6), cholesterol synthesis rates were highly correlated with both excess body weight and with adipose cellularity, with correlation coefficients of 0.66 and 0.72 respectively. Analysis of the data reported by these workers reveals that an even slightly stronger correlation ($r = 0.73$) exists between total body weight and cholesterol synthesis rate in the 8 patients studied. In morbid obesity, as the degree of adiposity increases relative to body surface area, the adipose organ may play an increasingly important role in influencing total body cholesterol production. This role can, however, be considered at least as well in terms of total weight rather than excess weight. Moreover, recent studies (7) have indicated that adipose tissue cholesterol synthesis per se contributes very little, if at all, to the enhanced cholesterol synthesis of obesity.

Cholesterol PR after adjustment for body size variation was not correlated with the serum cholesterol concentration, but was probably ($p < 0.05$) correlated with the triglyceride concentration. In 22 of the 24 subjects triglyceride levels fell between 80 and 300 mg/dl, while 2 patients had concentrations of 464 and 691 mg/dl. When the 2 patients with very high triglyceride levels were excluded, no correlation between adjusted PR and triglyceride level was observed. Our interpretation of these data is that patients with extremely high triglyceride levels may represent a different population with regard to the regulation of cholesterol turnover from those with normal or moderately elevated triglyceride levels. This conclusion is consonant with Grundy's suggestion (8) that a subgroup of hypertriglyceridemic patients may well exist who show an increased synthesis of cholesterol, although this is not found in most patients with hypertriglyceridemia.

Interesting differences and correlations were observed with regard to the sizes of the three pools. M_1 (normal 25.9 ± 2.8 g, mean $\pm$ SD) was correlated with all body size variables, but most strongly with excess weight. After adjusting for the effects of body size, M_1 was also correlated with the serum concentrations of both cholesterol and triglyceride. Major differences were found in the relationships between the physiological variables and the sizes of pools 2 and 3. M_2 was correlated neither with any of the indices of body size or adiposity, nor with the serum levels of either cholesterol or triglyceride. In contrast, all estimates of M_3 were correlated with indices of adiposity (but not of overall body size), and with the serum cholesterol concentration. These findings suggest that the amounts of cholesterol in slowly equilibrating tissue sites (which comprise pool 3) increase in relation to elevations in the serum cholesterol level. The increased accumulation of cholesterol in atherosclerotic arteries in patients with hypercholesterolemia may represent one aspect of this phenomenon. The results also confirm previous data (7) that adipose tissue cholesterol is an important part of pool 3.

In recent months we have been carrying out both computer simulation and patient studies in order to try to determine the simplest and most effective sampling schedule for defining the parameters of the three-pool model. We are currently testing a procedure which utilizes our accumulated information on long-term turnover to predict sampling times that minimize the sum of squared coefficients of variation of the parameter estimates. The optimal theoretical strategy for a total of 36 samples is to sample 6 times, collecting 6 samples at each time. We have compared the results of this simplified sampling strategy with those of the usual strategy in 5 normal subjects. The first 3 sampling times in each of the subjects were chosen from previous information (from the 24 long-term studies described above) and were the same for all 5 subjects. Prior information was combined with the actual specific radioactivity data from the first 3 times in order to choose the 4th sampling time; the 5th and 6th sampling times were chosen similarly. Preliminary model parameter estimates generated with the simplified strategy were not significantly different from those estimates for the same individual given by the usual strategy. However, the residual error of the data at the 6 times about their best fit was smaller than that of the data at the 36 times. The meaning of these findings is not clear, since the apparent increase in precision may mainly reflect the existence of significant day-to-day biological variation. Further studies with normal subjects and subjects with hyperlipidemia are necessary in order to evaluate fully the potential usefulness of the simplified strategy.

BIBLIOGRAPHY

1. Goodman, DeW. S., and R. P. Noble. 1968. Turnover of plasma cholesterol in man. J. Clin. Invest. 47: 231-241.

2. Nestel, P. J., H. M. Whyte, and DeW. S. Goodman. 1969. Distribution and turnover of cholesterol in humans. J. Clin. Invest. 48: 982-991.

3. Samuel, P., and W. Perl. 1970. Long-term decay of serum cholesterol radioactivity: body cholesterol metabolism in normals and in patients with hyperlipoproteinemia and atherosclerosis. J. Clin. Invest. 49: 346-357.

4. Goodman, DeW. S., R. P. Noble, and R. B. Dell. 1973. Three-pool model of the long-term turnover of plasma cholesterol in man. J. Lipid Res. 14: 178-188.

5. Miettinen, T. A. 1971. Cholesterol production in obesity. Circulation 44: 842-850.

6. Nestel, P. J., P. H. Schreibman, and E. H. Ahrens, Jr. 1973. Cholesterol metabolism in human obesity. J. Clin. Invest. 52: 2389-2397.

7. Schreibman, P. H., and R. B. Dell. 1975. Human adipocyte cholesterol. Concentration, localization, synthesis, and turnover. J. Clin. Invest. 55: 986-993.

8. Grundy, S. M. 1975. Effects of polyunsaturated fats on lipid metabolism in patients with hypertriglyceridemia. J. Clin. Invest. 55: 269-282.

(4)

GENETIC STUDIES IN OUTPATIENTS: PLASMA CHOLESTEROL IN FAMILY AND TWIN STUDIES

Joe C. Christian, Ph.D., M.D.

Department of Medical Genetics
Indiana University School of Medicine
Indianapolis, Indiana, U.S.A.

INTRODUCTION

Probably the most difficult problem in the study of atherosclerosis is that the primary disease process is not readily accessible for observation and quantitation. This is extremely critical for family studies because at any one time the vast majority of individuals in a family do not have signs of atherosclerosis such as angina pectoris or myocardial infarction. Genetic studies have therefore concentrated upon risk factors which may be quantitated in individuals of all age groups. The tools available and the long-term nature of the disease have also virtually limited the genetic studies of atherosclerosis to outpatient studies.

This paper will review the results of family and twin studies of plasma cholesterol, as an example of the methods used and the problems in the genetic study of risk factors for atherosclerosis.

QUANTITATIVE GENETICS

At the present time there have been over 2,000 diseases ascribed to mutations of single genes (McKusick, 1975). Most of these so-called Mendelian disorders are relatively rare. In contrast the genetics of many of the common disease processes such as atherosclerosis do not fit the simple Mendelian ratios of single gene effects. There is however evidence pointing to the conclusion that genetic factors are important in pathogenesis of atherosclerosis and other multifactorial diseases. Most of the studies of genetic factors in common diseases therefore use the methods of quantitative genetics.

The basic use of quantitative genetic methods is to partition variation of a quantitative trait into genetic versus environmental sources. The field of quantitative genetics has strong roots in agricultural research, where the study of quantitative variation of traits such as food and fiber production led to strains of plants and animals that are extremely productive in the right environments. Most of the progress was made through selection and controlled matings, techniques not generally applicable to humans. Human quantitative genetics, in contrast to agricultural quantiative genetics, is an observational rather than an experimental science.

FAMILY STUDIES OF PLASMA CHOLESTEROL

Family studies of plasma cholesterol are summarized in Table 1. Studies of families selected because they had some disease process such as myocardial infarcation or familial hypercholesterolemia have not been included in Table 1. The basic statistic used to study family relationships is the intra-family correlation coefficient. If family members are significantly correlated the trait can be considered to be familial. Of the 4 studies in Table 1 that tested the significance of sibling-sibling correlations, all 4 found highly significant correlations and 6 of the 7 which tested the correlations of parents and offspring found highly significant correlations. It appears therefore that in most populations plasma cholesterol levels run in families.

Families share genes in common but also share environments in common so these significant correlation coefficients could be due either to genetics, environment or a combination of both. In other words familial is not synonymous with genetic. Because spouses share environments but in general are genetically unrelated, spouse correlations are often used as a measure of the effects of a common environment. Here the results of the studies summarized are mixed; of 8 testing spouse correlations, 3 found significant correlations and 5 did not. Spouses only share part of their adult environments in common and therefore are far from a perfect measure of the effects of common environment. At best they only provide a minimum estimate of adult environmental effects.

A second commonly used means of separating the common environment from genetic effects is to study populations where all families share a communal environment, hopefully leaving correlations of relatives which are due only to genetic factors. Two of the studies in Table 1 were designed in this manner. The study of Brunner _et al._ 1971 was done on collective farms in Israel and the study of Martin _et al._ of the North American Hutterites. Both groups have similar communal life styles. Brunner _et al._ found no significant correlations while Martin _et al._ found significant correlations with the exception of the spouse correlation, leaving the question far from resolved.

TABLE 1

SUMMARY OF PLASMA CHOLESTEROL FAMILY STUDIES

REFERENCE	SIB-SIB	FATHER-CHILD	MOTHER-CHILD	MOTHER-FATHER
		CORRELATION	COEFFICIENTS	
SCHAEFFER *et al*. 1958	.37**	.16-.26**	.34-.39**	.01
STEINBERG, 1963	.58**	.42**	.58**	.02
JOHNSON *et al*. 1965	.35**	.22-.26**	.26-.28**	.01
CHERASKIN & RINGSDORF, 1970	--	--	--	.46**
GODFREY *et al*. 1972[a]	--	SIG**	SIG**	SIG**
BRUNNER *et al* 1971	--	.01	.10	.06
SING & EGGLESTON, 1973	--	(PARENT-OFFSPRING	.34**)	.11*
MARTIN *et al*. 1973	.29-.30**	.25-.29**	.12-.31**	.0-.09
MIMURA, 1975[b]	.28	(PARENT-OFFSPRING	.26)	--

*P < 0.05
**P < 0.01
[a]chi square analysis used so correlation coefficients were not available, where significant relationships were found they were recorded as SIG.
[b]significance levels or numbers of subjects not given.
--not reported.

Another mechanism for separating environmental from genetic effects is to study adopted children who share an environment with their parents but do not share genes in common. This method has been used extensively with psychological variables but not to study plasma cholesterol.

Studies of individuals with hypercholesterolemia have revealed families in which hypercholesterolemia is segregating in a manner compatible with a single gene effect (Frederickson and Levy, 1972). This has been called familial hypercholesterolemia and accounts for approximately 10% of individuals with hypercholesterolemia, indicating that this fraction of total population variation of plasma cholesterol is genetic. However most quantitative genetic studies are not sensitive enough to detect this small fraction of total variation.

TWIN STUDIES OF PLASMA CHOLESTEROL

Twin studies are commonly used to separate environmental from genetic effects based upon the comparison of monozygotic (MZ) and dizygotic (DZ) twins. MZ twins are genetically identical and DZ twins share, on the average, 50% of their genes in common. If the total variances of MZ and DZ twins are equal and the assumption is made that MZ twins have no more or less similar environments than DZ twins then an estimate may be made of the genetic variability of a trait by subtracting the within MZ twin-pairs variation from the within DZ twin-pairs variation.

Table 2 summarizes early twin studies of plasma cholesterol. Seven of these 8 studies had significant estimates of genetic variance when the within DZ-pair variation was compared to the within MZ-pair variations. However, all of these studies assumed that the total variance of plasma cholesterol was equal for MZ and DZ twins.

Recently a large collaborative study of 514 sets of adult male twins was sponsored by the United States National Heart and Lung Institute. In the NHLI study the total variances of plasma cholesterol were compared and DZ twins estimated to have a total variance 140% that of MZ twins ($P<0.001$). When this difference in total variance was adjusted for by the methods of Christian *et al*. (1974), there was no significant genetic variance of plasma cholesterol. This difference in total variance was ascribed to environmental factors, unique to twins, that influence the level of plasma cholesterol (Christian *et al*. 1975).

TABLE 2

EARLY TWIN STUDIES OF PLASMA CHOLESTEROL

AUTHORS	NUMBER OF SETS DZ	MZ	WITHIN PAIR MEAN SQUARES W_{DZ}	W_{MZ}	F RATIO W_{DZ}/W_{MZ}
Osborne *et al.*, 1959	28	43	670	338	2.0*
Gedda & Poggi, 1960	50	50	78	6	11.6**
Meyer, 1962	17	24	745	297	2.5*
Jensen *et al.*, 1965	17	31	2,661	1,110	2.4**
Lundman & Blomstrand, 1966	102	91	2,046	1,592	1.3
Pikkarainen *et al.*, 1966	54	65	1,374	793	1.7*
Rifkind *et al.*, 1968	41	67	632	306	2.1**
Kang *et al.*, 1971	37	45	1,641	433	2.8**

*P < 0.05
**P < 0.01

SUMMARY

Quantitative genetic studies have much potential in partitioning the causes of variation of quantitative traits such as risk factors for atherosclerosis. Only if specific causes of variation are identified can specific therapy be developed to modify risks.

There have been extensive family studies of plasma cholesterol which reveal that the level of plasma cholesterol is correlated in family members. However, except for the relatively rare familial hypercholesterolemia the evidence is not convincing that correlations of relatives are due to genetic rather than environmental factors. Early twin studies were interpreted as supporting the hypothesis that levels of plasma cholesterol were strongly influenced by genetic factors. However a recent large study of twins cast doubt upon this hypothesis by finding no significant genetic variance of plasma cholesterol after correcting for differences in total variance of monozygotic and dizygotic twins.

REFERENCES

Brunner, D., Altman, S., Rosner, L., Bearman, J.E., Label, K. and Levin, S. (1971) Heredity, environment, serum lipoproteins and serum uric acid: A study in a community without familial eating patterns. J. Chron. Dis., 23:763-773.

Cheraskin, E. and Ringsdorf, W.M., Jr. (1970) Familial biochemical patterns part 1. Serum cholesterol in the dentist and his wife. Atherosclerosis, 11:247.

Christian, J.C., Kang, K.W. and Norton, J.A., Jr. (1974) Choice of an estimate of genetic variance from twin data. Am. J. Hum. Genet., 26:154-161.

Christian, J.C., Feinleib, M., Castelli, W., Fabsitz, R., Garrison, R., Hulley, S., Rosenman, R. and Wagner, J. (1975) Genetics of plasma cholesterol and triglycerides: A study of adult male twins. Acta Genet. Med. Gemellol. (in press)

Frederickson, D.S. and Levy, R.I. (1972) Familial hyperlipoproteinemia, in The Metabolic Basis of Inherited Disease, by Stanbury, J.B., Wyngaarden, J.B. and Fredrickson, D.S., McGraw-Hill, New York, pp. 545-614.

Gedda, L. and Poggi, D. (1960) Sulla regolazione genetica del colesterolo ematico (uno studio su 50 coppie gemellar: MZ e 50 coppie DZ). Acta Genet. Med. Gemellol., 9:135.

Godfrey, R.C., Stenhouse, W.S., Cullen, K.J. and Blackman, V. (1972) Cholesterol and the child: Studies of the cholesterol levels of Busselton school children and their parents. Australian Paediatric Journ., 8:72-78.

Jensen, J., Blankenhorn, D.H., Chin, H.P., Sturgeon, P. and Nare, A.G. (1965) Serum lipids and serum uric acid in human twins. Journal of Lipid Res., 6:193-205.

Johnson, B.C., Epstein, F.H., Kjelsberg, M.O. (1965) Distributions and familial studies of blood pressure and serum cholesterol levels in a total community - Tecumseh, Michigan. Journal of Chronic Dis., 18:147-160.

Kang, K.W., Taylor, G.E., Greves, J.H., Staley, H.L. and Christian, J.C. (1971) Genetic variability of human plasma and erythrocyte lipids. Lipids, 6:595-600.

Lundman, T., and Blomstrand, R. (1966) Serum lipids, smoking and heredity. Acta Medica Scandinavica, 180: Suppl. 455 pp. 51-60.

Martin, A.O., Kurczynski, T.W. and Steinberg, A.G. (1973) Familial studies of medical and anthropometric variables in a human isolate. Amer. J. Hum. Genet. 25:581-593.

McKusick, V.A. (1975) Mendelian Inheritance in Man. Johns Hopkins University Press, Baltimore and London.

Meyer, K. (1962) Serum cholesterol and heredity: A twin study. Acta Medica. Scandinavica 172:401-404.

Mimura, G. (1975) Genetic control of fatty acid metabolism, especially study of genetic control of cholesterol. Jap. Circ. 39:303-309.

Osborne, R.H., Adlersberg, D., DeGeorge, F.V. and Wang, C. (1959) Serum lipids, heredity and environment: A study of adult twins. Am. J. of Med. 26:54-59, January.

Pikkarainen, J., Jakkunen, J. and Kulonen, E. (1966) Serum cholesterol in Finnish twins. Amer. J. Hum. Genet., 18:115-126, March.

Rifkind, B.M., Boyle, J.A., Glae, M., Greig, W. and Buchanan, W.W. (1968) Study of serum lipid levels in twins. Cardiovascular Research, 2:148-156.

Schaeffer, L.E., Adlersberg, D., Steinberg, G. (1958) Heredity, environment and serum cholesterol. Circulation, 17:537-542.

Sing, C.F. and Eggleston, B.K. (1973) The inheritance of hypercholesterolemia in Tecumseh, Michigan. Amer. J. Hum. Genet. 25/6:72a.

Steinberg, A.G. (1963) Dependence of the phenotype on environment and heredity. In The Genetics of Migrant and Isolate Populations, ed. E. Goldschmidt, Williams and Wilkins, Baltimore.

This is publication #75-33 from the Indiana University Department of Medical Genetics and was supported in part by Contract number 71-2307 with the National Heart and Lung Institute of the National Institutes of Health, by PHS P01 GM21054, the John A. Hartford Foundation, Inc., and the Indiana Heart Association.

(5)

DISCUSSION (LIPID CLINIC II)

Discussion Following Papers of Drs. Klimov and Miettinen

Dr. Kritchevsky reported that a dose of pyridinolcarbamate of 20mg/kg/day had not affected the course of experimental atherosclerosis in rabbits but Dr. Klimov said that in his hands 10 mg/kg was effective.

In response to queries by Drs. Lewis and Mishkel, Dr. Miettinen said that the major side effect of probucol therapy was diarrhea and that long term neomycin therapy had to be closely monitored only in cases of renal abnormalities.

Dr. Sirtori reported that tibric acid was effective in treatment of triglyceridemias and questioned the dosage (single daily versus split) doses. He also revealed that propranolol administered following tibric acid or clofibrate produced a large triglyceride rebound effect. Drs. Mishkel and Carlson both commented that tibric acid was not especially efficacious in Type II patients and in Type IV cases it had no advantages over clofibrate.

Dr. Olsson reported on experiments with a new Parke Davis drug (C1719) in 12 patients with Type IV hyperlipidemia. The doses were either 450 or 750 mg/day. The drug gave a 25% decrease in lipid levels. The major decreases were in VLDL and LDL triglyceride. There was no change in total cholesterol but it seemed to be redistributed from VLDL to LDL. The drug is an aryloxyaliphatic acid (2,2 dimethyl-5(2,5-xylyloxy) valeric acid.

Dr. Sirtori reported on experiments with Metformin, a drug which reduces atherosclerosis in rabbits. In man, Metformin is an effective hypoglyceridemic agent in Type IV patients who are resistant to clofibrate. In some cases it exerts a hypoglycemic effect.

Discussion Following Papers of Drs. Krause* and Smith

Many of the questions were directed to Dr. Krause and concerned the methodology which his presentation had introduced. The technique involves simultaneous injection of (^{14}C)-mevalonate and (^{3}H)-cholesterol and measuring the radioactivity of the (^{14}C)-squalene synthesized from the mevalonate. Serum is sampled every 100 minutes over a 10 hour period. Later the ratio of (^{14}C)-cholesterol to (^{3}H)-cholesterol specific activities are measured. Dr. Little asked about correction for diurnal variation. Dr. Krause replied that this method tallied well with the balance method. Dr. Cooper asked about variations in blood volume but these would not affect the specific activity of squalene.

Dr. Angel asked about possible active and inactive pools of squalene. These apparently exist but no data were given. Squalene is transported primarily in the VLDL but also occurs in chylomicrons and other lipoproteins. One questioner asked about mixing of (^{14}C)-squalene with skin lipids, but none was observed. Dr. Paoletti reminded the audience that, in rabbits, squalene tends to be metabolized by the lungs. Dr. Krause replied that the presence of (^{14}C) in urine and feces had been determined, but not in breath. Dr. Miettinen voiced concern over the large amounts of isotope which are used.

Dr. Angel asked about the possible inclusion of muscle cholesterol into Pool 3. Dr. Smith replied that his data showed that adipose tissue was part of the third compartment, but that they had no data on muscle.

* Dr. Krause was unable to submit the manuscript relating to his presentation.

Discussion Following Dr. Christian's Paper

Dr. Kritchevsky asked if a finer estimate could be drawn by measuring cholesterol levels in different lipoprotein fractions rather than total serum cholesterol.

Dr. Christian replied that VLDL, LDL and HDL cholesterol levels had been quantitated and they all showed the same pattern of variance as did total cholesterol. All showed that the total variance in DZ twins was greater but when corrected using an unbiased estimate for genetic variance there was no significant genetic variance. If one examines his data using a "biased" estimate (biased by the difference in the total variance) then the Heart and Lung Institute Twin Studies bears out the earlier studies, namely a greater variance in DZ twins.

In reply to a question by Dr. Mishkel, Dr. Christian referred to his earlier study in young twins which indicated genetic variance in serum lipids but not erythrocytic lipids. Re-analysis of the data using their new estimate for variance shows the same result as found in the adult twins. The differences between families, which are greater than those within families suggest that the results may not only be due to genes in common but also to a common environment.

CHAPTER 6
ATHEROSCLEROSIS AND CHILDHOOD

(1)

EPIDEMIOLOGY AND RISK FACTORS IN CHILDHOOD

Shiela C. Mitchell, M.D.
Division of Heart and Vascular Diseases
National Heart and Lung Institute
Landow Building, Room C808
Bethesda, Maryland, U.S.A.

By now everyone is familiar with the risk factors of premature coronary heart disease: elevated serum cholesterol, hypertension, and cigarette smoking (1) - the big three, followed closely by obesity and diabetes. Age, sex, and inheritance are equally potent risk factors, but since they are beyond the individual's control in the preventive sense, they are rarely included in risk factor lists.

However, for every individual who is conversant with atherosclerotic or coronary heart disease risk factors, there are at least 10 who are not too sure what constitutes epidemiologic proof, and what it is, that is at the root of the reluctance, on the part of some, to make general recommendations as to effective preventive measures. Epidemiology - the study of disease in the community or among large numbers of potential patients - is not fundamentally a difficult discipline, nor need it be enveloped in mystique. However, it does have, as does any Science, its own rules and requirements that are violated at the investigator's and user's peril. Let me identify two or three of these so that you may see what I mean; and also see how relatively simple the rules are.

First, to understand the nature of epidemiologic proof (2), it is essential to recognize that all sciences are of one or two types. The first type contains such sciences as physics, where all phenomena are reducable to a small number of fundamental principles and constants. The second group contains such sciences as geography wherein no amount of knowledge of general principle will disclose the depth of Lake Erie, the head waters of the Athabascan River, or the shape of the Bay of Fundy. As one biostatistician has remarked, the continent of North America is not the shape that Pythagoras would have chosen. Epidemiology is like geography. One must get out and look.

Having decided to get out and look, the epidemiologist needs to give some thought as to what he is going to look at, or for (3). Two things should be uppermost when deciding upon the characteristics to be measured. One wants to measure something which can be accurately measured, so that measurements can be repeated, and real changes not be lost among measurement errors; and one wants to measure something that is directly related to the disease being studied or an outcome of it. Hoping to keep clear of some of the sand traps, death may be selected as the best indicator of disease. After all, "Stone cold hath no fellow." But a decrease in deaths from other causes may spuriously increase the number of deaths due to atherosclerosis and failure be accepted when success, in a clinical trial, or the actual identification of new risk factors, be almost at hand (4).

Selecting reliable, valid nonfatal expressions of disease to measure is not easy either. It is not just that "skim milk masquerades as cream" although in fact it does - so does coconut milk, soybean, and a host of other "fillers" for milk. But, in the physician's office angina may be indistinquishable from hiatus hernia, gastric ulcer, or anxiety neurosis. And those electrocardiograms so diagnostic of a myocardial infarction at this visit may be entirely normal 5 years later (5).

So one opts to look at, and measure, blood pressure or serum cholesterol. But these are not necessarily synonymous with disease. Possessing a statistical abnormality (being in the 95th percentile, i.e., having blood pressure or serum lipids higher than 95% of your "normal" friends) does not necessarily mean that you will inevitably become ill. Not everyone with high blood pressure suffers a heart attack or a stroke. Nor does everyone who falls victim to either of these have hyperlipidemia.

Indeed one of the most intriguing findings in the epidemiology of atherosclerosis is the marked difference in the clinical expression of what appears to be comparable underlying pathology, or pathological processes, among different racial groups. For example, death due to cerebral arteriosclerosis is very common in the Japanese (6) while coronary heart disease is very rare. Similarly blacks in

North America commonly succumb to hypertension but coronary heart disease in the black is relatively rare. Why these differences occur is not yet known, but occur they certainly do.

A recent report from this same study population in Georgia shows that, in those 15-19 years of age, except for the black male, the degree of obesity as measured by height/weight index, and skinfold thickness, is as good a predictor as is the blood pressure itself, in the black female and in both white men and white women, of blood pressure levels five to ten years later (7).

So picking obesity as something to look at, and for, was not a mistake. Determining its predictive value was not easy, but it could be done. Making sure that doing it would produce medically valid results, as well as statistically valid ones, is part of the art, the science, and the serendipity, needed in epidemiology.

Having faced up to these uncertainties of what to measure and how, which end points or signs of disease to look for, and how to deal with all the logistical problems along the way, is it then possible to apply epidemiologic studies to their proper end, which is prevention.

Prevention is so intertwined with epidemiology that we sometimes forget that descriptive epidemiology is also essential. So far, it has been the descriptive studies that have uncovered the currently accepted risk factors. These need now to be tested; in a clinical trial, or by further observational studies of natural history. Compounding other epidemiologic problems, is the ease with which these verification studies can be jeopardized by an earnest desire to prevent disease. If, for example, the recommendations are premature and wide spread, they can preclude the successful completion of a clinical trial. If this happens the necessary data are never obtained and we are doomed to stumble on in the dark.

It is also possible, while attempting to do good and save lives, to condemn an individual patient to a change in eating habits, an alteration of lifestyle, or a life time of drug therapy which may do him little biological good and much psychological harm.

Physicians accustomed to treating patients with acute disease rarely consider why their patients follow their advice. In actual fact it is not through understanding, not in alliance with their doctor, but through fear of more disease, more pain or immediate death. However, using fear as a preventive measure is risky. For one thing, people can get used to almost anything, even the total fear of war and death. For another, fear of a continuing and not yet painful sort has a certain attraction; at least it is not dull.

But it is most unlikely that any patient will change his or her way of eating and eat less, or take blood pressure pills throughout an entire lifetime, for fear of what may happen sometime in the future (8). Patients will do these things when they want to do them for a positive reason, not thru a negative goal. The positive reason for the small child may be pleasing Mommy. For the immortal teenager, and all teenagers expect to live forever (and most do since "forever" is 10 years), compliance may only come with recognition of the Responsible I.

It is all these considerations that have led at least a segment of the scientific community, to recommend that only those at unusual risk take unusual measures.

For the pediatrician this means, a child in a "high risk" family. A high risk family is one where brothers or sisters, or mother or father have markedly elevated serum lipids, or blood pressure; or one where a first degree relative has suffered a premature coronary event, such as a heart attack, before age forty. As a child of such a family you are much more likely than your classmates or friends to have abnormal serum lipids, abnormally elevated blood pressure and suffer heart disease at an early age.

Accordingly, some public health pediatricians have been recommending a giant step backward: a complete and detailed family history at every visit (9). If such a history is elicited, or if on routine physical the child himself, or herself, is found to have blood pressure, serum cholesterol, or ponderal index which seems high, then a detailed inquiry as to the health of other family members is certainly in order. Equally in order is a repeat reading of the blood pressure, or the blood lipid level, if this was the presenting abnormal sign.

Many youngsters can be cured of their high blood pressure by a repeat measurement, particularly by a repeat measurement with the proper size cuff. Here the rule of thumb is to use the largest possible cuff that can be placed on the patient's arm without squeezing the axilla or overlapping the antecubital fossa. A repeat of an apparently elevated serum cholesterol or triglyceride level is absolutely mandatory, for serum cholesterol levels can vary as much as 20 milligrams per ml, up or down, taken on the same child, in the same state, and in the same way, and determined in a highly skilled, standardized laboratory.

All of these "risk factors" will be gone into in more detail by the other speakers but the necessity for repeated examination and scrupulous care in physical measurements cannot be over emphasized in a disease with such far reaching implications as atherosclerosis. Mislabeling a child, as being at increased risk of this disease, is inexcusable, (1) because it is readily avoided and (2) because the price to the child is so high.

Epidemiology as a medical science and behavioral art is here to stay. So, at least for the next decade, is the risk factor concept. It behooves us all to understand both of them so that we can use them effectively for the benefit of our patients.

REFERENCES

1. Truett, J., et al: A Multivariate Analysis of the Risk of Coronary Heart Disease in Framingham, J. Chron. Dis. 1967, Vol. 20, pp 511-524.
2. Cornfield, J., Principles of Research, American Journal of Mental Deficiency, Vol. 64, No. 2, Sept. 1959.
3. Schneiderman, M. and Krant, M.: What Shall We Measure on Whom: Why?, Cancer Chemotherapy Reports, Vol. 50, No. 3, March 1966.
4. Cornfield, J.: The Estimation of the Probability of Developing a Disease in the Presence of Competing Risks, American Journal of Public Health, Vol. 47, No. 5, May 1957.
5. Keys, Ancel: Coronary Heart Disease in Seven Countries. American Heart Association Monograph No. 29, April 1970, pp. I-186-187.
6. Nakamura, M. et al: Cerebral Atherosclerosis in Japanese. I. Age Related to Atherosclerosis. Stroke, Vol. 2, July-August, 1971.
7. Johnson, Arnold J. et al: Influence of Race, Sex and Weight on Blood Pressure Behavior in Young Adults, The American Journal of Cardiology, 1975.
8. Leventhal, H.: Changing Attitudes and Habits to Reduce Risk Factors in Chronic Disease, The American Journal of Cardiology, Vol. 31, May 1973.
9. Mitchell, S.C., et al: Commentary: The Pediatrician and Atherosclerosis, Pediatrics, Vol. 49, No. 2, February, 1972.

(2)

THE LESION IN CHILDREN

Henry C. McGill, Jr., M.D.

Department of Pathology
The University of Texas Health Science Center
San Antonio, Texas, U.S.A.

The conventional concept of the initiation of atherosclerosis begins with the fatty streak, a deposit of lipid in the intima and inner media of elastic and large muscular arteries. More lipid is deposited and is encapsulated by smooth muscle and connective tissue to form the fibrous plaque. The fibrous plaque undergoes a series of changes to result finally in stenosis or thrombosis, and thereby occludes the blood supply to a vital organ.

Fatty streaks have long been recognized in the aortas of children as young as a few months of age. Zinserling (1925) described Sudan IV-stained fatty streaks in the aortas of children from Europe following World War I. The prevalence and extent of fatty streaks in these children were similar to those in the aortas of children in the United States 30 years later (Holman *et al.*, 1958). In a subsequent study of arterial specimens collected from 19 different geographic and racial population groups from different parts of the world (McGill *et al.*, 1968), fatty streaking in the aortas of young humans was nearly universal. Not only were aortic fatty streaks ubiquitous, but they were similar in degree of intimal surface involved in all geographic and ethnic groups examined, regardless of socioeconomic status or nutritional background.

Between 10 and 20 years of age, the percent of aortic intimal surface involved by fatty streaks increased rapidly, with wide individual variability ranging from less than 5% involvement to nearly 100% involvement (Eggen and Solberg, 1968). It has not been possible to find any consistent association between aortic fatty streaks in children and diet, obesity, geographic residence, terminal or complicating illness, or other conditions or characteristics commonly associated with severe adult atherosclerosis or with clinically manifest disease due to atherosclerosis. Furthermore, fatty streaks appeared first in the proximal portion of the aortic arch and later in the thoracic and abdominal aorta, while adult atherosclerosis typically is most severe in the abdominal aorta. Negro children, on the average, had a greater proportion of aortic intimal surface involved with fatty streaks than did white children, and females had a greater proportion of aortic intimal surface involved with fatty streaks than did males. The Negro/white difference occurred in populations from widely different geographic areas living under different environmental conditions, and particularly with different dietary habits. Both of these racial and sex differences were the reverse of that anticipated if childhood fatty streaks were invariable precursors of advanced adult lesions.

Fatty streaks occurred also in the coronary arteries of persons from all populations represented, but followed aortic fatty streaks by about a decade. By the age of 10 years, only about half of all children examined had detectable coronary artery lesions of any kind. The extent of these lesions in the coronary intima increased gradually with age to involve, on the average, 5-15% of the coronary artery intimal surface by age 20 years. As with the aorta, Negro children had more extensive coronary artery fatty streaks than did white children, and females had more extensive coronary artery fatty streaks than did males.

No atherosclerotic lesions appeared to any appreciable frequency or extent in the cerebral arteries, either extracranial or intracranial, before age 20 years. The age at which lesions begin to appear in the peripheral vessels is unknown.

Fibrous plaques, which typically consist of a core of necrotic debris and extracellular lipid surrounded by a capsule of connective tissue and smooth muscle, began to appear in the aortas of adolescents in the latter part of the second decade, particularly in populations likely to have a high incidence of coronary heart disease in middle age and later (Tejada *et al.*, 1968; Strong and McGill, 1969). Fibrous plaques occasionally appeared in the coronary arteries of persons under 20 years of age, but they became much more frequent in 20-29 year old males from populations with a high incidence of coronary heart disease.

Histologic examination of fatty streaks in the aortas and coronary arteries of adolescents showed differences in lipid and cellular infiltration among the different populations (Robertson *et al.*, 1963; Geer *et al.*, 1968; Restrepo and Tracy, 1975). Lesions of young persons from populations with severe atherosclerosis in middle age contained more lipid, more inflammatory cells, and more foci of extracellular lipid and necrotic debris than did lesions from populations with less severe atherosclerosis in middle age. Thus, differences exist in atherosclerotic lesions as early as the second decade of life, before gross differences in extent become apparent. These differences predict the average severity of advanced atherosclerotic lesions and clinical disease in that population in later life.

Fatty streaks in the aorta and coronary arteries of children contain lipid in the intracellular spaces, within smooth muscle cells, and in phagocytic mononuclear cells (Geer and Haust, 1972).

Chemical analysis has established that the lipid in fatty streaks is predominently cholesterol and cholesteryl esters combined with lesser quantities of triglycerides and phospholipids (Cornwell *et al.*, 1973). The principal fatty acid esterified to cholesterol is oleate. The finding of an absolute increase in the concentration of total lipid in the fatty streak as compared with adjacent uninvolved intima indicates that the lesion represents a localized accumulation of lipid and is not solely unmasking of tissue lipid (Geer *et al.*, 1958).

The relationship of the childhood fatty streak to the fibrous plaque that begins in late adolescence and young adulthood remains a controversial issue. It is apparent that not all fatty streaks become fibrous plaques, but at least some fatty streaks become fibrous plaques (Montenegro *et al.*, 1968). It is not certain that all fibrous plaques arise from pre-existing fatty streaks. There is much suggestive evidence, both from human observations and animal experimentation, that the simple fatty streak can regress leaving at most an intima thickened with smooth muscle and connective tissue, and possibly with no observable stigmata (Eggen *et al.*, 1974).

The absence of correlation of childhood fatty streaks with the usual risk factors for adult coronary heart disease, and the lack of geographic variations paralleling the incidence of coronary heart disease and related diseases cast further doubt on this association. On the other hand, the origin of the fatty streak itself in childhood remains an enigma. It may be hypothesized that the fatty streak of large muscular and elastic arteries arose at some point in primate evolution. Only when the human life span increased and man was exposed to other environmental influences such as hyperlipidemia, hypertension, cigarette smoking, and other related conditions were changes induced in the fatty streak which led eventually to clinical disease. If this concept is correct, prevention should be aimed not at the fatty streak, but at the conversion of fatty streaks to fibrous plaques.

It also is possible that there may be different kinds of fatty streaks, some of which may have the capacity for progression and others of which may remain static or regress. The critical difference may be in the type of lipid deposited, although no consistent differences have been found. The difference also may lie in the nature of cells of the arterial wall, as suggested by Benditt and Benditt (1973).

Although the mechanism of lipid deposition in the arterial intima remains an important issue in the pathogenesis of atherosclerosis, a more urgent question is the origin of the fibrous plaque. This lesion occurs infrequently in children, but its precursor is found in childhood or at least in adolescence. It seems certain that environmental conditions responsible for the differences in advanced atherosclerosis among different populations begin their effects in childhood.

References

Benditt, E.P. and Benditt, J.M. Evidence for a monoclonal origin of human atherosclerotic plaques. Proc. Natl. Acad. Sci. USA, 70: 1753-1756, 1973.

Cornwell, D.G., Geer, J.C., and Panganamala, R.V. Development of atheroma and the lipid composition of the deposit. In Pharmacology of Lipid Transport and Atherosclerotic Processes, Encycl. Pharmacol. Ther., Sect 24, chpt. 9, pp. 445-483. Pergamon Press, Oxford, 1973.

Eggen, D.A. and Solberg, L.A. Variation of atherosclerosis with age. Lab. Invest. 18:571-579, 1968.

Eggen, D.A., Strong, J.P., Newman, W.P., III, Catsulis, C., Malcolm, G.T. and Kokatnur, M.G. Regression of diet-induced fatty streaks in rhesus monkeys. Lab. Invest. 31:294-301, 1974.

Geer, J.C., Strong, J.P., McGill, H.C., Jr., Nyman, M.A., and Werthessen, N.T. Correlation of intimal sudanophilia and cholesterol anaylses of 3 layers of human aorta. Proc. Soc. Exp. Biol. Med. 98:260-263, 1958.

Geer, J.C., McGill, H.C., Jr., Robertson, W.B., and Strong, J.P. Histologic characteristics of coronary artery fatty streaks. Lab. Invest. 18:565-570, 1968.

Geer, J.C. and Haust, M.D. Smooth muscle cells in atherosclerosis. Monogr. Atheroscler., 2:1-140, 1972.

Holman, R.L., McGill, H.C., Jr., Strong, J.P., and Geer, J.C. The natural history of atherosclerosis. The early aortic lesions as seen in New Orleans in the middle of the 20th Century. Am. J. Pathol. 34:209-235, 1958.

McGill, H.C., Jr. Fatty streaks in the coronary arteries and aorta. Lab. Invest. 18:560-564, 1968.

Montenegro, M.R. and Eggen, D.A. Topography of atherosclerosis in the coronary arteries. Lab. Invest. 18:586-593, 1968.

Restrepo, C. and Tracy, R.E. Variations in human aortic fatty streaks among geographic locations. Atherosclerosis 21:179-193, 1975.

Robertson, W.B., Geer, J.C., Strong, J.P., and McGill, H.C., Jr. The fate of the fatty streak. Exp. Mol. Pathol. 2 (Suppl. 1): 28-39, 1963.

Strong, J.P. and McGill, H.C., Jr. The pediatric aspects of atherosclerosis. J. Atheroscler. Res. 9:251-265, 1969.

Tejada, C., Strong, J.P., Montenegro, M.R., Restrepo, C., and Solberg, L.A. Distribution of coronary and aortic atherosclerosis by geographic location, race, and sex. Lab. Invest. 18:509-526, 1968.

Zinserling, W.D. Untersuchungen über Atherosklerose. I. Über die Aortaverfettung bei Kindern. Virchow Arch. Pathol. Anat. 255:677-705, 1925.

(3)

GENETICS OF THE HYPERLIPIDEMIAS AND CARDIOVASCULAR IMPLICATIONS

Peter O. Kwiterovich, Jr., M.D.

Department of Pediatrics, Johns Hopkins University

School of Medicine, Baltimore, Md., U.S.A.

Among the risk factors implicated in the development of atherosclerotic cardiovascular disease, one of the most important is hyperlipidemia, i.e., an increased plasma concentration of either cholesterol or triglycerides or both. A variety of epidemiological studies have shown that both hypercholesterolemia and hypertriglyceridemia are associated with increased risk of developing ischemic heart disease (IHD); the association of hyperlipidemia with premature IHD is even more striking. Longitudinal, prospective data from the general population on the presence of hyperlipidemia early in life and its effect on the development of premature IHD in adulthood are not currently available. One approach is therefore to concentrate on those families in which inherited disorders of lipid and lipoprotein metabolism and IHD co-exist. The thrust of this discussion will therefore be on these familial diseases and their early biochemical, genetic and clinical presentations with an emphasis on their cardiovascular implications.

A large number of genetic loci are involved in the complex control of the plasma level of any lipid or lipoprotein species. Product of the genes, e.g., the concentration of the plasma cholesterol or triglycerides, is distributed over a range of values from which an arbitrary cutpoint is selected. A subset of patients thus defined represent a heterogeneous group, from which different monogenic models have been developed to describe the expression of familial elevations of plasma lipids and lipoproteins. Models have been generated according to plasma lipid levels by Goldstein and co-workers (1). Others, most notably Fredrickson and colleagues, developed genetic hypotheses using the concentrations of plasma lipoproteins (2). The classification schemes have been summarized in Table I and tentatively arranged according to their prevalence early in life. Regardless of the schemes of classification, the degree of genetic heterogeneity underlying these models remains unknown.

Table I. Classification and Prevalence of Hyperlipidemia and Hyperlipoproteinemia in Childhood.

Prevalence	Lipids	Lipoproteins
Common	Hypercholesterolemia	Hyperbetalipoproteinemia (type IIa hyperlipoproteinemia)
Relatively Uncommon	Hypertriglyceridemia	Hyperprebetalipoproteinemia (type IV hyperlipoproteinemia)
	Hypercholesterolemia Hypertriglyceridemia	Hyperbetalipoproteinemia Hyperprebetalipoproteinemia (type IIb hyperlipoproteinemia)
Rare	Hypertriglyceridemia (severe)	Hyperchylomicronemia (marked) (type I hyperlipoproteinemia)
Very Rare	Hypercholesterolemia Hypertriglyceridemia	1) Hyperchylomicronemia Hyperprebetalipoproteinemia (type V hyperlipoproteinemia) 2) Increased very low density lipoproteins with beta mobility and abnormal triglyceride to cholesterol ratio (type III hyperlipoproteinemia)

Familial hypercholesterolemia (FH) or "classic type II hyperlipoproteinemia" is the most commonly recognized form of familial hyperlipidemia in childhood, with an estimated prevalence of 1/200 to 1/500 (1-3). FH is characterized by significant increases in the plasma concentrations of both the total and low density lipoprotein (LDL) cholesterol. The phenotypic presentation may include tendon xanthomas, arcus corneae and premature IHD. FH is transmitted as a Mendelian dominant trait (or group of similar traits) with complete expression at birth (1-5). A single dose of the mutant gene(s) typically produces total plasma and LDL cholesterol levels above 300 and 240 mgs% respectively, and children and adults affected in this way are termed "heterozygotes". The heterozygote child is clinically asymptomatic in the first decade; approximately 10-15% of the children develop tendon xanthomas in the second decade but IHD is still rare (5). The natural history of premature IHD in their affected parents is so striking that significant atherosclerosis is probably already present in the children (5). In the offspring of two heterozygotes, one out of four children, on the average, receives a double dose of the mutant allele(s). These "homozygote" children usually have a plasma cholesterol between 600 and 1,000 mg% and are diagnosed early in life because of the appearance of planar xanthomas (2,6). Atherosclerosis, particularly of the coronary vessels and aortic valve, can present as IHD and aortic stenosis before age six but their expression is ordinarily "delayed" to the second decade of life (2,6). Brown and Goldstein (7) have recently described a lack of functional LDL receptors in fibroblasts grown in tissue culture from homozygous children. This deficiency of LDL receptors is associated with decreased proteolysis of LDL protein and faulty regulation of both the rate limiting enzyme of cholesterol biosynthesis, hydroxy methyl glutaryl CoA reductase and the intracellular content of free and esterified cholesterol (7). The capability of the parental cells to perform the above functions is only 50% of that of control cells (7).

In some families the presence of endogenous hypertriglyceridemia (type IV hyperlipoproteinemia) appears to be inherited as an autosomal dominant trait,characterized by significant increases in the plasma concentrations of triglycerides and very low density lipoproteins (1,2). Half of the children of an affected parent are expected to be affected. However, only 1 of 5 rather than 1 out of 2 children presented before the age of 20 with hypertriglyceridemia (1,2). The frequency of the disorder(s) in the general population is estimated to be 0.2 to 0.3% (1). With this frequency and reduced penetrance, only 1 of 2,500 children will present with this "monogenic form" of hypertriglyceridemia. The glucose intolerance, hyperuricemia, premature IHD and peripheal vascular disease seen in adults with hyperglyceridemia is not ordinarily seen in children with endogenous hypertriglyceridemia (1,2). The expression of hypertriglyceridemia, with or without hypercholesterolemia in childhood, as part of the syndrome of "familial combined hyperlipidemia" is likewise delayed (1).

Disorders of exogenous hyperglyceridemia (type I hyperlipoproteinemia) are rare with approximately 40 cases in the world literature (2). The massive increase in chylomicrons, accompanied by marked hypertriglyceridemia (as high as 10,000 mg%) present in childhood with abdominal pain. Other features include eruptive xanthomas, hepatosplenomegaly and lipemia retinalis. Premature IHD is not present (2). The disorder is due to a double dose of a mutant allele which causes a deficiency in the enzyme lipoprotein lipase (2).

The expression of type V hyperlipoproteinemia in a patient before the age of 20 is very rare (Table I). There are actually less pediatric cases of type V hyperlipoproteinemia in the literature than type I hyperlipoproteinemia (2). We have recently observed the complete expression of type V hyperlipoproteinemia in a nine year old girl. Despite marked hypertriglyceridemia (> 6,000 mg%), there was no history of abdominal pain, pancreatitis or fat intolerance. The child manifested both the fat and carbohydrate intolerance seen in affected adults. The somewhat increased predilection to vascular disease, observed in adults with the disorder, is not detectable in children (2).

Familial type III hyperlipoproteinemia is defined by the presence of a plasma VLDL which has an abnormal chemical composition and migrates as beta rather than prebeta lipoproteins (2). Both hypercholesterolemia and hypertriglyceridemia occur, but the underlying metabolic defect and mode of inheritance are unknown. Premature vascular disease involves both the coronary and peripheal vessels. Tendon and tuberous xanthomas may occur; however, the clinical hallmark of the phenotype(s) is the unusual yellow deposits in the creases of the palms (2). The above phenotype has been ascertained in only two patients less than the age of twenty (8,9). The first was in a nine year old Canadian boy, who presented with obesity and both hypercholesterolemia and hypertriglyceridemia of approximately 400 mg%. The second case is more complicated and was recently described by Kwiterovich et al (9). This 15 year old girl has xanthoma striata palmaris, beta VLDL, and elevated LDL; her mother and two siblings had tendon xanthomas and hyperbetalipoproteinemia, a clinical picture indistinguishable from FH. This pediatric patient probably represents a genetic variant of the standard type III phenotype, the heterogeneity of which has been recently suggested by Fredrickson et al (10).

It has yet to be proven that treatment of susceptible patients at any given stage of atherosclerotic development will change or reverse the natural history of the disease process. Nevertheless, treatment of these predisposed children and young adults appears judicious and prudent in view of the current information available.

1. Goldstein, J.L., Schrott, H.G., Hazzard, W.R., Bierman, E.L. & Motulsky, A.G. Hyperlipidemia in coronary heart disease. II. Genetic analysis of lipid levels in 176 families and delineation of a new inherited disorder, combined hyperlipidemia. J. Clin. Invest. 52:1544-1568, 1973.

2. Fredrickson, D.S. & Levy, R.I. Familial hyperlipoproteinemia. In The Metabolic Basis of Inherited Disease. ed. Stanbury, J.B. Wyngaarden, J.B. & Fredrickson, D.S. 3rd Edn. Ch.26, New York: McGraw-Hill, p.545-614, 1972.

3. Glueck, C.J., Hickman, F., Schoenfeld, M., Steiner, P. & Pearce, W. Neonatal familial type II hyperlipoproteinemia: Cord blood cholesterol in 1880 births. Metabolism 20:597-608, 1971.

4. Kwiterovich, P.O., Levy, R.I. & Fredrickson, D.S. Neonatal diagnosis of familial type II hyperlipoproteinemia. Lancet 1: 118-122, 1973.

5. Kwiterovich, P.O., Fredrickson, D.S. & Levy, R.I. Familial hypercholesterolemia (One form of familial type II hyperlipoproteinemia). A study of its biochemical, genetic and clinical presentation in childhood. J. Clin. Invest. 53:1237-1249, 1974.

6. Khachadruian, A.K., Uthman, S.M. Experiences with the homozygous cases of familial hypercholesterolemia. A report of 52 patients. Nutr. Metabol. 15:132-140, 1973.

7. Brown, M.S., Faust, J.R., Goldstein, J.L. Role of the low density lipoprotein receptor in regulating the content of free and esterified cholesterol in human fibroblasts. J. Clin. Invest. 55:783-793, 1975.

8. Godolphin, W.J., Conradi, G., Campbell, D.J. Type III hyperlipoproteinemia in a child. Lancet, 209-210, January 22, 1972.

9. Kwiterovich, P.O., Neill, C., Margolis, S., Thamer, M. & Bachorik, P. Allelism, non-allelism, and genetic compounds in familial hyperlipoproteinemia. Clin. Res. 23:262A, 1975.

10. Fredrickson, D.S., Morganroth, J., & Levy, R.I. Type III hyperlipoproteinemia: An analysis of two contemporary definitions. Ann. Int. Med. 82:150-157, 1975.

(4)

DIETARY MANAGEMENT OF FAMILIAL TYPE II - HYPERLIPOPROTEINEMIA IN CHILDREN AND ADOLESCENTS - A FEASIBILITY STUDY

G. Schlierf, C.C. Heuck, P. Oster, H. Raetzer,
B. Schellenberg, G. Vogel

Department of Medicine, University of Heidelberg
D-6900 Heidelberg, Bergheimer Strasse 58, Germany

Studies in the USA (Glueck et al, 1971), South Africa (Stein et al, 1974) and Germany (Greten et al, 1974) suggest 0.9 to 3 % familial type II hyperlipoproteinemia in the newborn. According to Slack (1969) more than 50 % of the heterozygous subjects will have clinically manifest coronary heart disease by the age of 50. Homozygous children rarely reach the age of 20. Thus, early identification and treatment of this disorder appears to be mandatory.

While infants appear to react very favorably to appropriate diets (Glueck and Tsang, 1972), reports in children are equivocal. Andersen and Claussen (1972), and Glueck and co-workers (1973) were able to normalize elevated cholesterol levels on an out-patient basis in affected children. Lloyd (1974), in contrast, had moderate results with dietary management and therefore initiates early drug treatment, particularly when there is a family history of premature atherosclerosis.

Material and methods. The first part of this report concerns a feasibility study in 38 children and adolescents with type II hyperlipoproteinemia from 17 families, 14 girls and 24 boys, age range 3 to 22 years, with a cholesterol lowering diet (P/S-ratio 1.5 - 2.0 daily, cholesterol intake less than 300 mg). The families were instructed on several occasions by an experienced dietician who also visited them at monthly intervals. Adherence was monitored by shopping lists and meal records. Plasma total cholesterol and beta- and alpha-lipoprotein cholesterol was measured every 3 months. Two samples had been obtained before treatment 4 to 8 weeks apart. The patients were started on the diet in 1972/1973 - the duration of the study has, therefore, been two to three years in most of them.

When it became apparent, that out-patient management was quite unsatisfactory in most cases, 8 children were admitted to a metabolic ward to obtain data on maximum diet responsiveness with fat modified, low cholesterol and low fat diets, respectively. This study lasted for 1 month.

Results. Figure 1 shows the time course of plasma total cholesterol levels in 29 children who completed a minimum of 1.5 years on the diet as out-patients. Data are plotted for half-year periods, each point being the mean of 2 determinations at three-months intervals. The mean cholesterol level fell by about 10 % early in the study and remained at this level. In only 3 of 29 children plasma cholesterol levels fell below 250 mg/100 ml.

Figure 2 shows, for 8 children, the plasma cholesterol responses to a 4-week inpatient period. In every case, the cholesterol level fell within a few days. The mean decrease of plasma cholesterol levels was 27 %. 5 of the 8 now showed cholesterol levels at or below 250 mg/100 ml. There was no obvious difference between a fat modified, low cholesterol formula diet, a low fat formula diet and a fat-modified, low cholesterol diet consisting of mixed foods.

Discussion. In accordance with Lloyd (1974) we have found out-patient dietary management of type II hyperlipoproteinemia in children and adolescents unsuccessful in spite of dietary councelling which far exceeded the routine for patients with metabolic disorders. Of the initial 38 patients, 9 were drop-outs after a few months. Food recording was successful in 9 of 17 families and indicated satisfactory P/S-ratios in 4 families only. Since good diet responsiveness was demonstrated in all patients who could be admitted to the metabolic ward, dietary adherence appears to be the main problem. Contrary to the USA, fat-modified foods are not yet available in West Germany and low fat foods are not readily accepted or are rather expensive. Skimmed milk, for instance, to many is a reminder of food shortage during the war and post-war-period. Children, in addition, are quite successful to get the food they want out of their homes, even if the parents try for suitable diets.

Although a 10 % cholesterol lowering obtained with the out-patient children is comparable to results of feasibility studies in adults (National Diet Heart Study, 1968) attempts of reduction of risk for coronary heart disease should aim at a better cholesterol lowering effect. Then, according to the estimation

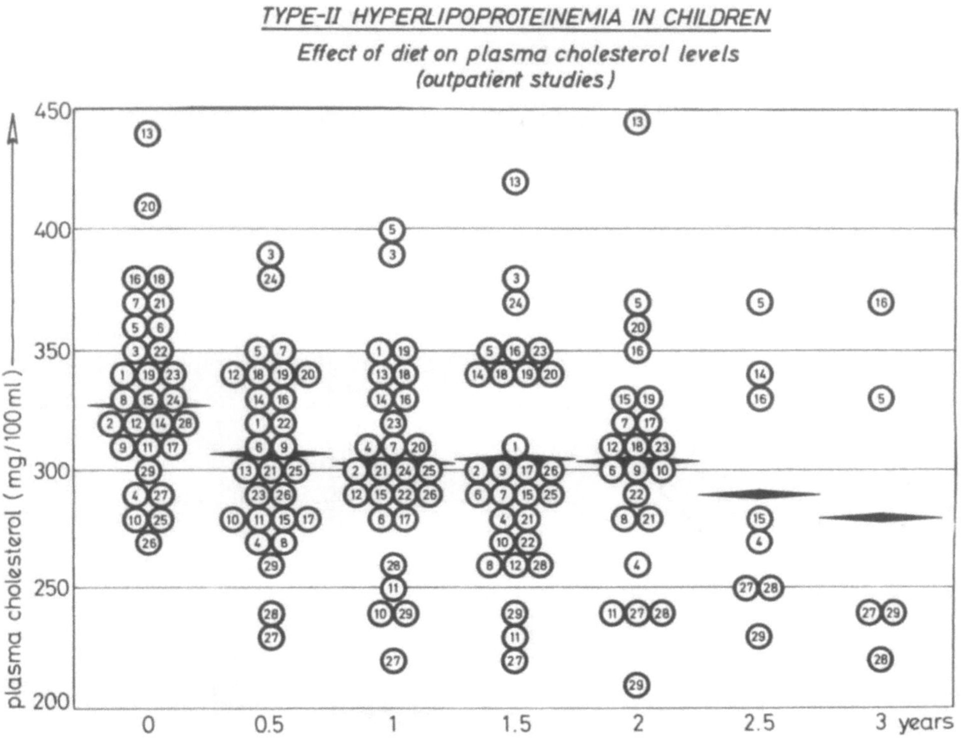

Fig. 1 Circles represent mean values for two cholesterol determinations per 1/2 year. The course of individual patients can be identified by the patient numbers. Note that not all patients have completed 2, 2 1/2 and 3 years.

of the Intersociety Commission of Heart Disease Resources, reduction of risk could amount to as much as 50 %.

The study was supported by Deutsche Forschungsgemeinschaft - Sonderforschungsbereich 90.

The assistance of Dr. Wachtel, Maizena GmbH and Mr. Scherf, Wander GmbH, who supplied constituents of the formula diets is gratefully acknowledged.

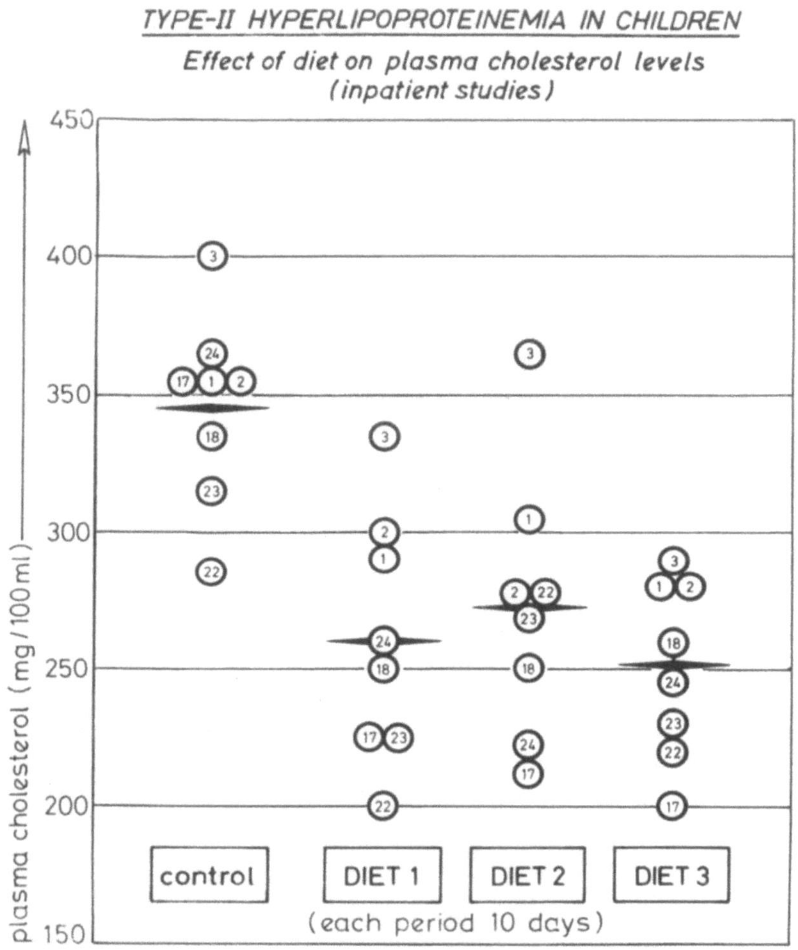

Fig. 2 Circles represent values for two cholesterol determinations at the 8th and 10th day of each dietary period.
Diet 1: 37 % polyunsaturated fat formula diet.
Diet 2: 8 % (low fat) formula diet.
Diet 3: 37 % polyunsaturated fat mixed food diet.

REFERENCES

Andersen, G.E., J. Clausen
Tracing and treatment of children with essential familial hypercholesterolemia.
Zeitschrift für Ernährungswissenschaft 11:120, 1972

Glueck, Ch. J., F. Heckman, M. Schoenfeld, P. Steiner, W. Pearce
Neonatal familial type II hyperlipoproteinemia: cord blood cholesterol in 1800 births.
Metabolism 20: 597, 1971

Glueck, Ch. J., R.C. Tsang
Pediatric familial type II hyperlipoproteinemia: effects of diet on plasma cholesterol in the first year of life.
The American Journal of Clinical Nutrition 25:224, 1974

Glueck, Ch. J., R. Fallat, R. Tsang
Pediatric familial type II hyperlipoproteinemia, treatment with diet and cholestyramine resin.
Pediatrics 52:669, 1973

Greten, H., M. Wagner, G. Schettler
Frühdiagnose und Häufigkeit der familiären Hyperlipoproteinämie Typ II.
Deutsche Medizinische Wochenschrift 99:2553, 1974

Lloyd, J.K.
Dietary management of type II familial hyperlipoproteinemia in children.
Atherosclerosis III, Ed. G. Schettler and A. Weizel, page 765, Springer Verlag, Berlin, 1974

Slack, J.
Risk of ischemic heart disease in hyperlipoproteinemic states.
Lancet II:1380, 1969

Stein, E.A., D. Mendelsohn, I Bersohn
Detection of familial hyperlipoproteinemia by cord blood analysis.
Atherosclerosis III, Ed. G. Schettler and A. Weizel, page 479, Springer Verlag, Berlin, 1974

The National Diet Heart Study, Final Report.
American Heart Association Monograph Number Eighteen, 1968

Report of Inter-Society Commission for Heart Disease Resources.
Primary prevention of the atherosclerotic diseases.
Circulation, XLII, 1970

(5)

TREATMENT OF HYPERLIPIDEMIAS IN CHILDHOOD

C.J. Glueck, R.W. Fallat, R.C. Tsang, and M.J. Mellies

General Clinical Research and Lipid Research Centers, and the Fels Division of Pediatric Research and Newborn Division, University of Cincinnati, College of Medicine, Cincinnati, Ohio, U.S.A.

INTRODUCTION

Coronary heart disease risk factors can easily be recognized in school children, and even in infancy[1,2]. It has been proposed that the primary prevention of atherosclerosis might best begin in childhood, a period during which the actual vascular lesion is probably either absent or reversible[2]. This report is focused on therapy of hyperlipidemias in childhood, with the recognition that there are several effective approaches to normalization of elevated cholesterol and triglyceride. There is as yet, no prospective, longitudinal evidence that normalization of cholesterol and triglyceride levels in childhood will prevent the development and progression of atherosclerosis[2].

DISCUSSION

Evaluation of treatment regimens in children with hyperlipidemia should begin with a most careful definition of the nature of the disorder, including a distinction between familial and acquired. We suggest at least two separate determinations of cholesterol and triglyceride after a 12-14 hour fast. Where possible, measurement of total, low density lipoprotein, very low density lipoprotein (LDL and VLDL) cholesterols, and triglyceride will give the most accurate and meaningful diagnosis[2,3]. In every child with elevated cholesterol and/or triglycerides laboratory evaluation to screen for secondary hyperlipidemia should be carried out[2-5], including urinalysis, liver function tests, thyroid function tests, and fasting blood sugar. After exclusion of secondary hyperlipidemia, a nutritional history, drug intake history (including where appropriate, intake of oral

TABLE 1. TREATMENT OF FAMILIAL AND ACQUIRED HYPERTRIGLYCERIDEMIA

	Diet, Drug Therapy	Effects of Therapy on Triglyceride and VLDL Cholesterol.
FAMILIAL HYPERTRIGLYCERIDEMIA:		
All ages	Weight reduction to ideal body weight NIH,NHLI Type IV diet at ideal body weight	95% or more of children should normalize
Drugs of Choice	No published experience, but of limited need since diet alone should normalize most children	
	Limited experience shows that clofibrate 1-2 gm/day is uniformly effective in older teenagers unresponsive to diet	
ACQUIRED HYPERTRIGLYCERIDEMIA: (Dietary)		
All ages	Restriction of alcohol, caloric, carbohydrate intake	All children should normalize
ACQUIRED HYPERTRIGLYCERIDEMIA: (Secondary to poorly controlled diabetes, hypothyroidism, nephrotic syndrome, liver disease, oral contraceptives, etc.)		
All ages	Treatment of primary disease state	If primary disease can be cured, triglyceride will normalize. If primary disease state cannot be cured, limited information on treatment of secondary hypertriglyceridemia.

TABLE 2. TREATMENT OF FAMILIAL AND ACQUIRED HYPERCHOLESTEROLEMIA

	Diet, Drug Therapy		Effects of Therapy on Total and LDL Cholesterol
FAMILIAL HYPERCHOLESTEROLEMIA: (Heterozygote)			
Birth - Age 1	Low cholesterol, saturate restricted diet		90% of infants normal at age 1
Age 1 - Age 3	Low cholesterol, saturate restricted diet		80% of children normal at age 3
Age 3 - Age 7	Low cholesterol, saturate restricted diet enriched in polyunsaturates		Variable response. About 40% normal, 30% moderately elevated, 30% high.
Age 7 - Age 19	Low cholesterol, saturate restricted diet enriched in polyunsaturates		Variable response. About 30% normal, 20% moderately elevated, 50% high.
Drugs of Choice	Cholestyramine resin	12-20 gm/day	60% of children normal, 15% moderately elevated, 20-40% reduction in cholesterol.
	Colestipol	10-15 gm/day	
Drugs or Surgical Procedures with Limited Experience	Clofibrate	1-2 gm/day	33% reduction in cholesterol
	Ileal bypass		30-40% reduction in cholesterol

(continued)

TABLE 2 (con't): TREATMENT OF FAMILIAL AND ACQUIRED HYPERCHOLESTEROLEMIA

	Diet, Drug Therapy		Effects of Therapy on Total and LDL Cholesterol
FAMILIAL HYPERCHOLESTEROLEMIA: (Homozygote)			
All ages	Low cholesterol, saturate restricted diet enriched with polyunsaturates		<5% reduction in cholesterol
Drugs of Choice	Cholestyramine resin	20-40 gm/day	Variable response. About 10-30% reduction in cholesterol.
(usually given as combination therapy)	Nicotinic Acid Clofibrate	2-6 gm/day 1-2 gm/day	
Drugs or Surgical Procedures with Limited Experience	Portacaval Shunt		-
	Ileal bypass		-
ACQUIRED HYPERCHOLESTEROLEMIA: (Dietary)			
All ages	Low cholesterol, saturate restricted diet		All children should normalize.
ACQUIRED HYPERCHOLESTEROLEMIA: (Secondary to hypothyroidism, nephrotic syndrome, liver disease, etc.)			
All ages	Treatment of primary disease state		If primary disease can be cured, cholesterol will normalize.
	Low cholesterol, saturate restricted diet, enriched in polyunsaturates		If primary disease state cannot be cured, limited information on treatment of secondary hypercholesterolemia.

contraceptives) and alcohol intake history may be useful. Family study, including at a minimum, measurement of cholesterol in parents and siblings, is necessary to define the presence, or absence of any familial component of the hyperlipidemia. Only after all of the above steps do we then make plans for therapy of the hyperlipidemia, and for discussion of its implications with the family. Since the diagnosis of hyperlipidemia in a child usually raises well warranted concerns in the family, it is very important to have a well defined diagnosis, prior to treatment. Outlines for a suggested approach to treatment of familial and acquired hyperlipidemias are given in Tables 1 and 2.

Hypertriglyceridemia

Although familial and acquired hypertriglyceridemias are much less common in children than hypercholesterolemia[1,2,3], they are important to recognize, since essentially all children with familial hypertriglyceridemia will normalize triglyceride levels with weight reduction and the NIH type IV diet[3] (Table 1). Hypertriglyceridemia acquired through excess alcohol intake or through oral contraceptives (the two most common acquired hypertriglyceridemias in the general population) should normalize when the diet or drug regimen is changed (Table 1).

Hypercholesterolemia

In infants and young children with familial hypercholesterolemia diet alone should suffice in most cases to reduce total and LDL cholesterol to normal levels (Table 2)[4-7]. In older children with familial hypercholesterolemia who maintain persistently elevated total and LDL cholesterol on the best diet, cholestyramine resin[7-9] or Colestipol[10] provide major additional cholesterol reduction with normalization of about 2/3 of the children treated (Table 2). While both resins may produce some constipation or diarrhea, no systemic side effect have been reported, save for folic acid deficiency on high dises (30-40 gm/day of cholestyramine resin)[9], which is reversed by addition of 5 mg folic acid/day. There has been limited experience with Clofibrate which may, however, provide substantial additional cholesterol lowering. The ileal bypass[11] has been advocated as an effective approach towards treatment of pediatric familial hypercholesterolemia, but neither confirmatory reports of its safety nor comparisons with cholestyramine resins have yet appeared.

For the children homozygous for familial hypercholesterolemia, diet alone has no effect. Combination therapy of cholestyramine resin, nicotinic acid and clofibrate has been used[12] but with variable response and little apparent reduction in the accelerated rate of atherosclerosis (Table 2). An entirely new approach to the homozygote, the portacaval shunt [13], appears to have great promise, but there is no prospective data on utility, safety, and effectiveness, particularly in children.

For children with hypercholesterolemia acquired due to dietary excess (Table 2), all should normalize on diet (Table 2). The earliest dietary intervention possible might be useful in such children, prior to development of persistently bad eating habits.

In the treatment of either the familial or the acquired hyperlipidemias in children, a series of conservative and apparently safe approaches now are available for normalizing cholesterol and triglyceride levels. There is as yet, however, no prospective data to indicate that successful longitudinal treatment of hyperlipidemia from childhood will retard or prevent the development of atherosclerosis in adulthood.

REFERENCES

1. Lauer RM, Connor WE, Leaverto PE, et al: Coronary heart disease risk factors in school children. Muscatine study. J Pediatr 86:697-706, 1975.

2. Glueck CJ, Fallat RW, Tsang R: Hypercholesterolemia and hypertriglyceridemia in children. A pediatric approach to primary atherosclerosis prevention. Am J Dis Child 128: 569-577, 1974.

3. Glueck CJ, Tsang R, Fallat R, et al: Familial hypertriglyceridemia: studies in 130 children and 45 siblings of 36 index cases. Metabolism 22: 1287-1309, 1973.

4. Tsang RC, Glueck CJ, Fallat RW, et al: Neonatal familial hypercholesterolemia. Am J Dis Child 129:#1, 83-91, 1975.

5. Tsang RC, Fallat RW, Glueck CJ: Cholesterol at birth and age 1: Comparison of normal and hypercholesterolemic neonates. Pediatrics 53:458-470, 1974.

6. Glueck CJ, Tsang RC: Pediatric familial type II hyperlipoproteinemia: effects of diet on plasma cholesterol in the first year of life. Amer J Clin Nutr 25:224-230, 1972.

7. Glueck CJ, Fallat R, Tsang R: Pediatric familial type II hyperlipoproteinemia, therapy with diet and cholestyramine resin. Pediatrics 52:669-679, 1973.

8. West RJ, Lloyd JK: Use of cholestyramine in treatment of children with familial hypercholesterolemia. Arch Dis in Childhood 48:#5, 370-374, 1973.

9. West RJ, Lloyd JK: Effect of cholestyramine on intestinal-absorption. Gut 16:93-98, 1975.

10. Glueck CJ, Fallat RW, Mellies M, et al: Pediatric familial type II hyperlipoproteinemia: therapy with diet and Colestipol resin. Pediatrics, in press, 1975.

11. Buchwald H, Moore RB, Varco RL: Ten years clinical experience with partial ileal bypass in management of hyperlipidemias. Ann Surg 180:384-392, 1974.

12. Moutafis CD, Myand NB, Mancini M, et al: Cholestyramine and nicotinic acid in the treatment of familial hyperbetalipoproteinemia in the homozygous form. Atherosclerosis 14: 247-258, 1971.

13. Stein EA, Mieny C, Spitz L, et al: Portacaval-shunt in four patient with homozygous hypercholesterolemia. Lancet 1: 832-835, 1975.

(6)

DISCUSSION (ATHEROSCLEROSIS AND CHILDHOOD)

Dr. Silverberg: (Edmonton) We have been carrying out screening for hypertension in Edmonton school children and find that our systolic readings are 27 mmHg higher, and diastolic readings 11 mmHg higher, than those obtained by their family doctors. We use the blood pressure cuffs as recommended by the American Heart Association, while the family physicians use regular adult cuffs.

Dr. Shiela Mitchell: (Bethesda) This problem of the proper blood pressure cuff for children is a difficult one. Few pediatricians use them although they are available.

Dr. Kidd: (Baltimore) It is very difficult to see how a proper cuff could give you a higher blood pressure reading, on basic physiological grounds. Too narrow a cuff will give too high a reading, a proper cuff and a broader cuff will give you the same reading. Possibly the higher reading you obtain is due to excitement and unfamiliarity with the procedure.

Dr. Silverberg: I don't think so. Using the same cuffs as the family doctors use, we still got a difference, but it was smaller.

Dr. Mitchell: Dr. Berenson, what do you do in your study in New Orleans.

Dr. Berenson: (New Orleans) Our objective was trying to get good, basic blood pressures on children and we spent a whole year studying methods of how to do this; we arrived at a set protocol for the cuff size based on both width and arm comfort, and you can get both proper bladder size and comfort. One important thing is to have a bladder that completely encircles the arm circumference, and the same width measurements that are recommended by the American Heart Association (AHA). But, the standard cuff recommended by the AHA is a little too short, it doesn't cover the whole arm circumference. So, you are apt to get into the seriously high level. And one of the problems that I think Dr. Silverberg might be running into is that he is taking mass readings on these children, just running them in, and taking their blood pressure, without any preparatory examination. Now, these are apt to give very high values. In our screening program, again, which is rather rigid, examination is the last thing that we do to the children. They get their blood drawn, we give them breakfast, they see other children get their blood pressures taken and then we take blood pressure readings. Our readings tend to be lower than those published in the textbooks, like Moss and Adams.

Member of the Audience: Dr. Kwiterovich, you showed heterogeneity of lipoprotein and lipid disorders in a single family. This gives rise to the possibility that we do not really have the nice genetic situation that we like to think we do. Isn't it possible that these disorders are not as closely related to a specific gene and maybe there is some more generalized lipid disorder which can manifest itself in several ways?

Dr. Kwiterovich: I think that's a very good point; lipoproteins and lipids are gene products that are very far removed from the genes, so it is not like an enzyme. If one looks at, for example, the distribution of the enzyme involved in galactose metabolism and galactosemia: in the distribution curve between normals and heterozygote carriers, one will find an overlap between those two, similar to the overlap that is present in the distribution of LDL in children. So that even within such a condition, in which the gene product is an enzyme, there is an overlap between normal and heterozygotes. I think that the recent work of Dr. Goldstein starts defining these things in biochemical terms. Even there, we are still one step removed; we do not understand whether what has been observed in tissue culture explains the situation in vivo, and exactly what is wrong with the receptor is not known. Is it that the receptor doesn't work, or is it completely absent, or is it protein that's modified, or what is the receptor? We are just now beginning to appreciate how little we really know and I think that's the first step to advancement.

Dr. Glueck: I believe this monolithic or pseudomonolithic structure is going to be further fragmented. The response to diet and treatment varies widely in families, which is an indication of the differences in the families themselves.

Member of the Audience: Do you agree with Goldstein's analysis that there are five models, 3 monogenic, one polygenic and the sporadic model?

Dr. Kwiterovich: Well, what one does is build up a model and then make a hypothesis. The biostatistical tools for doing this are not very well developed, so that there are certain inherent limitations. The models for familial hypercholesterolemia and familial hypertriglyceridemia are more convincing than that for familial combined hyperlipidemia. In familial combined hyperlipidemia, Joan Slack, for example, believes that the whole thing is a statistical artifact, because of the way in which the propositi were selected: they had to have a second affected propositus who was included in the segregation ratio analysis. The interpretation becomes very difficult. However, I feel it was very worthwhile to build these models, because they provide the framework within which one can work and look for basic defects. In other words, if you don't have a framework within which to work, it is very difficult to concentrate in terms of potentially revealing exactly what the biochemical defects are.

Dr. McGill: I have a question for the last three members of the panel. It's pretty well established that the children of North America have, on the average, higher serum cholesterols than those of other countries in the world. This is associated with their higher risk of coronary heart disease. I think all three of you in your presentations directed your attention to the severely hyperlipidemic children. Are you willing to go on to the mass of children in North America and suggest that they modify their diets?

Dr. Glueck: I believe that recommendations should be made in a proven and restricted sense but not necessarily in an evangelistic sense for all American children. One of the things we tried to do is to test the feasibility of a moderate restriction of cholesterol intake by approximately 50% in children, whose average cholesterol intake was about 800 to 1000 milligrams a day. This was a diet that we hoped they would follow. We have studied about 120 of such children and they have had a very dramatic response to this restriction.

Dr. Schlierf: I believe that such a widespread dietary restriction would be very difficult since it wouldn't involve a few children but many children. For practical purposes, because children eat at school at the middle of the day, this is very difficult.

Dr. Kwiterovich: I think this problem is a difficult one. I do not believe it is clear that a child at age ten is going to track his cholesterol, that is, a child in the upper fifth percentile in infancy or childhood is going into a high risk group when he becomes an adult. If this <u>is</u> so, I think we should consider recommending prudent diets for these children. But whether that will prevent heart disease, I don't know. Perhaps if we could first show that one could prevent heart disease, then it might be worthwhile making that recommendation.

Dr. McGill: I think that there is evidence from Evans county that suggests that from age 15 to the early 20's the serum lipids do track.

Dr. Connor: (Iowa City) I also have noted, along with Dr. Glueck, what I would call progressive decompensation to dietary management with age. We also find this in adults, that is, the susceptibility to dietary factors in lowering blood-lipid levels becomes less and less as the person ages. So I think this bears upon the question that Dr. McGill raised, that if we wait too long, we are going to have a population that will not respond very well to diet. So that maybe we should think rather seriously about the lower ages in which to recommend this so-called prudent diet.

Dr. Stamler: (Chicago) With reference to Dr. Kwiterovich's lipid distribution curves and his concern with the upper fifth percentile, what would be wrong with shifting the whole distribution to the left, ten or fifteen percent, by making some improvements in regard to what might be called the high consumption of junk by American children. By junk, I mean high caloric, empty calorie foods of a variety of types, which we all know American children are eating in larger quantities than any other population of children in the world. It results in a prevalence rate of ten or twenty percent of obesity, in particular when accompanied by a lack of physical activity. Why do we need to wait ten or twenty or thirty years to reach the obvious conclusion that this is not an optimal diet for children. Here is the reverse question: Are you prepared to say this is an optimal diet for children which should not be changed? I think that anyone who says we must wait to do something about this diet is essentially taking this position: "From everything that I know in science, this is the optimal diet for children today." I challenge everybody that takes that position.

Dr. Mitchell: One of the things about that terrible ghastly diet that everybody talks about is that is has produced, apart from coronary heart disease, a pretty healthy-looking group of kids that don't get rheumatic fever or rickets, and some of this is probably due to this ghastly diet.

Dr. Glueck: I find myself in general agreement with Dr. Stamler's position. I don't believe there would be any harm from a moderate and prudent diet and I am willing to wait to determine whether or not major benefits will accure. If no harm is inferred, I would be in favor of a moderate restriction, particularly in that group of children who are in the upper five percent of the range.

Dr. Kwiterovich: I personally feel that the emphasis should be on children who are genetically susceptible to developing premature ischemic heart disease and I feel that we have neither the right nor the scientific back-up to recommend, across the board, that there should be changes for all Americans. While it is true that we want to change the diet of American children, I think it is questionable whether we should do so in the justification of trying to cure coronary heart disease. I'd like to raise a basic question. I am wondering whether the basic defects which produce the fatty streaking and the plaques carry elevated cholesterol and triglyceride as a symptom and whether by lowering the cholesterol by diet and drugs we're not treating the symptom rather than the disease and whether it is going to be shown, similar to some of the drug trials, that what we're working at is not really altering the basic risk factors for coronary heart disease.

Dr. Connor: I just wanted to respond to Dr. Mitchell's point. At the present time we do apply nutritional measures for deficiencies that only afflict a small portion of the population. For instance, we treat all children with Vitamin D and iodine, and the epidemiology of rickets is that not too many children got it and not too many people got iodine deficient goiter either. So I think we can modify the diet of the child, keeping all the good things, Dr. Mitchell, that may have helped to improve health, but taking out the things that may have some implications for poor health in adult life. I think we can still keep a good diet.

Member of the Audience: There are abnormalities associated with plant sterol intake documented. Such things as β-sitosterolemia and xanthomatosis. Dr. Glueck has also observed that plant sterol elevation does occur in infants that are given diets high in polyunsaturated fats. So I think the recommendation, at least that I would be interested in having discussed, would be a diet low in dietary cholesterol and saturated fats, which gets away from some of the junk foods that Dr. Stamler mentioned producing obesity but which does not increase the intake of polyunsaturated fat.

Dr. Glueck: I agree; if we push polyunsaturated fat this could have serious consequences later on.

Member of the Audience: I would like the panel to go back even further and give comments on feeding during pregnancy as it might influence the offspring.

Panel: We have no information on that.

Dr. Stamler: We have just been conducting studies concerning smoking, another risk factor, and the expenditures since the Surgeon General's report on antismoking education. We've sent questionnaires to all the Federal Agencies and to a random sample of state, county, and metropolitan area agencies. I was unable to get any information on how much had been spent. My working hypothesis is that the expenditure on antismoking education has been, if I may use the proverbial word, peanuts, compared to the smoking expenditure by the tobacco industry to perpetuate the habit. And it turns out that every public agency that has so far returned our questionnaire (and we have an 80% response) indicates that next to nothing or nothing has been spent. There is a small expenditure by the Clearing House on Public Education. And there has been virtually no effective public education efforts except for the limited resources of voluntary agencies and despite the continued communication of the tobacco industry the figures for the National Clearing House are that since the 1950's some 20 million adult men have quit cigarette smoking in the United States. If the per capita consumption overall is up, which it is unfortunately, this is primarily due to two phenomena, which must be of grave concern. Firstly, the continued smoking by women and the very much lower quit-rate in adult women than in men. Secondly, the progressive taking up of the habit by teenagers, including in the last ten or fifteen years, teenage girls. So that by now in the schools, the prevalence rate of cigarette smoking in the United States is about equal among boys and girls. I think that a reasonable working hypothesis, and with all the noise in the system and all the limitations in the effort to communicate, the message, understandably has not gotten through except to a segment of the male population. It is interesting that in this situation with the limited changes in America for some reason or another that we can not explain, the coronary rates are beginning to decline. I would like, hypothetically, to relate this to the limited improvements we have brought about, not only in care for sick people but also in the lifestyles of the American people. I know I can't prove that, but its part of my belief that leads me to the conviction that it is better to change and improve the diet on the whole. I would challenge Dr. Kwiterovich: I am sure you advocate cessation of cigarette smoking, or not picking it up, among children. We have no proof that that does any good either. Are you not inconsistent?

Dr. Kwiterovich: I still believe that the recommendation of radical dietary changes should be confined to those children who are known to be at risk.

CHAPTER 7
PLASMA LIPIDS AND THROMBOSIS

(1)

INTRODUCTION

Dr. A. G. Shaper

MRC Social Medicine Unit
London School of Hygiene and Tropical Medicine
Keppel Street, London, England

My role this morning is to define the function of this workshop within the overall frame-work of the whole conference. Having read all the papers to be presented, there is a considerable temptation simply to present you with a summary by way of introduction; however, the speakers this morning are perfectly capable of presenting their own material, and my Co-Chairman, Dr. Renaud, will comment on their papers in his summing-up of this workshop. We are focusing on the relation between the plasma lipids and thrombosis, an area that may be fundamental to atherosclerosis and to its complications, in particular coronary heart disease (CHD), peripheral vascular disease (CVD) and possibly stroke (CVA).

Whatever one's beliefs concerning the factors initiating atherosclerosis, there is little doubt that the plasma lipids play a major role in the development of the vascular lesions. Much will be said about plasma lipids and hyperlipidaemia during this meeting and about the factors involved in mural lipid accumulation. There will be considerable concern with the permeability of vascular endothelium and with the evolution and the regression of the arterial lesions both in man and experimental animals. But apart from this session, there is likely to be very little discussion about the relationship between plasma lipids and the formation of thrombus and its subsequent dissolution or incorporation.

The role of thrombosis in the development of atherosclerosis has a long history of debate, and its precise place in the initiation of clinical events is also controversial. Later in this Workshop - Conference (on Wednesday afternoon) Dr. Wissler will review current concepts of coronary thrombosis as related to atherosclerosis and myocardial infarction, and perhaps our session will provide some basic information for the discussion on the role of thrombus in the development of atherosclerosis and whether thrombosis precedes or follows myocardial infarction.

In 1963 Merskey and Marcus reviewed the subject of "Lipids, coagulation and fibrinolysis" and noted that "Much energy and effort has been expended in an attempt to show that dietary ingestion of fat significantly alters blood coagulation and fibrinolysis and promotes a hypercoagulable state" and they concluded that up to that date this thesis remained unproved (1). Ten years later in 1973 a symposium was held in Lyon, France, to see whether a more definite conclusion could be reached (2). The symposium was almost entirely concerned with dietary fats and plasma lipids and their effect on platelet composition and behaviour. Apart from one brief mention of fibrinolytic activity in Bolivians living in the Andes, the symposium did not discuss this enzyme system. In the concluding remarks at that symposium, Dr. Renaud considered that there was good evidence that dietary fats, apparently due to their content of long chain saturated fatty acids, predisposed to arterial and venous thrombosis partly through their effect on platelets. There were however, those in that symposium who were unconvinced of any vital link between plasma lipids and platelet behaviour. No conclusions were drawn regarding fibrinolysis.

Today, the major part of our workshop will again be devoted to platelet problems, and because of this, I feel constrained to draw attention to some aspects of fibrinolysis which may not be more fully discussed in this session. Almost 70 years ago, Nolf (3) suggested that the lining of vessels contributed components of the fibrinolytic system and that disturbance of this system could lead to a deposition of fibrin on the vessel wall. Since then, it has been demonstrated by the use of fibrinolysis autography, that most of the plasminogen activator in tissue is related to the endothelium of blood vessels (4). This knowledge has allowed the development of hypotheses relating the fibrinolytic capacity of vessels and the condition of the intimal lining and has also raised the possibility that plasminogen activator in endothelium can affect the flow arrangements in the vessel, with a layer of defibrinated plasma lubricating the movement of the blood (5). This latter theory may have relevance to the distribution of fibrin within the walls of blood vessels. In normal vessels, fibrinogen would be degraded by shearing and fibrinolysis before it could penetrate the wall. Where these arrangements were disturbed by changes in fibrinolytic capacity or blood coagulation, fibrinogen could penetrate the wall and establish lesions (6).

Today, we are 12 years on from the Merskey and Marcus review and we will briefly examine the current position regarding plasma lipids, thrombus formation and the fibrinolytic process. The implications of our conclusions are of importance not only because there are drugs now available which are known to affect platelet behaviour and fibrinolytic activity. They are important because a knowledge of the factors affecting the behaviour of platelets and fibrinolysis may lead to measures which could prevent thrombosis or accelerate clot dissolution and thus possibly retard the development of atherosclerosis and its complications.

If we have learnt anything at all from the many conferences and workshops we have all attended over the past decade or more, it is that the development of atherosclerosis and its clinical complications is a complex problem involving a large number of pathogenic pathways and a fair number of aetiological factors. It seems highly unlikely that some single aspect of thrombus formation or dissolution will supply us with all the answers. On the other hand, it seems likely that the dynamics of thrombus formation play some role in the story of atherosclerosis and CHD and we shall attempt to approach a definition of that role in this workshop.

REFERENCES

1. Merskey, C., and Marcus, A. J.: Lipids, coagulation and fibrinolysis. Annual review of Medicine 14:323, 1963.
2. Renaud, S., Nordøy, A. (Eds.): Dietary fats and thrombosis. S. Karger Basel, 1974.
3. Nolf, P.: La fibrinolyse. Arch. Int. Physiol. 6:306-359, 1908.
4. Todd, A.S.: Endothelium and fibrinolysis. Bibliotheca Anatomica 12:98-105, 1973.
5. Todd, A.S.: Endothelial fibrinolysis and blood flow. Lancet 1:1179, 1971.
6. Lendrum, A.C.: Deposition of plasmatic substances in vessel walls. Path. Microbiol. 30:681-684, 1967.

(2)

FIBRINOLYTIC ACTIVITY AND RISK FACTORS FOR ATHEROSCLEROSIS

* N.A. MARSH and ** A.G. SHAPER

* Dept. of Physiology, Queen Elizabeth College, London W.8.

** MRC Social Medicine Unit, London School of Hygiene & Tropical Medicine, Keppel Street, London, England

Introduction

Our interest in the fibrinolytic enzyme system arises from its possible relation to atherosclerosis and its complications. However, there is at present no clear evidence which relates a disturbed fibrinolytic system to the aetiology or pathogenesis of atherosclerosis or which indicates that established arterial disease is associated with a deficient fibrinolytic system. It has been suggested that the conflicting results from various studies may arise from the usual practice of only measuring resting fibrinolytic levels which some workers regard as an inadequate measure of overall fibrinolytic capacity. Increased amounts of plasminogen activator are present after stress of many kinds including exercise, adrenaline administration and venous occlusion, the latter procedure increasing the fibrinolytic activity of blood within the occluded segment. Some individuals respond poorly to these various stimuli and "poor responders" to one stimulus are likely to be poor responders to others. It is clearly of considerable importance to know whether the response of the fibrinolytic system to stimulation (i.e. the fibrinolytic capacity) is related to plasma fibrinolytic activity at rest and to determine the relationship between fibrinolytic activity and the known risk factors for atherosclerosis.

Study

We have examined the fibrinolytic response to stress in a group of 59 healthy men aged 45-53 years. Venous occlusion was chosen as a more acceptable and convenient stimulus than exercise or adrenaline injection in these middle-aged men. The men were participating in a longterm dietary programme and their resting fibrinolytic activity had been measured on four previous occasions over a three-year period. We deliberately selected men who had consistently shown low or high levels of fibrinolytic activity over these previous four visits in order to determine whether such extreme groups differed in their response to stress. Fibrinolytic activity was measured by the euglobulin lysis (ELT) method and results expressed in units of fibrinolytic activity using the reciprocal of the square of the lysis time, multiplied by 10^6 for convenience of expression.

Results

When the resting levels are plotted against the increment in fibrinolytic activity (FA) produced by venous occlusion there is a good relationship between resting activity and the increment on occlusion (Figure 1). This relatively small group of men is of particular interest because of the consistency with which the individuals have remained in the low or high activity group over a long period of time. It is therefore of interest to examine the status of the high and low activity groups with regard to the known risk factors for atherosclerosis (Table 1). There is clearly a marked difference between the two groups in the levels of cardiovascular risk factors. The group with high resting fibrinolytic activity (all having a good response to stress) have significantly lower levels of plasma cholesterol and triglycerides, a lower Quetelets index, lesser skinfold thickness and lower blood pressure. This high FA group also includes more non-smokers and more physically active subjects although neither the smoking nor the physical activity findings achieve statistical significance. It is of considerable interest to note that those subjects who had never smoked were clustered in the high response area of the figure.

As low resting levels of fibrinolytic activity (< 100 units) are associated with considerable variation in fibrinolytic response, we have compared subjects showing low resting FA and poor response to stress with those showing equally low levels at rest but with a much greater response to stress. For this purpose, the low activity group has been equally divided on the basis of response to venous occlusion. The table shows the median fibrinolytic response in these two groups contrasted with the high activity group and also shows the mean levels of cardiovascular risk factors. Plasma cholesterol and triglycerides are lower in the high response group and there are more non-smokers and fewer heavy smokers in this group but the findings are not statistically significant.

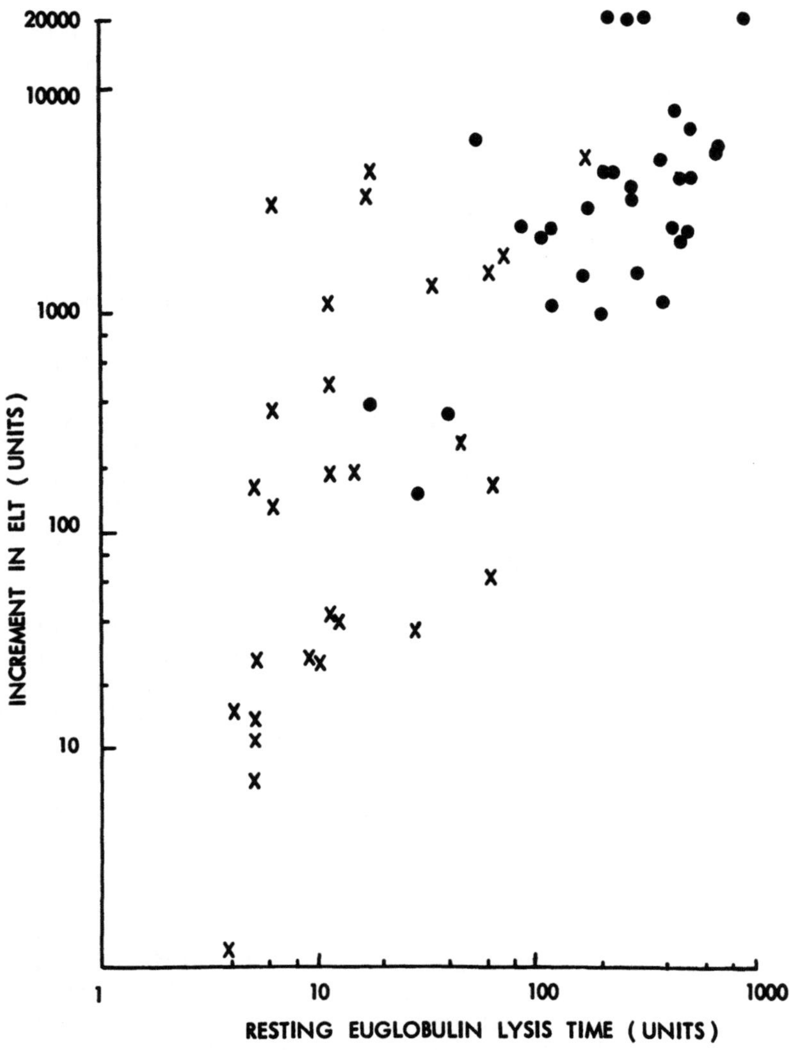
20000
10000
1000
100
10
INCREMENT IN ELT (UNITS)
1
10
100
1000
RESTING EUGLOBULIN LYSIS TIME (UNITS)

Figure 1

Table 1. Fibrinolytic activity (median resting and response levels) and cardiovascular risk factors in high resting and low resting groups. Figures in brackets represent mean levels for the low resting activity group. Significance levels (** = P $<$ 0.01; * = P $<$ 0.05) refer to the differences between high resting and low resting groups.

	High Resting		Low Resting		
	High Response		High Response		Low Response
Number of men	31		14		14
Resting (units)	260		28		6
Response (units)	3646		1220		26
Cholesterol (mg %)	165	**	178	(186)	195
Triglycerides (mg %)	60	**	98	(109)	121
Quetelets Index	238	**	257	(258)	259
Total Skinfolds (mm)	46	*	52	(52)	53
Diastolic B.P. (mm Hg)	76	*	82	(81)	80
Systolic B.P. (mm Hg)	127	n.s.	133	(132)	132

Discussion

There are a number of hypotheses relating FA to atherosclerosis, two of which warrant discussion. In the first hypothesis, the level of plasminogen activator in the blood vessels is adversely affected by atherosclerosis resulting in an increased tendency to fibrin accumulation and thrombosis. Subjects with high resting levels of FA and a good response to stress would be assumed to have the least atherosclerosis. In agreement with this supposition, the high activity group does have levels of all the measured risk factors for atherosclerosis which are lower than those of subjects with low resting FA. In the latter group (defined as less than 100 units in this study) the hypothesis indicates a greater degree of atherosclerosis and suggests that those subjects with low resting FA and a good response to stress have less atherosclerosis than those with low resting FA and a poor response to stress.

An alternative hypothesis is that the cardiovascular risk factors exert an adverse effect on fibrinolytic activity by some inhibitory effect on plasminogen activator. This could lead to an increased tendency to fibrin accumulation, thrombosis and ultimately to atherosclerosis. The differences in cardiovascular risk factors between the low activity and high activity groups would fit this concept but within the low activity group, the small and non-significant differences in risk factor levels between low and high responders seem inadequate to explain the striking differences in fibrinolytic response to venous occlusion.

Unfortunately for assessment of the hypotheses, we do not know the relative contribution of veins and arteries to the total systemic fibrinolytic capacity and we know remarkably little about the function of the veins in subjects with atherosclerosis. It is possible that both hypotheses are operating but whichever is the more important, there is little doubt that the recognised risk factors for CVD are closely associated with fibrinolytic activity and it is possible that in the response to stress (venous occlusion) we may have an indicator of the degree of atherosclerosis present.

Reference

Shaper, A.G., Marsh, N.A., Patel, I., Kater, F. Response of fibrinolytic activity to venous occlusion. British Medical Journal, 3, 1975.

(3)

DIETARY FATTY ACIDS AND ARTERIAL THROMBOSIS: EFFECTS AND MECHANISM OF ACTION WITH SPECIAL REFERENCE TO LINOLEIC ACID

G. Hornstra

Unilever Research, Vlaardingen

Olivier van Noortlaan 120, Vlaardingen, The Netherlands

SUMMARY

In rats dietary long-chain saturated fatty acids with more than 14 carbon atoms promote arterial thrombus formation, whereas dietary linoleate has a specific antithrombotic effect. The dietary fat effects are not mediated by changes in coagulation but are most probably caused by changes in the aggregation tendency of blood platelets.

In man dietary linoleic acid decreases platelet aggregation and the plasma fibrinogen content. Indications have been obtained for a long-term protective effect of adipose tissue linoleic acid on platelet aggregatibility when feeding thrombogenic diets.

The postulated role of platelet arachidonate and cholesterol is discussed in relation to the findings reported. It is concluded that, because of the antithrombotic activity of linoleic acid and of its decreasing effect on plasma lipid concentrations, an ample intake of dietary linoleic acid is recommendable as a preventive measure against atherosclerosis.

Atherosclerosis is a multifactorial disease with a generally accepted thrombotic component, both in the development of the disease and in its complications (1,2,3). Since dietary fats have been shown to strongly affect the course of the atherosclerotic process (4,5), the (anti)thrombotic effects of dietary fats are being studied rather extensively.

As has recently been reviewed (6,7), dietary long-chain

saturated fatty acids are thrombogenic, whereas (poly-)unsaturated fatty acids are not, or may even be anti-thrombotic. We showed that in rats the thrombogenicity of a dietary fat is mainly determined by the content of saturated fatty acids with 14 or more carbon atoms. Consequently, unsaturated fatty acids would be antithrombotic only, if they replace saturated fats in the diet. However, when oleic and linoleic acid were compared for this "passive" antithrombotic effect, it appeared that linoleic acid is significantly more antithrombotic than oleic acid (8).

It is highly probable that in the model used, the effects of dietary fats on arterial thrombosis are not mediated through differences in blood coagulability. In rats fed antithrombotic sunflowerseed oil or thrombogenic coconut fat, no differences were observed in the recalcification times of platelet-free and platelet-containing plasma, whole blood clotting time (measured in Chandlers rotating loop), platelet factor 3 (PF_3) content and activity while PF_3 availability in response to collagen was even significantly reduced in the thrombogenic group (9). These findings are different from those, reported by Renaud and Gautheron (7) who showed dietary-induced hyperlipidemia to be associated with increased thrombosis tendency and hypercoagulability, due to enhanced PF_3 activity. This discrepancy is most probably the result of dietary and methodological differences and needs further clarification.

Although platelet aggregation in platelet-rich plasma in response to adenosine diphosphate (ADP), collagen and thrombin was the same in both groups, ADP- and collagen-induced platelet shape change was significantly enhanced in the thrombogenic group, as was the spontaneous- and ADP-induced aggregation in circulating blood. Since platelet counts are invariably higher in rats fed the thrombogenic diet, it is highly probable that changes in the thrombotic properties of blood platelets are the basis of the dietary fat induced changes in arterial thrombosis tendency (9). Therefore, we investigated the effect of dietary linoleic acid on spontaneous platelet aggregation in flowing blood in man, using a newly developed device, the Filtragometer (10).

Measurements were carried out in two groups of male subjects taking part in the Helsinki primary prevention trial. One group received the normal Finnish diet, comprising only 4 cal% linoleic acid, whereas the other group a modified diet containing 12 cal% linoleic acid was offered. In a 12-year period, mortality due to coronary heart disease had decreased by 50% in men on the high linoleic acid diet (11). In this group platelet aggregation appeared to be significantly depressed also by about 50% (12).

Later studies by the Atherosclerosis Research Group in Montclair, N.J., USA, confirmed the aggregation-inhibiting effect of dietary linoleic acid in man. Moreover, they showed this effect to appear very quickly and to be readily reversible on re-feeding a low linoleic acid diet (13). However, in a group of Trappist monks, having a rather high linoleic acid intake (about 11 cal%), no effect on platelet aggregation was observed on decreasing the linoleic acid content, for 6-8 weeks, to less than 4 cal% by replacing dietary sunflowerseed oil by olive oil or butterfat.

This finding might have important implications as it points to a possible long-term protecting effect of the linoleic acid body stores on pro-thrombotic dietary changes. This seems reasonable since the composition of the adipose tissue changes less readily on dietary changes than does that of the plasma lipids (14,15). From studies in rats we already knew that the increase of the arterial thrombosis tendency on feeding a thrombogenic fat occurs more slowly, the longer the animals had been pre-fed with antithrombotic sunflowerseed oil (9). From the Helsinki study, mentioned earlier, we got the same impression since, three months after replacing the experimental by the normal diet, the degree of aggregation was still significantly depressed in people who had been on the high linoleic acid diet for 4-6 years, whereas it was not different from normal in subjects whom had been offered the high linoleic acid diet for less than 1 year only.

A high content of linoleic acid in the adipose tissue might also be benificial for another reason. Rapid mobilization of free fatty acids (FFA), occurring in stress situations, may present a hyperthrombotic state, especially when the amount of FFA released exceeds the binding capacity of the plasma proteins and when the FFAs are of the long-chain saturated type (16). Thrombotic risks, associated with FFA mobilization might be expected to be low, provided the body fat contains a high amount of linoleic acid since this fatty acid has low thrombogenic potency in vitro as well as in vivo (17,18). Moreover, since fatty acids require fibrinogen as a cofactor to induce aggregation in the presence of albumin (18), our finding that a diet rich in linoleic acid decreases the plasma fibrinogen content (Table 1) is also relevant.

Linoleic acid, the main essential fatty acid, is metabolized via di-homo-γ-linoleic acid (19) the precursor of prostaglandin E_1 (PGE_1) (20) a very active inhibitor of platelet thrombotic functions (21). Since the platelet lipid composition reflects to some extent the dietary fatty acid intake (22), it was tempting to speculate that the mechanism by which dietary linoleate decreases arterial thrombosis tendency, is through an increased PGE_1 synthesis in the blood platelets and the vessel wall. However, linoleic acid is also converted into arachidonic acid (19) which causes platelet aggregation after enzymatic conversion into the endoperoxides PGG_2 and PGH_2, intermediates in the biosynthesis of PGE_2 (23,24). Stimulation of platelets with thrombin also causes the production of these platelet endoperoxides (24,25) which lends further support to the suggested regulatory role of platelet arachidonic acid metabolism in thrombogenesis (26,27,28).

Table 1 Effect of a diet rich in linoleic acid on plasma fibrinogen levels (mean ± s.e.m, n=22)

	Control	Experimental	$P_2(\Delta)$*
Triglyceride linoleate (%)	20.5 ± 1.34	32.9 ± 1.03	<0.001
Plasma fibrinogen (mg/100 g)	238 ± 11.8	206 ± 12.7	< 0.02

* Wilcoxon's signed rank test.

However, recent work on rats, made deficient in essential fatty acids (EFA), does not support this hypothesis. In EFA deficiency arachidonic acid is present in only small amounts (9), whereas the PG-synthesizing system is markedly depressed (29) leading to lower tissue PG-levels (29,30). Since thrombin was reported to stimulate endogenous PG-synthesis (25,26,31) - through which its aggregating effect has been explained - in EFA deficiency, a decreased thrombin-induced aggregation might be expected. However, EFA-deficient platelets appeared to be hypersensitive to thrombin. A more pronounced change in platelet shape in response to ADP and collagen also indicates an increased platelet reactivity in EFA deficiency (G. Hornstra and E. Haddeman, to be published). In EFA-deficient man, platelet retention in glass bead columns is reported to be enhanced (32) which also points to a hyperthrombotic state of blood platelets in EFA deficiency.

All these findings indicate that PG-endoperoxide production from platelet arachidonate is not the one and only thrombosis-regulating mechanism. Moreover, results obtained by Silver et al. (26) and Gerrard et al. (33) imply that the concept of thrombosis regulation by platelet arachidonate alone is too simple. They showed that polyunsaturated fatty acids other than arachidonate inhibit PG-endoperoxide formation in platelets. It might be expected that on platelet stimulation not only arachidonic acid is released from platelet phospholipids, but other fatty acids as well. Therefore, it seems reasonable to postulate that the ratio between arachidonic acid and the other polyunsaturated fatty acids in platelets might ultimately determine thrombosis tendency (26,34). Dihomo-γ-linolenic acid has already been shown to decrease platelet thrombotic functions (26,35), possibly through two mechanisms:

a. interference with endoperoxide production (26,33);
b. conversion into PGE_1 (20) which inhibits platelet aggreation and release induced by PGH_2 (27).

Since dihomo-γ-linolenic acid is synthesized from linoleic acid (19) and the platelet lipid composition can be influenced by dietary fatty acids (22,35), a high linoleic acid intake seems efficient in preventing and counteracting excessive pro-thrombotic endoperoxide production.

Since certain hyperlipoproteinemias predispose to fatal trombotic complications of atherosclerosis, the effect of plasma lipids - especially cholesterol and triglycerides - on platelet function is of interest. In platelets the major neutral lipid is cholesterol, which is almost exclusively present in the free form (36). Platelets are unable to synthesize cholesterol (37) but take it up from their medium. This process appears to be positively related to the cholesterol to phopsholipid mole ratio (C/PL-ratio) of the surrounding medium (38). Since increased platelet cholesterol uptake coincides with enhanced platelet aggregation in response to epinephrine and ADP (38,39), lowering the plasma cholesterol content might be useful to decrease the aggregation tendency of blood platelets.

Because of the antithrombotic effect of dietary linoleic acid and its well documented decreasing effect on plasma lipids, ample intake of linoleic acid can be recommended as a preventive measure against thrombosis.

REFERENCES

1. Mustard, J.F., M.A. Packham, S. Moore and R.L. Kinlough-Rathbone in: G. Schettler and A. Weizel: Atherosclerosis III, Berlin-Heidelber-New York, Springer Verlag, 1974 pp. 253-267.

2. Moore, S., *Thromb. Diath. Haemorrh.* Suppl. 60:205-212, 1974.

3. Chandler, A.B., *Thromb. Res.* 4, Suppl. 1:3-23, 1974.

4. Turpeinen, O., *J. Amer. Diet. Ass.* 52:209-213, 1968.

5. Malmros, H., *Lancet* ii:479-484, 1969.

6. Hornstra, G., *Haemostasis* 2:21-52, 1973/74.

7. Renaud, S. and P. Gautheron, *Haemostasis* 2:53-72, 1973/74.

8. Hornstra, G., and R.N. Lussenburg, *Atherosclerosis*, in press.

9. Hornstra, G., in: A.J. Vergroesen (Ed): The Role of Fats in Human Nutrition, Academic Press Inc. (London) Ltd., 1975 pp. 303-330.

10. Hornstra, G., and F. ten Hoor, *Thromb. Diath. Haemorrh.* in press.

11. Miettinen, M., O. Turpeinen, M.J. Karvonen, R. Elosuo and E. Paavilainen, *Lancet* ii:835-838, 1972.

12. Hornstra, G., A. Chait, M.J. Karvonen, B. Lewis, O. Turpeinen and A.J. Vergroesen, *Lancet* i:1155-1157, 1973.

13. Fleischman, A.I., M.L. Bierenbaum, D. Justice, A. Stier, A. Sullivan and M. Fleischman, *Amer. J. Clin. Nutr.* 28:601-605, 1975.

14. Dayton, S., *J. Lipid Res.* 7:103-111, 1966.

15. Fleischmann, T. Hayton and M.L. Bierenbaum, *Amer J. Clin. Nutr.* 20:333-337, 1967.

16. Connor, W.E., J.C. Hoak and E.D. Warner, in: S.Sherry et al. (Eds): Thrombosis, Nat. Acad. Sci. Washington D.C., 1969 pp. 355-373.

17. Hoak, J.C., A.A. Spector, G.L. Fry and E.D. Warner, *Nature* 228:1330-1332, 1970.

18. Prost-Dvojakovic, R.J., and M. Samama, *Haemostasis* 2:73-84, 1973/74.

19. Mead, J.F., *Fed. Proc.* 20:952-955, 1961.

20. Van Dorp, D.A., R.K. Beerthuis, D.H. Nugteren and H. Vonkeman, *Nature* 203:839-841, 1964.

21. Kloeze, J., in: S. Bergström and B. Samuelsson (Eds): Prostaglandins, Stockholm, Almkvist and Wiksell, 1967 pp. 241-252.

22. Nordöy, A., and J.M. Rödset, *Acta Med. Scand.* 190:27-34, 1971.

23. Nugteren, D.H., and E. Hazelhof, *Biochim. Biophys. Acta,* 326: 448-461, 1973.

24. Hamberg, M., J. Svensson, T. Wakabayashi and B. Samuelsson, *Proc. Nat. Acad. Sci. USA* 71:345-349, 1974.

25. Hamberg, M., J. Svensson and B. Samuelsson, *Proc. Nat. Acad. Sci. USA* 71:3824-3828, 1974.

26. Silver, M.J., J.B. Smith, C. Ingerman and J.J. Kocsis, *Prostaglandins* 4:863-875, 1973.

27. Willis, A.L., F.M. Vane, D.C. Kuhn, C.G. Scott and M. Petrin, *Prostaglandins* 8:453-508, 1974.

28. Malmsten, C., M. Hamberg, J. Svensson and B. Samuelsson, *Proc. Nat. Acad. Sci. USA* 72:1446-1450, 1975.

29. Tan, W.C., and O.S. Privett, Biochim. Biophys. Acta 296:586-592, 1973.

30. Van Dorp, D.A., *Ann. N.Y. Acad. Sci.* 180:181-199, 1971.

31. Smith, J.B., and A.L. Willis, *Brit. J. Pharmacol.* 40:545-546 P, 1970.

32. Press, M., H. Kikuchi, T. Shimoyama and G.R. Thompson, *Brit. Med. J.* 2:247-250, 1974.

33. Gerrard, J.M., J.G. White and W. Krivit, *Blood* 44:918, 1974.

34. Pace-Asciak, C., and L.S. Wolfe, *Biochim. Biophys. Acta* 152:784-787, 1968.

35. Willis, A.L., K. Comai, D.C. Kuhn and J. Paulsrud, *Prostaglandins* 8:509-519, 1974.

36. Marcus, A.J., L.B. Safier and H.L. Ullman in: G.J. Nelson (Ed.): Blood lipids and lipoproteins, Wiley Interscience, 1972 pp. 417-439.

37. Derksen, A., and P. Cohen: *J. Biol. Chem.* 248:7396-7403, 1973.

38. Shattil, S.J., R. Anaya-Galindo, J. Bennett, R.W. Colman and R.A. Cooper, *J. Clin. Invest.* 55:636-643, 1975.

39. Bennett, J.S., S.J. Shattil, R.A. Cooper and R.W. Colman, *Blood* 44:918, 1974.

(4)

UPTAKE OF LABELLED CHOLESTEROL BY ORGANIZING THROMBUS

Bernard I. Weigensberg and Robert H. More

Department of Pathology, McGill University

Montreal, P.Q., Canada

In previous studies (1- 7) it was shown that non-occlusive white mural thrombus induced by a catheter inserted into the abdominal aortae of rabbits organized into raised fibrofatty type atherosclerotic lesions which have also been referred to as thromboatherosclerotic lesions, a term denoting their origin. Histological and chemical studies in normolipidemic rabbits (4,5, 7) showed that the lesions contained appreciable amounts of various lipids including anisotropic clefts and needles of cholesterol. Ouantitative analysis of these raised lesions at various time intervals show the free cholesterol and cholesterol ester tissue concentrations summarized in Figure 1 (8).

The object of this study was to determine the origin and the time that this cholesterol accumulated. The data depicted in Fig.1 is not sufficient to indicate the time that this cholesterol accumulated since it is likely that the rise and fall of the data depicted are partly artifacts caused by the great dilution of cholesterol concentration caused by the large amounts of connective tissue. Expressing the data in terms of DNA introduces difficulties since it also rises and falls as the lesion evolves and does not remain constant.

To investigate the origin of this cholesterol in this lesion two types of experiments were conducted. In the first type, C^{14} labelled cholesterol(25 μCi in olive oil per kg body weight) was administered by stomach tube on the same day the catheter was inserted (Day 0) and the rabbits were sacrificed at various time (N) intervals up to 60 weeks. Four days prior to sacrifice (Day N-4) a second dose containing a similar amount of H^3 labelled cholesterol

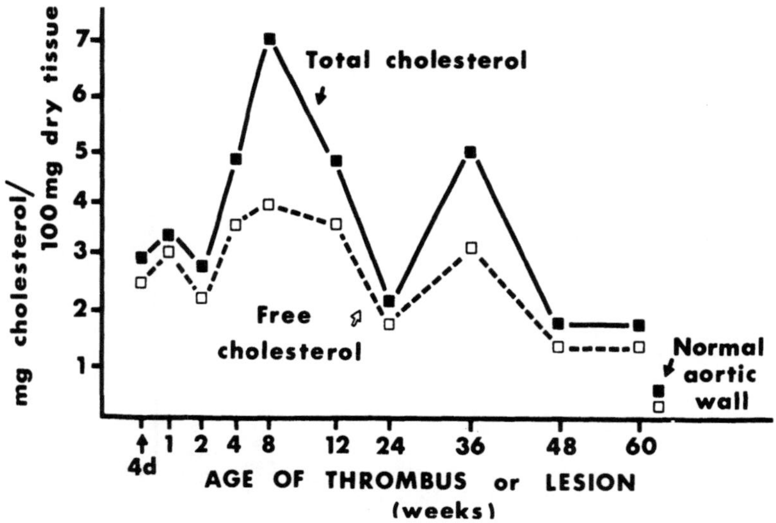

Figure 1. This figure shows the mean accumulation of unlabelled cholesterol in organizing thrombi as they evolve into fibrofatty type atherosclerotic lesions in normolipidemic rabbits. Each point represents the mean of at least 20 rabbits. Further details of the lipid chemistry of these lesions are described in another paper (8).

was administered in order to measure the accumulation of new cholesterol by permeation into these lesions during a 4-day interval between Day N and Day N-4. The fresh thrombus or organized thrombus or fibrofatty lesions were removed and separated from the aortic wall, lipids extracted, chromatographed on silicic acid columns and the radioactivity in the free and esterified cholesterol fractions was counted. It was also of some interest to simultaneously measure the cholesterol accumulating in the Evans blue positive injured abdominal aortic wall and the normal non-injured thoracic aorta of the same rabbits. The data were expressed as DPM per 100 mg dry tissue, or as specific activity (DPM per cholesterol).

In Fig. 2 the open squares show the cholesterol uptake after its administration on Day 0 by organizing thrombus while the black squares show the cholesterol uptake by the lesions when administered 4 days prior to sacrifice (Day N-4). It should be noted that the scale in Fig. 2 is 10 times the scale of Fig. 3 for the injured aortic wall. It may be seen in Fig. 2 that the cholesterol uptake by the organizing thrombus is about 10 times higher than the injured wall shown in Fig. 3, and was more than 30 times the uptake by the normal aortic wall. In the organizing thrombus, shown in Fig. 2, there is decline with time in the DPM per 100 mg

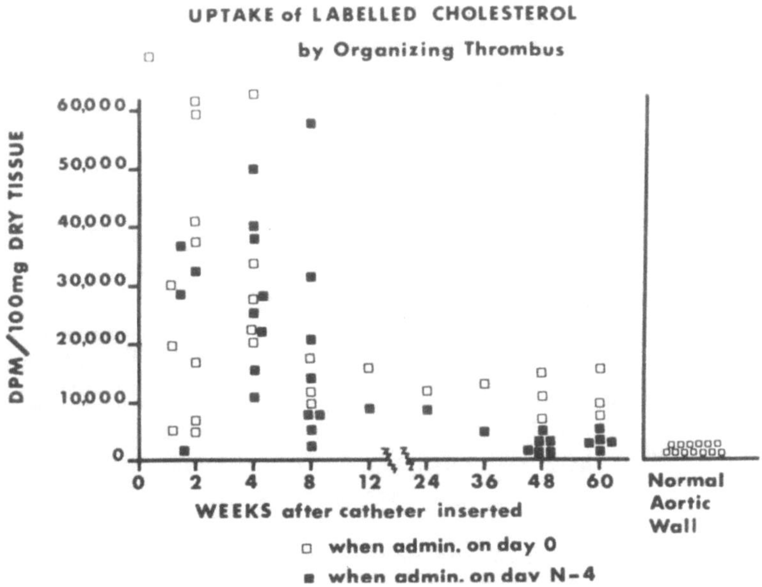

Figure 2

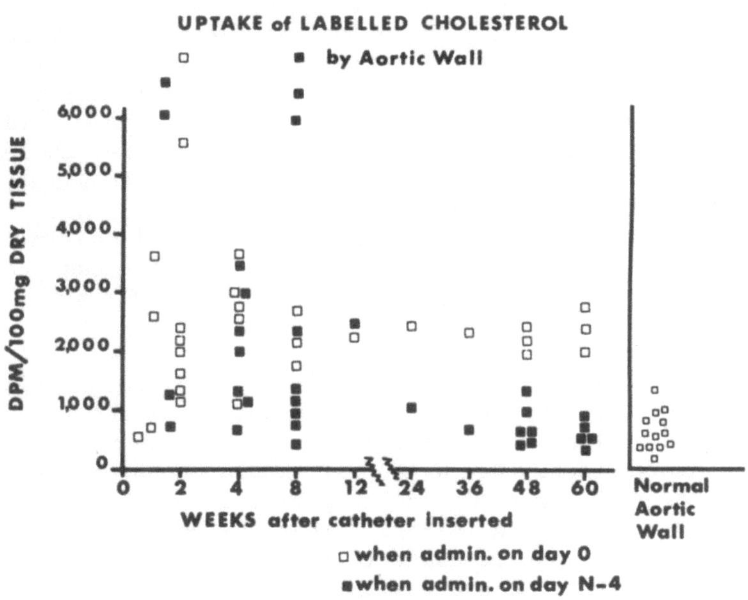

Figure 3

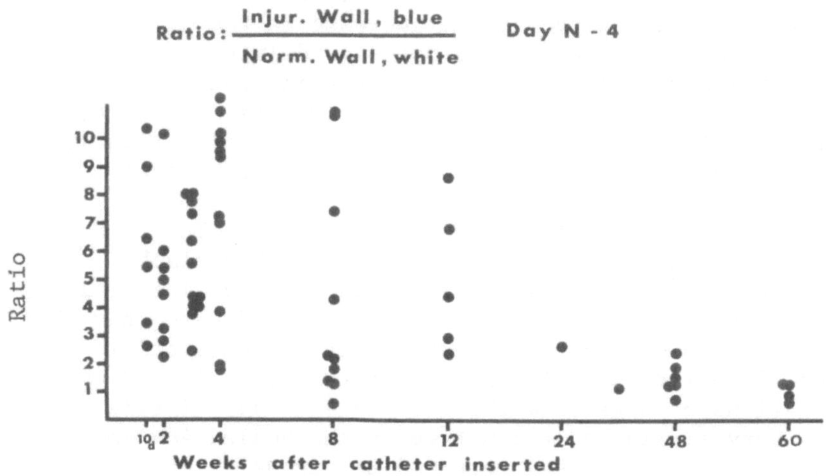

Figure 4. Ratio of labelled cholesterol in injured wall to normal wall of the same rabbit.

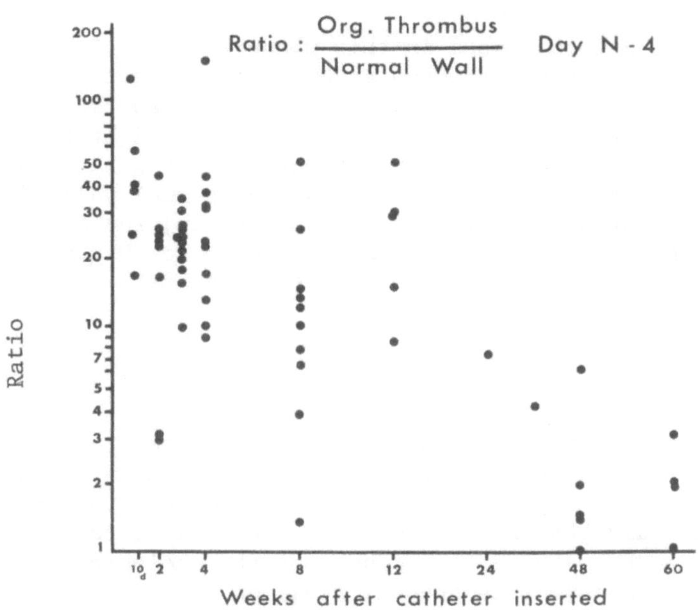

Figure 5. Ratio of labelled cholesterol in organizing thrombus to normal wall of the same rabbit.

dry tissue in the white open squares, originating from the cholesterol trapped in the thrombus on Day 0. Some of this decline can be partly explained by the increase in the size and growth of the lesions. Since the isotope was administered at the time when thrombosis was first initiated, the lipoprotein plasma cholesterol trapped in the thrombus at thisttime was diluted by the subsequent growth of the resulting lesions and this probably caused a dilution of the labelled cholesterol by more tissue.

Another explanation for this decline is that the labelled cholesterol is exchanging or leaving the lesion. The black squares which show the uptake of tritiated labelled cholesterol administered 4 days prior to sacrifice (Day N-4) indicate that the organizing thrombus at 4 and 8 weeks takes up substantial amounts of new labelled cholesterol. In contrast, at 48 and 60 weeks these lesions of organized thrombus take up very little new cholesterol. Very similarly, the uptake by the healed 48- and 60-week injured aorta in Fig. 3 has returned to virtually the same range of values found in the normal wall.

In view of the wide scatter it appeared to be of interest to determine the scatter if the data for each rabbit-injured wall or thrombus were expressed as a ratio of uptake to the normal aortic non-injured arch and thoracic aorta of the same rabbit.

When the data are expressed in this manner in Fig. 5, it may be seen that the organizing thrombus accumulated between 30 and 100 times more labelled cholesterol than the normal aortic wall (shown in Fig. 5) during the first 4 days on a dry weight basis. At 12 weeks this ratio declined somewhat but still has between 10 and 50 times more labelled cholesterol than the normal wall of the same rabbit. In contrast, Fig. 4 shows that the injured abdominal aortic wall (Evans blue positive) takes up from 3 to 10 times more labelled cholesterol than the uptake of the normal wall of the same rabbit.

Discussion and Conclusions

Smith (9), in a comparative study of mural thrombi, plasma and atherosclerotic lesions, noted firstly that the cholesterol in platelets themselves cannot account for the cholesterol of atherosclerotic lesions, and secondly that human organizing thrombi do not trap sufficient plasma cholesterol to account for the cholesterol in atherosclerotic lesions. This present study of the uptake of labelled cholesterol by organizing thrombi in rabbits indicates firstly, that cholesterol originating from plasma is trapped in the thrombus when it forms, and secondly, that the organizing thrombus, in particular during the first 8 weeks, has an exceptionally strong capacity to take up and accumulate new cholesterol. The injured aortic wall takes up between 3 and 10 times more labelled cholesterol than the non-injured normal aortic wall, however, organizing thrombus takes up 10 times more cholesterol than the injured aortic wall and takes up between 30 and 100 times more cholesterol than the normal aortic wall. The results suggest that a significant amount of labelled cholesterol is trapped in the thrombus and remains in the organizing thrombus and this may constitute something more than half of the cholesterol found in the late lesion. The remainder of the cholesterol appears to arise by permeating into the lesion during the period between 4 days and 12 weeks.

This work suggests that clinically <u>if</u> arterial thrombosis is diagnosed it would be desirable to maintain low serum cholesterol levels during the first critical 8-week period in order to reduce the cholesterol uptake by the organizing thrombus. If the cholesterol uptake of the organizing thrombus can be reduced there are many reasons to believe that the progression of the resulting lesions to complicated atherosclerotic lesions may also be reduced and this may slow down the vicious circle of atherosclerosis and thrombosis.

References

1. Friedman, M. and Byers, S.O. Experimental thromboatherosclerosis. J. Clin. Invest. 40: 1139, 1961.
2. Friedman, M., Byers, S.O. and George, S.S. Origin of lipid and cholesterol in experimental thromboatherosclerosis. J.Clin. Invest. 41: 828, 1962.
3. Friedman, M. Pathogenesis of Coronary Artery Disease. McGraw-Hill, N.Y., 1969.
4. Sumiyoshi, A., More, R.H. and Weigensberg, B.I. Aortic fibro-fatty type atherosclerosis from thrombus in normolipidemic rabbits. Atherosclerosis 18: 43, 1973.
5. Moore, S. Thromboatherosclerosis in normolipidemic rabbits. A result of continued endothelial damage. Lab. Invest. 29: 478, 1973.
6. Weigensberg, B.I., More, R.H., Sumiyoshi, A. and Mullen, B. Effects of a surfactant on two types of atherosclerosis. Exp. Molec. Pathol. 20: 422, 1974.
7. Day, A.J., Bell, F.P., Moore, S. and Friedman, R. Lipid composition and metabolism of thromboatherosclerotic lesions produced by continued endothelial damage in normal rabbits. Circ. Res. 34: 467, 1974.
8. Weigensberg, B.I., More, R.H., Sumiyoshi, A. Lipid profile in the evolution of experimental atherosclerotic plaques from thrombus. Lab. Invest. 33: 1975.
9. Smith, E.B. Quantitative and qualitative comparison of the lipids in platelets, aortic intima and mural thrombi. Cardiovas. Res. 1: 111, 1967.

(5)

MURAL THROMBOSIS AND PLAQUE GROWTH

Dr. Neville Woolf

Department of Histopathology
Bland-Sutton Institute
Middlesex Hospital Medical School
London, England

The suggestion that thrombosis may play a part in the growth of atherosclerotic plaques is by no means new since it was first put forward by Rokitansky some 130 years ago. Duguid in 1946 revived interest in what has been called the "thrombogenic hypothesis" a poor term since it appears to carry for some the connotation that mural thrombosis is the initiating factor in atherogenesis. Assessment of the possible role of mural thrombosis in plaque growth can be carried out, basically in two ways. The first of these depends on identification of thrombotic residua in atherosclerotic plaques, the determination of the frequency with which this occurs and the relationship, if any, to the presence of clinically significant occlusive arterial disease. The second approach to the problem lies in a study of the natural history of experimentally induced thrombosis in a variety of animal species.

IDENTIFICATION OF INCORPORATED MURAL THROMBUS IN HUMAN ATHEROSCLEROTIC LESIONS

Thrombotic residua may often be identified with ease in conventionally prepared histological material stained with H & E by the presence of bands of brightly eosinophilic material moulded to the outlines of the plaque cap or appearing within the substance of the plaque cap well below the luminal surface of the vessel. The use of appropriate special stains such as the Lendrum Picro-

Mallory technique may be of further assistance and in the case of recent thrombi the platelet and fibrin components can be distinguished from each other.

Conventional staining techniques for fibrin and platelets are capricious and dependent, at least in part, on the age of the thrombi and more consistent results have been obtained by the application of the Coens fluorescent antibody technique.

Treatment of frozen sections of human atherosclerotic lesions with sera prepared against human fibrin has revealed two basic distribution patterns (Woolf, 1961). The first of these, found most frequently in gelatinous elevations, fatty streaks and small predominantly fatty plaques, is characterized by diffuse fluorescence in the thickened intima occasional flecks of fluorescent material being present in the media as well. In the second, which is found most frequently in raised lesions (fibrolipid plaques) with a well-formed connective tissue cap, the antigen appears in the form of coarse band-like aggregates. These tend to be roughly parallel to the luminal surface of the vessel wall and are often multilayered. (Fig. 1). When sequential sections of these lesions are treated with anti-human platelet sera consistently negative results are obtained when the DIFFUSE pattern of anti-fibrin binding has been observed. In contrast the presence of the BANDED pattern of anti-fibrin binding is associated with the presence of platelet antigens in approximately half the plaques studied. (Fig. 2). It seems likely to us that this banded pattern of anti-fibrin binding represents the residuum of incorporated mural thrombosis. (Woolf and Carstairs, 1967).

FREQUENCY OF IDENTIFICATION OF THROMBOTIC RESIDUA AND ITS RELATIONSHIP TO OCCLUSIVE ARTERIAL DISEASE

For technical reasons it is easier to carry out studies of the INCIDENCE of plaque with the banded pattern of anti-fibrin binding in the aorta rather than in the coronary arteries. In the latter site, prevalence studies have shown plaques of this type to be present in 27/38 patients dying with coronary artery occlusion as opposed to 14/51 patients without occlusion.

In the aorta published data suggest that incorporated mural thrombus may be present in 41-45% of plaques.

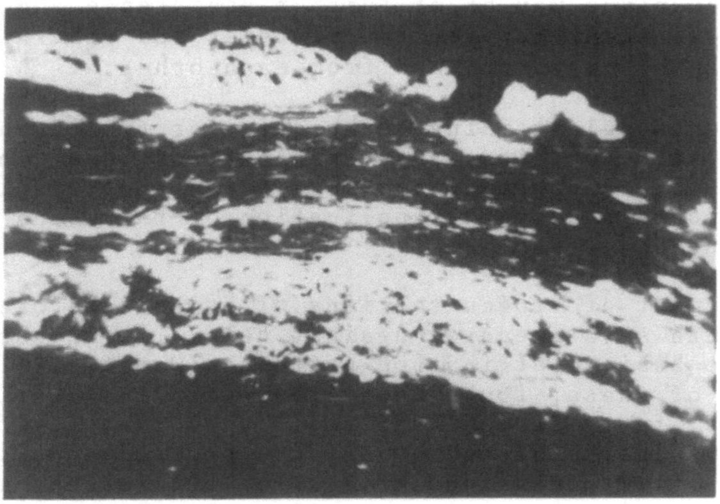

Figure 1.
Aortic atherosclerotic plaque. Frozen section treated with fluoresceinated anti-fibrin serum. Fluorescent material appears in thick focal bands suggesting incorporation of mural thrombus (UVL x600).

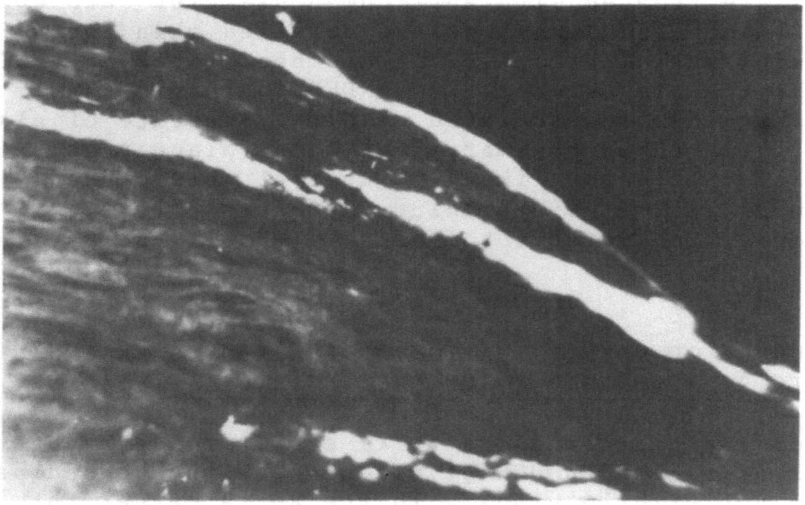

Figure 2.
Aortic atherosclerotic plaque. Frozen section treated with fluoresceinated anti-human platelet serum. Fluorescent material is present within the thickened intima in the form of isolated layers suggesting multiple episodes of thrombosis with subsequent incorporation (UVL x1200).

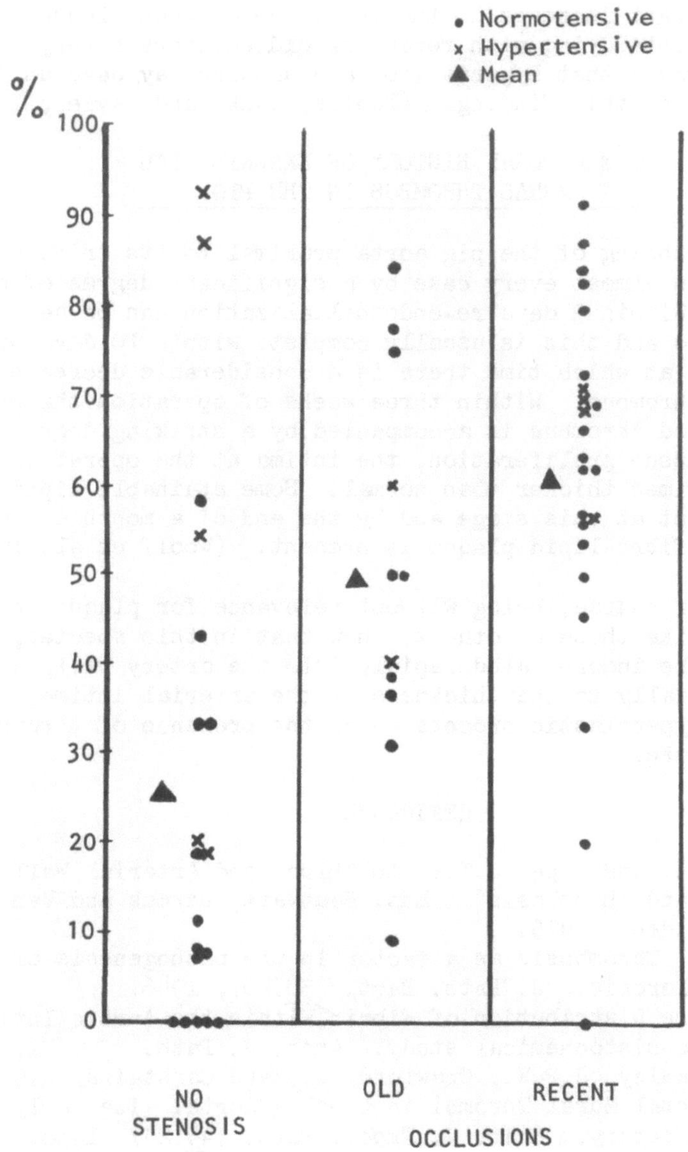

Figure 3
This diagram illustrates the proportion of plaques from each case showing the banded pattern of fibrin distribution. Each dot represents one case. The proportions are expressed as percentages of plaques examined per case. The cases have been divided into three groups: (1) those with no stenosis; (2) those with old occlusions and (3) those with recent occlusions.

(Chandler and Pope, 1974). Our own data (Fig. 3) show a statistically significant increase in the incidence of such plaques in the aorta of patients dying with recent or old coronary artery occlusion, and suggest that hypertension and smoking may have an incremental effect on this finding. (Woolfe, Sacks and Davies, 1969).

THE NATURAL HISTORY OF EXPERIMENTAL MURAL THROMBUS IN THE PIG

Gentle rubbing of the pig aorta proximal to its trifurcation is followed in almost every case by a significant degree of mural thrombosis. Within 3 days re-endothelialization can be seen to have commenced and this is usually complete within 10 days of internal abrasion, at which time there is a considerable decrease in the bulk of the thrombus. Within three weeks of operation the presence of incorporated thrombus is accompanied by a striking degree of connective tissue proliferation, the intima at the operation sites being 10-15 times thicker than normal. Some stainable lipid is usually present at this stage and by the end of a month a small but definite fibro-lipid plaque is present. (Woolf et al. 1968).

While, of course, being without relevance for plaque initiation these data (like those of others) show that in this species, mural thrombus can be incorporated rapidly into the artery wall, and add very substantially to the thickness of the arterial intima, chiefly through the hyperplastic process which the presence of thrombus appears to evoke.

REFERENCES

Chandler, A.B., and Pope, J.T.: In "Blood and Arterial Wall Atherogenesis and Thrombosis". Eds. Hautvast, Hermus and Van der Haar, Leiden. 1975.

Duguid, J.B.: Thrombosis as a factor in the pathogenesis of coronary atherosclerosis. J. Path. Bact. 58:207, 1946.

Woolf, N.: The Distribution of Fibrin Within the Aortic Intima: An immuno-histochemical study. Amer. J. Path. 39:521, 1961.

Woolf, N., Bradley, J.P.W., Crawford, T., and Carstairs, K.C.: Experimental Mural Thrombi in the Pig Aorta. The Early Natural History. Brit. J. Exper. Path. 49:257, 1968.

Woolf, N., and Carstairs, K.C.: Infiltration and Thrombosis in Atherogenesis - a study using immuno-fluorescent techniques. Amer. J. Path. 51:373, 1967.

Woolf, N., Sacks, M.I. and Davies, M.J.: Aortic Plaque Morphology in Relation to Coronary Artery Disease. Amer. J. Path. 57: 487, 1969.

(6)

DYNAMICS OF THROMBUS FORMATION

M.A. Packham and J.F. Mustard

Department of Biochemistry, University of Toronto and Department of Pathology, McMaster University Hamilton, Ontario, Canada

In the arterial circulation, thrombi may form in response to vessel wall injury, or in response to intravascular agents such as antigen-antibody complexes, viruses or bacteria. Vessel injury is believed to be related to the development of atherosclerosis and its complications and thrombosis also appears to have a role in these processes. These subjects have been reviewed recently (1, 2, 3).

When a vessel wall is injured, subendothelial structures to which platelets can adhere are exposed. These are collagen, basement membrane, and the microfibrils around elastin. Collagen also activates factor XII of the blood coagulation sequence. Activated factor XII promotes reactions leading to thrombin generation but also causes the conversion of plasminogen to plasmin and the formation of plasma kinins. Tissue thromboplastin may also become available at an injury site and activate the intrinsic pathway of blood coagulation.

When platelets adhere to collagen, or interact with the thrombin that is generated, they release the contents of their storage granules (4). Among the released materials is adenosine diphosphate (ADP) which causes platelets flowing past the injury site to adhere to the platelets that are already adherent to exposed subendothelial structures. Thus a mass of aggregated platelets forms. Its growth is governed mainly by blood flow, the concentration of released ADP, and the amount of thrombin that is generated. Thrombin generation is accelerated by the platelet phospholipoprotein (platelet factor 3) which becomes available during the release reaction (5). In addition to causing the platelet release reaction and thus promoting further platelet aggregation, thrombin also causes fibrin to polymerize around the aggregated platelets. Platelets adhere to polymerizing fibrin around and under the thrombus (6), and fibrin helps to stabilize the thrombus (7). Platelet aggregates formed in response to ADP break up rapidly unless fibrin forms and prevents their immediate dissolution. If sufficient fibrin forms around the initial mass to stabilize it, the thrombus may persist and eventually be incorporated into the vessel wall, producing an intimal thickening. However, if proteolysis of the fibrin occurs as the result of the action of the fibrinolytic enzyme plasmin, the platelet-fibrin thrombus will be broken up within a few hours.

The growth of a thrombus will be greatest in areas of disturbed blood flow; the forces that influence this have been studied in detail by Goldsmith (8). In areas where flow is slow or disturbed large amounts of fibrin may form and red cells will be trapped in the thrombus.

The platelet-fibrin thrombus generates factors that are chemotactic for leukocytes (9), and the platelets release materials which promote thrombus growth and affect the vessel wall. Among the released materials (10) are ATP, ADP, serotonin, adrenaline, lysosomal enzymes, cationic proteins, mucopolysaccharides, fibrinogen, platelet factor 4, factors that increase vessel permeability (11), and a factor that stimulates the growth of smooth muscle cells (12) and fibroblasts (13). Elastase (14) and collagenase (15) also appear in the medium around platelets which have undergone a release reaction. In addition, the response of platelets to release-inducing agents is associated with the formation of prostaglandins E_2 and $F_{2\alpha}$ from platelet arachidonic acid; some of the short-lived intermediates and by-products of this pathway themselves cause platelet aggregation and the release reaction (16-18). Materials from platelets may be responsible for the vessel wall changes and vasculitis that can develop at sites where platelet aggregates are in contact with a vessel wall (19).

Direct observation of the microcirculation has shown that thrombi are not static structures. Although they form rapidly at sites of vessel wall injury, they tend to break down, the emboli are swept away by the flowing blood, and the thrombi may reform. Baumgartner (20) has shown that removal of the endothelium of the rabbits' aorta results in immediate formation of thrombi on the subendothelium. However, forty minutes after the injury, much of the thrombus material has been dislodged and only a thin layer of adherent platelets remains. The platelets which have taken part in thrombus formation and then have been dislodged can return to the circulation and survive normally; this has been shown for platelets aggregated by ADP (21) or extensively degranulated by thrombin (22). It is not known whether platelets that have adhered to subendothelial structures can return to the circulation, but new thrombus material does not tend to adhere to areas where thrombi have been dislodged. It is understandable, therefore, that areas of vessel injury can be found that do not appear to have platelets or fibrin associated with them (23-25).

The emboli that pass downstream when a thrombus is dislodged, or the platelet aggregates that form in response to intravascular agents such as antigen-antibody complexes, viruses, and bacteria, may injure the organs downstream where the emboli impact in the microcirculation. Mural thrombi at the bifurcation of the internal carotid artery can fragment and shower the cerebral circulation with micro-emboli; these have been observed passing through the retinal circulation and are considered to be responsible for transient monocular blindness and cerebral dysfunction (26, 27). Moore (28, 29) has provided evidence that mural thrombi above the renal arteries may shower the kidney with micro-emboli, causing chronic renal disease and elevated blood pressure. There is less evidence concerning this mechanism in the coronary circulation where thrombi may form in association with atherosclerotic lesions. It has been shown experimentally in animals that transient platelet aggregates in the microcirculation of the myocardium can lead to arrhythmia and sudden death (30). These aggregates could only be found in histological sections removed immediately; after thirty minutes the aggregates had broken up and could not be observed. Moschos et al. (31) have shown that experimentally induced thrombi in the coronary artery of dogs embolize into the distal circulation. Since the time before human post-mortem material can be examined is much longer than in animal experiments, histological evidence of this process in man is difficult to obtain, although Haerem (32) has reported finding a slightly higher incidence of platelet aggregates in the microcirculation of individuals with coronary heart disease who died suddenly than in persons who died suddenly of other causes. It seems likely that thromboemboli which impact in the microcirculation may be responsible for some of the sudden deaths that occur in association with coronary artery disease but we do not know what proportion of the sudden deaths in this condition are attributable to this mechanism.

Intravascular platelet aggregates may also be responsible for organ disfunction in some cases. Haft and his colleagues (33, 34) have shown that noradrenaline infusion or stress cause the formation of platelet aggregates in the microcirculation of the myocardium under conditions in which mural thrombi did not form in the main coronary artery.

It should also be pointed out that some types of dietary fat, smoking and some hormones such as oestrogens have been shown to enhance thrombosis in experimental animals and man (1).

Thus thrombi are generally not static structures. There is a balance between the effects of the factors promoting their growth and those causing their dissolution. Many thrombi are unstable, break up immediately or after fibrinolysis, and shower the distal circulation with thrombo-emboli. Other thrombi are only partially removed by flowing blood and remain to become incorporated into the vessel wall.

1. Mustard, J.F., Packham, M.A., Moore, S. and Kinlough-Rathbone, R.L. In: Atherosclerosis III, eds. G. Schettler and A. Weizel, Springer-Verlag, New York, pp. 253-267, 1974.

2. Mustard, J.F., Kinlough-Rathbone, R.L. and Packham, M.A. Thromb. Diath. Haemorrh. Suppl. 59, 157-188, 1974.

3. Mustard, J.F. and Packham, M.A. Thromb. Diath. Haemorrh. Suppl. (in press).

4. Hovig, T. Thromb. Diath. Haemorrh. 9, 264-278, 1963.

5. Joist, J.H., Lloyd, J.V. and Mustard, J.F. J. Lab. Clin. Med. 84, 474-482, 1974.

6. Niewiarowski, S., Regoeczi, E., Stewart, G.J., Senyi, A. and Mustard, J.F. J. Clin. Invest. 51, 685-700, 1972.

7. Hirsh, J., Buchanan, M., Glynn, M.F. and Mustard, J.F. Blood 32, 726-737, 1968.

8. Goldsmith, H.L. In: Progress in Hemostasis and Thrombosis, Vol. 1. ed. T.H. Spaet, Grune and Stratton, New York, pp. 97-139, 1972.

9. Weksler, B.B. and Coupal, C.E. J. Exp. Med. 137, 1419-1430, 1973.

10. Holmsen, H., Day, H.J. and Stormorken, H. Scand. J. Haemat. Suppl. 8, 1-26, 1969.

11. Packham, M.A., Nishizawa, E.E. and Mustard, J.F. Biochem. Pharmacol. Suppl. 171-184, 1967.

12. Ross, R., Glomset, J., Kariya, B. and Harker, L. Proc. Nat. Acad. Sc. U.S.A. 71, 1207-1210, 1974.

13. Kohler, N. and Lipton, A. Exptl. Cell Research 87, 297-301, 1974.

14. Robert, B., Robert, L., Legrand, Y., Pignaud, G. and Caen, J. Ser. Haemat. 4, 175-185, 1971.

15. Chesney, C.M., Harper, E. and Colman, R.W. J. Clin. Invest. 53, 1647-1654, 1974.

16. Willis, A.L., Vane, F.M., Kuhn, D.C., Scott, C.G. and Petrin, M. Prostaglandins 8, 453-507, 1974.

17. Smith, J.B., Ingerman, C., Kocsis, J.J. and Silver, M.J. J. Clin. Invest. 53, 1468-1472, 1974.

18. Hamberg, M., Svensson, J., Wakabayashi, Y. and Sammuelsson, B. Proc. Nat. Acad. Sc. U.S.A. 71, 345-349, 1974.

19. Jørgensen, L., Hovig, T., Rowsell, H.C. and Mustard, J.F. Amer. J. Pathol. 61, 161-170, 1970.

20. Baumgartner, H.R. Microvascular Res. 5, 167-179, 1973.

21. Mustard, J.F., Rowsell, H.C., Lotz, F., Hegardt, B. and Murphy, E.A. Exptl. Molec. Pathol. 5, 43-60, 1966.

22. Reimers, H.J., Packham, M.A., Kinlough-Rathbone, R.L. and Mustard, J.F. Brit. J. Haematol. 25, 675-689, 1973.

23. Jørgensen L., Packham, M.A., Rowsell, H.C. and Mustard, J.F. Lab. Invest. 27, 341-350, 1972.

24. Gutstein, W.H., Farrell, G.A. and Armellini, C. Lab. Invest. 29, 134-149, 1973.

25. Björkerud, S. and Bondjers, G. Atherosclerosis 18, 235-255, 1973.

26. Fisher, C.M. Neurology (Minneap.) 9, 333-347, 1959.

27. Jørgensen, L. In: Thrombosis eds. S. Sherry, K.M. Brinkhous, E. Genton and J.M. Stengle, Nat. Acad. Sc., Washington, D.C. 506-533, 1969.

28. Moore, S. J. Path. Bact. 88, 471-478, 1964.

29. Moore, S. Geriatrics 24, 81-90, 1969.

30. Jørgensen, L., Rowsell, H.C., Hovig, T., Glynn, M.F. and Mustard, J.F. Lab. Invest. 17, 616-644, 1967.

31. Moschos, C.B., Lahiri, K., Lyons, M., Weisse, A.B., Oldewurtel, H.A. and Regan, T.J. Amer. Heart J. 86, 61-86, 1973.

32. Haerem, J.W. Atherosclerosis 15, 199-213, 1972.

33. Haft, J.I., Kranz, P.D., Albert, F.J. and Fani, K. Circulation 46, 698-708, 1972.

34. Haft, J.I. and Fani. K. Circulation 47, 353-358, 1973.

(7)

SUMMARY (PLASMA LIPIDS AND THROMBOSIS)

Dr. S. Renaud

Director, INSERM, U63
22, Avenue du Doyen-Lépine
69500 Lyon-Bron, France

More than a century ago, Virchow postulated that three main factors were essential for thrombosis to occur. It seems that today the Virchow's triad is still valid with minor additions as follows :

1- Stasis or as emphasized by Dr. Packham (1), modifications of blood flow.

2- Endothelial lesions or in a more general way, a triggering event. Dr. Packham in this workshop (1) has underlined what could be the mechanisms involved in that event.

3- An alteration in blood coagulation. Since we have now some deeper knowledge, than in the middle of the 19 th century, on the mechanisms involved in thrombus formation, we can foresee that the alteration in blood, susceptible to predispose to thrombosis, might take place at different levels. In brief, it might be due to

a) an increase in the susceptibility of platelets to form aggregates, the earliest phase of a thrombus.
b) an increase in the speed or the quantity of fibrin formed to stabilize the platelet aggregates. This might result from an increase in the activity of the clotting factors or a decrease in the activity of antithrombin.
c) a decrease in the removal of fibrin resulting from a decrease in fibrinolytic activity.
d) a combined effect occuring at the three levels, mentioned above.

We will not make any attempt to determine which of these parameters might be more important for the predisposition to thrombosis induced by lipids. It seems that, at the present time, we have more knowledge of the mechanisms involved in the effect of lipids on platelet aggregation and platelet clotting activity and that most of the animal experiments we have performed did not indicate that by blocking fibrinolysis, we can predispose to thrombosis. However, further work on the role of fibrinolysis in thrombosis, is certainly needed to determine the entent of its participation in that event.

Dr. Marsh and Dr. Shaper (2) have reported data indicating that the fibrinolytic activity in response to venous occlusion, was decreased in patients prone to coronary heart disease. This suggests that fibrin can be more easily deposited on vessel walls and that thrombosis has more chances to occur.

Dr. Hornstra (3) and several other investigators including ourselves (4) have shown that saturated dietary fats predispose to thrombosis in animals. Hornstra has also reported (5) that the thrombogenic fatty acids were increasing the susceptibility of platelets to aggregation, a result we had also noted in our experimental conditions in animals (4,6,7). In fact, feeding rats for 3 months physiologic diets containing 25% fat and only 0.1% cholesterol conduced according to the type of fat fed, to marked differences in the susceptibility of platelets to thrombin induced aggregation, as we observed recently in still underway experiments.

We have previously reported (8) that this increase in the platelet susceptibility to aggregation was also associated with an increase in the activity of the so-called platelet factor 3. This factor 3 activity is in fact an activity of the platelet phospholipids (9). It seems that by changing the fatty acid composition of these platelet phospholipids as it results from various fats feeding, one changes both the susceptibility to aggregation and the clotting activity of platelets.

Many other clotting factors appear to have an increase in their activity in hyperlipemic animals, but platelet factor 3 is probably of special interest since as compared to the other clotting factors which even normally, are largely in excess, platelet factor 3 might be the limiting factor of coagulation, and therefore an increase in its activity appears to result in the acceleration of blood clotting (8).

In support of the animal experiments, human studies have conduced to similar results. Dr. Carvalho and her collaborators in Boston (10) have recently reported that in hyperlipoproteinemic patients, particularly in type II, a marked increase in the susceptibility of platelets to aggregation could be observed. In **normo-lipidemic** coronary patients, we found that it was mostly to thrombin that the platelets were suceptible (7). In addition, these patients presented a marked increase in their platelet factor 3 clotting activity.

Those results emphasize some of the mechanisms by which blood lipids and dietary fats, might predispose to thrombosis, either occluding or mural. In coronary heart disease, this lipid induced predisposition to thrombosis appears to be highly significant not only because coronary thrombosis is most of the time, the final occluding event, but also because there is more and more evidence that mural thrombosis contributes significantly to the atherosclerotic plaque formation. We do not know so far whether all the fibrous plaques derive from an organized thrombus but as emphasized by Dr. Chandler, to-day we do know that a large proportion of them contain platelets and fibrin, and probably result from the organization of a mural thrombus as indicated several years ago by Haust and colleagues (12). The role of mural thrombosis has been substantiated in this workshop by the presentation of Dr. Woolf following the pionner work of Duguid (11), and of the Canadian investigators (12) mentioned above. Some of the mechanisms involved in the lipid accumulation during the organization of the mural thrombus into a fibro-fatty type atherosclerotic lesion have been emphasized by the work of Dr. Weigensberg (13).

Also of interest here regarding the relationship between platelets, thrombosis and atherosclerosis is, as mentioned by Dr. Packham, the recent results of Ross and his colleagues on a platelet substance able to stimulate the proliferation of smooth muscle cells, the cells found to be, as emphasized yesterday by Dr. Haust, in large number, in fibrous plaques.

I **would** like to conclude by saying that we have now some evidence from human as well as from animal studies, that dietary fats and blood lipids seem to be predisposing to thrombosis per se, apart from the atherosclerotic lesions they might induce. In fact we have even evidence that lipids might induce atherosclerotic fibrous plaque formation through thrombosis.

Changing the type of dietary fat eaten, might be the cheapest and the most effective way to eliminate thrombosis, one of the most significant contributing event to coronary heart disease.

REFERENCES

1- Packham, M.A. and Mustard, J.F. Dynamics of thrombus formation; **this book.**

2- Marsch, N.A. and Shaper, A.G. Fibrinolytic activity and risk factors for atherosclerosis; **this book.**

3- Hornstra, G. Dietary fatty acids and thrombosis : Effects and mechanism of action with special reference to linoleic acid; this book.

4- Renaud, S. and Godu, J. Induction of large thrombi in hyperlipemic rats by epinephrine and endotoxin. Lab. Invest. 21: 512 1969.

5- Hornstra, G. Dietary fats and arterial thrombosis. In "Dietary fats and thrombosis" S. Karger publ., Basel, 1974, p. 21

6- Renaud, S., Kinlough, R. and Mustard, J.F. Relationship between platelet aggregation and the thrombotic tendency in rats fed hyperlipemic diets. Lab. Invest. 22: 339, 1970.

7- Renaud, S., Kuba, K., Goulet, C., Lemire, Y. et Allard, C. Relationship between platelet fatty acid composition and platelet aggregation in rat and man, in connection with thrombosis. Circulat. Res. 26: 553, 1970.

8- Renaud, S. and Lecompte, F. Hypercoagulability induced by hyperlipemia in rat, rabbit and man. Role of platelet factor 3 Circulat. Res. 27: 1003, 1970.

9- Gautheron, P., Dumont, E. and Renaud, S. Clotting activity of platelet phospholipids in rat and man. Thromb. Diath. Haemorrh. 32: 382, 1974.

10- Carvalho, A.C.A., Colman, R.W. and Lees, R.S. Platelet function in hyperlipoproteinemia. N. Engl. J. Med. 290: 434, 1974.

11- Duguid, J.B. Thrombosis as a factor in the pathogenesis of coronary atherosclerosis. J. Path. Bact. 58: 207, 1946.

12- Haust, D., More, R.H. and Movat, H.Z. The mechanism of fibrosis in arteriosclerosis. Amer. J. Path. 35: 265, 1959.

13- Weigensberg, B.I. and More, R.H. Uptake of cholesterol by organising thrombi; this book.

(8)

OPENING REMARKS TO DISCUSSION

A. B. Chandler, M.D.
Eugene Talmadge Memorial Hospital
Medical College of Georgia

Augusta, Georgia, U.S.A.

In opening the general discussion of this session on the interrelationships of plasma lipids and thrombosis, I would like to focus on the thrombotic build-up of atherosclerotic plaques. From the outset, I would join Dr. Woolf in emphasizing the role of thrombosis in contributing to the growth and progression of atherosclerotic lesions. Thrombosis is less likely to be a significant factor in the initiation of the disease, even though embolic thrombi can give rise to plaques in a previously normal artery (1). Lipids are related to the pathogenesis of thrombotic plaques essentially through two pathways: 1) dietary and plasma lipids may influence both the formation and lysis of thrombi, and 2) the lipids in thrombi may directly contribute to the lipid content of the plaques.

There is a long history of experimental studies on the association of dietary and plasma lipids with thrombosis (2). Today, we heard from Dr. Hornstra some of the ways dietary long-chain saturated fatty acids enhance platelet reactivity and promote experimental arterial thrombosis. Of particular interest is the evidence presented for a long-term protective effect against thrombosis through the intake and storage of unsaturated fatty acids. Observations in man on the thrombogenic effects of dietary and plasma lipids are limited mainly to in vitro assessment of platelet reactivity and coagulability, not to actual thrombotic events within an artery.

Another important determinant of the fate of thrombi discussed by Dr. Packham is the balance between those factors that promote thrombosis and those factors that favor the dissolution of thrombi. Marsh and Shaper have correlated high fibrinolytic activity with low levels of plasma lipids and cholesterol. Other experimental studies indicate that hyperlipemia may directly interfere with thrombolysis, and lead to the formation of a more stable and larger thrombus (1).

Thus, plasma lipids could act as a two-edged sword in the thrombotic growth of plaques by promoting thrombosis and inhibiting thrombolysis.

The lipid content of thrombi might be expected to affect the lipid composition of a thrombotic plaque (3). Platelets are a major source of lipid in thrombi. They are especially rich in cholesterol, which seems to be present in platelets in proportion to plasma levels (4). One mechanism whereby platelets acquire lipid after release from the marrow is by phagocytosis of lipid particles in plasma (5). The contribution of platelet and other cellular lipids of thrombi must be weighed against that of the plasma lipids that are incorporated during and after thrombus formation. Woolf, Pilkington and Carstairs (6) first showed some years ago that plasma lipoproteins are incorporated in thrombi. Now, Weigensberg and More, by their quantitative experimental studies, have fully corroborated that plasma lipids, specifically cholesterol, may be entrapped by a forming thrombus and continue to be absorbed as it organizes.

What is the role of endothelial regeneration in the development of thrombotic plaques? As long as the thrombus is uncovered, absorption of plasma, and either lysis or growth might occur. Hence, the rate of endothelial overgrowth could markedly affect the ultimate size of the thrombotic-vascular lesion. In man, it takes 6-8 days for endothelium to cover a small arterial needle puncture (7). It is of interest to note that Davies et al. (8) have shown that hyperlipemia does not influence the rate of endothelial regeneration over thrombi in the experimental animal.

Lastly, I wish to comment on the quantitative studies in man that indicate the frequency with which thrombi can be found incorporated in plaques. Most work over the past 40 years has been reported on aortic lesions, and in older age groups. Since thrombi, in time, lose their identity as they are organized and converted to plaque tissue, the published data indicating a frequency of 41-45% incorporated thrombi in aortic plaques would seem to be an underestimate of the true incidence (3). These observations would suggest that the relative contribution of thrombosis to plaque growth is substantial.

REFERENCES

1) Chandler, A.B.: Thrombosis and the development of atherosclerotic lesions. In: Second International Symposium on Atherosclerosis, Jones, R.J. (ed.), New York, Springer-Verlag, 1970, pp. 88-93.

2) Hornstra, G.: Dietary fats and arterial thrombosis. Haemostasis 2: 21-53, 1973-1974.

3) Chandler, A.B. and Pope, J.T.: Arterial thrombosis in atherogenesis A survey of the frequency of incorporation of thrombi into atherosclerotic plaques. In: Blood and Arterial Wall in Atherogenesis and Arterial Thrombosis, Hautvast, J.G.A.J., Hermus, R.J.J. VanDerHaar, F. (eds.) Leiden, E.J. Brill, 1975, pp. 110-118.

4) Shattil, S.J., Anaya-Galindo, R., Bennett, J., et al.: Platelet hypersensitivity induced by cholesterol incorporation. J. Clin. Invest. 55: 636-643, 1975.

5) Hovig, T. and Grottum, K.A.: Lipid infusions in man - Ultrastructural studies on blood platelet uptake of fat particles. Thromb. Diath. Haemorrh. 29: 450-460, 1973.

6) Woolf, N., Pilkington, T.R.E. and Carstairs, K.C.: The occurrence of lipoprotein in thrombi. J. Pathol. Bacteriol. 91: 383-387, 1966.

7) Crawford, T.: The healing of puncture wounds in arteries. J. Pathol. Bacteriol. 72: 547-552, 1956.

8) Davies, M.J., Woolf, N. and Bradley, J.P.W.: Endothelialisation of experimentally produced mural thrombi in the pig aorta. J. Pathol. 97: 589-594, 1969.

CHAPTER 8
ANIMAL MODELS IN THE STUDY OF ATHEROSCLEROSIS

(1)

GENETIC STUDIES OF ATHEROSCLEROSIS IN ANIMALS

H. B.Lofland and T. B. Clarkson

Arteriosclerosis Research Center
Bowman Gray School of Medicine of Wake Forest University
Winston-Salem, N. C., U. S. A.

Genetic factors may influence the extent of atherosclerosis by determining the degree of hypercholesterolemia resulting from the daily ingestion of a given amount of cholesterol, by determining the susceptibility of various arteries to the atherosclerotic process, by the co-existence of a primary dyslipoproteinemia or other "risk factor" diseases such as hypertension, or perhaps in other ways not yet understood. In this brief report an attempt is made to review the literature concerning any of these genetic mechanisms as they occur in nonhuman animal populations.

CHICKENS

Chickens have been used in several studies designed to determine the extent of genetic control of plasma control homeostasis. The studies thus far reported have dealt with breeds consuming a grain (low fat-cholesterol free diet (1, 2, 3). The results of the studies are summarized in Table I. The data suggest that about 30% of the variation in plasma cholesterol concentration of chickens is determined by genetic factors.

CATTLE

A single study has been reported concerning genetic control of plasma cholesterol concentration of beef cattle (4). The results of their study are summarized in Table II. During the first year of life it would appear that about 80% of the variation among individuals in plasma cholesterol concentration is determined

TABLE I. GENETIC CONTROL OF PLASMA CHOLESTEROL HOMEOSTASIS IN CHICKENS

Heritability Estimate		Reference
Sire	0.19	Cherms et al. (Poultry Sci. 39: 889-892, 1960)
Dam	0.41	
Sire & Dam	0.30	
Sire	0.34	Wilcox et al. (Poultry Sci. 42: 37-42, 1963)
Dam	0.17	
Sire & Dam	0.25	
Sire	0.26	Estep et al. (Poultry Sci. 48: 1908-1911, 1963)
Dam	0.04	

TABLE II. GENETIC CONTROL OF PLASMA CHOLESTEROL HOMEOSTASIS IN BEEF CATTLE.[a]

Number of Animals	143
Plasma Cholesterol Concentration (mg/dl) ± S.D.	109 ± 18
Heritability Estimate ± S.E.	0.80 ± 0.42

Correlation coefficient between two measurements made at beginning and end of second year was 0.23 suggesting large environmental effect.

[a] Adapted from data of Stufflebean and Lasley (J. Heredity 60: 15-16, 1969).

by genetic factors. It is of interest that there was a rather poor correlation between individual plasma cholesterol concentrations taken early in life and at the end of the second year of life, suggesting to the authors that rather large environmental effects became important with increasing age.

RATS

Considerable information is available on the genetic control of plasma cholesterol concentrations of rats. Kohn (5) examined the plasma cholesterol concentrations of the progeny produced from stocks of rats having similar and dissimilar mean concentrations. The data derived from this study are summarized in Table III. In situations in which F_1 progeny were derived from stocks with dissimilar plasma cholesterol concentrations, their plasma cholesterol concentrations were very nearly at the midpoint of the two parental stocks. When stocks were used with similar cholesterol concentrations the offspring resembled their parents in that regard.

Kohn extended these studies in an attempt to determine the organ system associated with genetic control in rats. He selected a stock of rats with a high plasma cholesterol concentration (Sprague-Dawley) and a stock with a low cholesterol concentration (Holtzman). The animals were hypophysectomized and after 30 days the phenotypic differences in plasma cholesterol concentrations were no longer prevalent. These data are summarized in Table IV. The author interpreted the data as suggesting the mechanisms of genetic control in the rat may, in some way, reside in one of the functions of the pituitary gland.

A particularly valuable contribution to the use of rats in the study of lipid metabolism has been the work of Adel and coworkers (6). By selective breeding of Carworth Farms Nelson Strain rats, these investigators have established two distinctive substrains, one being hyporesponsive to dietary cholesterol while the other is hyperresponsive to the cholesterol containing diet. Descriptive information on these substrains appears in Table V.

Several strains of rats have been selected with genetically determined obesity (for example, the Zucker and Koletsky rats). These animals are said to be hypercholesterolemic and usually hypertriglyceridemic. Unfortunately, no studies of the lipoproteins of these animals could be found to substantiate the usual presumption that the hypercholesterolemia is associated with a hyperbetalipoproteinemia or that the hypertriglyceridemia is associated with an increased plasma cholesterol concentration of prebetalipoproteins.

TABLE III. GENETIC CONTROL OF PLASMA CHOLESTEROL HOMEOSTASIS IN RATS.[a,b]

Parent strain	Parent strain	F1 Progeny	F2 Progeny
Sprague-Dawley (120 ± 6)	Tumblebrook Hooded (68 ± 3)	→ F_1 Progeny (89 ± 5)	→ F_2 Progeny (88 ± 14)
Osborne-Mendel (132 ± 4)	Tumblebrook Hooded (68 ± 3)	→ F_1 Progeny (93 ± 5)	→ F_2 Progeny (93 ± 13)
Osborne-Mendel (132 ± 4)	Holtzman (65 ± 3)	→ F_1 Progeny (94 ± 3)	
Osborne-Mendel (132 ± 4)	Sprague-Dawley (120 ± 6)	→ F_1 Progeny (123 ± 4)	

[a] All plasma cholesterol values are expressed as mean mg/dl ± S.D.

[b] Adapted from data of Kohn (Am. J. Physiology 163: 410-417, 1950).

TABLE IV. EFFECT OF HYPOPHYSECTOMY ON PLASMA CHOLESTEROL PHENOTYPE OF RATS.[a,b]

		Hypophysectomy	
Sprague-Dawley	(120±6) ———	↓ 30 days ——→	(192±5)
Holtzman	(65±3) ———	30 days ——→	(188±8)

[a]Plasma cholesterol values expressed as mg/dl ± S.D.

[b]Adapted from data of Kohn (Am. J. Physiology 163: 410-417, 1950).

TABLE V. GENETIC CONTROL OF PLASMA CHOLESTEROL AND TRIGLYCERIDE CONCENTRATIONS AMONG RATS FED FAT AND CHOLESTEROL.[a,b]

Strain	Sex	Plasma Cholesterol (mg/dl)	Plasma Triglyceride (mg/dl)
Hyperresponder	M	182 (range 151-237)	201
	F	156 (range 136-203)	---
Hyporesponder	M	89 (range 76-113)	132
	F	76 (range 57 - 89)	---

[a]All rats were fed 0.1% cholesterol and 11% fat added to chow.

[b]Adapted from data of Adel *et al*. (Circ. Suppl. 39-40: III-1, 1969).

MICE

In view of the ready availability of large numbers of well defined inbred strains of mice it is surprising that only a few studies have been done on genetic influences on cholesterol metabolism in these animals. Bruell and his coworkers (7) observed differences in plasma cholesterol concentration among inbred strains of mice. Later, Bruell examined the genetic aspects of plasma cholesterol concentration and determined that the trait was neither dominant or recessive but instead intermediate.

Yamamoto et al. (8) have examined genetic variations in plasma lipid concentration of mice. In their studies, genetic control of variation in plasma cholesterol concentrations was suggested since within litter variation was greater in F_2 than in F_1 progeny. Further exploration of mouse strains could be useful to future research.

Like rats, there are several obese strains of mice. These animals are said to have abnormal lipoprotein phenotypes but no careful studies have been reported.

RABBITS

Laird and his coworkers (9) have reported on rather large differences in the mean plasma cholesterol concentration of 11 strains of rabbits. Additionally, Wang et al. (10) reported differences in plasma lipid concentrations within three strains of rabbits. More recently Roberts et al. (11) have attempted to measure the strength of genetic control of the plasma cholesterol increase of rabbits fed a diet containing about 0.5 milligrams of cholesterol per Calorie. Their findings are summarized in Table VI. It is suggested that about 50% of the variability in the response of rabbits to a cholesterol containing diet is under genetic influence.

TABLE VI. GENETIC CONTROL OF PLASMA CHOLESTEROL HOMEOSTASIS OF RABBITS.[a,b]

	Heritability [c] ($h^2 \pm$ SE)
Sire	0.49 ± 0.08
Dam	0.95 ± 0.08
Mid-Parent	0.50 ± 0.05

[a]Adapted from data of Roberts et al. (Atherosclerosis 19: 369-380, 1974).

[b]Response of progeny and parents to diet containing about 0.5 mg of cholesterol/Cal.

[c]h^2 was calculated as 2 times the regression co-efficient for the sire and dam effect and was equal to the regression co-efficient for the mid-parent calculation.

PIGEONS

Naturally occurring atherosclerosis in several breeds of pigeons has been described by our group (12). Among White Carneau pigeons, older than three years, 100% of birds have aortic atherosclerosis. There is no sex difference. The raised yellow plaques cover 10 to 15% of the aortic surface and usually occur in the distal thoracic aorta near the bifurcation of the celiac artery. Coronary artery atherosclerosis occurs in about 70% of adult grain fed White Carneau pigeons. In contrast, Show Racer pigeons have virtually no naturally occurring aortic or coronary artery atherosclerosis. We have examined these atherosclerosis susceptible and resistant pigeons to determine if any consistent differences could be found in plasma lipid concentrations. No differences could be found to explain the presence or absence of this naturally occurring atherosclerosis and the accumulated data would support the conclusion that the genetic differences may be operative at the level of the artery wall (13, 14, 15).

Since the original publications on pigeons as animal models of atherosclerosis, interest has been directed primarily toward attempts to develop substrains of pigeons with greater use for research. Patton and his coworkers (16) studied the variability in plasma cholesterol concentrations among grain fed White Carneaux. They were able to select for increased plasma cholesterol concentrations and to establish that the trait was familial. Later, we examined the offspring of about 75 pairs of pigeons in an attempt to identify parental pairs producing progeny susceptible to the induction of selected atherosclerosis characteristics (17). Based on the atherosclerosis characteristics of progeny the following strains were selected:

1. A strain of White Carneau with severe aortic atherosclerosis having mean aortic cholesterol concentrations of 60.42 mg/g aorta while about 24 mg/g of aorta is usual for the bird.

2. A strain of Show Racer with very little aortic atherosclerosis having a mean aortic cholesterol concentration of 2.40 mg/g aorta while about 5 mg/g of aorta is usual for the bird.

3. A strain of F_2 with concomitant severe coronary artery atherosclerosis (mean coronary artery index of 38) and very little aortic atherosclerosis (mean aortic cholesterol concentration of 6.13 mg/g aorta).

4. A Show Racer and an F_2 strain with a frequency of myocardial infarction of 43 and 60%, respectively, while about 12% is usual for these strains.

In subsequent studies it was determined that Show Racers with the least atherosclerosis were hyporesponsive to dietary cholesterol (having cholesterol concentrations 319-457 mg/dl) while the Show Racer strain with a high frequency of myocardial infarctions was hyperresponsive to dietary cholesterol (plasma cholesterol concentrations 1417-2253 mg/dl) (18). Metabolic studies were undertaken in an attempt to determine the mechanisms of the genetic control of plasma cholesterol in these selected lines of Show Racer pigeons. Some of the results are summarized in Tables VII and VIII. The study failed to clarify the way in which cholesterol metabolism of the strains differ. It is our presumption that clear differences could not be shown because the animals were in the cholesterol steady state at the time the studies were done and that the differences between the strains probably relates to the time consuming the cholesterol added diet or the plasma cholesterol concentrations required to induce metabolic compensation.

TABLE VII. CHOLESTEROL TURNOVER IN HYPER- AND HYPORESPONDER SHOW RACER PIGEONS.

	M_A (mg)	PR_A (mg/day)	k_A
Hyperresponders	841[a] ± 51	70.3 ± 1.4	0.084[a] ± 0.004
Hyporesponders	413 ± 70	75.5 ± 6.4	0.190 ± 0.015

[a]$P < 0.05$
Adapted from Wagner, W.D. and Clarkson, T.B. (Proc Soc Exp Biol Med 145: 1050-1057, 1974).

TABLE VIII. CONTRIBUTIONS OF DIET AND ENDOGENOUS SYNTHESIS TO PLASMA CHOLESTEROL IN HYPER- and HYPORESPONDER PIGEONS.

	Absorption %	Absorption mg/day	Synthesis %	Synthesis mg/day
Hyperresponders	83[a] ± 1	58 ± 1	17[a] ± 1	12[a] ± 1
Hyporesponders	63 ± 2	48 ± 5	37 ± 2	28 ± 1

[a]$P < 0.001$
Adapted from Wagner, W.D. and Clarkson, T.B. (Proc Soc Exp Biol Med 145: 1050-1057, 1974).

The strain of White Carneau pigeons with enhanced susceptibility to diet aggravated atherosclerosis has been of special interest to us since they may reflect genetically controlled differences in susceptibility at the mesenchymal level. The differences in extent of atherosclerosis in this strain, which we have designated as the WC-2 strain, and that of random bred WC are summarized in Table IX. While large differences exist in atherosclerosis susceptibility we have not been able to find differences in the usual risk factors. These observations are summarized in Tables X and XI. It is our feeling that these birds will be of increasing importance in arteriosclerosis research.

TABLE IX. ATHEROSCLEROSIS IN WC-2 PIGEONS.

Strain	No.	Diet	Atherosclerosis Index	Aortic Cholesterol mg/gm
WC-2	30	Atherogenic	57 ± 6	25.7
RBWC	30	Atherogenic	23 ± 4	9.7
WC-2	30	Control	5 ± 1	2.6
RBWC	30	Control	2 ± 1	1.7

Adapted data from Wagner and Clarkson (Fed. Proc. 34: 876, 1975)

PRIMATES

Among both human and nonhuman primates there is considerable individuality in the extent to which plasma cholesterol concentrations are increased when a given amount of dietary cholesterol is consumed. Figure 1 is an illustration of the variability in response of human primates to a cholesterol containing diet. While the majority of both males and females had plasma cholesterol concentrations between 160 and 300 mg/dl, significant numbers of individuals had concentrations below 160 and greater than 300 mg/dl.

Among squirrel monkeys fed a diet containing 1 mg/Cal of cholesterol there is even more marked individuality in the hypercholesterolemic response of these animals (Figure 2). Among squirrel monkeys fed cholesterol, certain individuals (hyperresponders) develop severe hypercholesterolemia while others

TABLE X. PLASMA CHOLESTEROL AND TRIGLYCERIDE CONCENTRATIONS TWO THROUGH EIGHT MONTHS OF STUDY.

Strain	No.	Diet	Cholesterol mg/dl	Triglyceride (mg/dl)
WC-2	30	Atherogenic	1065 ± 93	74 ± 2
RBWC	30	Atherogenic	1144 ± 92	87 ± 4
WC-2	30	Control	362 ± 11	79 ± 4
RBWC	30	Control	316 ± 8	77 ± 2.0

Adapted data from Wagner and Clarkson (Fed. Proc. 34: 876, 1975)

TABLE XI. BLOOD PRESSURE, PLASMA GLUCOSE, AND PLASMA URIC ACID CONCENTRATIONS OF WC-2 PIGEONS.

Strain	No.	Diet	Mean Blood Pressure (mm Hg)	Plasma Glucose (mg/dl)	Uric Acid (mg/dl)
WC-2	30	Atherogenic	150 ± 4	228 ± 4	3.3 ± 0.2
RBWC	30	Atherogenic	143 ± 3	222 ± 4	3.4 ± 0.3
WC-2	30	Control	158 ± 4	242 ± 4	3.3 ± 0.4
RBWC	30	Control	146 ± 3	228 ± 3	3.7 ± 0.2

(hyporesponders) fed the same diet maintain plasma cholesterol concentrations near that of controls. We have conducted an experiment to determine the importance of genetic influence on plasma cholesterol concentrations and, additionally, the extent and severity of the atherosclerotic lesions associated with hypercholesterolemia among the hyperresponder squirrel monkeys (19).

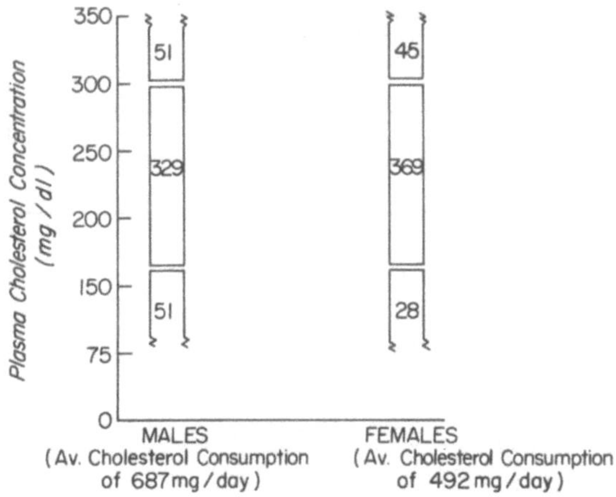

Fig. 1. Variability in response of human primates to a cholesterol containing diet. Adapted from data of Kannel, W.B. and Gordon, T., The Framingham Study. Section 24, 1970.

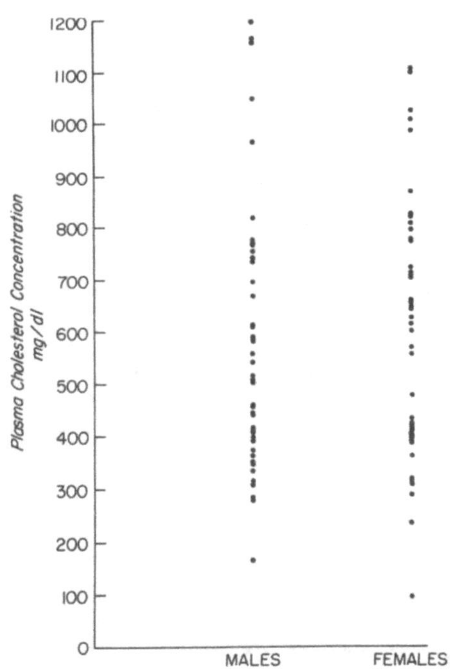

Fig. 2. Variability in response of squirrel monkeys to a cholesterol containing diet (1.0 mg/Cal).

Data derived from this and subsequent studies suggest that about 65% of the variability in plasma cholesterol concentration of cholesterol fed squirrel monkeys is attributable to genetic factors. Since such a large percent of the variability is genetically determined, it has been possible by selective breeding to develop colonies of hypo- and hyperresponder squirrel monkeys (Figure 3) (20).

Of additional interest, particularly to students of pediatric atherosclerosis, has been the observation that the response of an infant squirrel monkey to its mothers milk has strong predictive value in determining the response of the animal to a high cholesterol containing diet in later life. These observations are summarized in Figure 4.

Hyporesponder squirrel monkeys fed cholesterol containing diets, even for long periods, have only minimal arterial lesions. In contrast, the same lesions resemble qualitatively those described previously for cholesterol fed monkeys, except that they are now more extensive and severe. Lesions frequently associated with hyperlipidemia are seen in organs other than arteries (19). The coronary artery atherosclerosis of cholesterol fed hyperresponders is extensive, often calcified, and frequently affects the proximal main branches.

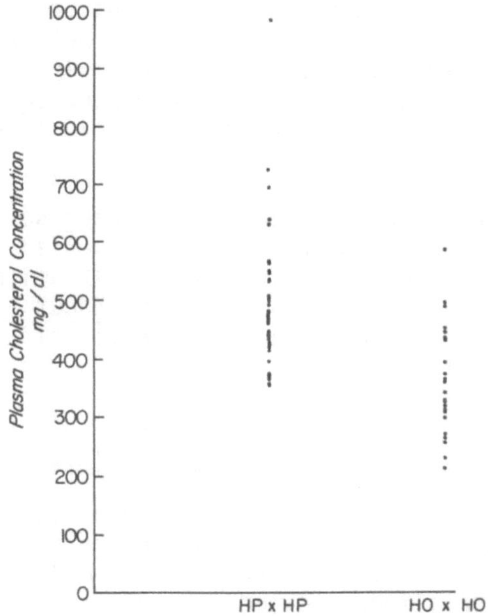

Fig. 3. Variability in response to a cholesterol containing diet (1.0 mg/Cal) of squirrel monkeys produced by hypo- and hyperresponder sires and dams.

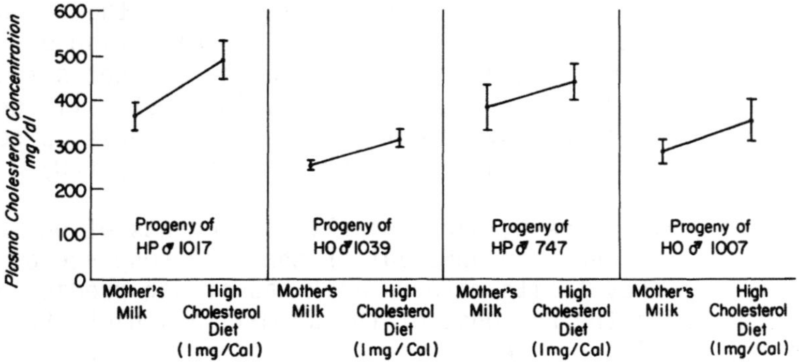

Fig. 4. Genetic differences in the response of squirrel monkeys to mother's milk and a high cholesterol containing diet.

Arterial lesions in other vascular beds are common among hyperresponders and about one-half of the hyperresponders have cutaneous xanthomatosis. Xanthelasma is infrequent. Foam cell lesions are often seen in the aortic valve leaflets and at the base of the aortic valves. Similar foam cell lesions are seen in the choroid plexus of some of the animals (19).

We have conducted cholesterol balance studies on hyper- and hyporesponder squirrel monkeys in an attempt to better understand the biochemical processes that are under genetic influence (21). The data derived would suggest that hyperresponder squirrel monkeys have a lesser ability to enhance bile acid excretion after cholesterol feeding.

Variability among nonhuman primates in response to dietary cholesterol (also presumably under genetic influence) is in no way unique to squirrel monkeys. By way of illustration, some observations on African green monkeys (Cercopithecus aethiops) and Cynomolgus macaques (Macaca fascicularis) are illustrated in Figures 5 and 6 respectively.

DYSLIPOPROTEINEMIAS OF NONHUMAN PRIMATES

Naturally occurring primary dyslipoproteinemias among nonhuman primates are quite rare. In 1961 Greenberg and Moon (22) reported on a single male rhesus monkey (Macaca mulatta) presumed to have primary hyperbetalipoproteinemia. Unfortunately, the animal died before breeding studies could be completed. Later, in 1968, Morris and Fitch (23) reported on the discovery of naturally occurring hyperbetalipoproteinemia in two male rhesus monkeys. The animals also had rather high concentrations of

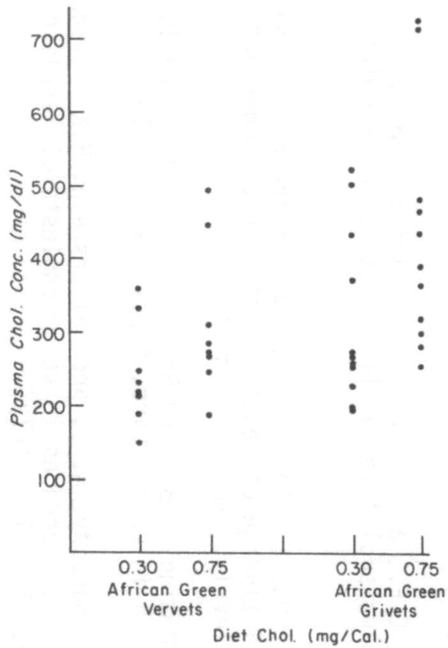

Fig. 5. Variability in response of African green monkeys to a cholesterol containing diet (0.75 mg/Cal).

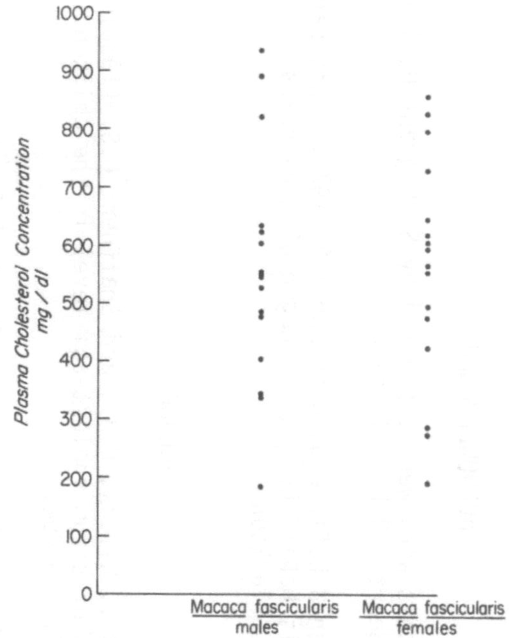

Fig. 6. Variability in response of <u>Macca fascicularis</u> monkeys to a cholesterol containing diet (0.56 mg/Cal).

prebetalipoproteins and their lipoprotein phenotype was interpreted as being Type IIB by the criteria of Fredrickson and Levy (24). Both of these animals have progeny and studies on the offspring are currently under way.

ACKNOWLEDGMENT

Portions of this work were supported by SCOR grant HL 14164 from the National Heart and Lung Institute.

Professor Hugh B Lofland died on April 2, 1975. This paper was presented in his behalf by his colleague of many years, Professor Thomas B. Clarkson.

REFERENCES

1. Cherms, F.L., Jr., Wilcox, F.H., and Shaffner, C.S. (1960). Genetic studies of serum cholesterol level in the chicken. Poultry Sci. 39, 889-892.

2. Wilcox, F.H., Cherms, F.L., Jr., VanVleck, L.D., Harvey, W.R., and Shaffner, C.S. (1963). Estimates of genetic parameters of serum cholesterol level. Poultry Sci. 42, 37-42.

3. Estep, G.D., Fanguy, R.C., and Ferguson, T.M. (1963). The effect of age and heredity upon serum cholesterol levels in chickens. Poultry Sci. 48, 1908-1911.

4. Stufflebean, C.E., and Lasley, J.F. (1969). Hereditary basis of serum cholesterol level in beef cattle. J. Heredity 60, 15-16.

5. Kohn, H.I. (1950). Changes in plasma of the rat during fasting and influence of genetic factors upon sugar and cholesterol levels. Am. J. Physiology 163, 410-417.

6. Adel, H.N., Deming, Q.B., and Brun, L. (1969). Genetic hypercholesterolemia in rats. Circ. Suppl. 39-40: III-1.

7. Bruell, J.H., Daroczy, A.F., and Hellerstein, H.K. (1962). Strain and sex differences in serum cholesterol levels of mice. Science 135, 1071-1072.

8. Yamamoto, R.S., Crittenden, L.B., Sokoloff, L., and Jay, G.E., Jr. (1963). Genetic variations in plasma lipid content in mice. J. Lipid Res. 4, 413-418.

9. Laird, C.W., Fox, R.R., Schultz, H.S., Mitchell, B.P., and Blau, E.M. (1970). Strain variations in rabbits: biochemical indicators of thyroid functions. Life Sciences 9, II: 203-214.

10. Wang, C.I., Schaefer, L.E., Drachman, S.R., and Adlersberg, D. (1953). Plasma lipid partition of the normal and cholesterol-fed rabbit. J. Mt. Sinai Hospital N. Y. 20, 19-25.

11. Roberts, D.C.K., West, C.E., Redgrave, T.G., and Smith, J.B. (1974). Plasma cholesterol concentration in normal and cholesterol fed rabbits. Atherosclerosis 19, 369-380.

12. Clarkson, T.B., Prichard, R.W., Netsky, M.G., and Lofland, H.B. (1959). Atherosclerosis in pigeons. Arch. Path. 68, 143-147.

13. Lofland, H.B, Clarkson, T.B., Prichard, R.W., and Netsky, M.G. (1959). Further studies on spontaneous atherosclerosis in pigeons. Circ. 20, 973.

14. Lofland, H.B, and Clarkson, T.B. (1959). Biochemical study of spontaneous atherosclerosis in pigeons. Circ. Res. 7, 234-237.

15. Lofland, H.B, Jr., and Clarkson, T.B. (1960). Serum lipoproteins in atherosclerosis-susceptible and resistant pigeons. Proc. Soc. Exp. Biol. Med. 103, 238-241.

16. Patton, N.M., Brown, R.V., and Middleton, C.C. (1974). Familial cholesterolemia in pigeons. Atherosclerosis 19, 307-314, 1974.

17. Wagner, W.D., Clarkson, T.B., Feldner, M.A., and Prichard, R.W. (1973). The development of pigeon strains with selected atherosclerosis characteristics. Exp. Mol. Pathol. 19, 304-319.

18. Wagner, W.D., and Clarkson, T.B. (1974). Mechanisms of the genetic control of plasma cholesterol in selected lines of Show Racer pigeons. Proc. Soc. Exp. Biol. Med. 145, 1050-1057.

19. Clarkson, T.B., Lofland, H.B, Bullock, B.C., and Goodman, H.O. (1971). Genetic control of plasma cholesterol. Arch. Pathol. 92, 37-45.

20. Clarkson, T.B., Lehner, N.D.M., Bullock, B.C., Lofland, H.B, and Wagner, W.D. (1974). Atherosclerosis in New World Monkeys. In Atherosclerosis in Primates. Strong, J.P. ed. Karger, New York. In Press.

21. Lofland, H.B, Clarkson, T.B., St. Clair, R.W., and Lehner, N.D.M. (1972). Studies on the regulation of plasma cholesterol levels in squirrel monkeys of two genotypes. J. Lipid Res. 13, 39-47.

22. Greenberg, L.D., and Moon, H.D. (1961). Blood lipid studies in a rhesus monkey with essential hypercholesterolemia. Fed. Proc. 20, A256d.

23. Morris, M.D., and Fitch, C.D. (1968). Spontaneous hyperbetalipoproteinemia in the rhesus monkey. Biochem. Med. 2, 209-215.

24. Fredrickson, D.S., and Levy, R.I. (1972). Familial hyperlipoproteinemia. In The Metabolic Basis of Inherited Disease. Stanbury, J.B., Wyngaarden, J.B., and Fredrickson, D.B. eds. McGraw-Hill, New York. pp. 545-614.

(2)

THE BABOON AS AN EXPERIMENTAL MODEL IN DRUG TESTING

A. N. Howard

Department of Medicine, University of Cambridge,

Cambridge, England

CHOLESTEROL CONTAINING DIETS

All non-human primates respond to cholesterol feeding, but there is a great variation in response. Figure 1 shows results obtained by several investigators using different species. By far the greatest response in serum cholesterol is given by the rhesus monkey and chimpanzee, whilst the baboon gives relatively low values. Likewise, the extent of arterial disease seen in the baboon is small and is confined chiefly to sudanophilic streaks in the aorta, whereas in the rhesus monkey, extensive coronary lesions have been reported.

Studies using baboon fed cholesterol diets are often disappointing. Baboons fed diets containing cholesterol gave a fairly large initial rise and then a few weeks later the serum cholesterol fell to considerably lower values (about two thirds maximum). Presumably, the animals have adapted to the increased cholesterol load by either greatly diminishing synthesis and/or decreasing absorption and/or increasing excretion of cholesterol and its metabolism such as the bile acids. The ability of the baboon to compensate appears to be much greater than other non-human primates.

Groups of baboons receiving cholesterol containing diets were given cholestyramine (400 mg/kg) or clofibrate (200 mg/kg). After four weeks no change was seen with clofibrate but cholestyramine produced a 15% decrease in serum cholesterol. The effect of cholestyramine is similar to that seen with anion exchange resins in the cholesterol fed chick and rabbit,

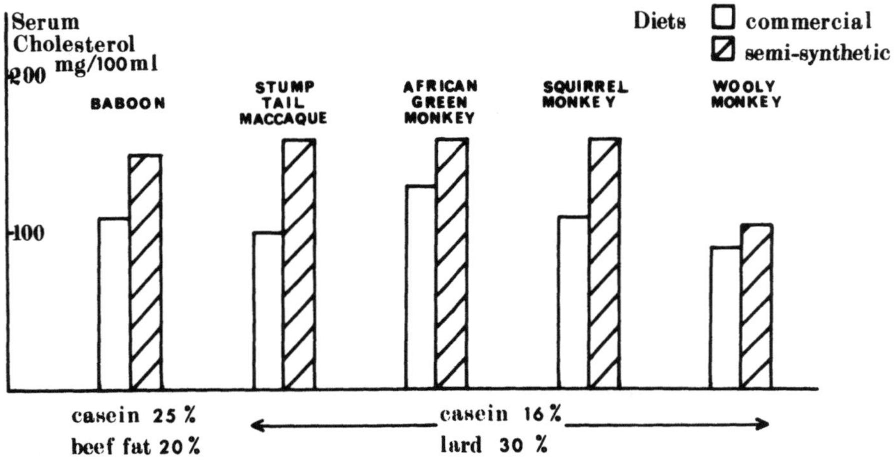

Fig. 1

Hypercholesterolaemia in non-human primates (1 - 5)

although the magnitude of the effect is not so great in the baboon. Clofibrate has only been reported to lower cholesterol in animals fed normal diets.

SEMI-SYNTHETIC DIETS

Rabbits, when given a semi-synthetic diet, develop hypercholesterolaemia and atherosclerosis. Although Malmros and Wigand (6) claimed that the syndrome could be explained on the basis of an essential fatty acid deficiency, this appeared not to be the whole explanation. The situation has been clarified by Carroll (7), who compared commercial and semi-synthetic diets to which were added fat of different unsaturation. The hypercholesterolaemia was found to be due to a combination of factors: low polyunsaturated fatty acids and a high animal protein content.

Seven baboons were maintained on a semi-synthetic diet containing 20% beef tallow and 25% casein for nine months. Two of the animals had serum cholesterol above the normal range (8). Likewise, Kritchevsky et al (9) reported on studies in which baboons were maintained for a year on cholesterol free semi-synthetic diets containing different carbohydrates. Serum cholesterol rose approximately 35% in all groups and at autopsy fatty streaks were observed in all animals.

In recent experiments a comparison was made between two commercial diets containing a moderate (12%) and high (20%) animal protein content but otherwise very similar. After four weeks the serum cholesterol was elevated by 30 mg/100 ml (33%). Such results provide evidence of the importance of animal protein in influencing the serum cholesterol levels of primates. At the present, the mechanism seems obscure but the problem represents a challenge which is not insoluble using modern cholesterol-balance techniques.

Animals given commercial diets without added cholesterol do not give a hypocholesterolaemic response to cholestyramine (400 mg/kg) but clofibrate (200 mg/kg) gives a 25% decrease in serum cholesterol.

The results closely parallel those seen in the rat given a normal diet. Presumably, the baboon is also able to completely compensate for the loss of cholesterol as bile acids when cholestyramine is fed.

COMBINATION OF HYPERCHOLESTEROLAEMIC AND IMMUNOLOGICAL INJURY

Because the extent of arterial disease is disappointing in baboons given hypercholesterolaemic diets, attempts were made to accelerate the disease by injuring the vessel wall by injecting protein antigens (1). This technique has been already employed successfully in the rabbit using bovine serum albumin or horse serum.

Baboons given a diet of egg yolk and butter had an elevation of serum cholesterol to 280 mg/100ml and in the space of six months no aortic disease was evident. Likewise, the injection of bovine serum albumin (BSA), a substance which causes immunological injury, had no demonstrable effect on vascular pathology. However, the combination of hypercholesterolaemia and BSA produced extensive aortic sudanophilia and atherosclerosis. Neither the mild lipaemia nor injury alone were sufficient but both factors acted synergistically.

This method of producing atherosclerosis in baboons has been extensively useful in studying drugs which may be anti-atherogenic without affecting blood lipid levels, especially EPL solution (soya bean lecithin dissolved in deoxycholic acid solution) which shows a beneficial effect prophylactically (1) but does not influence the regression of lesions (2).

REFERENCES

1. Howard, A.N., J. Patelski, D.E. Bowyer and G.A. Gresham. Atherosclerosis 14:17 (1971).
2. Howard, A.N. and J. Patelski. Atherosclerosis 20:225 (1974).
3. Howard, A.N. et al. In, Protides of the Biological Fluids, Edit. H. Peeters. Oxford: Pergamon Press, p.341 (1972).
4. Fraser, R. et al. Atherosclerosis 16:203 (1972).
5. Newman, W.P., D.A. Eygen and J.P. Strong. Atherosclerosis 19:75 (1974)
6. Malmros, H. and G. Wigand. Lancet 2:749 (1959).
7. Carroll, K.K. Atherosclerosis 13:67 (1971).
8. Howard, A.N., G.A.Gresham, C.N. Hales, F.T. Lindgren and A.A. Katzberg. In, The Baboon in Medical Research, Edit. H. Vagtborg, Vol.2, p.333. Univ. of Texas Press, Austin (1967).
9. Kritchevsky, D. et al. Am. J. clin. Nutr. 27:29 (1974).

(3)

ADVANCED CORONARY ATHEROSCLEROSIS IN SWINE PRODUCED BY COMBINATION OF BALLOON-CATHETER INJURY AND CHOLESTEROL FEEDING

K.T.Lee and W.M.Lee

Department of Pathology, Albany Medical College

Albany, New York, U.S.A.

INTRODUCTION

In recent years a considerable amount of research effort has been devoted to the development and characterization of experimental animal models for the study of atherosclerosis. We have been using swine fed high fat-cholesterol diets as a model for the study of various aspects of the pathogenesis of atherosclerosis. With diets alone a year or longer is required to produce advanced coronary atherosclerosis with a significant luminal narrowing. These slowly developing coronary artery lesions have not been associated with myocardial infarction, sudden death or other manifestations of coronary heart disease.

In another approach to the development of suitable models for the study of atherosclerosis we have investigated possible synergism of a high fat-cholesterol diet and direct injury to the artery in the production of lesions. In a recent study deep x-irradiation was given as a form of injury to the coronary arteries of swine. A combination of x-irradiation and atherogenic diets produced occlusive coronary artery disease with myocardial infarction and sudden death from fatal cardiac arrhythmia in swine.

In a more recent study we were able to produce rapidly developing advanced atherosclerosis in the aorta of swine by a combination of an atherogenic diet and a balloon-endothelial cell denudation procedure. In the current study we have extended this combined procedure to coronary arteries of swine in an attempt to produce advanced coronary atherosclerosis. We were able to produce occlusive coronary artery lesions, myocardial infarction and sudden death in these swine within a relatively short time and the results are presented in this report.

MATERIALS AND METHODS

Forty-two male Yorkshire swine, approximately 12 to 15 weeks old, weighing 12 to 16 kg were used in this study. They were housed in individual slat-bottomed cages in temperature controlled animal quarters. The swine were divided into two groups; one group of 26 swine was fed a high-cholesterol diet (Table I) following the balloon-endothelial cell-denudation procedure, and the other group of 16 swine fed a high-cholesterol diet alone without the denudation procedure.

TABLE 1

Completion of Daily Diet Given Each Experimental Swine

Ingredients	Amount in Grams
Casein	160
Sucrose	225
Butter	200
Peanut Oil	40
Salt mix, Wesson	32
Vitamin Mix	28
Cellulose	88
Cholesterol	16
Sodium cholate	11
Total	800
Total Calories	3700 calories

Balloon-Endothelial Cell Denudation Procedure-The swine were anesthetized with Halothane followed by Katamine HCl and the procedure was carried out under sterile conditions. An incision was made to expose the right carotid artery. A nick was made in the artery and a 2F Fogarty Arterial Embolectomy Catheter was introduced and passed into either the left or right coronary artery under the guidance of fluoroscopy. For most swine one or two of the three main coronary arteries were ballooned. During the procedure electrocardiogram and blood pressure were monitored continuously and lidocain (70 mg/kg/min) was infused intravenously. In our previous study we found that lidocain increased significantly the ventricular fibrillation threshold.

The balloon was carefully inflated by 0.4 ml of air and then pulled back quickly to minimize the blockage of coronary blood flow and occurrence of ventricular fibrillation. In our preliminary *in vitro* tests with swine of similar size to those used in this experiment, 0.4 ml of air introduced in the balloon was sufficient to denude most of endothelial cells in the proximal portion of the coronary artery up to 2 cm from the origin without excessive damage or rupture of the vessels. After the balloon-endothelial cell denudation procedure all swine were fed a high-cholesterol diet shown in Table I throughout the experiment.

TABLE 2

Number of Swine, Body Weight, and Serum Cholesterol Levels of Ballooned and Control Swine

Group (Survival after ballooning in weeks)	Number of Swine	Weight (Kg)		Serum Cholesterol (mg/100 ml)	
		Initial	Final	Initial	Final
Sudden Death Group (6-12)	7	15.76* ± 1.97	20.08 ± 0.97	67.3 ± 8.1	554.5** ± 30.4
Controls for Sudden Death Group (8-13)	6	14.88 ± 1.66	19.95 ± 1.79	74.6 ±10.5	842.8 ±104.4
Sacrificed Group (24-38)	15	14.28 ± 1.25	45.66 ± 6.72	72.1 ± 4.3	503.9 ± 22.1
Controls for Sacrificed Group (25-37)	9	12.82 ± 0.88	38.44 ± 2.01	97.3 ± 8.1	410.8 ± 45.1

*Mean ± S.E.M.

**These figures represent interim cholesterol values

Autopsies were performed on all swine. The heart and aorta were removed intact, and all major organs were examined routinely. The heart was examined systematically both grossly and microscopically for the presence of myocardial infarcts or other abnormalities. After the heart was fixed in 10% formalin, a series of cross sectional cuts along the first 2 cm of the three main coronary arteries were made with 3 mm intervals and every other block was processed for light microscopy. The amount of coronary atherosclerosis was measured with an ocular micrometer. The diameters of the artery and its lumen, the wall thickness at its thickest point, and the area of the lumen at its smallest were measured. All other microscopic observations such as hemorrhage into a plaque, calcium deposits, necrosis and virtual or complete occlusion of the lumen were also recorded.

Electrocardiograms were obtained monthly from all swine, to determine the presence of myocardial damage.

Serum cholesterol levels were determined in all swine before the experiment, and periodically thereafter to assess the effect of the atherogenic diet.

RESULTS

These swine generally tolerated the diet well and usually ate the entire amount of food given. However, 5 swine, four from the ballooned group and one from the control group, died very early in the experiment.

Between 6 and 12 weeks after the procedure, 7 swine died in their cages rather suddenly without noticeable preceding signs of sickness. Fifteen swine survived 24-38 weeks until they were sacrificed to assess the degree of coronary atherosclerosis produced. Of the 15 control swine 6 were killed between 8-13 weeks to serve as controls for those that died suddenly during the same period and 9 were sacrificed between 25-38 weeks to serve as controls for the experimental swine sacrificed during this period.

TABLE 3

Maximal Wall Thickness, Minimal Cross-Sectional Area of Lumen and Other Data on Coronary Arteries of Ballooned and Control Swine

Group	No. of Swine	L A D*			L C			R C			hemo-rrhage	Cal. Dep.	Myo. Infarct
		No. of Swine Bal-looned	Mean max wall thick (mm)	Mean minim lumen (mm^2)	No. of Swine Bal-looned	Mean max wall thick (mm)	Mean minim Lumen (mm^2)	No. of Swine Bal-looned	Mean max wall thick (mm)	Mean minim Lumen (mm^2)			
Sudden Death Group	7	2	0.63** ±0.08	0.48 ±0.09	7	0.78 ±0.18	0.31 ±0.15	3	0.77 ±0.14	1.19 ±0.30	3	2	6
Controls for Sudden Death Group	6	0	0.28 ±0.03	0.65 ±0.13	0	0.26 ±0.05	1.11 ±0.47	0	0.31 ±0.02	1.12 ±0.24	0	0	0
p value			<0.01	NS		<0.01	<0.01		<0.01	NS			
Sacrificed Group	15	9	1.05 ±0.16	0.96 ±0.16	5	1.14 ±0.21	1.29 ±0.23	10	1.46 ±0.14	1.31 ±0.28	3	5	4
Controls for Sacrificed Group	9	0	0.52 ±0.03	2.82 ±0.25	0	0.45 ±0.05	1.41 ±0.33	0	0.79 ±0.09	2.90 ±0.44	0	0	0
p value			<0.01	<0.01		<0.01	NS		<0.01	<0.01			

* L A D = Left Anterior descending L C= Left circumflex R C= Right coronary

** Mean ± S.E.M.

Out of 22 swine subjected to the balloon-denudation procedure and the high-cholesterol diet, 10 had myocardial infarcts that were either acute, old or both. Of these 10 infarcts, 6 were from the swine that died suddenly between 6-12 weeks of the experiment and 4 were from the swine that were sacrificed between 24-38 weeks. The size of the infarcts varied greatly ranging from 2-6 cm in the greatest dimension and some involved large portions of the left ventricle. The proximal portions of the coronary arteries that had been subjected to the balloon-denudation procedure showed advanced atherosclerosis with marked luminal narrowing whereas the remainder of the coronary arteries that had not been subjected to the balloon procedure showed only a minimal to moderate degree of atherosclerosis. None of the 15 control swine showed advanced coronary atherosclerosis nor myocardial infarction.

Histological appearance of coronary lesions varied depending upon the length of time the swine were on the diet. In most instances the proximal portions of one or two main coronary arteries showed the wall thickened by smooth muscle cell proliferation and many of the cells were filled with lipid. The narrowed lumen was frequently eccentric and irregular in shape. Necrosis, calcification and hemorrhage in the plaque were also present to a variable extent. Surprisingly none of these experimental animals had thrombosis. Complete or virtual occlusion of one or two main coronary arteries were observed in 7 animals. The histologic appearance of the myocardial infarct was similar to that of a human infarct.

DISCUSSION

Advanced occlusive coronary artery disease was induced rapidly in swine by using a combination of injurious and atherogenic agents. The occlusive arterial disease produced in these swine has many similarities to and some difference from that observed in man. The most important feature from the standpoint of the objective of the study is that the lumen of the coronary artery is narrowed and the blood flow to parts of the myocardium is reduced. The swine frequently developed ischemic heart disease with myocardial infarction and sudden death. Sudden death in the current group of swine was similar to that frequently seen in man, in that observers usually were not able to recognize signs of impending disaster by visual inspection before the terminal collapse and the occurrence of death within minutes. We have observed in previous studies extensive coronary artery disease with myocardial infarction and sudden death in swine subjected to x-irradiation and atherogenic diets. The immediate cause of death in these swine was found to be a fatal cardiac arrhythmia, either ventricular fibrillation or ventricular asystole. The immediate cause of death in swine dying suddenly in the current study was not determined, but judging from the extent of the coronary artery disease and the myocardial damage it is reasonable to assume that pathophysiological cause of death in some of the swine in the current study was also a fatal cardiac arrhythmia.

Extensive atherosclerotic lesions were limited to the proximal portions of major coronary arteries that were subjected to the balloon-denudation. Hemorrhage into plaques was more frequent than in man. Histologically the prominent cells making up atherosclerotic plaques were smooth muscle cells as in man and much lipid was present both intra- and extracellularly. However, the cellular component was more prominent and the necrotic debris and calcification were much less prominent than in advanced coronary atherosclerosis seen in man. This is to be expected in rapidly developing lesions in the current experiment since the early phase in both men and experimental animals appears to be largely cellular proliferation, with extensive fibrosis and large regions of necrotic debris developing later.

Possible advantages of the current model over the previous one developed by using x-irradiation and atherogenic diets are that primary lesions are mainly in the proximal portions of coronary arteries as in man, and there are no direct irradiation effects on the myocardium. This model would appear to be useful for studies of physiological derangements resulting from ischemic myocardium and for studies of regression of extensive coronary atherosclerosis.

SUMMARY

There has been a constant demand for an animal model of advanced coronary atherosclerosis produced in a short period. It was well known that mild atherosclerosis could be produced in various vascular beds by high cholesterol diets. However, it requires considerable time to produce advanced atherosclerotic lesions by diets alone. The current study was designed to investigate effects of combination of a balloon-denudation procedure and high cholesterol diet in swine. We could produce advanced atherosclerotic lesions in coronary arteries in cholesterol-fed swine within a short period of time by inserting a balloon-catheter via carotid artery into the coronary artery, inflating it so as to distend the lumen and pulling it back quickly which resulted in extensive denudation of the endothelium of coronary arteries. An athero-slcerosis-like lesion develops at the site with eventual narrowing of the lumen leading to myocardial ischemia, myocardial infarction and occasionally sudden death thus resembling in many aspects human coronary artery disease. Among 22 swine studied, 10 had severe atherosclerosis with virtual occlusion of proximal portion of either, or both, coronary arteries, and developed myocardial infarction within two to three months. Seven of these died suddenly probably due to arrhythmia. This model should be appropriate for studies where advanced coronary atherosclerosis with its complications is needed.

(4)

EVOLUTION AND REGRESSION OF AORTIC FATTY STREAKS IN RHESUS MONKEYS

Jack P. Strong, Herbert C. Stary, and Douglas A. Eggen

Department of Pathology, Louisiana State University

Medical Center, New Orleans, Louisiana, U.S.A.

The rhesus monkey, Macaca mulatta, has now been used extensively in atherosclerosis research to study both the development of experimental arterial lesions and the regression of these lesions. Recent reviews by Armstrong (1) and Strong (2,3) have included material on the evolution and regression of experimental atherosclerosis in rhesus monkeys. This report will be confined to aortic lesions in the rhesus monkey model. The aorta is chosen for special emphasis because it is large enough to be studied by both morphologic and chemical methods in a single animal.

The purpose of this report is 1) to describe the evolution of experimental aortic atherosclerosis in rhesus monkeys after they have been fed an atherogenic diet for varying periods of time and 2) to describe the regression of experimentally induced atherosclerosis in this species after 8 and 12 weeks of atherogenic diet and varying periods of time after returning the animals to a low cholesterol basal diet.

Investigators have studied the rhesus model for both the production of atherosclerotic lesions (4-15) and the regression of experimentally induced lesions (16-24). Experimental diets and periods of diet feeding vary widely among these studies. This report will describe the progression and regression of lesions in experiments conducted in our laboratory where time intervals of feeding the atherogenic diet and the regression periods have varied, but the atherogenic diets used have been similar. The atherogenic diets fed to all of the monkeys in this report contained monkey chow, casein, butter, beef tallow, cholesterol, salt mixture and vitamin mixture with fat contributing 40% of calories and cholesterol at 1 mg per kcal or 0.37% by weight. Thus, we are evaluating features of experimental lesions produced by an atherogenic diet of moderate severity with a combination of methods - gross morphology, histology, electron microscopy, chemical analysis, and radioautography.

PROGRESSION OF EXPERIMENTAL LESIONS

Atherogenic Diet for 4 Weeks

Two rhesus monkeys were studied after only 4 weeks on the atherogenic diet (20). Serum cholesterol levels rose to 320 and 560 mg/dl, and at autopsy a few sudanophilic fatty streaks were present in the aortas (2 and 9% of the intimal surface covered by lesions). Lesions were more extensive than in control animals for this experiment, however, we have had other rhesus monkeys fed only monkey chow who had approximately this level of lesions. Nevertheless, after one month of cholesterol feeding, electron microscopy showed foam cells in the intima of the aorta (15) and an increased number of lipid inclusions in intimal smooth muscle cells. Radioautographs of the aorta showed an increased tritiated thymidine labeling frequency of endothelial cells, intimal spindle cells and medial smooth muscle (14).

Atherogenic Diet for 8 Weeks

Three rhesus monkeys were fed our standard atherogenic diet for 8 weeks and autopsied at that time (17). The elevation of serum cholesterol was variable (terminal values 322, 900 and 1100 mg/dl); however, sudanophilic aortic lesions were produced. The extent of lesions in these animals exceeded the small amount of lesions in control animals and covered an estimated 17,30, and 36% of the aortic intimal surface.

The intimal lesions were 1 to 5 cell layers thick and contained both intracellular and extracellular lipid. Ultrastructurally the lesions were composed principally of lipid-filled foam cells (which we believe to be macrophages), smooth muscle cells containing lipid, and extracellular lipid. No striking increase in connective tissue elements was observed. The foam cells were frequently located directly below the endothelium in a sheet-like arrangement. Many of the foam cells had degenerative changes and some were disrupted and were spilling their contents into the extracellular spaces. While only a small number of animals were examined, the qualitative features of the lesions were constant from animal to animal and were clearly different from the controls.

Atherogenic Diet for 12 Weeks

We have studied arterial lesions induced with a 12-week period of atherogenic diet in several experiments and have used this period in all recent experiments on regression (22). Some of these animals were fed the atherogenic diet for 12 weeks and then returned to the basal diet for 2, 3 or 4 weeks before autopsy. Lesions in these animals are probably still in the progression phase since the elevated serum lipid levels remain above baseline levels for some time after diet change. The findings in these animals will be considered with the evolving lesions. Monkeys fed the atherogenic diet for 12 weeks and basal diets for 8 weeks are probably just at the interface of progression and regression and have not yet been studied sufficiently to be included in this report.

Aortas from some of these groups were stained grossly with Sudan IV and evaluated grossly for extent of lesions; in others, the aortas were used for histology, electron microscopy, chemical analysis and tritiated thymidine radioautography, and were not available for gross evaluation.

Aortic lesions.--Lesions were produced in all animals. There was, however, considerable variablilty in extent of lesions which appeared to be correlated with mean serum cholesterol levels during atherogenic diet periods. Only an occasional "resistant animal" failed to exceed the baseline level of lesions observed in control animals. Many of the animals had half or more of the intimal surface covered by sudanophilic lesions. The average per cent of the intimal surface covered by lesions in 6 animals examined after 2 weeks on basal diet was 57% of the thoracic aorta and 29% of the abdominal aorta.

Serum cholesterol.--The serum cholesterol concentration of all animals fed the atherogenic diet increased rapidly at first, and then more slowly. The mean concentration increased from a basal level of 128 mg/dl to 536 mg/dl at 12 weeks.

Histologic evaluation.--The 12-week atherogenic diet period produced lesions characterized by accumulation of stainable lipid in a slightly thickened intima with a small but variable amount of lipid sometimes occurring in the underlying media. One micron sections of Maraglas-embedded tissue examined by light microscopy, and fine sections examined by electron microscopy showed that the lesions typically consisted of foam cells below the endothelium, lipid droplets in intimal smooth muscle cells beneath this layer, and moderate amounts of extracellular lipid.

Aortic intimal lipid.--The total cholesterol content of the aortic intima-media preparation increased more than twofold during the hypercholesterolemic period. The relative increase in the ester cholesterol fraction was greater than that of the free cholesterol fraction. There was an increase in all major fatty acid fractions of the cholesteryl esters during the 12 weeks on atherogenic diet. Cholesteryl oleate was present in greatest concentration. The largest proportional increase was in stearic and oleic esters and the least proportional increase was in linoleic and arachidonic esters.

Cell proliferation.--Selected animals were injected with tritiated thymidine and studied by radioautography of aortic specimens (14,25). Control animals on the basal diet had no intimal lesions, and endothelial cells and intimal smooth muscle cells were labeled infrequently. Four animals killed after 12 weeks on the atherogenic diet and two animals given the atherogenic diet for 12 weeks and killed 3 weeks later had many intimal lesions consisting mainly of foam cells and intimal smooth muscle cells with lipid. There was frequent labeling of both foam cells and smooth muscle cells in the intimal lesions. Endothelial cells on the surface of lesions also showed more frequent labeling than endothelial cells in control animals.

Ultrastructure.--Electron microscopic examination of the aorta revealed that the lipid of the developing fatty streak was both intracellular and extracellular. Intracellular lipid was in foam cells and in intimal smooth muscle cells. Foam cell lipid was in the form of lipid droplets of variable electron density, cholesterol clefts, and residual bodies. Intimal smooth muscle cells contained lipid inclusions which were mainly of the electron-dense type. Intimal smooth muscle cells were usually below the foam cell layer and extended as far as the internal elastic lamina.

Many foam cells and a smaller number of smooth muscle cells were necrotic. Cell fragments and lipid inclusions released from necrotic cells accumulated in the extracellular space. The extracellular space also contained elastic fibrils of varying size and appearance, collagen fibers, and finely reticulated ground substance. Necrotic cell debris and lipid had a tendency to accumulate in pools between the foam cell layer and the internal elastic lamina.

Atherogenic Diet for 40 Weeks

Six monkeys were fed the atherogenic diet for 40 weeks (11,20). These animals had predominantly intimal fatty streaks in the aorta. Two animals with most extensive involvement also showed features suggestive of early fibrous plaques in the descending thoracic aorta. No complicated or calcified lesions were present. Four animals had from 35 to 69% of the aortic intimal surface involved by lesions; another had only 19%; and the remaining animal had only 2%, well within the range of lesions found in control animals. This animal was also resistant to the development of hypercholesterolemia.

Electron microscopic examination showed that intracellular and extracellular lipid accumulation was most extensive in the intima. At some points it extended into the adjacent media, and foam cells were seen among medial smooth muscle cells adjacent to large intimal lesions. Tritiated thymidine radioautography showed a larger number of cells labelled in the aortic intimal lesions after ten months than after shorter periods of cholesterol feeding.

Atherogenic Diet for 18 Months

Monkeys were fed the atherogenic diet for 18 months in a study designed to compare the response of three primate species to an identical atherogenic diet. The serum lipid response and certain parameters of cholesterol metabolism have been reported (26). This group of rhesus monkeys was on the atherogenic diet longest of any we have studied. The lesions produced were extensive and were considered to be advanced fatty streaks. By light and electron microscopy the intimal lesions had further increased in extent and in thickness compared to 40 week lesions. Furthermore, in animals with the highest serum cholesterol levels, lesions involved the adjacent aortic media.

REGRESSION OF EXPERIMENTAL LESIONS

There is little doubt that lesions in animals that resemble fatty streaks in children can regress (27). Armstrong (1) and Strong (2,3) have reviewed regression of experimental atherosclerosis in primate models. Wissler recently reviewed regression of atherosclerosis in experimental animals and man (28).

Atherogenic Diet for 8 Weeks; Basal Diet for 16 Weeks

When basal diet was fed for 16 weeks following induction of lesions with the atherogenic diet for 8 weeks, marked qualitative changes occurred in the lesions (19). These changes occurred even though the lipid content of the intima and gross extent of lesions did not change appreciably. The main difference was in the distribution of lipid in the intima.

After the atherogenic diet most of the intimal lipid was in foam cells and smooth muscle cells. After regression for 16 weeks, only rare foam cells were present and smooth muscle cells contained fewer lipid inclusions; most of the lipid was extracellular. Even though these striking qualitative changes in the distribution of lipid in the lesions occurred, the findings in this study indicate that fatty streaks in rhesus monkyes require more than 4 months at low serum lipid levels before the gross extent and lipid content of lesions is reduced appreciably.

Atherogenic Diet for 12 Weeks; Basal Diet for 12,16,24,32,40 or 64 Weeks

While we have now obtained some information on animals fed the atherogenic diet for 12 weeks and then returned to low cholesterol basal diet for periods varying from several weeks to 64 weeks after the serum lipid levels have returned to baseline levels, we have most complete information and the largest number of animals per group for those monkeys fed the atherogenic diet for 12 weeks and then returned to the basal diet for 32 and 64 weeks. After some general comments on the entire group of "regression" animals, more specific data will be described for the two latter groups.

General Comments.--In two separate experiments, groups of animals were fed the basal diet after an atherogenic diet for 12 weeks. All of the animals responded to atherogenic diets with elevations of serum cholesterol. Shortly after return to a basal diet serum cholesterol levels began to drop. In one of the experiments the serum cholesterol concentration dropped and had attained basal levels in most of the animals after 3 to 4 weeks (22). In the other experiment cholesterol levels in some animals remained elevated well above baseline levels for longer than 8 weeks. Twelve weeks after return to the basal diet all of the serum cholesterol levels were near normal baseline values.

Arterial lesions.--After the first 32 weeks of regression the intimal sudanophilia which developed during 12 weeks on the atherogenic diet had decreased markedly. A further reduction occurred after an additional 32 week period of regression; however, even after 64 weeks the monkeys had slightly more aortic intimal sudanophilia than the control group fed basal diet throughout. Comparing the extent of the aortic surface covered with sudanophilic lesions, lesions in the thoracic aorta dropped from a mean of 57% after the atherogenic period to 15% after an additional 64 weeks on basal diet. The mean extent of lesions in the abdominal aorta dropped from 29% to 9%.

Histologic evaluation.--After 32 weeks of regression the total amount of intimal lipid was greatly decreased and foam cells were difficult to detect. After 64 weeks of regression, foam cells had almost completely disappeared, lipid droplets were much less numerous in smooth muscle cells and the residual lipid (decreased in amount) was almost entirely extracellular. Lipid in residual lesions frequently extended into the media. Quantitative microscopic grading of intimal lipid also decreased dramatically from the levels observed after 12 weeks on the atherogenic diet.

Aortic intimal lipid.--In the animals undergoing regression for 32 and 64 weeks most of the increase in free and esterified cholesterol which developed in the intima during the atherogenic diet disappeared during the first 32 weeks of regression. During the second 32 week regression period cholesterol in the intima decreased until the free and ester fractions were only slightly greater than in control animals.

Cholesteryl esters of all major fatty acids decreased after 32 weeks on the basal diet; cholesteryl stearate and cholesteryl arachidonate had returned to approximately baseline levels. Cholesteryl esters of palmitic, palmitoleic, oleic, and linoleic acids remained elevated during this period and were still elevated above baseline levels after 64 weeks. Cholesteryl linoleate made up a somewhat higher proportion of the total cholesteryl esters in the regression animals than in progression or control animals.

Aortic connective tissue.--A collaborative investigation of the connective tissue concentration of the intima-media residue left after lipid extraction was conducted with members of the LSU SCOR-A (24). While total collagen concentration of the aortic media did not change significantly there was a qualitative change. Non-autoclavable collagen concentration decreased during production of lesions and increased again to control levels after regression. There were dramatic qualitative changes in glycosaminoglycan (GAG) components although total GAG concentration did not change significantly. The hyaluronic acid component increased greatly during regression while chondroitin sulfate C decreased during regression.

Cell proliferation.--Two groups of two animals given the atherogenic diet for 12 weeks and killed 16 weeks and 40 weeks after return to the basal diet were studied by radioautography after tritiated thymidine injections and compared to animals killed at 0 and 3 weeks after return to basal diet. The first group still had numerous intimal lesions which showed decreased cellularity due to loss of the majority of foam cells. Some of the residual foam cells were still labeled. There appeared to be an overall reduction in the labeling frequency of all cell types in the intimal lesions. The two animals which received the atherogenic diet for 12 weeks and were killed 40 weeks later had a few, small intimal lesions consisting of extracellular debris, some intimal smooth muscle cells with lipid, and rare solitary foam cells. None of the foam cells were labeled. The labeling frequency of smooth muscle cells and endothelial cells was similar to that of two control monkeys given the basal diet only and also injected with tritiated thymidine.

Ultrastructure.--Two animals examined 16 weeks after changing to the basal diet were found to have a pronounced decrease in the number of foam cells. In many of the remaining foam cells, lipid inclusions were associated with peripheral tubular structures of lysosomal nature. The number of intimal smooth muscle cells with lipid did not seem to be greatly decreased at that time, and the nature of the intracytoplasmic lipid did not differ from the group examined following the 12-week atherogenic diet period.

After 32 weeks of regression, there was a further striking decrease in the number of foam cells. Intact foam cells were infrequent. Persisting intracellular lipid was mainly within intimal smooth muscle cells, although the number of lipid-containing smooth muscle cells was also decreased. After 40 weeks the changes were similar to those at 32 weeks. After 64 weeks foam cells were as rare as in normal control animals and lipid-containing smooth muscle cells were infrequent and lipid inclusions were small. Extracellular lipid remained the predominant form of visible lipid, but it was greatly reduced as compared to the earlier periods.

CONCLUSIONS

Our findings clearly indicate regression of diet-induced fatty streaks in the aorta of rhesus monkeys. While fatty streaks in the rhesus monkey require more than four months at low serum lipid concentrations before their gross extent is reduced appreciably, grossly visible sudanophilic lesions in the aorta can regress to nearly initial levels after 64 weeks on a basal diet.

The histologic characteristics of lesions change dramatically during regression. After 64 weeks of regression, essentially all foam cells and most of the lipid inclusions in smooth muscle cells disappeared, and extracellular lipid in the intima decreased markedly.

The selective accumulation and depletion of certain cholesteryl esters in the aorta demonstrates the dynamic nature of arterial cholesterol ester metabolism in this experiment model.

We did not determine the mechanism by which the intimal lipid was removed. The lipid may have been metabolized *in situ* into a product no longer recognizable as lipid. It is more likely, however, that the lipid was transported out of the artery wall either through the endothelium or through the adventitia via the lymphatics or vasa vasora.

Chemical studies of connective tissue components of the aortic wall suggest that there is a decrease of some connective tissue components during production of lesions (perhaps by dilution) and return to control level or greater during regression. The most intriguing findings are qualitative changes in GAG components.

The number of animals used in the radioautographic studies was small, nevertheless the results indicate that increased intimal cell proliferation induced by hypercholesterolemia can return to normal levels. This change is attributed solely to removing the stimulus of high serum cholesterol levels. Thus, it seems unlikely that a permanent proliferative impulse is induced in arterial cells by a short period of hypercholesterolemia.

In these studies we have shown that regression of early diet-induced fatty streaks occurs in rhesus monkeys when the dietary stimulus is removed and the serum cholesterol is allowed to return to basal levels. We have not shown a complete regression since certain residual changes remain for as long as 64 weeks after removal of dietary stimulus.

REFERENCES

1. Armstrong, M.L. 1975. Atherosclerosis in rhesus and cynomolgus monkeys. In J.P. Strong (ed.) Atherosclerosis in Primates. Vol. 9 of Primates in Medicine. pp.16-40. Karger, Basel.

2. Strong, J.P. 1975. Introduction and overview. In J.P. Strong (ed.) Atherosclerosis in Primates. Vol. 9 of Primates in Medicine. pp.1-15. Karger, Basel.

3. Strong, J.P., D.A. Eggen, and H.C. Stary. 1975. Reversibility of experimental fatty streaks in rhesus monkeys. In J.P. Strong (ed.) Atherosclerosis in Primates. Vol. 9 of Primates in Medicine. pp.299-320. Karger, Basel.

4. Mann, G.V., and S.B. Andrus. 1956. Xanthomatosis and atherosclerosis produced by diet in an adult rhesus monkey. J. Lab. Clin. Med. 48:533-550.

5. Cox, G.E., C.B. Taylor, L.G. Cox, and M.D. Counts. 1958. Atherosclerosis in rhesus monkeys. I. Hypercholesteremia induced by dietary fat and cholesterol. Arch. Path. 66:32-52.

6. Taylor, C.B., D.E. Patton, and G.E. Cox. 1963. Atherosclerosis in rhesus monkeys. VI. Fatal myocardial infarction in a monkey fed fat and cholesterol. Arch. Path. 76:404-412.

7. Scott, R.F., E.S. Morrison, J. Jarmolych, S.C. Nam, M. Krams, and F. Coulston. 1967. Experimental atherosclerosis in rhesus monkeys. I. Gross and microscopic features and lipid values in serum and aorta. Exp. Molec. Path. 7:11-33.

8. Manning, J.P., and T.B. Clarkson. 1972. Development, distribution, and lipid content of diet-induced atherosclerotic lesions in rhesus monkeys. Exp. Molec. Path. 17:38-54.

9. Newman, W.P. III, D.A. Eggen, and J.P. Strong. 1974. Comparison of arterial lesions and serum lipids in spider and rhesus monkeys on an egg and butter diet. Atherosclerosis 19:75-86.

10. Vesselinovitch, D., G.S. Getz, R.H. Hughes, and R.W. Wissler. 1974. Atherosclerosis in the rhesus monkey fed three food fats. Atherosclerosis 20:303-321.

11. Stary, H.C. 1975. Coronary artery fine structure in rhesus monkeys: The early atherosclerotic lesion and its progression. In J.P. Strong (ed.) Atherosclerosis in Primates. Vol. 9 of Primates in Medicine. pp.359-395. Karger, Basel.

12. Mohan, A.P., and R.N. Chakravarti. 1975. Serum and aortic lipid profiles in spontaneous and cholesterol-induced atherosclerosis in rhesus monkeys. Atherosclerosis 22:39-46.

13. Goldfischer, S., B. Schiller, and H. Wolinsky. 1975. Lipid accumulation in smooth muscle cell lysosomes in primate atherosclerosis. Amer. J. Path. 78:497-504.

14. Stary, H.C. 1969. Radioautographic observations on DNA synthesis of aortic cells in rhesus monkeys. Circulation 40 (Suppl. 3):25.

15. Stary, H.C. 1970. Electron microscopic observations on the progression of aortic atherosclerosis in rhesus monkeys. Circulation 42 (Suppl. 3):9.

16. Armstrong, M.L., E.D. Warner, and W.E. Conner. 1970. Regression of coronary atheromatosis in rhesus monkeys. Circulation Res. 27:59-76.

17. Armstrong, M.L., and M.G. Megan. 1972. Lipid depletion in athermatous coronary arteries in rhesus monkeys after regression diets. Circulation Res. 30:675-680.

18. DePalma, R.G., W. Insull, E.M. Bellon, W.T. Roth, and A.V. Robinson. 1972. Animal models for the study of progression and regression of atherosclerosis. Surgery 72:268-278.

19. Tucker, C.F., C. Catsulis, J.P. Strong, and D.A. Eggen. 1971. Regression of early cholesterol-induced aortic lesions in rhesus monkeys. Amer. J. Path. 65:493-514.

20. Stary, H.C. 1972. Progression and regression of experimental atherosclerosis in rheusu monkeys; in Medical Primatology 1972, part 3, pp.356-367. Karger, Basel.

21. Vesselinovitch, D., R. Hughes, L. Frazier, and R.W. Wissler. 1973. Studies of the reversal of advanced atherosclerosis in the rhesus monkey. Amer. J. Path. 70:41a.

22. Eggen, D.A., J.P. Strong, W.P. Newman, III, C. Catsulis, G.T. Malcom, and M.G. Kokatnur. 1974. Regression of diet-induced fatty streaks in rhesus monkeys. Lab. Invest. 31:294-301.

23. Kokatnur, M.G., G.T. Malcom, D.A. Eggen, and J.P. Strong. 1975. Depletion of aortic free and ester cholesterol by dietary means in rhesus monkeys with fatty streaks. Atherosclerosis 21: 195-203.

24. Radhakrishnamurthy, B., D.A. Eggen, M.G. Kokatnur, S. Jirge, J.P. Strong, and G.S. Berenson. 1975. Composition of connective tissue in aortas from rhesus monkeys during regression of diet-induced fatty streaks. Lab. Invest. 33: 136-140.

25. Stary, H.C. 1974. Cell proliferation and ultrastructural changes in regressing atherosclerotic lesions after reduction of serum cholesterol. In G. Schettler and A. Weizel (eds.) Atherosclerosis III. pp.187-190. Springer-Verlag, Berlin.

26. Eggen, D.A. 1974. Cholesterol metabolism in rhesus monkey, squirrel monkey, and baboon. J. Lipid Res. 15:139-145.

27. McMillan, G.C. 1973. Development of arteriosclerosis. Amer. J. Cardiol. 31:542-546.

28. Wissler, R.W., and D. Vesselinovitch. 1975. Regression of atherosclerosis in experimental animals and man. Proc. 81 Mtg. German Soc. Int. Med., Wiesbaden, p. 269.

(5)

COMPARISON OF PRIMATES AND RABBITS AS ANIMAL MODELS IN EXPERIMENTAL ATHEROSCLEROSIS

Dragoslava Vesselinovitch and Robert W. Wissler

University of Chicago, Department of Pathology

Chicago, Illinois, U.S.A.

"It takes a genius to say new and surprising things about old subjects."

--Aldous Huxley

The need for a satisfactory animal model in experimental atherosclerosis arises from the fact that it is very difficult to study this multifactorial disease in man. It develops slowly, and accurate and easy measurement of the extent and severity *in vivo*, as well as controlled investigations of human subjects are very difficult. The essence of a satisfactory study is reproducibility - a formidable problem in human studies because of variant environments and lifestyles.

However, various animal species show differential susceptibilities to both spontaneous and experimental atherosclerosis. These differences between species can actually be advantageous, making it possible to choose particular animal models for specific research objectives.

RABBIT

The rabbit was one of the first animals to be used in experimental studies of atherosclerosis and it has continued to be used for a number of reasons, the most important being that is very susceptible to rapid lesion induction. This species is plentiful, easily handled, inexpensive, and biologically well-characterized.

This study was supported by HL 15062 USPHS (SCOR).

However, rabbits are physiologically unprepared to dispose of ingested cholesterol, making the validity of experimental observations in this species questionable.

In the fashion in which rabbits have usually been used, they not only develop a "cholesterol storage disease" with huge pools of cholesterol in the reticuloendothelial system, but also large deposits of cholesterol in the interstitial cells of the heart, kidney and lungs. Furthermore, they develop large numbers of cholesterol-laden circulating cells and deposits of arterial lipids in many small sized arteries usually not affected by atherosclerosis in humans (1).

However, the criticism that blood-derived foam cells are the primary constituents of rabbit lesions is not valid in all cases. "Foamy type" cells are indeed predominant in early rabbit lesions and there is considerable evidence that they come from the blood stream, but several ultrastructural studies indicate that smooth muscle cells may become the most numerous cells (2,3). However, monocytes and macrophages remain much more common than in human lesions. Furthermore, beef-fat fed rabbits develop lesions with extensive extracellular lipid deposition and only a few foam cells (4).

In fact, since Ignatowsky's studies in 1908, numerous investigators have used nutritional, physical, chemical or immunological stimuli to induce in rabbits the entire spectrum of atherosclerotic lesions observed in humans (summarized in Fig. 1 - 1, 2, 4 to 28).

Another problem with the rabbit model concerns the nature of the hyperlipemic LDL. Rabbits fed a cholesterol-rich diet become extremely hypercholesterolemic. The resultant hyperlipidemia is of an unusual pattern and composition. Fraser _et al._ (29) suggest that some of the predominant serum lipoproteins may be "remnant" chylomicrons which have been partially stripped of their triglycerides. This proposed "remnant particle" hyperlipidemia in rabbits may have its parallel in Type III human hyperlipidemia. Recently Stange _et al._ (30) found reduced electrophoretic mobilities of VLDL and LDL and a different apoprotein pattern in rabbits fed an atherogenic diet.

PRIMATES

Ever since the early stages of biological research, scientists have been seeking animal models similar to humans. This is probably the reason for Galen's experiments with monkeys.

Out of 192 living species of monkeys and apes, at least 9 old world and 9 new world species have been utilized in the study of atherosclerosis. The omnivorous monkey resembles man in many respects, including the similarities of nutritional and metabolic patterns; anatomical structure; cardio-pulmonary physiology; and

NUTRITIONAL	Semi-synthetic diets (cholesterol, high-fat)	Ignatowsky 1908, Malmros 1959, Gresham 1962, Imai 1966, Kritchevsky 1971
	Intermittent feeding	Deguid 1954, Constantinides 1960
PHYSICAL	Cauterization Freezing	Petroff 1922, Taylor, 1950
	Endothelial Abrasion Laceration	Prior 1956, Gutstein 1963, Bjorkerud 1969
	X-ray Irradiation	Rieser 1955, Tiamson 1970
	Balloon Catheter	Baumgartner 1963, Stemerman 1972
CHEMICAL	Epinephrine, Allylamine, Thyroxine, Calciferol, etc.	ERB 1905, Waters 1948, Hass 1961, Constantinides 1961, Giordano 1970
	Hypoxia	Astrup 1967, Helin 1969
	Nicotine	Hass 1961, Brinson 1974
IMMUNOLOGICAL INJURY	Infection	Waters 1955
	Homograph rejection	Fisher 1956, Bowyer 1974
	Allergic injury	Minick 1966

Figure 1. Methods for Induction of Atherosclerosis in Rabbits

INVESTIGATOR (year)	SPECIES INDUCTION PERIOD (Mos.)	SEVERITY OF LESIONS	REGRESSION DIET PERIOD (Mos.)	REGRESSION RESPONSE (degree of improvement)
Portman, Maruffo, et. al. (1967, 68)	Squirrel 3	2+	Chow (3,5)	1+
Armstrong, Warner Connor (1970, 72)	Rhesus 17	3+	Low Fat or Corn Oil (40)	3+
Tucker, Catsulis, Eggan, Strong (1971)	Rhesus 2	1+	Chow (4)	1+
Vesselinovitch, Jones, Wissler (1973)	Rhesus 18	3+	Low Fat Corn Oil + W (18)	3+
Stary (1972, 73, 74)	Rhesus 3	2+	Low Fat Basal (1,3,10)	3+
Wissler, Vesselinovitch, Borensztajn (1975)	Rhesus 12	3+	Low Fat Corn Oil + Choles	3+

Figure 2. Regression Studies in Primates

significantly for our purposes, the histogenesis and topography of atherosclerotic lesions, as well as comparable clinical complications of advanced disease. It is noteworthy that many macaques develop high serum lipid levels and atherosclerosis relatively easily and without the circulating lipophages and the severe generalized storage disease found in rabbits. Moreover, several monkey species are large enough to permit a variety of clinical and surgical manipulations.

However, monkey models of atherosclerosis do have certain disadvantages, including the expense, difficulties in procurement, and the necessity for special housing. Sex differences in severity of disease are also frequently not observed in monkeys.

However, despite these problems, the primates have been widely used for the study of atherosclerosis ever since the pioneering work of Hueper (31) with M. mulatta. Selected examples of choosing particular primate species for specific types of studies include using M. speciosa if a larger, but docile animal is desired (32), and M. irus if coronary artery occlusions - particularly of the proximal portion - and myocardial infarction are to be evaluated (33). M. mulatta is particularly useful for studies of nutritionally induced atherosclerosis and regression (34-37). Squirrel monkeys (S. sciurcus) have the interesting characteristic of being hypo- or hyper-responders to atherosclerotic diet, and can be used for studies of the genetic control mechanisms of cholesterol metabolism (38). M. nigra is recommended for studying the relationship between diet and atherosclerosis in diabetes (39). The baboon is very useful for studies of whole-body cholesterol metabolism because it absorbs and excretes cholesterol very much as humans do (40). Cebus monkeys develop more extensive lesions in the coronary arteries than in the aorta (41). M. nemestrina develops fibromuscular lesions after intra-arterial balloon injury (17). The cercopithecus aethiopes, one of the African green monkeys, appears to develop more fibrous and complex atheromatous lesions than several other species when fed a high-fat, cholesterol-rich diet. It may also have serum lipids most similar to Type II (42). Although not all 18 genera currently employed in atherosclerotic studies are fully characterized, the existing models afford the possibility of choosing the animal most suited to the particular problem under consideration.

CONTRASTING PATTERNS OF PATHOGENESIS

There may be at least two predominant pathogenetic patterns in atherosclerosis. The way the lesions develop may affect cellular composition of the plaques, the degree of cell necrosis and type of clinical complications. Rabbits fed an atherogenic diet readily develop intimal lesions - essentially foam cell lesions - which appear to contain a large portion of monocytes and macrophages, while most of the primates studied so far show a much slower development of lesions, composed largely of lipid-containing smooth muscle cells, probably derived from the arterial media. A three month period of cholesterol-rich diet will cause severe atherosclerosis in rabbits, while in most monkeys lesions will just be starting to develop. It was formerly believed that hypercholesterolemia caused inhibition of arterial fibrosis in rabbits, but not in primates; however, more recently it has been observed that moderate hypercholesterolemia stimulates predominantly collagenous responses both in rabbits and monkeys (7). In spite of continuous hyperlipemia, monkeys can develop collagen-rich lesions. In rabbits either an interruption of cholesterol feeding (1) or a high-fat diet without cholesterol (7) may result in lesions with a thick fibrous cap.

More thorough explication of genetically controlled species differences and the corresponding mechanisms through which the basic atherogenic processes are controlled would be valuable for our understanding of atherosclerosis. Perhaps the reasons for certain species' immunity to this disease could be used to develop new forms of treatment for humans.

REGRESSION

The possibility that experimental and spontaneous atherosclerosis could be reversed has long been suspected, but it is only within the last few years that a variety of basic animal experiments have verified this opinion. There is now abundant evidence indicating that rather simple dietary measures can cause regression of advanced atherosclerotic lesions in monkeys. In fact, it is likely that reversal can be achieved consistently in the Rhesus monkey if the cholesterol level is sustained at a level of 150 mg% or lower over a long time period.

There are, furthermore, significant differences between rabbits and primates in response to diet-induced regression of atherosclerotic lesions following removal of the dietary stimulus. Although primates show considerable sensitivity to regressive treatment, the same is not generally true for rabbits, in which cessation of cholesterol feeding may result in lesion consolidation (43), while withdrawal of the atherogenic diet leads to increased severity of disease (1). However, very mild rabbit lesions resulting from very brief feeding periods do show regression (1). Unfortunately, the rabbit was one of the first species in which regression studies were attempted, and this has probably delayed advancements in this important field. Studies now exist which indicate that substantial reversal of rabbit lesions can indeed be effected by rather complicated treatments - a low-fat, low-cholesterol diet combined with additional therapeutic manipulations such as hyperoxia, EDTA, surfactants, colcemid, estrogen or cholestyramine administration, or a combination of these factors (44-49). However, this animal is not ideal for studies of regression and experimental results should not be used to guide studies in patients.

In contrast, primates belong to an intermediate animal group as far as their sensitivity to experimental atherosclerosis is concerned. In comparison to species employed so far in regression studies (mainly squirrel and Rhesus monkeys), they are proving to be quite suitable for regression treatment (Fig. 2; 50-52). Simple dietary manipulations appear to be quite effective. Our most recent studies of diet and cholestyramine administration show considerable regression, even when the drug is accompanied by atherogenic diet (52). Recent studies with Rhesus monkeys show reversal, even in the most advanced atherosclerosis that is similar to advanced human atheromas. It is quite encouraging. Many of the lesions at the beginning of therapy were advanced and complicated with necrotic centers and fibrosis. Coronary arteries with severe lumenal narrowing improved greatly during the treatment period.

CONCLUSION

Admittedly, no animal model perfectly duplicates the human disease or satisfies all requirements of the "ideal" model, but intelligent choice of species will help achieve research objectives. There now exist a number of methods suitable for studying induction or regression of a wide variety of atherosclerotic lesions in both rabbits and primates. Some of these animal lesions appear to bear a striking resemblance to human lesions, even though the morphological componenets and rate of development may vary. Useful information can be gained by analysing and comparing the differential responses and the disease severity in several species.

It is very important to realize that although morphological similarities do exist between animal and human atherosclerosis, there are also differences which suggest different pathogenetic factors. Great caution should be used in extrapolating results obtained from the animal model to the human disease.

References:

1. Constantinides, P. Experimental atherosclerosis. Elsevier Publishing Co. New York, 1965.

2. Imai, H., Lee, K.T., Pastori, S., Panlilio, E., Florentin, R. and Thomas, W. A. Exp. Mol. Pathol. 5:273, 1966.

3. Geer, J. C. Circulation Vol. Suppl. 2-3, 13, 1965.

4. Gresham, G. A. and Howard, A. N. Arch. Pathol. 74: 13, 1962.

5. Ignatowsky, A. Tr. Military-Med. Acad. Petersburg, 16: 174,1908.

6. Malmros, H. J. and Wigand, G. Lancet 2: 749, 1959.

7. Kritchevsky, D., Tepper, A., Vesselinovitch, D. and Wissler, R.W. Atherosclerosis, 14: 53, 1971.

8. Duguid, J.B. Lancet 1, 891, 1954.

9. Petroff, J.R., Beitr. pathol. Anat. u. allgen. Pathol. 71: 115, 1922.

10. Taylor, C.B., Baldwin, D. and Hass, G.M. Arch. Pathol. 49: 623, 1950.

11. Christensen, B.C. and Garbarsch, C. Virchows Arch (Pathol. A nat) 360:93, 1973.

12. Prior, J.T. and Hartmann, W.H. Am. J. Path. 32: 417, 1956.

13. Gutstein, H., Lazzarini-Robertson, A. Jr., and LaTaillade, N. Amer. Journ. of Path. 42: 61, 1963.

14. Björkerud, S. Virchows Arch. (Pathol. Anat.) 347: 197, 1969.

15. Tiamson, E. et al. Exp. Mol. Pathol. 12: 175, 1970.

16. Baumgartner, H.R. and Studer, A. Pathol. Microbiol. (Basel) 26: 129, 1963.

17. Stemerman, B., Baumgartner, H.R., Spaet, T. H. Lab. Invest. 24: 179, 1971.

18. Spaet, T.H., Stemerman, M.B., Veith, F.J. and Lejnieks, I. Circulation Res. 36: 58, 1975.

19. Erb, W. Arch. f. Exper. Path. u. Pharmakol. 53: 173, 1905.

20. Hass, G.M., Trueheart, R.E. and Hemmens, A. Amer. J. Path. 38: 289, 1961.

21. Giordano, A.R., Spraragen, S.C., Hamel, H. Lab. Inves. 22: 94, 1970.

22. Astrup, P., Kjeldsen, K., and Wanstrup, J. J. Athero. Res. 7: 343, 1967.

23. Helin, P. and Lorenzen,J. Angiology, 20: 1, 1969.

24: Brinson, K. and Chakrabarti, B. K. Atheorsclerosis 20:527, 1974.

25. Waters, L.L. Symposium on Atherosclerosis, National Academy of Sciences, National Research Council Publication 338:91,1955.

26. Fisher, E.R., Fisher, B. Surgery 40: 530, 1956.

27. Bowyer, D.E., Dunn, D. and Gresham, G.A. Atherosclerosis III. eds. Schettler and Weizel, Springer-Verlag, New York p 348,1974.

28. Minick, C., Murphy, E. and Campbell, G. Jr. J. Exp. Med. 124: 635, 1966.

29. Fraser, R., Courtice, F.C., Vesselinovitch, D. and Wissler, R.W. In press. Atherosclerosis. 1975.

30. Stange, E., Agostini, B., Papenberg, J. Atherosclerosis 22: 125, 1975.

31. Hueper, W.C. Am. J. Path. 22 : 1287, 1946.

32. Wissler, R. W. and Vesselinovitch, D. Atherosclerosis III. eds. Schettler and Weizel, Springer-Verlag, New York p 319,1974.

33. Kramsch, D.M. and Hollander, W. Exp. and Mol. Pathol. 9:1,1968.

34. Armstrong, M.L., Warner, D.E. and Connor, W.E. Circ. Res. 27: 59, 1970.

35. Stary, H.C. Med.Primatology, Part III, eds. Goldsmith and Morr-Hankowsky. p 356, 1972.

36. Vesselinovitch, D., Wissler, R.W. Hughes, R. and Borensztajn, J. In Press. Atherosclerosis, 1975.

37. Jones, R., Vesselinovitch, D., Hughes, R. and Wissler, R. W. Fed. Proc. 32: 158, 1973.

38. Lofland, H. B., Clarkson, T. B., St.Clair, R. W. J. L. Res. 13: 39, 1972.

39. Howard, C.F. Diet and Atherosclerosis. Vol. 60. eds. Sistori, Ricci and Gorino, p 13, 1975.

40. Strong,J. P. and McGill, H.C., Jr. Am. J. Pathol. 50: 669, 1967.

41. Clarkson, T.B. Advances in Veterinary Science and Comparative Science. Vol. 16. p 151, eds. Bundly and Cornelius, New York Acad. Press. 1972.

42. Bullock, B.C., Lehner, D.N., Clarkson, T.B., Feldner, M.A., Wagner, W.D. and Lofland, H. B. Exp. and Mol. Pathol.22: 151, 1975.

43. McMillan, G.C., Horlick, L., Duff, G.L. AMA Archives of Path. 285, 1949.

44. Anitschkow, N. Verh. dtsch. Ges. Path. 23: 473, 1928. in Zbl. allg. Path. path. Anat., suppl. ad vol. 43, 1928.

45. Wartman, A., Lampe, T.L., McCann, D.S. and Boyle, A.J. J. Atheroscler. Res. 7: 331, 1967.

46. Vesselinovitch, D., Wissler, R.W., Dzoga, K., Hughes, R.H. and Dubien, L. Atheroslcerosis 19: 259, 1974.

47. Kjeldsen, K., Astrup, P. and Wanstrup., J., J. Atheroscl. Res. 10: 173, 1969.

48. Weigensberg, B.I. and Stary, H. Circulation, 48. Suppl.IV, 160, 1973.

49. Kramsch, D.M. and Chan, C.T. Fed. Proc. 235, abs. 93, 1975.

50. Portman, O.W., Alexander, M. and Maruffo, C.A. J. Nutrition, 91:35, 1967.

51. Tucker, C.F., Catsulis, C. Strong, J.P. and Eggen, D.A. Am. J. Pathol. 65: 493, 1971.

52. Wissler, R.W., Vesselinovitch, D., Borensztajn, J. and Hughes, R. Abstract accepted for AHA Ann. Scient. Meet.1975.

(6)

DISCUSSION (ANIMAL MODELS IN THE STUDY OF ATHEROSCLEROSIS)

DISCUSSION FOLLOWING DR. THOMAS B. CLARKSON'S PRESENTATION

An Unidentified Speaker: I would like to know please, if the response of the arterial wall to hypercholesterolemia is different between hypo-and hyperresponder animals.

Dr. Clarkson: I take it that you refer to differences between random bred and WC-2 White Carneau pigeons. Morphologically, we can find no differences other than simply exaggerated pathogenesis of the lesion. It may be that there is an early accumulation of greater amounts of glycosaminoglycans in the aorta. There may also be qualitative differences in the glycosaminoglycans composition, but these observations are tentative at this time.

Dr. Stein: My question concerns the genetic studies of cholesterol fed animals. Are their plasma cholesterol concentrations different when they are fed diets without added cholesterol?

Dr. Clarkson: The genetic differences that we have observed between these two strains of pigeons that are hyper-or hyporesponsive to dietary cholesterol concerns only their response to dietary cholesterol. They are not different in plasma cholesterol concentration when fed diets without added cholesterol. That is also true of hypo-and hyperresponder squirrel monkeys. It is probably true that there are differences between hyper-and hyporesponsive macaques on low cholesterol diets.

An Unidentified Speaker: Are there differences in the progression of atherosclerosis among WC-2's and random bred White Carneau pigeons when they are fed regular grain diets.

Dr. Clarkson: Yes. There are differences in the amount of plaque as measured grossly and in the cholesterol ester concentration, beginning at about 12 months of age with the WC-2's having more advanced disease.

DISCUSSION FOLLOWING DR. ALLEN HOWARD'S PRESENTATION

Dr. Kottke: Were your studies on cholesterol ester hydrolase made with a powder preparation or did you use a microsomal preparation?

Dr. Howard: The studies were done using acetone powder preparations.

DISCUSSION FOLLOWING DR. K. T. LEE'S PRESENTATION

Dr. Alonzo: Dr. Lee, from the pictures you showed, it appears that the media has disappeared as a result of balloon injury and the atherogenic diet. I wonder if balloon injury without the atherogenic diet would have affected the media?

Dr. Lee: The injury is rather superficial and does not extend significantly into the media. If one utilizes the method delicately it is possible to injure the endothelium without substantial injury to the underlying media.

Dr. Wissler: I should like to comment further on that question. Among most species healing of arterial injury is essentially complete if the animals are fed control rather than atherogenic diets. How reversible are these lesions produced by balloon injury in swine if the animals are fed a normal diet?

Dr. Lee: We have done some control studies in a number of swine. After a month, 2 or 3, one sees some thickening due to scar tissue but the lesions contained no lipid.

Unidentified Speaker: Do you have any evidence that injury to the coronary artery endothelium during coronary angiography hastens the development of lesions.

Dr. Lee: In our coronary angiographic studies we attempt to be very careful not to injure the endothelium. In swine cases, however, where the endothelium has been injured and the animals are fed an atherogenic diet, intimal thickenings do occur. It is probably true that the atherogenic diet that we feed to the swine is much worse than the diet consumed by human beings.

Dr. Constantinides: This is a beautifully presented study on vascular injury. I think it would perhaps be more interesting if you used the kinds of injury that might occur in man. I know of no injury that affects the entire endothelium for such a considerable segment. Examples of the kind of injury to which I refer might be immunologic injury or injury due to hypertension.

DISCUSSION FOLLOWING DR. S. DRAGA VESSELINOVITCH'S PRESENTATION

Dr. Rapacz: I would like to comment on the important role that genetics might play in atherosclerosis. The existence of hypo- and hyperresponders to atherogenic diets has often been observed in animal models but its basis has been shown to be genetic only during the last decade. This was demonstrated mainly by Clarkson and Lofland and co-investigators in monkeys and pigeons. It is well known to geneticists that environmental factors influence genetic traits to a greater or lesser degree depending upon the nature of the gene control and the load of environmental input. On the other hand environmentalists often completely disregard the role of genetics in affecting the phenotype being studied.

In the majority of animal models, investigators were very fortunate in having animals of the same age and sex tested with the same diet. Unfortunately, little attention was paid to the possible role of genetics in accounting for the observed variations. It is true that in most of these cases the mode of inheritance would be difficult to establish when a complex genetic polymorphism operates on one locus and yet could be much more complicated while two or more systems and gene regulatory mechanisms are involved.

From the data on the African green monkey presented by Dr. Clarkson, it seems clear that the responsiveness to the atherogenic diet is not to be explained by a single gene but rather it is a polygenic trait, by comparison similar to the weight-gain in animals. This species should be investigated because it is suggested as the closest to man as an experiment animal model to study atherosclerosis.

In this regard, I believe that the presentation of Dr. Vesselinovitch is very pertinent. She mentioned a few animal models for studying genetic factors in atherosclerosis. It is not clear to me why only these few species were suggested for genetic studies. It is because these species might have more simple modes of inheritance or is she concerned about the molecular mechanism involved in the expression of the "defective gene" (mutants)? Both approaches are interesting. However, the former may account only for a small number of genetic factors involved in atherogenesis, and the latter is still poorly understood, with the exception of hypercholesterolemia type II in man, where the mechanism leading to the development of the syndrome was explained but the number of mutants is unknown. My concern is that the complexity of atherosclerosis discourages many investigators from looking at genetics as an important discipline particularly if the genetic mechanism is more complex than simple Mendelian segregation. This approach may be misleading because of its oversimplification and omission of the important genetic role in atherosclerosis.

While I fully appreciate the difficulties in changing orthodox view of some investigators, I would respectfully plead that the role of genetics be more carefully evaluated.

DISCUSSION FOLLOWING DR. J. P. STRONG'S PRESENTATION

Dr. Kramsch: My question concerns the changes in the connective tissues during regression and how you have expressed the data.

Dr. Strong: Let me say something about that before you go further because that has been questioned before. The figures that I showed were concentrations in mg/g of dried defatted artery. After some criticism on that at the Dallas meeting, Dr. Murthy went on and recalculated the same data on a per aorta basis and it comes out very much the same way. Dr. Armstrong has also recalculated our data using some assumptions about dilutions and came up with a different conclusion. I know Prof. Zemplenyi has been puzzled by the fact that we can't decide about what we have got. I think we really don't know, we are doing other experiments at different periods of time. I hope that we will come up with something more conclusive. Would you make a suggestion?

Dr. Kramsch: Amongst small animals it is proper to express data as absolute amounts per aorta. In large animals like monkeys with more variation in body weight it might be a good idea to express the data per unit of protein and in that way you eliminate the error due to calcium or by mucopolysaccharides.

Dr. Wissler: I would like to make two very quick observations. One is that it is interesting that when you use the relatively brief period for induction, you do get topographically much more disease in the thoracic aorta than in the abdominal aorta, whereas in our longer experiment we almost always, not always, have considerably more disease in the abdominal area than in the thoracic.

Dr. Strong: May I say one word about that Dr. Wissler. The exact experience of the human fatty streak telescoped from about 15 years down to 1 or 2 years because the thoracic aorta is more extensively involved in early childhood and later on the abdominal aorta overtakes it.

Dr. Wissler: That is the reason I thought it would be interesting to bring that point out. The second comment concerns Elspeth Smith's observations on differences in fatty streaks and the question of how lesions progress, and what kind of lesions one starts with to get progressive lesions. I think it is very interesting that you have, in a very fine kind of model experiment, shown that if you produce a fair amount of regression you go from intracellular to extracellular lipid and produce a plaque very much like a gelatinous elevation. Having worked recently with Dr. Smith we have now looked at sections together which has been a great help to me and I think perhaps she benefited some too. I think maybe Dr. Constantinides some years ago put his finger on the key point, namely, that the disease in man is almost certainly episodic. It comes and goes and the reason Dr. Smith connects these elevations with progression is that people have more of this up and down kind of fluctuation and thus they show more extracellular lipid as this occurs several times in the progression of lesions. I think this is a very important observation.

Dr. Hauss: In addition to studying the amount of collagen did you study the type of collagen?

Dr. Strong: We did not study the type of collagen. We really don't have the final answer on this.

Dr. Hollander: If I understand correctly, you tried to recalculate your data on the basis of the absolute weight of the intima-media and you found that there was no difference in weight between the regressed aorta and the progressed aorta even though the lipid content was significantly lessened in the regressed aorta. From this calculation you concluded that concentrations of the fibrous proteins were not different.

The point I should wish to make about these data is that one must have available the entire aorta if one is to use an expression of aorta content of a given substance. In our laboratories, we no longer split aortas longitudinally using half for morphologic observations and the other half for biochemical determinations. When one splits aortas longitudinally, they are making the assumption that composition is exactly the same in both halves when they calculate aorta content. We have begun expressing biochemical measurements in terms of intimal surface area which we feel takes into account the thickness of the aorta and the thickness of the lesion.

With regard to the mucopolysacharrides, Dr. Schmidt and I have been examining atherosclerotic lesions from a variety of animal models and of human beings. We find that the predominant mucopolysacharride in the arterial wall is not Chondroitin sulfate B but is Chondroitin sulfate C. For this reason it is very difficult for us to comment on the quantitative differences that you observed in your experiment. We have also found that there is very little hyaluronic acid in the normal aorta and also in the atherosclerotic aorta.

Dr. Strong: I should like to respond to the comment about splitting aortas longitudinally. In our laboratories this has been useful as far as determinations of artery lipids are concerned probably because they increase so considerably and because the disease is symmetrical. I am sure that the next time we are concerned with measurement of arterial connective tissue proteins, we will elect to express them in all ways that are available to us.

Dr. Hayes: Related to these last two questions, were there any ultrastructural correlations between the changes in amorphous ground substance or connective tissue and elastin in the abdominal vs thoracic in the progression of the disease.

Dr. Strong: Biochemical quantitation is difficult and ultrastructural quantitation is even more difficult. We thought there was more collagen ultrastructurally, and perhaps more ground substance but we are uncertain about the significance of these changes quantitatively.

CHAPTER 9
LIPID CLINIC III
(The Effects of Nutrition and Treatment on Lipid Metabolism)

(1)

THE EFFECTS OF NUTRITION ON LIPID METABOLISM*

William E. Connor

The Department of Medicine
University of Oregon School of Medicine
Portland, Oregon, U.S.A.

Nutritional factors have important effects upon lipid metabolism in man and indeed play the dominant role in the pathogenesis of the hyperlipidemia and atherosclerosis so commonly found in populations of the Western World. Many past investigations have documented that certain dietary substances have decisive effects upon the serum lipid concentrations and the sterol balance of the body. These dietary factors are sterols, fats and total calories. This review will focus upon a discussion of their roles. Other substances whose effects are to date less well defined but which may have some influence especially in certain individuals, include carbohydrates, fiber and alcohol. Proteins, minerals and vitamins have little or no effect upon lipid metabolism in amounts and kinds typically consumed by the American population.

Cholesterol: The substance best known for its effects upon lipid metabolism is dietary cholesterol (1). In 1912 it was identified as the constituent of animal foods which would readily elevate the serum cholesterol levels and produce atherosclerosis in experimental animals. Subsequently, cholesterol-rich diets have regularly caused hypercholesterolemia, atherosclerosis and even at times, myocardial infarction in a large number of species of experimental animals, including primates. For a time, however, dietary cholesterol was considered of little importance in human lipid metabolism (2). By the early 1960s a decisive effect of cholesterol in the diet of man upon the serum lipid levels was clearly demonstrated in a series of metabolic ward experiments being carried out in normal volunteers (3,4,5,6,7). Dietary cholesterol is absorbed by the gut in amounts proportional to the intake up to a dietary level of perhaps 1200-1500 mg per day. Only about 40 percent of the intake is absorbed (8,9). In many, absorbed cholesterol is transported initially in chylomicrons, largely as ester cholesterol, reaches a peak concentration in the plasma some 48 hours after a given meal and then contributes its mass to the total body pools of cholesterol (10). Its subsequent transport from the chylomicron is not well understood in man. Presumably cholesterol-rich chylomicron remnants are metabolized by the liver. In the experiments now to be described, good evidence is provided that cholesterol of dietary origin is transfered ultimately into other lipoprotein classes, especially beta and very low density lipoproteins (11).

Twenty-five subjects previously consuming the usual American diet were given cholesterol-free diets for 3-4 weeks and then 1000 mg/day of dietary cholesterol for another 3-4 weeks. The diets were otherwise identical and contained 40 percent of the calories as fat. The resulting plasma cholesterol changes are depicted in Table 1. All subjects had a pronounced decline in plasma cholesterol concentration following the consumption of the cholesterol-free diet. The previous typically American diet had been high in cholesterol content and saturated fat. The mild and severe type II-a, and the normal and the type IV subjects responded similarly.

With the baseline cholesterol-free diet, the composite mean level of plasma cholesterol for the 25 subjects was 211 mg/dl. The inclusion of 1000 mg of dietary cholesterol in the diet which was added without changing the other constituents of the diet (calories, carbohydrates, fat, protein, minerals and vitamins) caused an increase in serum cholesterol to 247 mg/dl or a net change of +36 mg/dl. All subjects changed in the upward direction, even the type IV subjects. The severe type II subjects appeared to have the greatest change, an increase of 67 mg/dl.

The crucial question of this study was then to ascertain what lipoprotein fractions changed in response to the 1000 mg high cholesterol diet. Which lipoprotein carried the increase in plasma cholesterol concentration? For normal subjects and those with type II-a hyperlipidemia, the increase was almost entirely in the form of low density (beta) lipoprotein (LDL) with slight increases being seen in high density (alpha) lipoprotein (Figure 1). There were no significant increases in very low density lipoprotein (VLDL). In the type IV patients, however, a somewhat different result occurred. Both VLDL and LDL cholesterol increased. Each accounted for about 50 percent of the total increase. We interpret these findings as indicating that dietary cholesterol effects in most individuals will be reflected in an increase of LDL cholesterol concentration. This pertains even to normal subjects with baseline serum cholesterol levels quite low, 141 mg/dl as well as for the type II-a subjects with mild or severe hypercholesterolemia. In the type IV subjects the metabolic block in the usual conversion of VLDL to LDL becomes evident. Both VLDL and LDL cholesterol increased as a result of dietary cholesterol ingestion.

Table 1

THE PLASMA CHOLESTEROL LEVELS (mg%) AFTER A CHOLESTEROL-FREE AND HIGH CHOLESTEROL DIETS IN NORMAL AND HYPERLIPOPROTEINEMIC SUBJECTS

	Usual American Diet	Cholesterol-free Diet	Change	High Cholesterol	Change
Normal Subjects	171 ± 8	141 ± 14	-30	174 ± 20	+33
Type II-a Mild	258 ± 18	209 ± 27	-49	245 ± 29	+36
Type II-a Severe	376 ± 22	338 ± 43	-38	405 ± 17	+67
Type IV	251 ± 36	208 ± 23	-43	231 ± 23	+23
Composite		211		247	+36

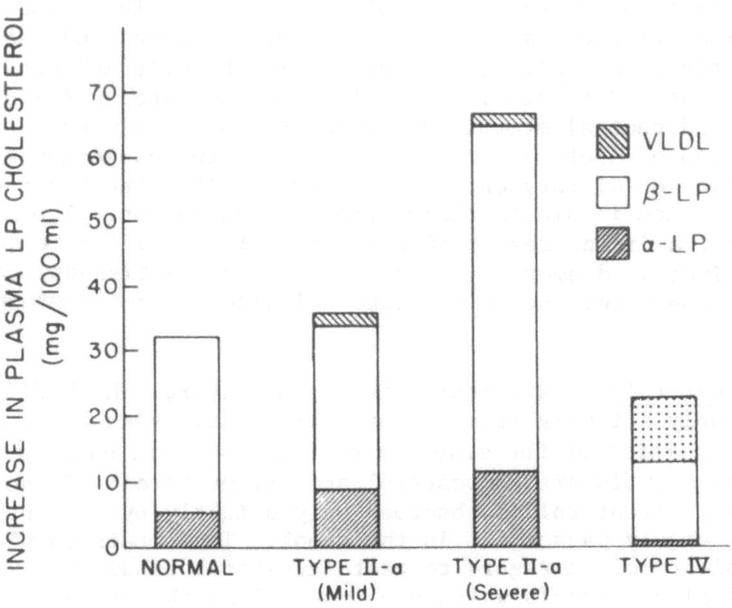

Figure 1. Effects of a 1000 mg Cholesterol Deit Upon the Plasma Lipoproteins in Hyperlipidemic and Normal Subjects.

This takes us to a consideration of the mechanism whereby dietary cholesterol increases the total serum cholesterol concentrations and also LDL cholesterol concentrations. The concept of the sterol balance suggests that dietary cholesterol may simply overload the disposal system. The input of sterols into the plasma-tissue pool is twofold: From dietary cholesterol (0 to 1500 mg/day) and from synthesized cholesterol derived from the liver and intestinal tract. The synthesis rate in man is not very labile and most studies have shown little or no effect upon synthesis from the ingestion of dietary cholesterol. This means that the total amount of sterol entering the body either from diet or by synthesis may be much greater in individuals consuming a high cholesterol diet than in individuals consuming a low cholesterol diet. The output of sterols from the body is largely by way of the feces and includes the cholesterol and bile acids excreted in the bile and not reabsorbed by the gut. Most studies to date have indicated a failure of bile acid and neutral steroid excretion to increase very much after the ingestion of dietary cholesterol. Thus, two consequences from the ingestion of dietary cholesterol may result. The first consequence is a rise in plasma cholesterol concentration. The second consequence, a direct result of the first, is the ultimate deposition of increased amounts of cholesterol in the tissues, particularly in the arteries, to initiate and sustain the atherosclerotic process.

<u>β-sitosterol</u>: β-sitosterol is a plant sterol which differs in structure only slightly from cholesterol in having an ethyl group at the 22 position of the side chain of the steroid nucleus. Other plant sterols are campesterol and stigmasterol. In normal individuals, sitosterol is absorbed only slightly by the intestinal tract and largely passes out in the stool. Thus it is completely unlike cholesterol in regard to gastointestinal handling. The amounts of plant sterols which are ingested in the normal American diet are not inconsiderable, perhaps 200-400 mg per day. In pharmacological doses, β-sitosterol has been shown to have an hypocholesterolemic effect because of interference with the absorption of cholesterol.

However, in some individuals with a genetic abnormality, β-sitosterol is absorbed in much greater amounts than is customary, twenty to thirty percent of an ingested dose, so that it and other plant sterols accumulate in the blood and tissues (12). Two sisters and one other woman with this disorder have been described to date. In these individuals, β-sitosterol contributes to a disease process. Xanthoma occurs and presumably atherosclerosis, so that its level in the diet for these susceptible persons is of paramount importance. Of unknown significance is the occurrence of considerable amounts of β-sitosterol in the blood of infants fed formula diets containing vegetable oils (13).

The important consideration is to appreciate that this entity does occur and that the administration of β-sitosterol is contraindicated either in the course of the consumption of vegetable oils or in the use of β-sitosterol as a hypocholesterolemic drug.

Dietary Fat; Amount and Saturation: The amount and kind of fat in the diet have a considerable effect upon the serum lipid concentrations. Saturated fat elevates and polyunsaturated fat decreases the serum cholesterol levels. Monounsaturated fat (i.e., oleic acid being the characteristic fatty acid) has a neutral effect and does not in itself either elevate or depress the serum lipids. For practical purposes, all animal fats are highly saturated except those derived from marine animals and fish. Many, but not all, of the currently marketed vegetable oil shortenings are only lightly hydrogenated and thus retain the basic unsaturated characteristics of vegetable oils in general. Coconut oil and chocolate, perhaps the only saturated vegetable fats commonly consumed, have a hypercholesterolemic effect.

Precisely why dietary fat affects the serum lipids is not completely known. Dietary fat facilitates cholesterol absorption from the intestinal tract, hence, its restriction may lessen the input of dietary cholesterol into the body. With very low fat diets it is known that cholesterol from the diet is poorly absorbed. Certainly in many individuals polyunsaturated fat enhances the excretion of cholesterol and its chief metabolite, bile acids, from the body and into the feces and thus creates a more negative cholesterol balance (14, 15). The enhanced fecal excretion of sterols and bile acids will more than account for the amount of cholesterol which leaves the plasma, with the concomitant lowering of plasma cholesterol levels. Large amounts of linoleic fatty acid in the diet alter the fatty acid composition of the serum lipoproteins. This change presumably lessens their capacity to carry lipids, in particular cholesterol, with a consequent lower serum cholesterol concentration.

Calories: Hypertriglyceridemia may result from excessive caloric consumption of any source of food with an associated weight gain. Caloric excesses are particularly significant when the serum triglycerides are already elevated and of lesser importance in the genesis of the hyperlipidemia when only the serum cholesterol level is increased. The excessive calories result metabolically in increased substrate for triglyceride synthesis in the liver. Further, reduced clearance of triglyceride from the blood may be partly responsible for the hypertriglyceridemia of the obese. Enlarged adipose tissue cells apparently have a reduced capacity to remove circulating triglyceride from the plasma.

Excessive caloires from whatever source (fat, carbohydrates, protein or alcohol), then, are responsible in some individuals for hyperlipidemia, especially hypertriglyceridemia. There is usually an associated hypercholesterolemia, resulting partly from the concomitantly increased intake of dietary cholesterol and saturated fat but also because the lipoproteins (VLDL) which carry the increased triglyceride content transport cholesterol as well. The typical American adult consumes excessive quantities of food containing en masse excessive calories, cholesterol and saturated fat. Reduction of caloric intake in hypertriglyceridemic patients and the subsequent loss of adiposity invariably leads to lower plasma lipid levels, perhaps even to a normal range (16, 17). Plasma cholesterol levels concomitantly fall also.

REFERENCES

1. Connor, W.E. and Connor, S.L. The Key Role of Nutritional Factors in the Prevention of Coronary Heart Disease. Prev. Med. 1:49, 1972.

2. Keys, A., Anderson, J.T., Mickelson, O., Adelson, S.F. and Fidanza, F. Diet and Serum Cholesterol in Man: Lack of Effect of Dietary Cholesterol. J. Nutr. 59:39, 1956.

3. Connor, W.E., Hodges, R.E. and Bleiler, R.E. The Effect of Dietary Cholesterol Upon the Serum Lipids in Man. J. Lab. Clin. Med. 57:331, 1961.

4. Connor, W.E., Hodges, R.E. and Bleiler, R.E. The Serum Lipids in Men Receiving High Cholesterol and Cholesterol-Free Diets. J. Clin. Invest. 40:894, 1961.

5. Connor, W.E., Stone, D.B. and Hodges, R.E. The Interrelated Effects of Dietary Cholesterol and Fat Upon the Human Serum Lipid Levels. J. Clin. Invest. 43:1691, 1964.

6. Beveridge, J.M.R., Connell, W.F., Mayer, G.A. and Haust, H.L. The Response of Man to Dietary Cholesterol. J. Nutr. 71:61, 1960.

7. Steiner, A., Howard, E.J. and Akgun, S. Importance of Dietary Cholesterol in Man. J. Am. Med. Assoc. 181:186, 1962.

8. Connor, W.E., and Lin, D.S. The Intestinal Absorption of Dietary Cholesterol by Hypercholesterolemic (Type II) and Normocholesterolemic Humans. J. Clin. Invest. 53:1062, 1974.

9. Grundy, S.M., Ahrens, E.H., Jr. and Davignon, J. The Interaction of Cholesterol Absorption and Cholesterol Synthesis in Man. J. Lip. Res. 10:304, 1969.

10. Bhattacharyya, A.K., Connor, W.E., Mausolf, F.A. and Flatt, A.E.

Turnover Xanthoma Cholesterol in Hyperlipoproteinemic Patients. J. Lab. and Clin. Med. (in press).

11. Connor, W.E. and Jagannathan, S.N. Increased Beta Lipoprotein Cholesterol from the Feeding of Dietary Cholesterol to Normal and Hyperlipoproteinemic Subjects. Submitted for publication.

12. Bhattacharyya, A.K. and Connor, W.E. Betasitosterolemia and Xanthomatosis: A Newly Described Lipid Storage Disease in Two Sisters. J. Clin. Invest. 53:1033, 1974.

13. Mellies, M., Glueck, C.J., Sweeney, C., Fallat, R., Tsang, R. andIshikawa, T.T. Plasma and Dietary Phytosterols in Children. Pediatrics. In press, 1975.

14. Connor, W.E., Witiak, D.T., Stone, D.B. and Armstrong, M.L. Cholesterol Balance and Fecal Neutral Steroid and Bile Acid Excretion in Normal Men Fed Dietary Fats of Different Fatty Acid Composition. J. Clin. Invest. 48:1363, 1969.

15. Moore, R.B., Anderson, J.T., Taylor, H.L., Keep, A. and Frantz, I.D., Jr. Effect of Dietary Fat on the Fecal Excretion of Cholesterol and its Degradation Products in Man. J. Clin. Invest. 47:1517, 1968.

16. Olefsky, J., Reaven, G.M. and Farquahr, J.W. Effects of Weight Reduction on Obesity. J. Clin. Invest. 53:64, 1974.

17. Galbraith, W.B., Connor, W.E. and Stone, D.B. Weight Loss and Serum Lipid Changes in Obese Subjects Given Low Calorie Diets of Varied Cholesterol Content. Ann. Int. Med. 64:268, 1966.

*This study was supported by U.S. Public Health Service Research Grants HL 19,130 from the National Heart and Lung Institutes and by the General Clinical Research Centers Program (RR-334) of the Division of Research Resources, National Institutes of Health.

(2)

INFLUENCE OF DIETARY FAT AND PROTEIN ON PLASMA CHOLESTEROL LEVELS IN THE EARLY POSTNATAL PERIOD

K. K. Carroll[1] and M. W. Huff

Department of Biochemistry,
University of Western Ontario,
London, Ontario, Canada

The adult human populations of industrialized countries have considerably higher levels of serum cholesterol than those observed in most common animal species (Fig. 1). These high levels appear to be an important risk factor in coronary heart disease. It is therefore important to determine the reasons for the elevated levels in humans and to investigate the role of environmental factors such as diet.

The differential in serum cholesterol levels between animals and humans is partly due to changes that occur during or after weaning. In animals the levels are generally low at birth, show a marked rise during the suckling period and then decline at or near the time of weaning (Fig. 2). The serum cholesterol level in humans is also low at birth (usually < 100 mg/dl) and increases during the first weeks or months of life to 125-175 mg/dl (1). However, instead of dropping at the time of weaning as in other animal species, it remains high throughout childhood, adolescence and adult life (2,3). Consequently, the adult levels are considerably higher than those of other common animal species.

The lipid ingested with the milk appears to be an important factor in the hypercholesterolemia that develops during the suckling period (3,4), and the decrease in animals at weaning coincides with a change from a high fat to a low fat diet. This raises the possibility that serum cholesterol levels remain elevated in humans because they are weaned to diets relatively high in fat.

[1]Research Associate of the Medical Research Council of Canada.

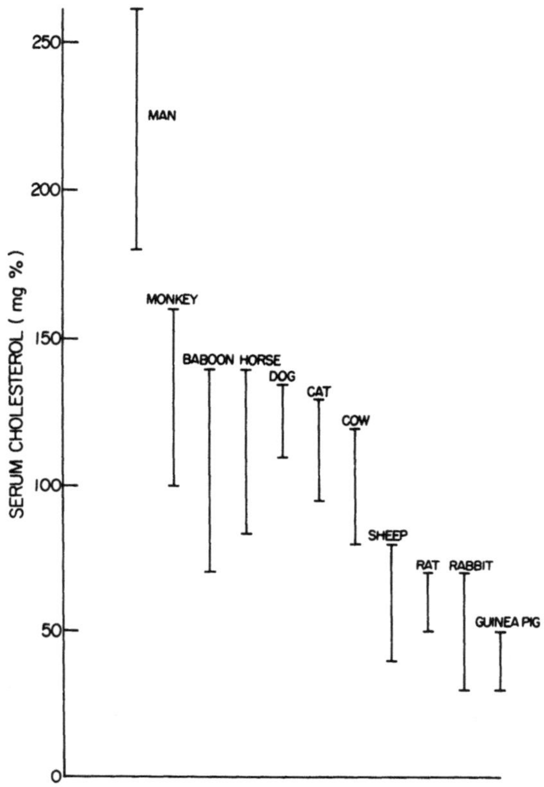

Fig. 1. Species variations in serum cholesterol levels. Data taken from Kritchevsky (2).

As in other animals, dietary fat appears to be responsible for the hypercholesterolemia in suckling rabbits (4). However, our studies with older rabbits indicated that dietary protein rather than dietary fat was exerting the major influence on plasma cholesterol levels (5). Animal proteins such as casein produced an elevation of plasma cholesterol when fed in a low cholesterol semisynthetic diet, whereas the level remained low when the dietary protein was derived from plant sources. Addition of butter to these semisynthetic diets or to commercial feed had little effect (5). The following experiments were therefore carried out to investigate the relative effects of dietary protein and dietary fat on plasma cholesterol levels in newly-weaned rabbits.

New Zealand White rabbits with litters were transferred from rabbit chow to low fat, semisynthetic diets over a period of two to three days, when the young were between one and two weeks of age.

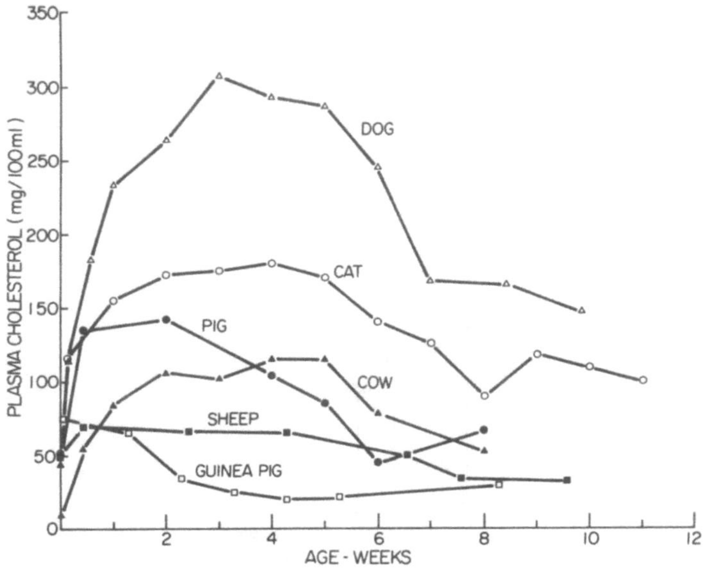

Fig. 2. Plasma cholesterol levels in young animals of different species. Results taken from Carroll, Hamilton and Macleod (3), and from unpublished experiments of R.M.G. Hamilton and K.K. Carroll.

The overall composition of the diets has been described previously (5). The plasma cholesterol levels of the young were then followed for a number of weeks and compared with controls whose mother was maintained on chow throughout. The young began to eat the mother's food at about three weeks of age, and were completely weaned by four weeks or shortly thereafter.

There was considerable variation in the level of plasma cholesterol of different litters prior to weaning, but in each case it dropped sharply when the animals were weaned (Fig. 3). The plasma cholesterol remained low in rabbits weaned to commercial feed, or to semisynthetic diet containing soy protein isolate, but it began to rise again in the rabbits on casein semisynthetic diet, so that this group was markedly different from the others by eight weeks of age. In another experiment designed to test the effect of dietary fat, a litter was weaned to a casein semisynthetic diet containing 15% butter. The results in this case were similar to those obtained with the low fat casein diet.

Since published data on the composition of rabbit milk (6) indicate that fat makes up 44% of total solids, a further experiment was carried out in which rabbits were weaned to semisynthetic

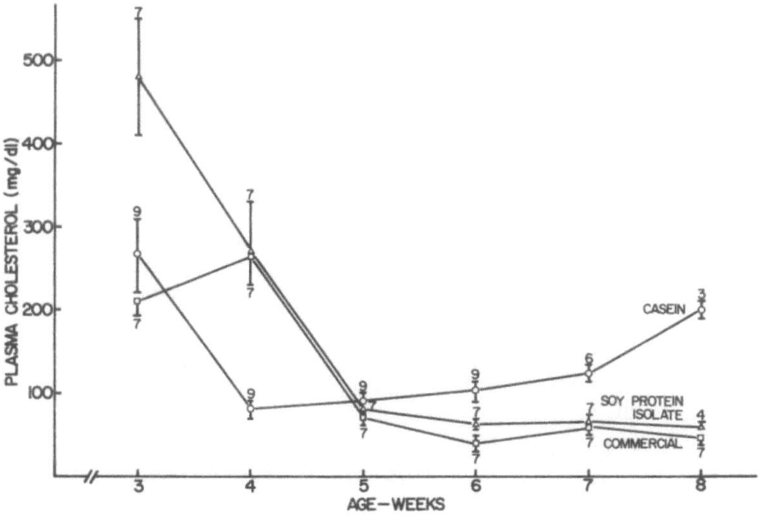

Fig. 3. Plasma cholesterol levels in young rabbits weaned to commercial diet (1 litter) or to semisynthetic diets containing casein or soy protein isolate as source of dietary protein (2 litters each). Each point represents the Mean ± S.E.M. for the number of animals indicated. Six animals on the casein diet died between 6 and 8 weeks of age and 3 animals on the soy protein diet were killed for analytical studies at 7 weeks. Mortality in these and other experiments appeared to be due to coccidiosis.

diets simulating more closely the composition of rabbit milk. These diets contained 41% protein, 7% dextrose, 44% butter and 8% salt mix, all calculated on a weight basis, with added vitamins. The salt and vitamin mixtures were the same as in previous experiments.

Results are shown in Fig. 4. Again there was a marked drop in plasma cholesterol, to about 200 mg/dl on the casein diet and 100 mg/dl on the soy protein diet, and this differential was maintained for the remainder of the experiment. It is evident from these studies that dietary fat and protein can both influence plasma cholesterol levels, but in weaned rabbits the protein appears to exert an overriding effect.

It is therefore of interest to consider the possible role of dietary protein in the control of serum cholesterol levels in humans. This seems especially relevant because the differential in levels between industrialized and non-industrialized countries appears to develop during the post-weaning period (7).

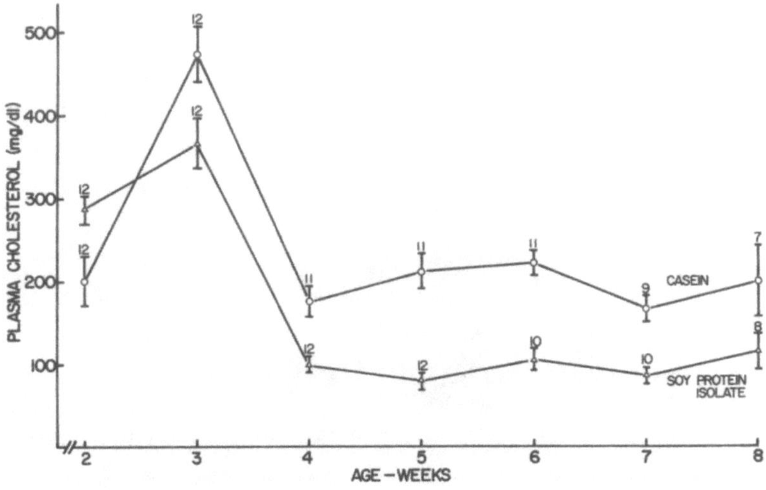

Fig. 4. Plasma cholesterol levels in young rabbits weaned to semi-synthetic diets containing 44% by weight of butter. Results are expressed as Mean ± S.E.M. for the number of animals indicated, from 2 litters in each case.

There is some evidence that diets rich in animal protein tend to produce hypercholesterolemia and that replacement of animal protein by vegetable protein can reduce the level of serum cholesterol in humans (5). It has also been found that vegetarians have low serum cholesterols (8), and Olson et al (9) observed that dietary amino acids can influence human serum cholesterol levels. In addition, epidemiological data show a strong positive correlation between animal protein intake and mortality from cardiovascular disease (10,11). These observations indicate that dietary protein may indeed be a significant factor in the etiology of hypercholesterolemia and atherosclerosis in humans.

ACKNOWLEDGEMENTS

This work was supported by the Ontario Heart Foundation and the Medical Research Council of Canada. Technical assistance by L. McPhee and R. Rasmussen is gratefully acknowledged. Soy protein isolate (Promine-R) was kindly provided for these studies by Dr. E. W. Meyer, Central Soya, Chemurgy Div., Chicago, Ill.

REFERENCES

1. Fomon, S. J. Infant Nutrition, 2nd Ed., W. B. Saunders Co., Philadelphia, 1974, pp. 172-173.

2. Kritchevsky, D. Cholesterol, John Wiley and Sons, Inc., New York, 1958.

3. Carroll, K. K., Hamilton, R.M.G. and Macleod, G.K. Plasma cholesterol levels in suckling and weaned calves, lambs, pigs, and colts. Lipids 8: 635-640, 1973.

4. Friedman, M. and Byers, S. O. Effects of diet on serum lipids of fetal, neonatal, and pregnant rabbits. Am. J. Physiol. 201: 611-616, 1961.

5. Carroll, K. K. and Hamilton, R.M.G. Effects of dietary protein and carbohydrate on plasma cholesterol levels in relation to atherosclerosis. J. Food Sci. 40: 18-23, 1975.

6. Altman, P. L. in Blood and Other Body Fluids. D. S. Dittmer, ed., Federation of American Societies for Experimental Biology, Washington, 1961, p. 466.

7. Whyte, H. M. and Yee, I. L. Serum cholesterol levels of Australians and natives of New Guinea from birth to adulthood. Aust. Ann. Med. 7: 336-339, 1958.

8. Sacks, F. M., Castelli, W. P., Donner, A. and Kass, E. H. Plasma lipids and lipoproteins in vegetarians and controls. New Engl. J. Med. 292: 1148-1151, 1975.

9. Olson, R. E., Nichaman, M. Z., Nittka, J. and Eagles, J. A. Effect of amino acid diets upon serum lipids in man. Am. J. Clin. Nutr. 23: 1614-1625, 1970.

10. Yudkin, J. Diet and coronary thrombosis. Hypothesis and fact. Lancet ii: 155-162, 1957.

11. Connor, W. E. and Connor, S. L. The key role of nutritional factors in the prevention of coronary heart disease. Prev. Med. 1: 49-83, 1972.

(3)

RESULTS OF TREATMENT OF HYPERLIPIDEMIAS; SHORT TERM EFFECT ON CHOLESTEROL METABOLISM

DR. M. A. MISHKEL AND MRS. L. HULL

H.G.H.-McMASTER LIPID RESEARCH CLINIC & LABORATORY

HAMILTON GENERAL HOSPITAL, HAMILTON, ONTARIO, CANADA

There has been a recent tendency to reduce the different forms of hyperlipidemia to fewer categories and to attempt a more unified approach to the dietary management of the hyperlipidemias(1). There is some justification for this approach, but the H.G.H.-McMaster Lipid Research Clinic still uses the internationally accepted World Health Organization classification(2) based on Fredrickson et al. This is because we believe that this classification of hyperlipoproteinemia(HLP) with all its imperfections has etiological, genetic, epidemiological, diagnostic and therapeutic potential. It should be remembered that in all 5 types of hyperlipoproteinemia that plasma cholesterol levels may be elevated, although this is most commonly seen in types IIa and b, III and IV HLP. The majority of this discussion will be devoted to the one parameter namely plasma lipids, which are routinely measured in the Lipid Clinic. No attempt will be made to elaborate on other important cholesterol pools--the liver, the intestine and its contents, adipose tissue and other tissue stores.

Is there any hard-core data available to suggest in the first instance that it is worthwhile lowering a raised plasma cholesterol? Most of the diet studies in this regard come up with a possible yes vote, which falls short of statistical significance. Should the results of the Coronary Drug Project(3) be interpreted as a vote of lack of confidence in the value of plasma lipid lowering? I would hope that the panel discussion will address this question. The two most promising studies that might provide answers are the European clofibrate study(4) and the North American cholestyramine study(5).

We believe to talk on the short term lowering of plasma lipids is almost an academic exercise. From a scientific point of view it is obviously important to know that a diet and/or drug safely lowers plasma cholesterol and preferably depletes the total cholesterol pool size, but if the therapy is unacceptable in the long-term to the patient, no benefit is likely to be derived. However, we have been given this title and must make an attempt to answer the question.

Plasma cholesterol can be lowered in almost all individuals on a short term basis by means of diet alone. There is a remarkable range of "susceptibility" to plasma cholesterol lowering in response to diet so that only a few generalisations can be made:

(i) homozygous type II individuals fare very poorly on combined diet and drug therapy;

(ii) pseudohomozygous type II individuals(6) and young heterozygous children often are very responsive to diet alone or in combination with drugs;

(iii) volunteers, found to have a raised plasma cholesterol by chance, appear to be much more diet-sensitive than the "hard-core" referrals to a Lipid Clinic;

(iv) weight reduction per se which initially (and even long-term) is almost always effective in lowering plasma cholesterol in type IV HLP patients, may produce a transient acute lowering of plasma cholesterol in patients with types IIa and b HLP;

(v) type III patients are exquisitively sensitive to dietary changes, both quantitative and qualitative, and most plasma cholesterol levels can be normalised by diet and/or drugs;

(vi) although patients with type II HLP and tendon xanthomas on the whole do poorly on diet alone, the exceptions to this rule suggest that we are dealing with a heterogeneous population;

(vii) unlike many other workers we have found subjects with type IIb HLP to be less responsive to diet and/or drugs than type IIa HLP.

The diet that we prescribe for types II, III and IV HLP has become similar over the years. The emphasis is on reduction to ideal body weight (with restriction of sucrose and alcohol intake); restriction of cholesterol intake; substitution of polyunsaturated for saturated fats. The relative emphasis on these dietary restrictions depends upon 3 major factors:

(i) the degree of obesity;

(ii) the diagnosis of the type of HLP (made by a minimum of 2 baseline fasting plasma cholesterol and triglyceride estimations, agarose gel electrophoresis, quantification of beta cholesterol, and ultracentrifugation in all suspected cases of type III HLP);

(iii) the responsiveness of the patient to the diet.

The patient should be instructed in the diet and asked to follow the principles for a minimum of 3 months before the diet is said to have failed to lower plasma cholesterol levels. The patient and his wife may sometimes require reinstruction before a decision is made to add a hypocholesterolemic drug to the regimen. The drugs used in our clinic have been clofibrate (Atromid S), cholestyramine (Questran), colestipol, tibric acid, d-thyroxine (Choloxin) and nicotinic acid. Oral calcium has been tried in a small study of normocholesterolemic subjects and no consistent fall in plasma lipids, no increased excretion of fecal bile acids nor change in biliary glycine/taurine ratio has been noted(7).

The overall short term (6 and 12 months) experience in plasma lipid lowering in more than 500 subjects seen in the HGH-McMaster Lipid Research Clinic is summarised in Table I. Men outnumbered women almost 4 to 1 and the average age of the clinic patient was 47 years (range 11 - 71 years). Although the vast majority were hyperlipidemic (with or without atherosclerotic vascular disease, hypertension, obesity, diabetes and other risk factors), a minority were obese, or had maturity onset diabetes with a bad family history of vascular disease, and were normolipidemic. Diet was given a minimum trial of 3 months, before a decision to commence one of the hypolipidemic drugs was made. In a small minority of patients (those with resistant type II HLP) a combination of drugs was tried, e.g. clofibrate plus cholestyramine or cholestyramine plus nicotinic acid. As a general rule, the patients treated with diet plus drugs had significantly higher cholesterol, but not necessarily higher triglyceride levels, than those treated by diet alone.

Even in such a heterogeneous population as seen in the Lipid Clinic, some generalisations can be made:

(i) the mean cholesterol lowering response, whether by diet or by diet plus drugs was disappointingly low (average 10.6%);

(ii) by contrast the fall in plasma triglyceride levels (average 36.0%) and reduction to ideal body weight (average 53.1% of patients) were very good;

(iii) although the numbers followed up at 12 months (305 patients) were less than at 6 months (509 patients) the average age, and plasma cholesterol, triglyceride and weight reduction, were very similar at the two time intervals;

(iv) women responded less well than men to therapy.

The greatest experience with short-term cholesterol lowering by means of combined drug and diet therapy has been obtained in the following subjects (some of whom are the same subjects as in Table I):

(i) the use of clofibrate and diet has been able to normalize the plasma cholesterol levels in 25 subjects with documented type III HLP;

(ii) more than 80% of 50 subjects with type IIa and b HLP

TABLE I

	6 MONTHS' TREATMENT DURATION		12 MONTHS' TREATMENT DURATION	
	Plasma Cholesterol mg/dl	Plasma Triglyceride mg/dl	Plasma Cholesterol mg/dl	Plasma Triglyceride mg/dl
DIET ONLY - MEN	n = 352	Average Age 48 yrs.	n = 195	Average Age 48 yrs.
Mean Initial Value±S.D.	234 ± 40	307 ± 243	238 ± 39	300 ± 206
(Mean % Reduction)	(9.0%)	(36.8%)	(14.5%)	(42.0%)
Mean Post-Rx Value±S.D.	213 ± 33	194 ± 98	212 ± 31	174 ± 70
% Attain Ideal Weight	54.5%		60.0%	
DIET ONLY - WOMEN	n = 74	Average Age 48 yrs.	n = 36	Average Age 48 yrs.
Mean Initial Value±S.D.	254 ± 52	244 ± 180	248 ± 39	260 ± 220
(Mean % Reduction)	(5.5%)	(26.2%)	(7.3%)	(28.8%)
Mean Post-Rx Value±S.D.	240 ± 51	180 ± 106	230 ± 35	185 ± 133
% Attain Ideal Weight	51.4%		63.9%	
DIET + DRUG - MEN	n = 49	Average Age 44 yrs.	n = 45	Average Age 45 yrs.
Mean Initial Value±S.D.	307 ± 65	391 ± 257	305 ± 66	408 ± 260
(Mean % Reduction)	(14.0%)	(35.3%)	(15.1%)	(41.7%)
Mean Post-Rx Value±S.D.	264 ± 57	253 ± 140	259 ± 54	238 ± 105
% Attain Ideal Weight	53.1%		42.2%	
DIET + DRUG - WOMEN	n = 34	Average Age 50 yrs.	n = 29	Average Age 46 yrs.
Mean Initial Value±S.D.	311 ± 74	199 ± 134	311 ± 72	186 ± 129
(Mean % Reduction)	(8.4%)	(22.1%)	(9.3%)	(28.0%)
Mean Post-Rx Value±S.D.	285 ± 71	155 ± 77	272 ± 65	134 ± 59
% Attain Ideal Weight	26.5%		27.6%	

have had at least a 20% lowering of plasma cholesterol levels with two bile acid sequestering resins, cholestyramine or colestipol;

(iii) clofibrate is more likely to lower cholesterol in type IIa than type IIb patients;

(iv) Tibric acid in a dose of 500 to 1500 mg/day had no hypocholesterolemic effect in 26 patients (type IIa - 6 patients; type IIb - 13 patients; type III - 2 patients; type IV - 5 patients) treated for a mean of seven months. By contrast, plasma triglyceride levels fell by 22%(8).

REFERENCES

1. Beaumont JL, Carlson LA, Cooper GR, et al: Classification of hyperlipidemias and hyperlipoproteinaemias. W.H.O. Bull. 43: 891 - 915, 1970.
2. Tabaqchali S, Chait A, Harrison R, et al; Experience with simplified scheme of treatment of hyperlipidaemia. Brit. Med. J. 3: 377-380, 1974.
3. The Coronary Drug Project Research Group: Clofibrate and Niacin in coronary heart disease. JAMA 231: 360-381, 1975.
4. Oliver MF: A primary prevention trial using Clofibrate (Atromid-S) in Drugs Affecting Lipid Metabolism (Ed. W.L. Holmes et al) Plenum Press, New York 1969 p. 339 - 344.
5. Little JA: The National Heart and Lung Institute Lipid Research Clinic program at Toronto-McMaster University. Canad. J. Pub. Health 65: 378-383, 1974.
6. Mishkel, MA: Pseudohomozygous and pseudoheterozygous type II hyperlipoproteinemia. Amer J. Dis. Children (in press).
7. Nazir DJ, Mishkel MA: The effect of calcium on plasma lipids and bile acid and fecal fat excretion in normolipidemic subjects. Clin.Chim.Acta 62: 117-123, 1975.
8. Mishkel, MA: Tibric acid. Its use in 26 hyperlipidemic subjects. Excerpta Medica (in press).

ACKNOWLEDGEMENT

The senior author wishes to acknowledge a grant from the Canadian Life Insurance Association and a grant from the Ontario Heart Foundation (grant # 15-10) without which this work could not have been accomplished.

(4)

RESULTS OF TREATMENT OF HYPERLIPIDEMIAS:

LONG-TERM COMPLIANCE AND EFFECT ON LIPID METABOLISM

Ivan D. Frantz, Jr.

From the Departments of Medicine and Biochemistry,
Medical School, University of Minnesota
Minneapolis, Minnesota, U.S.A.

Several of the more effective methods of treating hyperlipidemia were discovered by accident. In some cases the mode of action of the agents remains unknown. As long as this state of ignorance persists, one must harbor some misgivings that, despite a satisfying fall in blood lipid concentrations, the treatment may be doing more harm than good. The present discussion will begin with a brief, general consideration of the theoretical possibilities available to explain the action of hypolipidemic agents in metabolic terms, followed by an attempt to classify the commonly prescribed drugs according to the scheme.

POSSIBLE MODES OF ACTION OF HYPOLIPIDEMIC AGENTS

In hyperlipidemia several different lipids may be elevated, with more than one usually involved. Since the lipids are transported in combination as lipoproteins, it might be argued that the mechanisms of hyperlipidemia and the mode of action of lipid lowering agents should be approached as abnormalities and alterations of lipoprotein metabolism. It seems apparent, however, that, despite a common mode of transport, the components of the lipoproteins are manufactured and disposed of in relatively independent fashion. These processes undoubtedly interact. Indeed, they do so to such an extent that identification of the one primarily affected by a disease state or by a drug may be very difficult. Searching for the primary effect remains, nonetheless, the logical way to proceed.

A priori, blood cholesterol may be high because of increased synthesis, decreased excretion, or a shift in the equilibrium from tissues to blood. Ideally, treatment should be directed at correction of the abnormality. Currently, for lack of knowledge and of suitable agents, we must often be content to use any method that works. In some cases, this empiricism extends to the point of lowering the lipid which is primarily elevated by altering the metabolism of another.

We turn now to a discussion of the effect on lipid metabolism and, hence, the mode of action of the four most widely used lipid lowering drugs.

CHOLESTYRAMINE

This nonabsorbable resin is easiest to deal with, because its mode of action is abundantly clear. Many studies have shown that it combines with bile acids in the intestinal tract and carries them out of the body, thereby setting off a train of events which results in conversion of more cholesterol to bile acids and a fall in blood cholesterol (1-3).

Levy and Langer (4) have questioned this interpretation. They find it difficult to reconcile with the observation that the increased degradation is completely balanced by increased synthesis (5). In point of fact, such a balance is necessary if a steady state is to be restored. Otherwise, the concentration of cholesterol would fall to zero. If the flux outward from the blood compartment is increased, the flux into it must increase until it equals the flux outward. The concentration in the compartment will then become constant again, but at a lower level than existed before the system was disturbed. Levy and Langer found an increased turnover of the protein moiety of the low density lipoprotein, and suggested that cholestyramine acts by increasing the fractional catabolic rate of that component. Perhaps this viewpoint carries the usually desirable "translation of hyperlipidemia into hyperlipoproteinemia" one step too far. The effects of cholestyramine on the other components of LDL are undoubtedly secondary to its effect on cholesterol excretion.

Cholestyramine is currently recommended only for the treatment of Type II hyperlipoproteinemia, in which circulating LDL is increased (6). It is not consistently effective in Type IV.

Various possibilities have been considered as the primary abnormality in Type II hyperlipoproteinemia. One appealing concept is that excretion of cholesterol is impaired, so that a higher than normal concentration of cholesterol in the blood is maintained in the steady state. The work of Goldstein and Brown (7) implies, on the other hand, that it is the regulation of cholesterol synthesis that is defective. If this is so, our presently preferred treatment of Type II is not directed at the primary defect.

NICOTINIC ACID

Many diverse effects on lipid metabolism have been attributed to nicotinic acid. These have been reviewed by Kissebah, Adams, Harrigan, and Wynn (8). The most likely explanation of its lipid lowering action appears to be that proposed by Carlson et al. (9, 10), as confirmed by the authors referred to above (8). Their finding is that the primary effect is a decreased mobilization of free fatty acids from the tissues.

Nicotinic acid is useful in the treatment of Type II hyperlipoproteinemia, as well as in those types in which the triglycerides are primarily elevated, for which it would appear best suited. Presumably the reduction in cholesterol concentration is secondary to the reduction in triglycerides, which is due to decreased secretion of VLDL by the liver. This chain of events is set in motion by decreased availability of free fatty acids for triglyceride synthesis. Thus, nicotinic acid appears to interrupt or depress a cyclical process in which fatty acids are mobilized from the tissue triglycerides, transported to the liver, reesterified to triglycerides, secreted into the blood as a component of VLDL, liberated again as free fatty acids through the action of lipoprotein lipase, and returned to the tissues for storage again as triglycerides. Depression of this cycle reduces the need for lipid transport. Viewed from this narrow standpoint, the cycle appears to be without net effect, and moderate depression of it of no obvious harm to the organism.

CLOFIBRATE

Like nicotinic acid, clofibrate is most useful in treatment of those types of hyperlipoproteinemia in which the triglycerides are primarily elevated. Its mode of action is less clear. Kissebah et al. (8) have reviewed the many positive effects on lipid metabolism which have been attributed to clofibrate. These include reduction of lipolysis, fatty acid synthesis, glycerol esterification, apolipoprotein synthesis, and triglyceride release from the liver, and increased triglyceride clearance. Grundy et al. (11) demonstrated increased excretion of cholesterol into bile. Einarsson, Hellström, and Kallner (12) found, on the other hand, that the total daily formation of bile acids was greatly decreased when clofibrate was given to patients with Type IV. It seems necessary at present to withhold judgment as to the primary metabolic effect of clofibrate.

Strisower (13) has studied the effect of clofibrate on lipoprotein patterns, using the analytical ultracentrifuge. He found that as triglycerides fell in Type IV, the LDL concentration often rose, sometimes to abnormal levels, leading to a Type II pattern. The possibility of harm to the patient must be considered.

D-THYROXINE

More than half a century ago Epstein and Lande (14) reported that the blood cholesterol concentration is low in hyperthyroidism and high in myxedema. Rosenman et al. (15) showed that in rats rendered hyperthyroid, cholesterol synthesis and excretion were both increased, while they were decreased in the hypothyroid state. Starr et al. (16) found that the cholesterol lowering effect of the thyroid hormone was mimicked by dextrothyroxine, with a lesser effect on metabolic rate than that exerted by the natural hormone. Duncan and Best (17) showed that these properties were shared by a number of thyroxine analogues, but D-thyroxine has enjoyed the widest clinical application.

One might be inclined to speculate that the cause of the cholesterol lowering effect of thyroid hormone would be increased oxidation of cholesterol to bile acids. The work on steroid excretion by Miettinen (18) showed, however, that neutral steroid output is increased more consistently and to a greater degree. Simons and Myant (19) reached rather similar conclusions concerning the mode of action of D-thyroxine in Type II hyperlipoproteinemia. In two patients neutral steroid excretion was definitely increased, with no significant change in bile acid excretion. In a third patient, bile acid excretion was increased, accompanied by only a small increase in neutral steroid excretion. Simons and Myant suggested the D-thyroxine probably acts to increase cholesterol catabolism at some point prior to the divergence of the bile acid and neutral steroid pathways.

LONG-TERM EFFECTS

The best evidence points to the conclusion that none of the four cholesterol lowering drugs discussed above lose much if any of their effectiveness, regardless of the duration of treatment.

As early as 1965 Hashim and Van Itallie (3) reported a patient treated for more than 4 years with cholestyramine, without loss of the cholesterol lowering effect. This initial impression has been borne out by additional experience (20).

Good data for the three other drugs were accumulated in the Coronary Drug Project. With a 6 mg/day dose of D-thyroxine, the net fall in serum cholesterol level was 12 per cent and of triglyceride level, 15 to 20 per cent, with no deterioration in the effect after 3 years (21).

Niacin (3 g/day) and clofibrate (1.8 g/day) were about equally effective in their triglyceride lowering effect in the Coronary Drug Project (22), with a slight difference in favor of niacin. The average difference between the niacin and placebo groups was 26.1 per cent, and between the clofibrate and placebo groups, 22.3 per cent. These differences were maintained virtually constant for 5 years.

The cholesterol lowering effect of clofibrate was also maintained without change for 5 years, but the average difference from placebo was only 6.5 per cent. The difference for niacin was 9.9 per cent, with slight narrowing of this difference at the end of the 5 year study.

Clofibrate also showed no loss ot effectiveness over a 4 year period in the recent British coronary secondary prevention trials (23,24).

Long-term adherence to diet is more difficult to achieve than adherence to a drug. In the National Diet-Heart Feasibility Study (25), there was noticeable deterioration in the cholesterol response over a one year period in each of the 5 open centers, in spite of the advantage of commissary-supplied foods and intensive efforts by well trained nutritionists. In the sixth center, which worked with an institutionalized population for whom food was prepared centrally, no such deterioration occurred. This experience suggests that adherence is the critical factor, rather than a change in the subjects' metabolic responsiveness. In his dietary coronary secondary prevention trial, Leren (26) achieved a lowering of plasma cholesterol in his treated group to an average level that was 14.4 per cent below the average for the controls. The difference remained virtually constant for the entire 5 years of the trial. His superior response, as compared to the open centers in the National Diet-Heart Study, may have been due to the fact that his subjects had a higher cholesterol to begin with, or that they were more highly motivated by virtue of having already had a myocardial infarction, or that the nutritionists were able to perform more effectively without the restrictions imposed by a double-blind design.

Most investigators have found that all of the cholesterol lowering that can be achieved by diet takes place in the first 2 or 3 weeks. Keys et al. (27) have identified population groups in various parts of the world, however, whose cholesterol levels are lower than those seen in the United States even with radical dietary modification. Thus, middle-aged fishermen in the town of Ushibuka in Japan averaged only 140 mg/100 ml. These findings raise the possibility that consumption of a diet low in cholesterol and saturated fats from birth onward produces an effect which is greater than can be achieved by dietary modifications made later in life.

REFERENCES

1. Bergen, S.S. Jr., Van Itallie, T.B., Tennent, D.M., and Sebrell, W.H.: Effect of an anion exchange resin on serum cholesterol in man. Proc. Soc. Exp. Biol. Med. 102:676-679, 1959.
2. Tennent, D.M., Siegel, H., Zanetti, M.E., Kuron, G.W., Ott, W.H., and Wolfe, F.J.: Plasma cholesterol lowering action of bile acid binding polymers in experimental animals. J. Lipid Res. 1:469-473, 1960.
3. Hashim, S.A., and Van Itallie, T.B.: Cholestyramine resin therapy for hypercholesteremia. J. A.M.A. 192:289-293, 1965.
4. Levy, R.I., and Langer, T.: Hypolipidemic drugs and lipoprotein metabolism. Adv. Exp. Med. Biol. 26:155-163, 1972.
5. Goodman, D.S., and Noble, R.P.: Turnover of plasma cholesterol in man. J. Clin. Invest. 47:231-241, 1968.
6. Levy, R.I., Morganroth, J., and Rifkind, B.M.: Treatment of hyperlipidemia. New Eng. J. Med. 290:1295-1301, 1974.
7. Goldstein, J.L., and Brown, M.S.: Hyperlipidemia in coronary heart disease: a biochemical genetic approach. J. Lab. Clin. Med. 85:15-25, 1975.
8. Kissebah, A.H., Adams, P.W., Harrigan, P., and Wynn, V.: The mechanism of action of clofibrate and tetranicotinoylfructose (Bradilan) on the kinetics of plasma free fatty acid and triglyceride transport in Type IV and Type V hypertriglyceridaemia. Europ. J. Clin. Invest. 4:163-174, 1974.
9. Carlson, L.A., and Orö, L.: The effect of nicotinic acid on the plasma free fatty acids. Demonstration of a metabolic type of sympathicolysis. Acta Med. Scand. 172:641-645, 1962.
10. Carlson, L.A., and Nye, E.R.: Acute effects of nicotinic acid in the rat. 1. Plasma and liver lipids and blood glucose. Acta Med. Scand. 179:453-461, 1966.
11. Grundy, S.M., Ahrens, E.H. Jr., Salen, G., Schreibman, P.H., and Nestel, P.J.: Mechanisms of action of clofibrate on cholesterol metabolism in patients with hyperlipidemia. J. Lipid Res. 13:531-551, 1972.
12. Einarsson, K., Hellström, K., and Kallner, M.: The effect of clofibrate on the elimination of cholesterol as bile acids in patients with hyperlipoproteinaemia Type II and Type IV. Europ. J. Clin. Invest. 3:345-351, 1973.
13. Strisower, E.H.: Observations on the use of clofibrate in common hyperlipoproteinemias. Acta Cardiol. Supp. 15:139-150, 1972.
14. Epstein, A.A., and Lande, H.: Studies of blood lipoids. I. The relation of cholesterol and protein deficiency to basal metabolism. Arch. Int. Med. 30:563-577, 1922.

15. Rosenman, R.H., Byers, S.O., and Friedman, M.: The mechanism responsible for the altered blood cholesterol content in deranged thyroid states. J. Clin. Endocrin. 12:1287-1299, 1952.
16. Starr, P., Roen, P., Freibrun, J.L., and Schleissner, L.A.: Reduction of serum cholesterol by sodium dextrothyroxine. Arch. Int. Med. 105:830-842, 1960.
17. Duncan, C.H., and Best, M.M.: Thyroxine analogues as hypocholesterolemic agents. Am. J. Clin. Nutr. 10:297-309, 1962.
18. Miettinen, T.A.: Mechanism of serum cholesterol reduction by thyroid hormones in hypothyroidism. J. Lab. Clin. Med. 71:537-547, 1968.
19. Simons, L.A. and Myant, N.B.: The effect of D-thyroxine on the metabolism of cholesterol in familial hyperbetalipoproteinaemia. Atherosclerosis 19:103-117, 1974.
20. Levy, R.I., Fredrickson, D.S., Shulman, R., Bilheimer, D.W., Breslow, J.L., Stone, N.J., Lux, S.E., Sloan, H.R., Krauss, R.M., and Herbert, P.N.: Dietary and drug treatment of primary hyperlipoproteinemia. Ann. Int. Med. 77:267-294, 1972.
21. The Coronary Drug Project Group, The Coronary Drug Project. Findings leading to further modifications of its protocol with respect to dextrothyroxine. J.A.M.A. 220:996-1008, 1972.
22. The Coronary Drug Project Group. Clofibrate and niacin in coronary heart disease. J.A.M.A. 231:360-381, 1975.
23. Trial of clofibrate in the treatment of ischaemic heart disease. Physicians of the Newcastle-upon-Tyne Region. Br. Med. J. 4:767-775, 1971.
24. Ischaemic heart disease: A secondary prevention trial using clofibrate. Research Committee of the Scottish Society of Physicians. Br. Med. J. 4:775-784, 1971.
25. The National Diet-Heart Study Final Report. Circ. 37, Suppl. 1, 1-428, 1968.
26. Leren, P.: The effect of plasma cholesterol lowering diet in male survivors of myocardial infarction. Acta Med. Scand. Suppl. 466, 7-92, 1966.
27. Keys, A., Aravanis, C., Blackburn, H.W., van Buchem, F.S.P., Buzina, R., Djordjević, B.S., Dontas, A.S., Fidanza, F., Karvonen, M.J., Kimura, N., Lekos, D., Monti, M., Puddu, V., and Taylor, H.L.: Epidemiological studies related to coronary heart disease: Characteristics of men aged 40-59 in seven countries. Acta Med. Scand. Suppl. 460, 392, 1966.

(5)

THE DRUG TREATMENT OF HYPERLIPIDEMIA

Richard J. Jones, M.D.

University of Chicago

950 E. 59th Street, Chicago, Illinois, U.S.A.

There are three pharmaceutical compounds which are now popular in the U.S.A. for treatment of hyperlipidemia. At least two of these seem to have different mechanisms of action, insofar as we presently understand them, and may therefore be accepted as supplementary to each other in the treatment of hyperlipidemia. In fact, it is axiomatic that, if one affects the blood lipids by a different mechanism than the other, the combination will work better than either drug alone.

The current literature on the drug treatment of hyperlipidemia suggests investigators are seeking closely related compounds which may show a slight advantage in effectiveness (or therapeutic: toxic ratio) or are testing the gain from combining two compounds. As this sort of "applied" research goes forward, it sometimes contributes to our basic understanding. I shall therefore consider differences now appreciated between these drugs and the effectiveness of their combinations.

CLOFIBRATE

Ethyl-chlorophenoxyisobutyrate (CPIB) is probably the most widely used hypolipidemic drug in Europe and the U.S.A. at present. A recent review (1) has indicated its pharmacodynamics, toxicity and mechanism of action. Although there are few toxic manifestations in man, there is in rodents uniform hepatic enlargement with electron microscopic evidence for increased numbers of mitochondria, hypertrophy of the smooth endoplasmic reticulum and a proliferation of peroxisomes. The significance of these changes is not clear, but, turning to results in The Coronary Drug Project (2) on long term administration of the drug, an excess of 3.8% more men than in the placebo group did develop hepatomegaly, 1.3% splenomegaly, and 1.3% gallbladder disease. Although there were significant percentages of patients responding to the drug with elevations of blood urea nitrogen, SGOT and CPK, the percentage developing chemical jaundice, abnormal elevations of alkaline phosphatase, or significant hyperglycemia was smaller than in the placebo group. Thus, we still cannot explain what the rearrangement of hepatocyte architecture and metabolism by CPIB really means.

It has been well demonstrated that CPIB administration enhances hepatic mitochondrial glycerophosphate dehydrogenase and protein synthesis while reducing glycerophosphate concentration and triglyceride (TG) synthesis (1). This leads to a reduced very low density lipoprotein (VLDL) secretion further abetted by enhanced tissue disposal of VLDL and TG. The latter may be mediated through some sort of lipoprotein lipase stimulation, or through inhibition of cAMP synthesis (3). The hypocholesterolemic effect apparently arises from an increased fecal excretion of cholesterol (C) and bile acids, particularly in normolipidemic or hypertriglyceridemic subjects, without compensatory increase in cholesterol synthesis (4). The effects on VLDL and TG metabolism are independent of the changes in C metabolism. The lipid effects are patterned differently in normolipidemic subjects, in essential hypercholesterolemic, in hypertriglyceridemic or mixed hyperlipidemic patients. In any case, the mode of action of CPIB is obviously complex and still not satisfactorily explained.

It should perhaps be mentioned that the CDP results suggested, not only that there was no benefit in terms of mortality and morbidity in patients with advanced coronary disease, but also that this drug induced a greater incidence (2.8%) of pulmonary embolism and thrombophlebitis than was seen in the randomized placebo group (2). This plus a significant incidence of decreased libido and gynecomastia suggest estrogenic effects.

CHOLESTYRAMINE

If the action of clofibrate on lipid metabolism is complex, the action of cholestyramine is contrastingly simple. This non-absorbable cationic polystyrene resin sequesters bile acids in the intestinal tract for fecal excretion, thus inhibiting intestinal absorption of endogenous and exogenous cholesterol (5). Since the 7-α-hydroxylase enzyme system of the liver is stimulated by decreasing levels of bile acids, there is an increased conversion of the body's cholesterol pools to bile acids.

Aside from gastric fullness, the only undesirable effects attributable to this drug are related to retention in the fecal compartment of such substances as the fat soluble vitamins (K, A, D_3) and neutral fat. Absorption of many drugs, such as warfarin, digitoxin, thyroxin, tetracyclines and perhaps iron, has been impaired.

It is of interest that the lipid effects are almost the reciprocal of CPIB effects, when considered in lipoprotein terms. The LDL of the serum is primarily depressed, with minimal if any effect on the VLDL concentration: in certain susceptible people there may be an increase in the VLDL and hence TG of the serum (6). In addition, a reduction in the relative proportions of cholesterol to phospholipid and neutral fat are demonstrable in LDL and sometimes in VLDL (6, 7). This is compatible with the notion that reducing the availability of cholesterol for LDL production may inhibit its secretion by the liver.

NICOTINIC ACID

Niacin in pharmacological dosage has been one of the hardiest of hypolipidemic drugs, having thus far withstood the test of time better than any other agent. Although it also did not improve the mortality rates in The Coronary Drug Project, patients receiving it did enjoy a statistically significant reduction in recurrent myocardial infarctions, cerebrovascular accidents and development of new angina pectoris, as compared to the large placebo group, as well as a sustained 9.9% reduction of serum cholesterol (2). Thus, it may have a true deterrent effect upon atherogenesis which is not reflected in improved mortality rates this late in the disease process.

In addition to the acute flushing reaction, atrial fibrillation and other arrhythmias were more frequent in the niacin group than in the placebo group. Other side effects noted were an increased frequency of gouty arthritis, glucose intolerance, gastrointestinal distress and abnormal skin changes (ichthyosis, hyperpigmentation and acanthosis nigricans). Of particular interest, there was no unusual incidence of jaundice or elevation of liver enzymes. The earlier suspicions of hepatic dysfunction can now be laid to rest.

Niacin and its more potent derivative β-pyridyl carbinol apparently act to reduce serum C and TG levels by effecting reductions in both LDL and VLDL. There is no change in composition of LDL or VLDL lipids to suggest a depletion of one or more precursor lipid compounds. Although hepatic synthesis of cholesterol is inhibited there is no significant change in fecal excretion of cholesterol or bile acids (8). Study of LDL kinetics in man before and during treatment with niacin showed that the reduction in serum LDL was unaccompanied by any change in rate of removal of radio-labelled

LDL (9). On the other hand, maximum uptake of ^{14}C-threonine into both LDL and VLDL of the Rhesus Monkey is depressed by nicotinic acid administration, though its incorporation into HDL and albumin is not impaired (8). This confirms in the primate older data from other experimental animals and even purified systems that hepatic lipoprotein synthesis is indeed impaired. There has been remarkably little work on niacin with modern measurement of cholesterol pool size and metabolic balance in man.

COMBINATIONS

Occasional patients who show an incomplete serum lipid response to CPIB will show a greater response and even complete normalization of lipids when cholestyramine is added (6). Use of an anion exchange resin (DEAE Sephadex) combined with CPIB produced a cholesterol reduction of 30% in type II patients, whereas the resin alone effected only a 20% cholesterol reduction (10). Another study of clofibrate and penta-erythritol tetranicotinate combined showed, in a similar population of type II patients, a 20% reduction in serum cholesterol and 40% reduction in TG. However, the clofibrate or the nicotinate alone accomplished almost as much at appropriate dosage in terms of cholesterol reduction. In type IIa patients, clofibrate reduced serum TG while the nicotinate did not; in IIb patients, both effected TG reductions (11).

CONCLUSION

From the foregoing, it is clear that we have two modes of attack for the treatment of hyperlipidemia which are quite different in their lipid metabolic consequences. Clofibrate primarily reduces the VLDL and cholestyramine the LDL of the serum; the combination may produce nearly normal serum lipids. Comparing niacin and clofibrate, one is struck more by their similarities, both in lipoprotein response and in side effects, than by their differences. Their combination is apparently no more effective than nicotinate alone.

REFERENCES

1. Havel, R.J. and Kane, J.P.: Drugs and Lipid Metabolism in Elliot, H.W., Okun, R., and George, R. (Eds.) Annual Review of Pharmacology. 13:287, 1973.
2. The Coronary Drug Project Research Group. Clofibrate and Niacin in Coronary Heart Disease. J. Am. Med. Assoc. 231: 360, 1975.
3. D'Costa, M.A. and Angel, A.: Inhibition of Hormone Stimulated Lipolysis by Clofibrate. A Possible Mechanism for its Hypolipidemic Action. J. Clin. Invest. 55:138, 1975.

4. Grundy, S.M., Ahrens, E.H. Jr., Salen, G., Schreibman, P.H., Nestel, P.J.: Mechanisms of Action of Clofibrate on Cholesterol Metabolism in Patients with Hyperlipidemia. J. Lipid Res. 13:531, 1972.
5. Bergen, S.S. Jr., Van Itallie, T.B., Tennent, D.M., and Sebrell, W.H.: Effect of an Anion Exchange Resin on Serum Cholesterol in Man. Proc. Soc. Exp. Biol. Med. 102:676, 1959.
6. Jones, R.J., and Dobrilovic, L.: Lipoprotein Lipid Alterations with Cholestyramine Administration. J. Lab. and Clin. Med. 75:953, 1970.
7. Grundy, S.M., Ahrens, E.H. Jr., Salen, G.: Interruption of the Enterohepatic Circulation of Bile Acids in Man: Comparative Effects of Cholestyramine and Ileal Exclusion on Cholesterol Metabolism. J. Lab. Clin. Med. 78:94, 1971.
8. Magide, A.A., Myant, N.B., and Reichl, D.: The Effect of Nicotinic Acid on the Metabolism of the Plasma Lipoproteins of Rhesus Monkeys. Atherosclerosis 21:205, 1975.
9. Langer, T., and Levy, R.I.: The Effect of Nicotinic Acid on the Turnover of Low Density Lipoproteins in Type II Hyperlipoproteinemia. In Gey, K.F. and Carlson, L.A. (Eds.) Metabolic Effects of Nicotinic Acid and its Derivatives. pp. 641-647, Hans Huber Publishers, Bern, 1971.
10. Howard, A.N., Courtenay-Evans, R.J.: Secholex, Clofibrate and Taurine in Hyperlipidemia. Atherosclerosis 20:105, 1974.
11. Olsson, A.G., Orö, L., and Rössner, S.: Dose-Response Effect of Single and Combined Clofibrate (Atromidin) and Niceritrol (Perycit) Treatment on Serum Lipids and Lipoproteins in type II Hyperlipoproteinaemia. Atherosclerosis 22:91, 1975.

(6)

DISCUSSION (THE EFFECTS OF NUTRITION AND TREATMENT ON LIPID METABOLISM)

Dr. Blacket: Referring to Dr. Connor's experiments on the effects of different levels of dietary cholesterol on serum cholesterol, I think it would be valuable to know what happens when you go from an intake of from, say 300 to 600 mg/day; 600 mg being about the average in the Australian diet and 300 being a figure that could reasonably be obtained in attempting to reduce dietary cholesterol intake.

Dr. Connor: There are a number of experiments with intakes of 500-600 mg and it's interesting that in humans the effect is about the same as with 1,000 mg. There is one unpublished study that I know of, comparing 300 and 600 mg, and there, too, the effects were somewhat similar, so perhaps the real threshold is a little lower down, and then it may become linear from zero on up to whatever the threshold is.

Dr. Carlson: Dr. Connor, you referred to this as a sterol balance problem, but wouldn't you rather think that it is a sterol transport problem? The problem seems to be that you get raised levels of LDL in the plasma and that implies that the transport system is overloaded, or rather can't cope with the situation of the cholesterol load.

Dr. Connor: I think one could use that terminology as well, thinking of the balance equation for the whole animal, and then perhaps the arterial wall and the tissue culture cell. I think it's the transport system that goes awry in sterol balance, so I agree with you.

Dr. Carlson: Perhaps Dr. Zilversmit will tell us why LDL cholesterol rises when you eat more cholesterol.

Dr. Zilversmit: That isn't what I was going to do, but it probably is more of a transport phenomenon since cholesterol seems to circulate several times between liver and plasma; in the rabbit, for example, 3 or 4 times before it is finally excreted. I was actually going to ask Dr. Connor why the carbohydrate question seems to be so controversial, and why many people in England seem to think it is very important and yet I find very few people in the United States that believe this.

Dr. Connor: I can't answer your question except that it may be a case of blind men approaching different parts of the elephant. It seems to me that most of the data obtained from metabolic experiments in the United States do not indicate a clear cut difference between moderate amounts of sucrose in the diet and starch. This doesn't imply any pat on the back for sucrose because it is a form of empty calories. It may be that in large amounts some differences might exist in very hyperlipidemic subjects.

Dr. Zilversmit: I can't understand why there is such disagreement about sucrose vs starch. It seems like a relatively simple experiment and maybe there is something we are missing.

Dr. Connor: One of the factors I alluded to is that it is very hard to supply starch as a pure ingredient in a diet of mixed natural foods, because it comes along with protein. For example, if you are supplying bread or potato, you have a lot of other things coming in, so that if you try to compare bread with sucrose it can't really be balanced because of the fibre in bread, and because of the protein content, and because the caloric content may be different. That's one of the explanations.

Dr. Carlson: It seems that you also brought up another part of the story; that is, acute vs chronic effects of carbohydrate which not all investigators have realized.

Dr. Kritchevsky: With regard to dietary carbohydrate, in studies with rabbits, monkeys and baboons fed semipurified diets, starch was much less hypercholesterolemic than either sucrose or fructose.

Dr. Frantz: I'd like to go back to the cholesterol question and remind the audience that Drs. Hegsted and Stare did some very elegant and quantitative experiments with varying amounts of dietary cholesterol. I think they had around 600-700, 250 and 100 mg of cholesterol, with all the other conditions the same. On the average, a reduction of 5 mg serum cholesterol was obtained with a 100 mg reduction in dietary cholesterol. They used a high saturated fat diet with coconut oil, a mono-unsaturated fat diet with olive oil, and a third series with polyunsaturated fat.

Dr. Connor: I think those were very good studies.

Dr. Frantz: I think it's also very important to emphasize the interrelationship of the various factors in the diet. One cannot ignore all the other factors and consider just one, such as saturated fat or cholesterol. You have got to see how interdependent they are, and how important this interdependence is.

Dr. Shapcott: Do the polyunsaturated fats that were used contain added synthetic antioxidants, and if so, have there been control experiments to see what effect these may have?

Dr. Connor: I suppose I should know the answer to that, but I don't. Of course the natural antioxidant in most liquid vegetable oils is α-tocopherol, and there is a large quantity present in corn oil; I think much more than there would be in cocoa butter. We used redistilled corn oil rather than Mazola oil because we wanted the amounts of vitamins and plant sterols to be similar, so that we had less antioxidant in the corn oil we used than people would normally consume.

Dr. Carlson: Dr. Connor, you made a statement that the effect of alcohol was only a matter of calories; I don't think that is correct in all subjects, clearly not in those we recognize as hyperlipidemic.

Dr. Connor: I said, "In most people". We've done an alcohol study in which we have kept the caloric balance constant, and in most individuals we did not see any discreet effects of alcohol, except for intoxication. I agree there are some individuals who show discreet effects.

Dr. Sodhi: Hypercholesterolemia may not be an overload effect if one considers the effect of absorbed cholesterol on cholesterol biosynthesis. The overall yield appears to be about the same whether you take no cholesterol or 600-700 mg of cholesterol in the diet. Paul Nestel also did some studies with high carbohydrate diets with low or high cholesterol intake, and found that the total was more or less the same. There was really no difference in input into the system, indicating that the inhibition was appropriate to the amount of cholesterol absorbed. I just give you the possibility that this may not be entirely cholesterol overload.

Dr. Connor: I assume there is far less inhibition of synthesis in man than occurs in experimental animals such as the monkey, rabbit or rat. In other words, the inhibition is not very great, at least in the experiments that I know about.

Dr. Palmer: I'd like to ask Dr. Mishkel a question about the rapid response to diet. Is the serum concentration of cholesterol the only parameter to be thinking about? There is the tissue pool as well. Is this also unresponsive to diet? Secondly, I would like to refer to Dr. Connor's mention of the increased sterol excretion when he places people on polyunsaturates. Is there a lack of this response in the type of patients who do not respond to diet? Is this a Type II excretory problem related to the rapid fall in serum pools?

Dr. Mishkel: We are not doing metabolic studies on our patients. However, we do have some long-term dietary plus hypolipidemic drug studies in patients with resistant Type II hyperlipoproteinemia who have gross generalized xanthomatosis and they are having 3-monthly serum cholesterol, LDL cholesterol and other analyses. There have been a few patients where we are getting regression of all changes, both clinically and radiologically. If the plasma cholesterol level remains up, and tissue xanthomas regress, then one suspects that the cholesterol pool size may be decreasing.

Dr. Blacket: Last year we published some data showing the effect of weight loss in Type IIa and IIb. With a decline in weight of 13 kg and in relative body weight from 119 to 103 there was a 23% fall in serum cholesterol and 37% fall in serum triglycerides. Fall in calculated LDL cholesterol was similar in Types IIa and IIb. Since then we've collected further data. Fifty-four obese men who lost weight initially were compared with 28 who did not. In the steady weight state the diets were similar. In those who failed to lose weight the fall in serum cholesterol on a low fat low cholesterol diet high in polyunsaturates was 6.3%. The change in serum triglycerides was insignificant. The relationship between delta serum cholesterol and delta weight was as before. Stepwise regression analysis was done on cases with complete dietary data. After allowing for the change in weight, only the change in saturated fatty acid intake was significant. The net contribution of dietary polyunsaturates and cholesterol was insignificant. Change in weight and change in saturated fat accounted for 28% of the variance ($R = 0.53$).

In Type IV, weight reduction also brought about a dramatic fall in serum triglycerides in 20 healthy blood donors. This was maintained over 12 months of follow-up. It seems that hypertriglyceridemia can be controlled very well in a high percentage of subjects by reduction to truly ideal weight. What is ideal weight? We defined it as weight at age 20 in subjects who were not already obese at that age. The results of weight reduction are more impressive than those obtained with either clofibrate or nicotinic acid, whatever the initial level. The commonest impediment to a good result is alcohol. We took care of a man who obtained an excellent result but relapsed when he took 500 ml of beer a day. This is a small daily consumption by Australian standards.

Taking the results of weight reduction in Types IIa, IIb and IV and looking at the prevalence of weight gain after maturity in Western society we wonder whether we could do more for hyperlipidemia by controlling weight than by using low cholesterol low fat diets with polyunsaturates. This isn't to deny the great value of the low cholesterol, low fat diet, high in polyunsaturates, in lean Type II subjects.

Dr. Angel: A comment with respect to Dr. Frantz' paper. Dr. D'Costa in my laboratory has studied the mechanisms of action of clofibrate and has focussed attention on the level of cAMP in fat cells and its site of action. He has come to the conclusion that clofibrate is membrane-active, and has evidence to support that. More important, he recently demonstrated that in isolated human fat cells clofibrate acts in vitro to inhibit adenylate cyclase activity, at concentrations that correspond to the drug's therapeutic levels. Thus, the mechanisms of action of both clofibrate and nicotinic acid because of their antilipolytic actions are becoming more and more relevant, especially because of their therapeutic effectiveness in lowering blood lipids in man.

Dr. Frantz: I still use the same slide for clofibrate as for niacin.

Dr. Angel: He has also studied the effect of niacin in humans in fat cell ghosts and it's even more reactive than clofibrate, so both of them have parallel antilipolytic effects.

Dr. Frantz: That's very interesting. I'd like to add that there is experimental work on the Rhesus monkey showing that niacin, like clofibrate, does have an effect on LDL synthesis.

Dr. Carroll: I would like to ask about the occurrence of different genetic types in developing countries. Most of the studies on genetic typing seem to have been done in countries where hypercholesterolemia is a real problem.

Dr. Connor: From the literature and from personal experience, I would say that Type IIa is certainly found throughout the world. It is present in Pakistan, for example, in peasants; there are reports in the Japanese literature of Type IIa and I am sure there are others; China also.

Dr. Carroll: It seems to me that perhaps one can over-ride genetic differences by environmental factors, such as diet, and this provides encouragement for trying to find better ways of doing this.

Dr. Blacket: The dietary manipulation that might be required in practice may be unacceptable to the Western world. It is a tremendous problem.

Dr. Carroll: Diet may not be the only answer necessarily, but it seems to me at least possible that one could develop a satisfactory therapeutic diet that would be acceptable to the Western world if we knew a bit more about the variables involved. Perhaps that's being optimistic.

Dr. Little: I'd like to go back to Dr. Carroll's presentation where he showed the differences in different species with regard to cholesterol levels. Is it possible that the relative elevation of cholesterol in man indicates a greater need compared to other species, and is this the reason we are "superior" to other species? Therefore, I ask the question whether it is desirable for us to lower cholesterol too much.

Dr. Carroll: I don't know that I have an answer to that. One is impressed by the fact that the food provided by nature for young animals induces hypercholesterolemia pretty universally, and I think it suggests this is very appropriate, at least for that stage of life. There is probably good reason for it, but whether it is desirable to maintain hypercholesterolemia throughout life is another matter.

Dr. Connor: I just want to mention that the species with highest cholesterol level at the instant of birth is the newly hatched chick, which is living on egg yolk and has a level of about 400 mg, but this high level doesn't seem to last very long.

Dr. Shorland: Perhaps there is good reason to start off with a high cholesterol level because of the tissue needs, and this is why there is so much cholesterol in eggs.

Dr. Horlick: I was very impressed with Dr. Blacket's report, and I wonder if he would tell us a little more about how he recruits people and how he persuades them to lose this amount of weight, and how he achieves adherence for such long periods of time. This may be the most important thing I'm going to learn.

Dr. Blacket: The patients had suffered myocardial infarctions and that must provide strong motivation. The second group were healthy blood bank donors, who are perhaps rather unusual and not particularly representative samples of the population, and they cooperated very well. Now there are people who don't cooperate. I think the important thing in diet and heart disease is the delicacy of dietary counselling, and I think that is where most of us have been pretty weak. A great deal of effort goes into determining what the patient is eating in the first place, what changes can be made in order to fit in with one's concept of what they should be eating, and then there is the matter of good motivation by the dietician. It requires a good deal of the dietician's time, certainly no less than the doctor's time in the initial interview, and also in the follow-up. Subjects are seen twice at the initial encounter within two or three weeks prior to the start, and then on an average they are seen a month later, and then another three months later.

Dr. Shaper: May I just make a brief reference to a free-living group of 150 middle-aged men, about 40-50, in London, England, who were given very simple dietary conditions. No approach was taken to their wives; we didn't attempt to interfere with their family dietary habits, but only discussed it with the men themselves. We followed them over a period of 5 years, using very simple dietary recommendations. They were seen once every 6 months over the first 18 months, and then only once a year, so the pressure on them was very low and we tried to do it without weight loss. At the beginning this group of men had an average cholesterol of 250 mg and over a period of 4 years we achieved an overall reduction of about 15%. At 4½ years they'd begun to regress and whether this has somethings to do with our economic situation or the cost of polyunsaturates I'm not sure. Without undue pressure, there was only a change in weight of 1 kg overall, and the men had maintained a cholesterol reduction satisfactorily. They were volunteers from a civil service study and we approached them and asked if they would take part. There was an 86% response rate initially and they just stayed in the study. There was no carrot and no stick.

Dr. Carlson: I think it is time to end this Workshop, and I would like to close with two things of which perhaps the most important that was said in this Workshop according to my mind, was what Dr. Frantz said that we should look for drugs and means to correct metabolic errors behind the hyperlipidemias. I think too little attention has been paid to that. Secondly, perhaps those who participate tomorrow in the Workshop on Recommendations to the Public should extrapolate from what Dr. Carroll and Dr. Connor said and recommend rabbit chow rather than alcohol.

CHAPTER 10
CURRENT INVESTIGATIONS IN MYOCARDIAL PERFUSION

(1)

AN OVERVIEW OF MYOCARDIAL BLOOD FLOW

Colin M. Bloor, M. D.
Department of Pathology, School of Medicine
University of California, San Diego
La Jolla, California, U.S.A.

There are inherent difficulties in measuring myocardial blood flow because of several unique features of the coronary circulation. First, coronary blood flow is phasic, depending on phasic aortic pressure and the varying degree of resistance to flow offered by the myocardium during systole. Second, oxygen extraction of the myocardium is high while flow is relatively low, thus making coronary flow extremely sensitive to changes in myocardial oxygen requirements. Third, flow requirements and oxygen supply mechanisms can be simultaneously affected, often in opposite directions, by a single variable. Fourth, distribution of myocardial blood flow is not homogeneous across the ventricular wall. Since intramyocardial pressure exceeds intracavitary pressure, steadily increasing from the epicardium to the endocardium, coronary flow to the left ventricle occurs predominantly during diastole. Therefore, either prolonged systole or increased cardiac rate can encroach upon left ventricular coronary flow. The differences in the distribution of subendocardial and subepicardial flow can be accentuated under a variety of physiologic and pathologic conditions. Changes in perfusion pressure or in intramyocardial wall tension can alter these distribution patterns and render some layers of the myocardium more susceptible to tissue hypoxia. A fifth component of the myocardial circulation is the coronary collateral circulation which comprises anatomic structures present from early life. However, these structures vary in size and number and that, in turn, determines their functional effect. Thus each approach to the measurement of myocardial blood flow has as its inherent limitation the inability to account for all of these factors. Under experimental conditions each technique of measuring myocardial blood flow, however, has certain advantages.

DIRECT AND INDIRECT METHODS OF MEASURING MYOCARDIAL FLOW

Directly measuring myocardial blood flow via implanted flow devices in animals now makes it possible to measure its phasic variations continuously over long periods (1,2). Such animal models permit the continuous systemic and coronary hemodynamics to be continuously monitored during the progress of atherosclerotic disease. Thus as lesions develop it is possible to describe early changes in systemic and coronary hemodynamics which otherwise might not result in significant clinical features. This model also permits characterization of the phasic changes in myocardial blood flow. However, the direct measurement of flow has a significant limitation since it measures flow in the large epicardial branches. This flow represents total inflow to the coronary vascular bed but does not permit the distribution of myocardial flow throughout the different layers of the ventricular walls to be estimated in detail.

Other approaches have been used to monitor myocardial perfusion in the unanesthetized animal using various radiolabeled indicators, either diffusable indicators (3-5) or radioactive microspheres (6-10). These methods estimate the distribution of myocardial blood flow throughout the subendocardial and subepicardial layers. They also permit repeated measurements in the same animal over various periods, ranging up to several weeks. This has obvious advantages in any long term atherosclerosis studies, since the distribution of myocardial flow can be determined at different stages in the development of vascular wall lesions. The obvious disadvantage is that these measurements represent a summation of phasic flow over a period of time in which the labeled substance is homogeneously distributed into the general coronary circulation.

DISTRIBUTION OF MYOCARDIAL FLOW

Besides depending on aortic perfusion pressure, coronary blood flow is also influenced by changes in small vessel resistance, primarily at the arteriolar level. These arterioles respond strongly to many stimuli, and both constrict and dilate. In atherosclerotic coronary disease, resistance in large arteries can also change, but it is generally necessary to decrease the vessel lumen diameter by more than two-thirds to cause a significant pressure loss in a resting experimental animal. However, during augmented coronary flow, for example during physical exercise, the cross-sectional areas of a moderately compromised large vessel may impede adequate delivery of coronary flow, resulting in myocardial hypoxia.

Under normal circumstances myocardial flow is distributed relatively uniformly throughout the different layers of the heart in the unanesthetized, resting animal. When normal animals, in which the coronary vascular bed has no significant wall lesions, are subjected to severe physiologic stress, for example exercise, this homogeneous distribution of flow throughout the ventricular wall persists at all levels of exercise (Figure 1). When partial restriction of flow is induced in one large epicardial branch, mimicking minimal wall lesions seen in developing atherosclerosis, myocardial

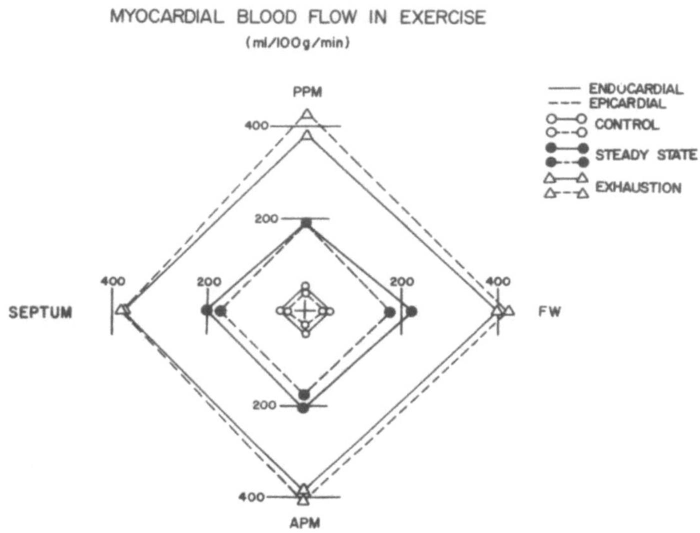

Figure 1. Myocardial blood flow distribution in the septum, free wall (FW) and papillary muscles (APM and PPM) of left ventricle of a dog at rest and during two levels of exercise stress. The plus is zero flow for the four coordinates. Endo- and epicardial blood flows increase homogeneously with increasing exercise stress.

flow continues to be homogeneously distributed, under resting conditions. However, when the animal is again subjected to severe physiologic stress, for example exercise, myocardial perfusion within the various layers of the ventricular wall become disproportionate (Figure 2). Thus, although such methods do not permit phasic determination of myocardial blood flow, they show some additional features that may change when early atherosclerotic lesions are present in the coronary vascular bed.

COLLATERAL CIRCULATION

Various approaches have been used to determine the functional development of the coronary collateral circulation. They include methods which directly measure blood flow in the unoccluded artery (11) or in a collateral branch (12), or which depended on indirect means such as measurement of peripheral coronary pressure, isotope washout, retrograde flow or anatomic evidence to estimate collateral blood flow (13-18). Other approaches have used diffusible indicators (5) or radioactive microspheres (19). Using such approaches, better insight can be gained into what factors affect coronary collateral development.

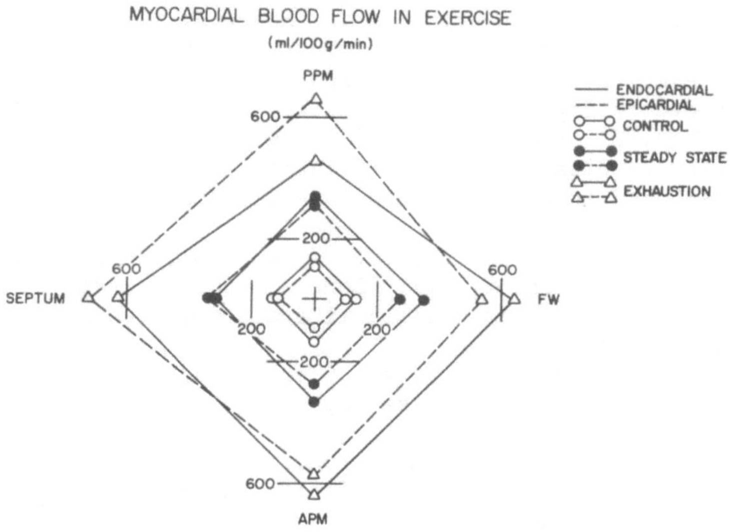

Figure 2. Myocardial blood flow distribution in left ventricle of a dog with fixed-diameter restriction of the left circumflex coronary artery. Plot is same as Fig. 1. With increasing exercise stress there is a skewing of blood flow distribution around the left ventricular wall, such that the zone most distal to the restriction, the posterior papillary muscle, suffers a reduction in total blood flow.

SUMMARY AND CONCLUSIONS

A variety of methods are available for measuring myocardial blood flow including collateral flow. Although each technique has as its inherent limitation its inability to account for all factors affecting the coronary circulation, each technique has certain advantages. Thus, appropriate selection of a method for measuring myocardial blood flow depends on the original questions posed in an individual investigation.

REFERENCES

1. Gregg, D.E., Khouri, E.M. and Rayford, C.R. Systemic and coronary energetics in the resting unanesthetized dog. Circ. Res. 16: 102-113, 1965.

2. Bloor, C.M., White, F.C. and Sobel, B.E. Coronary and systemic haemodynamic effects of prostaglandins in the unanaesthetized dog. Cardiovasc. Res. 7: 156-166, 1973.

3. Rees, J.R., Redding, V.J., Ashfield, R., Gibson, D. and Gavey, C.J. Myocardial blood flow measurements with Xenon-133. Effect of glyceryl trinitrate in dogs. Brit. Heart J. 28: 374-381, 1966.

4. Herd, J.A., Hollenberg, M., Thorburn, G.D., Kopald, H.H. and Barger, A.C. Myocardial blood flow determined with krypton-85 in unanesthetized dogs. Am. J. Physiol. 203: 122-124, 1962.

5. Linder, E. Measurements of normal and collateral coronary blood flow by close-arterial and intramyocardial injection of krypton-85 and Xenon-133. Acta Physiol. Scand. 68(272): 5-31, 1966.

6. Buckberg, G.D., Luch, J.C., Payne, D.B., Hoffman, J.I.E., Archie, J.P. and Fixler, D.E. Some sources of error in measuring regional blood flow with radioactive microspheres. J. Appl. Physiol. 31: 598-604, 1971.

7. Cobb, R.F., Bache, R.J. and Greenfield, J.C., Jr. Regional myocardial blood flow in awake dogs. J. Clin. Invest. 53: 1618-1625, 1974.

8. Domenech, R.J., Hoffman, J.I.E., Noble, M.I.M., Saunders, K.B., Henson, J.R. and Subijanto, S. Total and regional coronary blood flow measured by radioactive microspheres in conscious and anesthetized dogs. Circ. Res. 25: 581-596, 1969.

9. Fortuin, N.J., Kaihara, S., Becker, L.C. and Pitt, B. Regional myocardial blood flow in the dog studied with radioactive microspheres. Cardiovasc. Res. 5: 331-336, 1971.

10. Utley, J., Carlson, E.L., Hoffman, J.E., Martinez, H.H. and Buckberg, G.D. Total and regional myocardial blood flow measurements with 25μ, 15μ, 9μ and filtered 1-10μ diameter microspheres and antipyrine in dogs and sheep. Circ. Res. 34: 391-405, 1974.

11. Khouri, E.M., Gregg, D.E. and Lowensohn, H.S. Flow in the major branches of the left coronary artery during experimental coronary insufficiency in the unanesthetized dog. Circ. Res. 23: 99-109, 1968.

12. Elliot, E.C., Khouri, E.M., Snow, J.A. and Gregg, D.E. Direct measurement of coronary collateral blood flow in conscious dogs by an electromagnetic flowmeter. Circ. Res. 34: 374-383, 1974.

13. Elliot, E.C., Jones, E.L., Bloor, C.M., Leon, A.S. and Gregg, D.E. Day-to-day changes in coronary hemodynamics secondary to constriction of circumflex branch of left coronary artery in conscious dogs. Circ. Res. 22: 237-250, 1968.

14. Elliot, E.C., Bloor, C.M., Jones, E.L., Mitchell, W.J. and Gregg, D.E. Effect of controlled coronary occlusion on collateral circulation in conscious dogs. Amer. J. Physiol. 220: 857-861, 1971.
15. Pasyk, S., Bloor, C.M., Khouri, E.M. and Gregg, D.E. Systemic and coronary effects of coronary artery occlusion in the unanesthetized dog. Amer. J. Physiol. 220: 646-654, 1971.
16. Bloor, C.M. and White, F.C. Functional development of the coronary collateral circulation during coronary artery occlusion in the conscious dog. Amer. J. Pathol. 67: 483-500, 1972.
17. Blumgart, H.L., Zoll, P.M., Freedberg, A.S. and Gilligan, D.R. The experimental production of intercoronary arterial anastomoses and their functional significance. Circulation 1: 10-27, 1950.
18. Paul, M.H., Norman, L.R., Zoll, P.M. and Blumgart, H.L. Stimulation of interarterial coronary anastomoses by experimental acute coronary occlusion. Circulation 16: 608-614, 1957.
19. White, F., Bishop, S. and Bloor, C. Regional myocardial flow distribution during acute myocardial infarction in conscious dogs. Circulation 50(3): 104, 1974.

(2)

STUDIES OF REGIONAL MYOCARDIAL PERFUSION IN THE ANGINAL PATIENT

Attilio Maseri, Antonio L'Abbate, Antonio Pesola,
Mario Marzilli and Oberdan Parodi
Istituto di Patologia Medica e
Laboratorio di Fisiologia Clinica C.N.R.
Università di Pisa, Pisa, Italy

The pathogenesis of angina pectoris is currently related to a localized, acute imbalance between myocardial metabolic demands and coronary blood supply. An impairment of blood supply may be related: 1) to the presence of coronary artery obstruction which prevents the required increase of perfusion to meet increased myocardial demands; 2) to a sudden reduction of regional myocardial blood supply.

Angina secondary to increased myocardial demands is typically represented by angina in patients with critical coronary stenosis; angina constantly appearing any time a fixed work load of the heart is exceeded.

Angina secondary to reduction of myocardial blood supply is typically represented by angina occurring at rest, and not preceded by any increase in myocardial demands.

These patterns of acute myocardial ischemia may just be the two extremes of a continuous spectrum of the disease. The direct evaluation of myocardial perfusion during angina is one of the prerequisites for identifying the pathogenetic mechanism of angina and hence for a rationale approach to therapy. However, the study of myocardial perfusion in patients with coronary artery disease has been hampered by a basic methodologic problem. In fact while pathological and angiographic data on one side and electrocardiographic changes observed during angina on the other, indicate a localized character of the disease, the methods currently used to estimate coronary blood flow yield a value of average or of total myocardial perfusion. The recent development of radioisotopic methods for myocardial imaging opened the way to the study of myocardial perfusion on a regional basis (1-3).

In this presentation we wish to report the results of studies carried out in our laboratory during the past five years on regional myocardial perfusion in stress induced angina (4) and in spontaneous angina.

ANGINA CAUSED BY INCREASED DEMANDS

Material and Methods. In 12 patients with typical effort angina we determined the initial myocardial distribution and the regional washout curves of ^{133}Xenon (dissolved in saline) injected as a bolus into the left coronary artery. We used a gamma camera (Pho gamma III HP Nuclear Chicago) interfaced to a computer (2116 B Hewlett Packard).

The patients were selected on the following criteria: 1) long main stem of the left coronary artery (to insure adequate mixing of the indicator at the injection site); 2) presence of an isolated critical stenosis in one of the three main left coronary branches, but without detectable lesions in the anterior descending or circumflex branches (so that in each patient, in the left anterior projection, the behaviour of the tracer in the myocardial territory distal to the stenosed vessel could be compared with that observed in the control territory perfused by normal vessels); 3) typical ischemic ECG changes during stress testing.

The patients were studied at rest, during angina induced by atrial pacing and following nitroglycerin administration. In 4 patients who had a low threshold for angina, we also studied the alterations induced on the washout curves by suddenly beginning pacing above the angina threshold about 30 seconds after the injection of Xenon. In the last 8 studies the constancy of counting geometry during the course of the washout curves could be checked by the use of a dual counting apparatus accessory which allowed us to follow simultaneously the time activity curves of a constant reference indicator (^{99m}Tc human albumin microspheres injected at the beginning of the study into the left coronary). On the scintigram of Xenon in the initial studies and on that of the reference indicator in the others, a computer program identified 9 areas of interest and for each of them gave: 1) the fractional initial distribution of Xenon; 2) its time activity curves during the washout of 30% of the injected dose; 3) the initial slope of the curve down to 50% of the peak (as an indication of the washout in the better perfused myocardium in each area); 4) the percent of the peak at which it deviated from a monoexponential course (as an indication of non-homogeneous washout in each area); 5) the regional residual activity when 90% of the injectate was washed out (as an indication of slow washout areas); 6) the regional Xenon distribution 15 minutes after the injection (indicative of the epicardial fat distribution and helpful for the interpretation of the slow washout areas).

Results. At rest the perfusion in areas distal to stenosed vessels was characterized by a greater residual activity than areas perfused by normal vessels, at the time when 90% of the injected tracer was washed out. By contrast, although significant regional differences in initial washout slopes were observed as previously reported (5), they could not be consistently related to the location of the stenosis.

During angina the differences in residual activity became much greater distal to stenotic vessels in respect to control zones in all patients. In 8 patients, small but consistent differences in the initial washout slope appeared with a slower washout beyond the obstructed vessel. However, in the patients in whom the use of the technetium scintigram allowed the selection of the same areas in successive Xenon injections, the differences in the initial regional fractional distribution of the indicator were much larger than expected on the basis of the changes observed in the initial washout slopes (Figure 1). This suggested that perfusion to the ischemic areas was markedly non-homogenous, with some parts of the myocardium receiving too little indicator to contribute appreciably to the initial washout. This hypothesis was confirmed by inducing angina a second time about 30 seconds after a successive injection of Xenon. In fact, in all 4 patients while the washout become faster in the myocardium perfused by normal vessels it became slower than in resting conditions (Figure 2) in the ischemic areas, indicating that in some parts of the myocardium perfusion became impaired after the induction of angina by pacing (Figure 3). In the injection performed during angina these parts of the myocardium received little indicator therefore they could not be adequately represented in the initial washout curves.

Following nitroglycerin administration no consistent differences from the control curves were observed.

SPONTANEOUS ANGINA

Materials and methods. We studied the initial myocardial distribution of ^{201}Thallium in 6 patients who presented with very frequent episodes of rest angina and generally with ST segment elevation. Coronary angiography, performed in 5 revealed an extremely variable degree of obstruction ranging from normal vessels to triple vessel disease. One ml of ^{201}Tl was given intravenously at the patient's bed side in the coronary care unit, at the onset of ECG abnormalities. Scintigrams were obtained within 10-15 minutes of the cessation of pain utilizing a Jumbo Toshiba Gamma-camera in 3 projections with a high sensitivity collimator and I:I imaging on large size film. The same procedure was repeated several days later when the patient was free of clinical and ECG evidence of myocardial ischemia.

The analysis of the myocardial scintigrams was performed by visual inspection and by densitometric measurements on the film.

Results. In all six patients, the myocardial scintigram obtained during the attack of "spontaneous" angina showed a large transmural zone of reduced ^{201}Tl uptake (Figures 4A, 4B, 5A and 5B). Comparison of regional myocardial activity with that in the surrounding chest région revealed that the reduction of perfusion to the ischemic areas was not relative to an increased uptake in the healthy areas. Thus, an absolute reduction of tracer uptake in the ischemic areas and not a greater increase in the normal myocardium was responsible for the relative differences of perfusion observed in the scintigram.

CONCLUSIONS

Methodologic aspects. Regional myocardial blood flow studies make possible a semiquantitative evaluation of the severity of ischemia and indicate its location. In the presence of ischemia, the interpretation of Xenon washout curves requires the analysis of the tail of the washout curve and of the initial fractional redistribution of the tracer, because within the solid angle outlined by each area of interest, perfusion may be greatly non-homogenous (eg., endocardial in respect to epicardial layers). Thus, although exact quantitation of flow from ^{201}Tl uptake or from Xenon washout curves when perfusion is non-homogeneous is not warranted (6), the regional semiquantitative information provided by these methods may be of greater pathophysiologic significances than the exact determination of total or average myocardial blood flow.

Pathophysiologic aspects. The greater Xenon residual activity beyond stenosed vessels at rest (for comparable degree of fat accumulation at 15 min) indicates the presence of zones of ischemic myocardium within the solid angle of these areas. However, the absence of resting ECG alterations in most patients and the failure of nitroglycerin to abolish these differences, suggest local adaptations of myocardial oxygen requirements.

The reduction of washout rates in the ischemic zones when the angina was induced by pacing after Xenon injection indicates a severe impairment of perfusion secondary to the onset of ischemia. The observed increased pulmonary wedge pressure may be, at least in part, responsible for this phenomenon.

During "spontaneous" angina, the severe transmural reduction of perfusion documented with ^{201}Tl appears to confirm the hypothesis of a coronary artery spasm which reduces acutely regional myocardial blood supply in these patients (7). Indeed, in two patients of this series, hemodynamic monitoring of right and left ventricular pressures and of pulmonary artery oxygen saturation showed that no hemodynamic change indicative of increased myocardial demands appeared before the onset of the ischemic episode. In both patients, coronary angiography performed during one of the episodes revealed a spasm of the vessel perfusing the myocardium corresponding to the area of ST segment elevation and to the deficit of perfusion on the ^{201}Tl study.

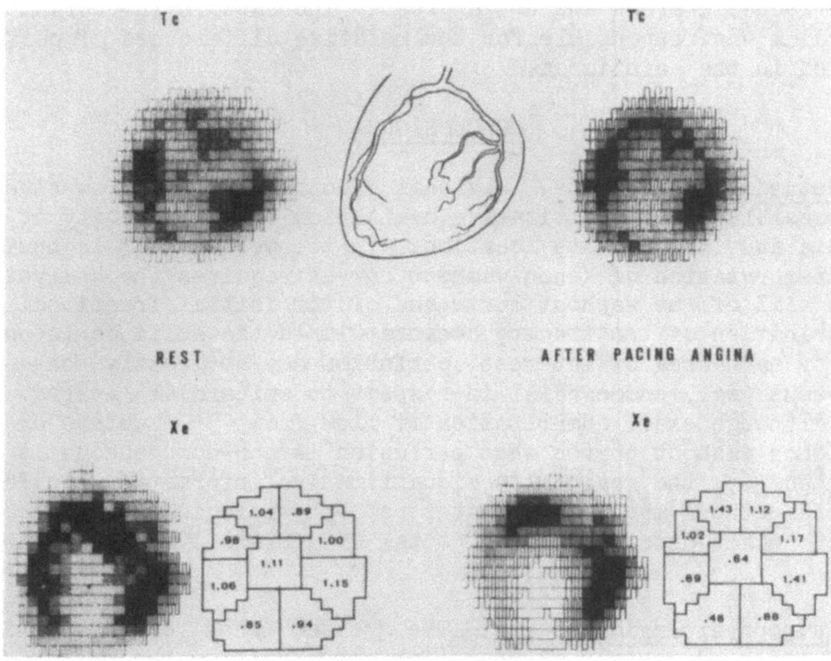

Fig. 1 Myocardial scintigrams in LAO position in a patient with typical angina but no previous infarction; proximal subocclusion of the LAD is the only angiographic abnormality. The ^{133}Xenon (Xe) left coronary scintigram obtained during angina is clearly different from that obtained at rest, with the development of a large cold area in the territory of the LAD. The scintigrams of ^{99m}Tc microspheres (Tc) (injected into the left coronary at the beginning of the study), recorded simultaneously with the two ^{133}Xenon scintigrams are practically unchanged. The average fractional distribution of Xenon to the elements of the matrix included into each area outlined on the reference ^{99m}Tc scintigram are indicated in the lower panels.

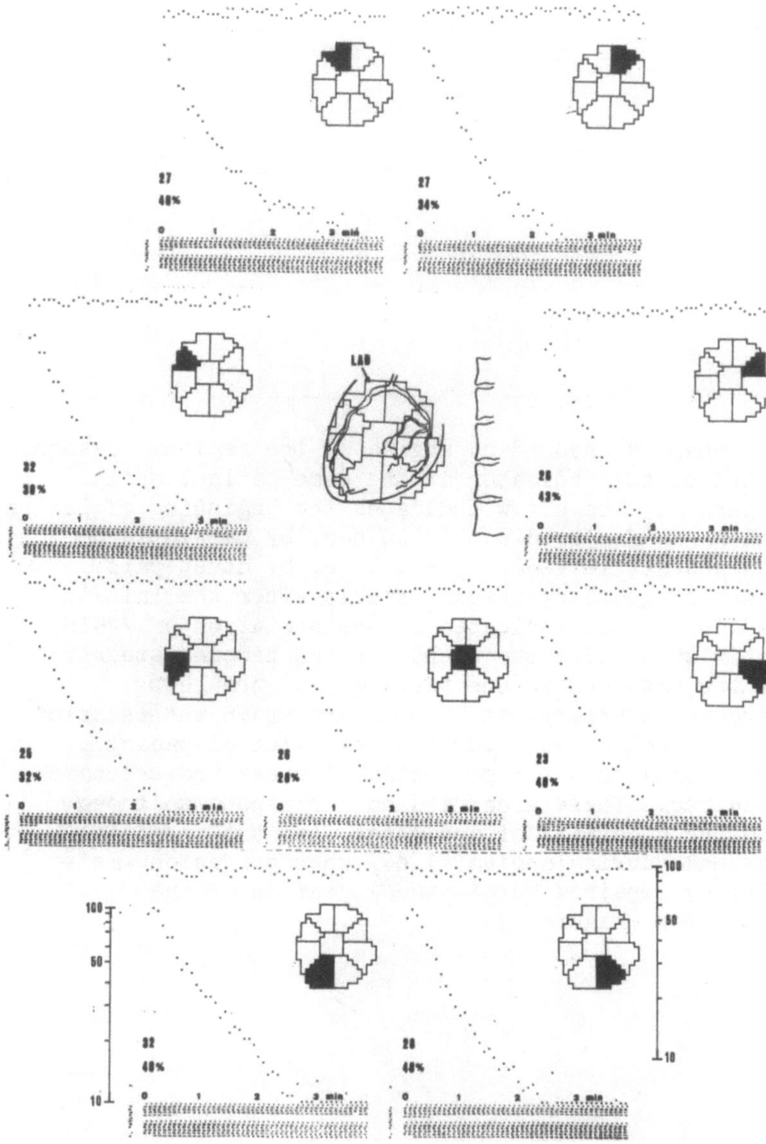

Fig. 2 Computer plot (of Figure 1) of the ^{99m}Tc microspheres time-activity curve and of the initial 90% washout curves in ^{133}Xenon at rest in semilogarithmic scale for the various areas (in black) in which the scintigram was subdivided. Each point is a 5 sec. interval. The half time of the curves and the per cent value up to which an exponential was fitted by the X^2 method are also shown. The patient as in Figure 1; the injection was the same as that of the scintigrams on the left of Figure 1.

Fig. 3 The changes induced by angina on the regional washout rates of the indicator in the same patient as in Figure 1. The arrow indicates the beginning of pacing, which was followed within 10 sec. by marked ischemic ECG changes in V_3 - V_5, and later by chest pain. Counting geometry remains stable after the initial sudden change, indicated by the variation of ^{99m}Tc activity. While the washout slope becomes steeper at the base and in the territory of the left circumplex artery, it becomes slower in the anterior and central areas after the beginning of pacing, indicating that the perfusion to these areas became impaired. These areas indeed correspond to those showing a deficit of indicator when the injection was made during angina, i.e., when perfusion was already impaired before the injection of the indicator (Figure 1).

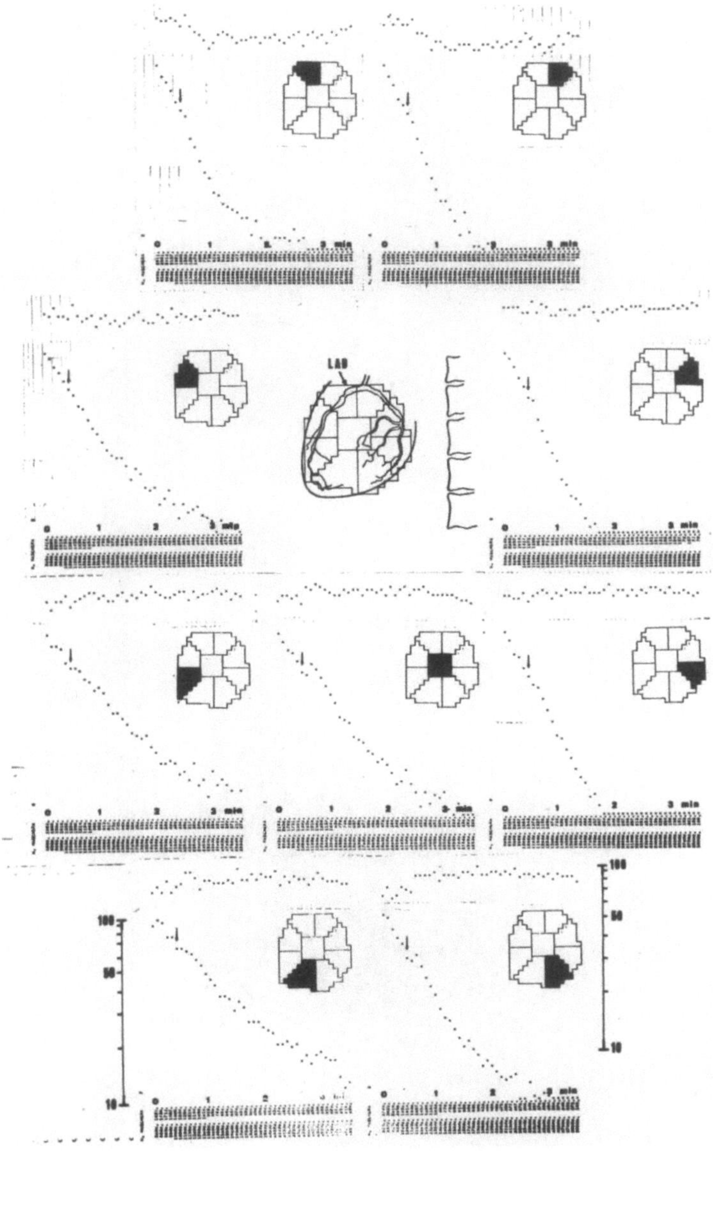

FIGURE 3

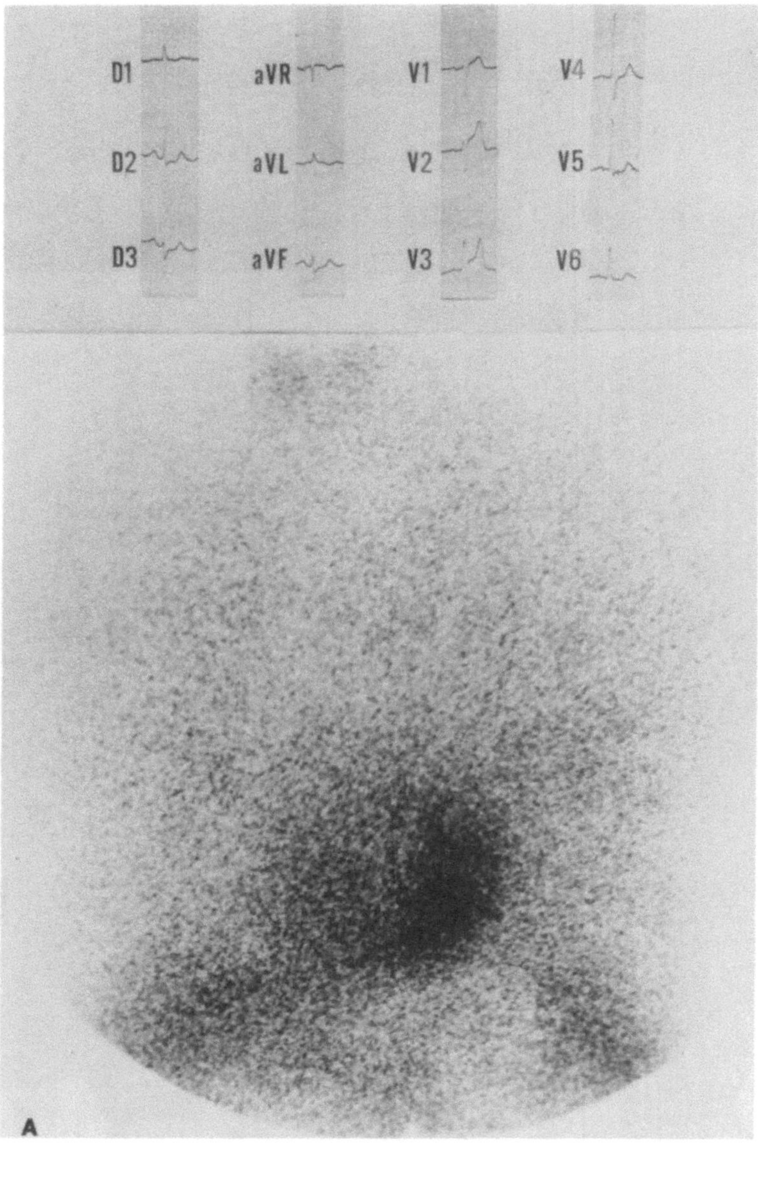
D1
aVR
V1
V4
D2
aVL
V2
V5
D3
aVF
V3
V6
A

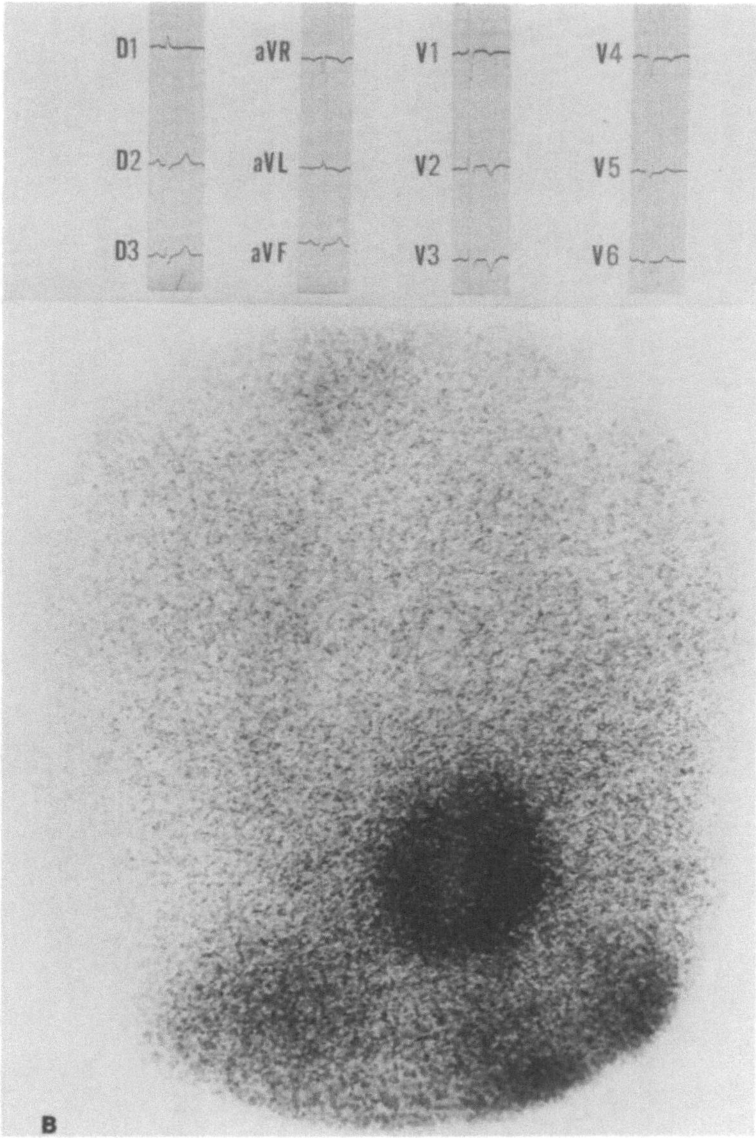

Fig. 4 ^{201}Tl myocardial scintigram in the 45° left anterior projection obtained during "spontaneous" angina (A) and under control conditions (B) together with the simultaneous 12-lead ECG. A severe transmural deficit of activity is observed in the anterior wall and septum during angina.

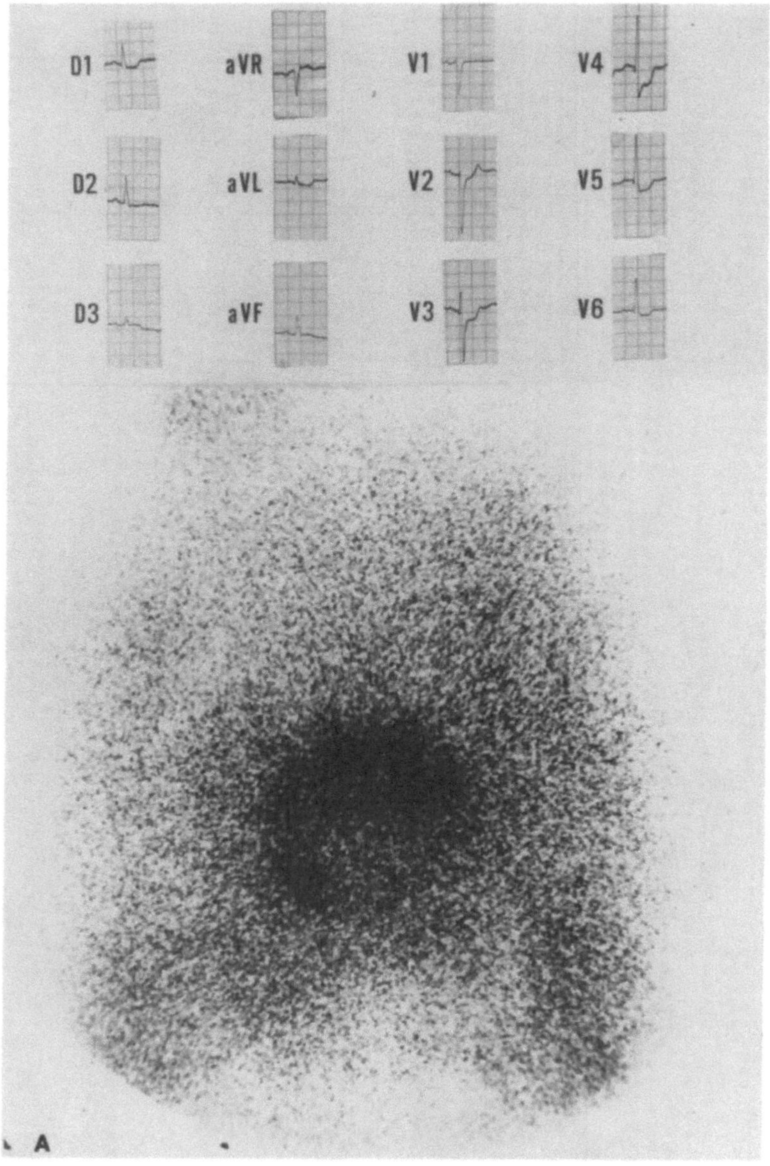

FIGURE 5A

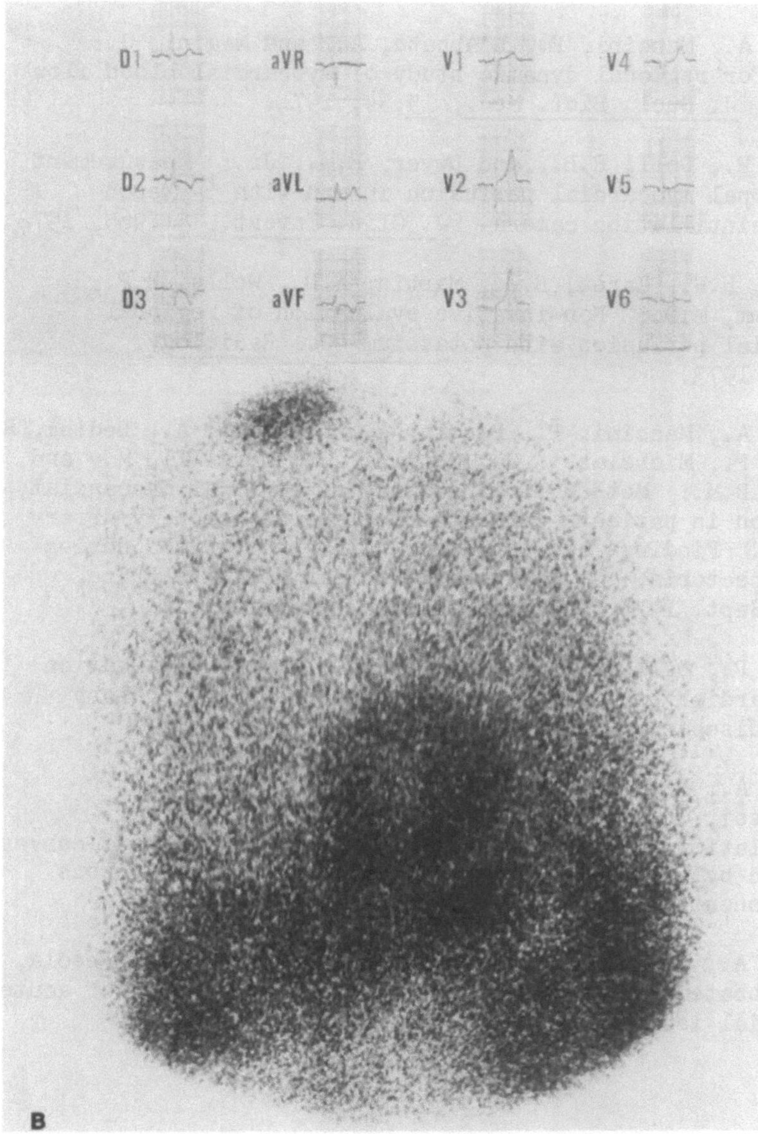

Fig. 5 The ^{201}Tl scintigram in a patient with ST segment elevation in lead D_2 during "spontaneous" angina (A). The control ECG and scintigram are shown for comparison in B. Coronary angiograms revealed triple vessel disease and a spasm completely occluding the left circumflex artery during a "spontaneous" attack.

REFERENCES

1. Maseri, A., Mancini, P., L'Abbate, A., and Magini, G.: Method for regional dynamic study of myocardial blood flow in man. J. Nucl. Biol. Med., 15:54, 1971.

2. Cannon, P., Dell, R.B., and Dwyer, E.M., Jr.: Measurement of regional myocardial perfusion in man with ^{133}Xenon and a scintillation camera. J. Clin. Invest., 51:965, 1972.

3. Strauss, H.W., Zaret, B.L., Martin, N.D., Wells, H.P., and Flamm, M.D.: Non-invasive evaluation of regional myocardial perfusion with potassium 42. Radiology, 108:85, 1973.

4. Maseri, A., Mancini, P., Pesola, A., L'Abbate, A., Bedini, R., Pisani, P., Michelassi, C., Contini, C., Marzilli, M., and De Nes, D.M.: Method for the study of regional myocardial perfusion in patients with atherosclerotic coronary artery disease. Findings at rest after nitroglycerin and during angina pectoris. G. Von Hevesy Nuclear Medicine Prize, Tokyo, Sept. 1974, Nuclear Medizine (in print).

5. Cannon, P., Dell, R.B., and Dwyer, E.M., Jr.: Evaluation of myocardial perfusion rates in patients with coronary artery disease. J. Clin. Invest., 51:978, 1972.

6. Maseri, A., Pesola, A., L'Abbate, A., Contini, C., Michelassi, C., and D'Angelo, T.: Contribution of recirculation and fat diffusion to myocardial washout curves obtained by external counting in man. Stochastic versus monoexponential analysis. Circ. Res., 35:826, 1974.

7. Maseri, A., Mimmo, R., Chierchia, S., Marchesi, C., Pesola, A., and L'Abbate, A.: Coronary artery spasm as a cause of acute myocardial ischemia in man. Chest (in print).

(3)

THE DETERMINANTS OF REGIONAL MYOCARDIAL BLOOD FLOW

G.A. Klassen, A. L'Abbate, F. Sestier, R.R. Mildenberger

Division of Cardiology, Royal Victoria Hospital

687 Pine Ave. W., Montreal, P.Q., Canada

INTRODUCTION

It is presumed that a region of myocardium does not always have the same blood flow. The purpose of this communication is to examine those factors which are determinants for changing regional flow. We have divided the determinants into three types. Those affecting a regional variation in blood flow which has a random distribution and a cyclic character which will be termed spatial and temporal heterogeneity (1). The second group are the determinants of the transmural distribution of coronary blood flow which were described by Griggs et al (2), Buckberg et al (3) and modified by L'Abbate et al (4). Finally, there are those determinants which are present when coronary artery obstruction occurs and collaterals develop which redistribute myocardial blood flow in a geographical sense (5,6).

METHODS

We have employed the microsphere technique (15±5μ) to measure regional myocardial blood flow. The measurements were performed using a canine preparation in which the left coronary artery was perfused by a pump from a bypass circuit. This system allowed us to vary systemic and coronary hemodynamic parameters independently and to inject the microspheres directly into the coronary circulation. The time from injection of microspheres to their impaction in the myocardium was less than 2 seconds. As well, we divided the myocardium into small pieces (less than 300 mg) each piece containing at least 800 microspheres. From these data we created a regional map of myocardial blood flow distribution both for time and for spatial distribution.

The variables we examined as possible determinants of myocardial blood flow distribution were time, autoregulation, coronary diastolic pressure, ventricular systolic pressure and ventricular diastolic pressure. The effect of time was assessed by injecting four varieties of microsphere either as a bolus (simultaneously) or in a time sequence (sequential). We then analyzed the regional variance in flow in a piece. The effect of autoregulation was examined by measuring regional distribution during its presence and when it had been abolished by either a 25 second period of stop flow or following administration of dipyridimole (0.1 mg intracoronary). Coronary diastolic pressure was altered by changing coronary blood flow, ventricular systolic pressure by aortic banding and ventricular diastolic pressure by increasing or decreasing preload (transfusion or bleeding).

RESULTS

I. Spatial and Temporal Heterogeneity

Following simultaneous injections of 4 types of microspheres (^{125}I, ^{141}Ce, ^{85}Sr, ^{95}Nb) we observed a variance in flow per gram of .005 which increased to .029 with 10 second sequential injections. These variances are statistically different at the 2.5% level. When autoregulation was abolished by dipyridimole the differences in variance between the two modes of injection was no longer present. From a series of timed injections we observed that the cycle time of a region from maximum to minimum flow was usually less than 90 seconds. Autoregulation is therefore a major component of a stochastic regional variation in myocardial blood flow. The determinants of this form of regional distribution of myocardial blood flow presumably relate to regional changes in myocardial oxygen consumption of functional units of myocardium.

II. Transmural Distribution of Myocardial Blood Flow

Histograms of the distribution of myocardial blood flow in the epicardium, midzone and endocardium are displayed in figure 1. In each instance the total weight of a layer was normalized to 100 percent. Each bar of the histogram is that percent of the layer having a flow per gram within a 0.2 ml range. In the first panel, coronary diastolic pressure was matched to aortic diastolic pressure. The distribution of flow pathways was gaussian with a narrow range about the mean. The ratio of flow distribution under these conditions as expressed by the ratio of mean endocardial flow to epicardial flow was 0.99. Coronary diastolic pressure was then increased by increasing pump flow so that it was greater than aortic

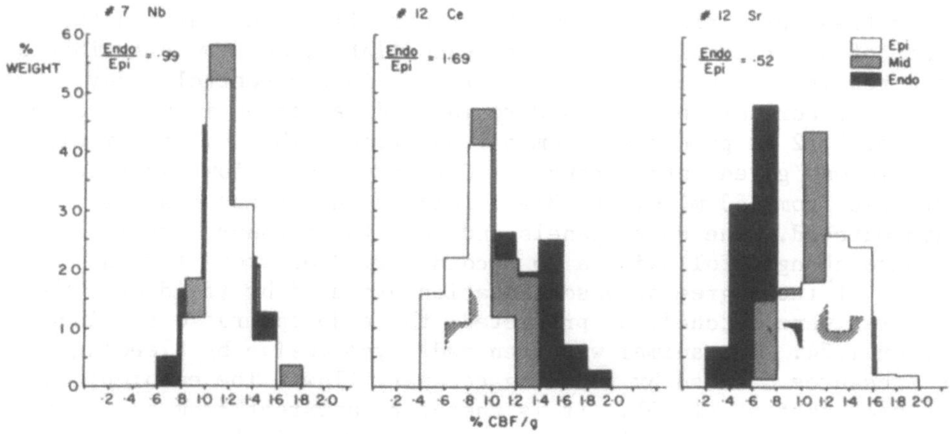

Figure 1. Flow per gram in the epicardium, midzone and endocardium. Each layers' weight is 100%. Conditions were for panel (1) coronary diastolic pressure equal to aortic diastolic pressure, (2) coronary diastolic pressure greater than aortic diastolic pressure and (3) coronary diastolic pressure less than aortic diastolic pressure. Type of microsphere used is indicated.

diastolic pressure (analogous to counterpulsation). Endocardial blood flow increased preferentially and the distribution profile flattened; epicardial flow tended to decrease resulting in an endo: epi ratio of 1.69. Coronary blood flow was then decreased (panel 3) so that coronary diastolic pressure was less than aortic. Endocardial blood flow decreased but remained gaussian in distribution; epicardial flow increased slightly with a wider range of flows. As well, some high flow pathways appeared in the epicardium. From this data and experiments where we kept coronary flow constant but changed left ventricular systolic and diastolic pressures, we arrived at a predictive formula for the endo:epi ratio (y)

$$y = 0.96x + 0.26 \quad (r=0.91)$$

where x is the ratio of coronary diastolic pressure to left ventricular systolic pressure. This equation is applicable when the left ventricular diastolic pressure is less than 10 mm Hg and is independent of autoregulation. When left ventricular diastolic pressure was increased above 10 mm Hg, the ratio decreased.

As a further test of the absence of an effect of autoregulation on the transmural distribution of coronary flow, we measured the effect of dipyridimole, a coronary vasodilator, on flow distribution; these results are presented in figure 2. In the control study, aortic and coronary pressures were matched resulting in an endo:epi ratio of 1.12 as predicted from our equation. Then 0.1 mg of dipyridimole was given intracoronary. Coronary blood flow was then increased from 153 ml/min to 385 ml/min so that pressures were again matched. The upper panels indicate the coronary artery pressure changes following a 25 second period of stop flow, a measure of the degree of vasodilatation produced by the drug. When pressures were matched, as predicted, the endo:epi ratio remained similar 1.24. The animal was then made hypotensive by bleeding and the pressures matched by reducing coronary flow. The endo:epi ratio remained constant (1.26). It is therefore apparent from our data that the coronary diastolic pressure, left ventricular diastolic and left ventricular systolic pressure are the determinants of transmural distribution of myocardial blood flow. Autoregulation per se is not a determinant. Heart rate was not controlled in our studies but within the range of 105 to 200 beats per minute, did not have an independent effect upon distribution.

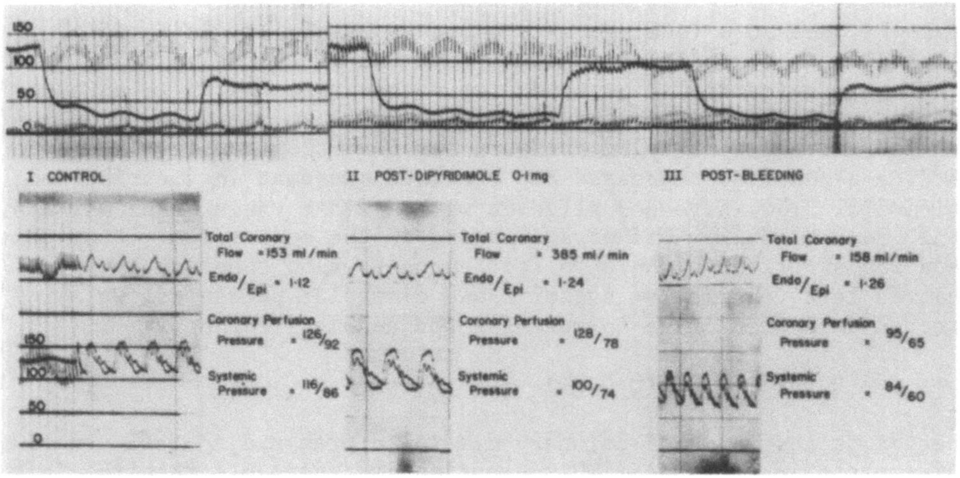

Figure 2. Effect of dipyridimole vasodilatation on the endo:epi flow ratio. In the top panels is the response of the mean coronary pressure to a 25 second stop flow (dark trace). The pressure present following restoration of flow is a reflection of the degree of coronary tone which is not metabolically determined.

The consequences of these determinants are shown in figure 3 where the average coronary diastolic pressure flow relationship for the left coronary system is illustrated (dotted line). Using our derived equation and an aortic pressure of 120/80 mm Hg we have calculated a pressure-flow relationship for the endocardium (A), midzone (B) and epicardium (C). It is apparent that as coronary diastolic pressure decreases (a consequence of coronary stenosis) regional myocardial blood flow in the endocardium decreases much more rapidly than does epicardial. Closure will therefore occur primarily in the endocardium as coronary perfusion pressure decreases. This is the reason why the endocardium is so vulnerable to undergo ischaemic necrosis.

III. Geographical Regional Differences

These differences in flow are the consequence of disease within the coronary arteries which cause differences in regional myocardial blood flow. These relate to both the distribution of the coronary arteries and the presence of a collateral circulation. These regional differences have been well described by the isotope mapping technique of Maseri et al (7) and Cannon et al (8). The deter-

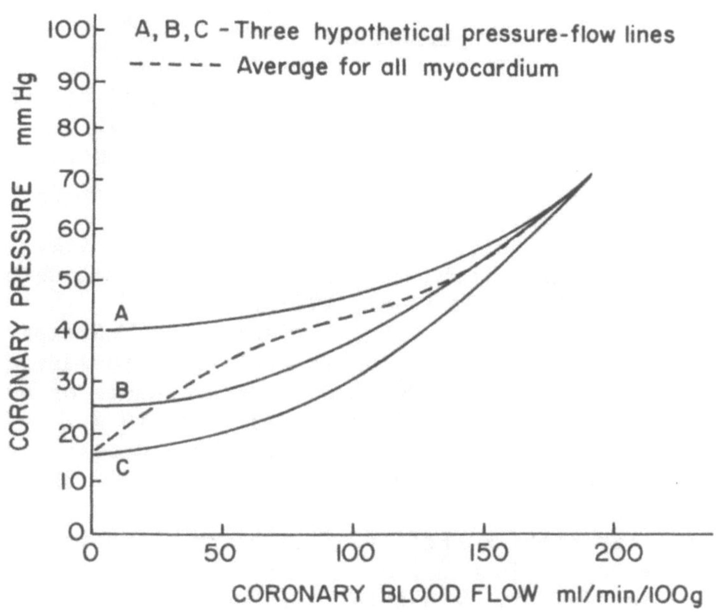

Figure 3. Coronary diastolic pressure, coronary blood flow relationship of the canine left coronary system. The dotted line is the measured value while A is the relationship for the endocardium, B for the midzone and C for the epicardium. A ventricular systolic pressure of 120 mm Hg is assumed.

minants are those described by Gould et al (5) for obstructions within the coronary circulation. The effect of coronary stenosis on transmural gradients will relate to changes in coronary diastolic pressure and consequent effects upon left ventricular systolic pressure and diastolic pressure. The presence or absence of collateral vessels will have an effect upon geographical regional distribution of coronary blood flow.

CONCLUSION

The determinants of regional myocardial blood flow on a microscopic level relate to the mechanism of autoregulation. The transmural distribution of myocardial blood flow relates to pressure gradients between the coronary circulation and ventricular cavity pressures. Obstruction within the coronary circulation and the development of collaterals are the major determinants of distribution of coronary blood flow on a geographical level.

ACKNOWLEDGEMENTS

Support of the MRC - MT 3238, Joseph Edwards Foundation and the Quebec Heart Foundation are acknowledged.

REFERENCES

1. Klassen, G.A. Coronary artery disease: A cause of heterogeneous myocardial perfusion. Cardiology 56: 343-346, 1971/72.
2. Griggs, D.M., Nakamura, Y. Effects of coronary constriction on myocardial distribution of iodoantipyrine ^{131}I. Am. J. Physiol. 215: 1082-1088, 1968.
3. Buckberg, G., Fixler, D., Archie, J.P., Hoffman, J.I.E. Experimental subendocardial ischaemia in dogs with normal coronary arteries. Circ. Res. 30: 67-81, 1972.
4. L'Abbate, A., Mildenberger, R.R., Christie, L., McGregor, M., Klassen, G.A. The role of coronary perfusion pressure and left ventricular intracavitary pressure as determinants of coronary blood flow distribution. Fed. Proc. 33: 414, 1974.
5. Gould, K.L., Lipscomb, K., Hamilton, G.W. Physiologic basis for assessing critical coronary stenosis. Am. J. Card. 33: 87-94, 1974.
6. Gould, K.L., Lipscomb, K. Effect of coronary stenosis on coronary flow reserve and resistance. Am. J. Card. 34: 48-54, 1974.
7. Maseri, A., Mancini, P., L'Abbate, A., Magini, G. Method for regional dynamic study of myocardial blood flow in man. J. Nucl. Biol. Med. 15: 54-57, 1971
8. Cannon, P.J., Dell, R.B., Dwyer, E.M. Jr. Measurement of regional myocardial perfusion in man with ^{133}Xenon and a scintillation camera. J. Clin. Invest. 51: 964-977, 1972.

(4)

REGIONAL MYOCARDIAL PERFUSION: STUDIES WITH ^{133}XENON AND A MULTIPLE-CRYSTAL SCINTILLATION CAMERA

Paul J. Cannon, M.D., Melvin B. Weiss, M.D., Kent Ellis, M.D. and William J. Casarella, M.D.
The Departments of Medicine and Radiology, College of Physicians and Surgeons, Columbia University
630 West 168th Street, N.Y.C., N.Y., U.S.A.

INTRODUCTION

Because it is impossible to measure the balance between coronary blood flow and the metabolic needs of the myocardium for oxygen by exclusively radiographic means, investigators in this laboratory developed a technique to make quantitative estimates of capillary blood flow in multiple areas of the human myocardium using ^{133}xenon and a multiple-crystal scintillation camera (1-3). The purpose of this report is to present preliminary results of studies of 175 patients who were studied at Columbia University. The regional myocardial perfusion rates obtained with the method were correlated with radiographic assessments of the degree and the extent of the coronary disease in each patient.

METHODS

Cardiac catheterization and coronary arteriography were performed only on patients for whom the studies were indicated clinically. Coronary arteriography was performed by a modified Judkin's technique. Images of contrast material injected into each coronary artery were recorded on a cine and/or serial cut films at a framing rate of 50 frames per second using a six inch image intensifier and 35 millimeter film. The coronary lesions were analyzed and coded by a modification of the scheme of Abrams (5).

Informed consent for the radioisotopic measurements of myocardial blood flow was obtained from each patient. The method has been described in detail elsewhere (3,6). In its current state of development, the approach consists of injection of ^{133}xenon selectively via a catheter into a coronary artery and the external measurements of isotope washout curves from multiple discrete areas of the myocardium with a multiple-crystal scintillation camera. ^{133}Xenon dissolved in saline is injected into the main right or left coronary artery as a bolus injection. All studies are done with the patient in the LAO position. The isotope rapidly passes by diffusion into myocardial tissue supplied by the artery; washout from the tissue is a direct function of capillary blood flow (3,7). The gamma radiation emitted by isotope within cardiac cells is collimated by a multichannel collimator and recorded externally by a multiple-crystal scintillation camera (294 separate crystals) which monitors ^{133}xenon washout from multiple areas of the myocardium. Scintillations produced by incident photons in each crystal are converted to an electrical signal, conditioned, stored in a digital memory and recorded on magnetic tape as counts per second (cps) for 4.5 - 7 minutes.

The data contained on magnetic tape are processed further by a digital computer (IBM 360/91). Crystals which record myocardial ^{133}xenon are identified by means of radiopaque-radioactive markers positioned along the cardiac margins and by a computer printout of the peak cps recorded by each crystal and the number of seconds after injection of tracer that the peak cps occurred. For each crystal, the computer calculates the slope (k) of the initial monoexponential portion of the isotope washout curve by the method of least squares and produces a second printout containing the clearance constants of ^{133}xenon washout from all of the crystals overlying the myocardium. A third printout contains calculations of regional myocardial blood flow rates/100g tissue in the different areas viewed by each crystal plus the standard deviation of each blood flow measurement. Myocardial blood flow in each region is calculated by the Kety formula (7): $F = K \times \lambda/\rho$ where F is myocardial blood flow in ml/100g·min, K is the rate constant of ^{133}xenon clearance from the myocardium determined experimentally, λ is the blood:myocardium partition coefficient for ^{133}xenon obtained by Conn in the normal dog (8) and ρ is the specific gravity of the tissue.

In performing these calculations monoexponential analysis of the initial portion of each curve and the λ of 0.72 were chosen because several studies (9-12) indicated that there was a close correspondence between left ventricular blood flow per 100 grams measured by a flowmeter and the blood flow per 100 grams measured simultaneously with radioxenon using this form of analysis. In addition, other data (11,12) suggested that initial slope mono-exponential analysis minimizes extraneous effects of cardiac fat or pulmonary xenon excretion which might otherwise influence the accuracy of the measurements.

A computer printout of the local myocardial blood flow rates is then superimposed upon a tracing of the patient's LAO left coronary arteriogram so that regions of myocardial perfusion can be localized by anatomical features of the coronary vasculature. Allignment and appropriate magnification of the two is facilitated by the presence of the radioactive-radiopaque markers present on both the arteriogram and the myocardial perfusion pattern. A mean left ventricular myocardial perfusion rate in each patient is calcuated by averaging the local blood flows recorded by all of the crystals overlying the left ventricle. The local perfusion rates of left ventricular subregions supplied by the anterior descending or the circumflex arteries are determined by averaging the perfusion rates of crystals in the appropriate areas of the perfusion pattern as determined from the tracing of the coronary arteriogram. In many studies, average perfusion rates in areas of myocardium distal to discrete coronary artery stenoses and in the remainder of the left ventricle are also estimated in a similar fashion.

Statistical analysis of the data is performed by standard techniques (13). Comparisons between the patient groups at rest and during atrial pacing are performed by an analysis of variance. Differences are deemed significant if the ρ value was <0.05.

RESULTS

Normal Coronary Arteriograms

Figure 1 shows the left and Figure 2 the right ventricular perfusion patterns in a patient with normal left and right coronary arteriograms. In 25 patients with normal arteriograms studied at Roosevelt Hospital (3) the average mean myocardial blood flow rate in the left ventricle (LV), 62±14 ml/100g·min, significantly exceeded that of the right ventricle 48±11 ml/100g·min and of the right atrial area, 34± ml/100g·min.

FIGURE 1

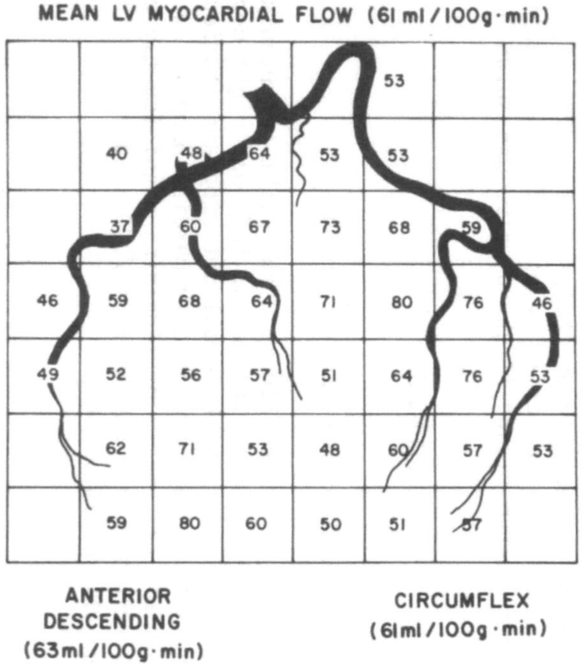

FIGURE 2

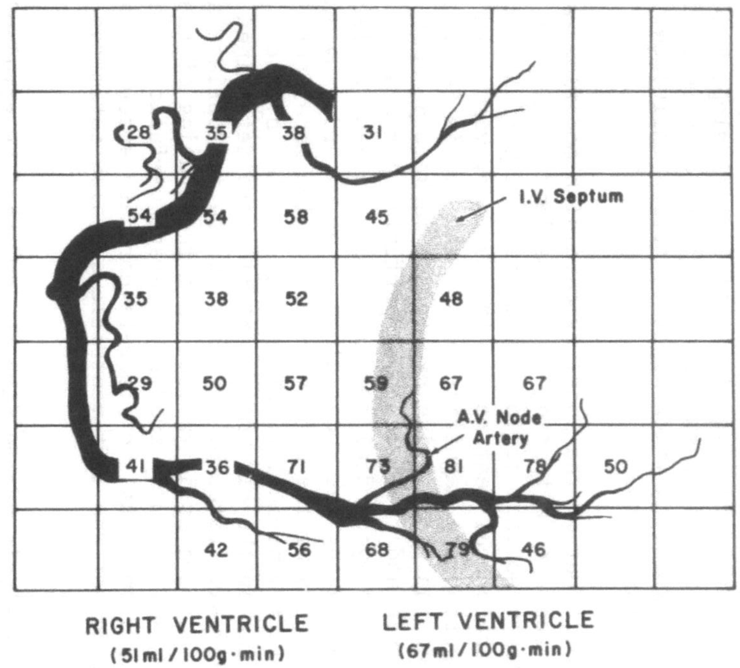

Figure 1: Left ventricular regional myocardial blood flow rate in ml/100g·min, in a patient with normal left coronary arteriogram.

Figure 2: Right ventricular regional myocardial blood flow rates in ml/100g·min, in a patient with a normal right coronary arteriogram.

The mean LV myocardial blood flow in 12 patients with normal intracardiac pressures, arteriograms and ventriculograms at Presbyterian Hospital was 61+6 ml/100g·min (14). The average blood flow rate in the myocardial subregions supplied by the left anterior descending artery, 61 ml/100g·min, was not significantly different from that of the circumflex regions, 62 ml/100g·min. In 17 patients the coefficient of variation of the multiple measurements of local LV perfusion was 15.8% (15). This includes both variation in perfusion rates and measurement error.

Mean Left Ventricular Myocardial Blood Flow/Unit Mass in Coronary Artery Disease

Mild Coronary Disease. In 10 patients (pts) with <50% lesions of one or more coronary arteries ("mild" disease), the average mean LV blood flow rate of 59±17 ml/100g·min was not significantly different from the control group with normal arteriograms and hemodynamics (14). Blood flow rates in the myocardial subregions supplied by the LAD and Circ, arteries were also not significantly lower than the controls. In four other types of heart disease: essential hypertension, 10 pts, mild aortic stenosis, 12 pts, aortic insufficiency, 7 pts, and cardiomyopathy, 20 pts, the presence of <50% coronary lesions was not associated with significant reduction of mean LV perfusion below the values found in the patients with the same four diseases who had normal coronary arteriograms.

Isolated LAD Lesions >50%. The average mean LV perfusion per unit mass of tissue was 59±14 ml/100g·min in 19 patients with isolated LAD obstructions >50% (16). This appeared to result from several factors: 1. the average degree of stenosis in the group corresponded to an 80% obstruction which may not have been sufficient to reduce resting flow distal to the lesion and 2. in individuals with a region of subnormal perfusion, much larger regions of higher blood flow brought the mean LV perfusion rate to within the range of normal.

LAD plus Right Coronary Disease. In 23 patients with >50% lesions of both the LAD and right coronary arteries, the mean LV myocardial blood flow rates averaged 47±11 ml/100g·min (16). This was significantly lower than the average mean LV blood flow observed in the control subjects and in those with "mild" coronary disease. In many of these patients regional LV perfusion was below control values not only in the LAD region but also in the circumflex area where the extent of radiographically apparent coronary artery disease was much less, i.e. normal or <50% obstruction.

LAD plus Circ. Coronary Artery Disease. Diffuse reductions of myocardial blood flow were observed at rest in patients with significant disease of both left coronary branches. In 8 patients with >50% obstruction of the LAD and Circ. arteries, the average mean LV myocardial blood flow rate of 53 ± 10 ml/100g·min, and the perfusion rates in the LAD (51 ± 11 ml/100g·min) and the Circ. (51 ± 11 ml/100g·min) subregions were reduced significantly below the corresponding values found in the control gorup (14).

Triple Vessel Disease. In 45 patients with >50% lesions of the LAD + Circ. + right coronary arteries, the average mean LV myocardial blood flow/unit mass was 45 ± 9 ml/100g·min (14). This is significantly lower than the values found in the controls, in those with "mild" disease and those with >50% isolated LAD lesions. This confirms our previous report (15) and is similar to data recently reported by Klocke et. al. (17) who measured mean LV perfusion/unit mass by the He washout technique with coronary sinus sampling.

Why perfusion/unit mass is reduced at rest in coronary disease patients who are free from angina and lack ECG evidences of ischemia is unclear. Perhaps reduced blood supply may be adequate for a reduced level of performance by the diseased ventricle in coronary disease. Weiss et. al. (18) found depressed mean LV blood flow/unit mass in patients with congestive and hypertrophic cardiomyopathy who had normal coronary arteriograms. In that study of 22 patients in which cardiac function was measured by quantitative ventriculography, multivariate regression analysis demonstrated that the level of resting LV perfusion was significantly related to heart rate, peak wall stress and performance (mean velocity of circumferential fiber shortening). Thus, it is possible that effects of individual coronary lesions upon regional perfusion may need to be interpreted against the relationship between myocardial blood flow and ventricular performance which exists in the individual patient.

Regional Myocardial Perfusion Differences at Rest: LAD Lesions >50%

Isolated LAD Disease. In 11 of the patients with isolated LAD lesions greater than 50% but less than 100% in whom the measurements could be made, the average degree of stenosis was equivalent to a 65% obstruction. In these patients the average mean regional myocardial blood flow rate distal to the LAD lesion, 58 ± 15 ml/100 g·min, was not significantly different from the average mean perfusion rate for the remainder of the ventricle, 58 ± 13 ml/100g·min, or from the average mean LAD regional perfusion rate for the control group. In 6 patients with 100% occlusions of the LAD, the average perfusion rate distal to the lesion was 53±8 ml/100g·min whereas it was 59± 6 ml/100g·min in the remainder of the LV.

LAD + Right Disease. In 11 of the patients with LAD + right coronary lesions of 50-95%, the average degree of stenosis was equivalent to 60% obstruction. In these patients the average regional perfusion at rest distal to the lesion, 45 ±17 ml/100g· min, was significantly lower than the LAD perfusion rates of the controls but it was not different from average perfusion in the remainder of the same ventricles, 45 ±15 ml/100g·min. In 11 others with 100% LAD obstructions, regional myocardial blood flow distal to the lesion was significantly depressed, 42±10 vs 49±8 ml/100g·min. Thus in this series of 42 left coronary studies selective depressions of average regional myocardial perfusion distal to coronary lesions below that of the rest of the LV were apparent at rest only in the group with 100% lesions (12).

RESPONSES OF MYOCARDIAL BLOOD FLOW DURING RIGHT ATRIAL PACING

In 48 patients the mean LV and regional myocardial blood flow/ unit mass, responses to right atrial pacing were studied (19). For the studies the heart rate was increased in graded increments until a heart rate of 150 or mild angina was produced. Measurements of regional myocardial perfusion were performed during a control period and in a steady state at the faster heart rate. The double product of heart rate times systolic blood pressure (DP) was used as an index of myocardial oxygen consumption (20). The responses of the control patients with normal coronary arteriograms were compared to those with >50% coronary lesions by an analysis of variance.

TABLE I

	ΔDP	Δ mean LV MBF ml/100g·min	Response Index $\frac{\Delta LV\ MBF \times 10^3}{\Delta DP}$
0 or <50 Lesions	8702	24.5	2.93
>50% Lesions	8539	15.4	1.76
	NS	*	*

* = Diff. signif with $p < 0.05$

TABLE II

	ΔRegional MBF ml/100g·min		
	LAD	Remainder of LV	
0 or <50% Lesions	24.8	24.3	N.S.
>50% Lesions	Distal to Lesion		
	11.7	17.9	*
	*	*	

	Regional Response Indexes		
	LAD	Remainder of LV	
0 or <50% Lesions	3.17	3.03	N.S.
>50% Lesions	Distal to Lesion		
	1.39	2.18	
	*	*	*

* = Diff. signif with p 0.05

None of the 24 patients with normal coronary arteriograms developed chest pain or ECG changes of ischemia during pacing, whereas 20 of the 24 with >50% did. Although the index of $M\dot{V}O_2$ rose similarly in the two groups of patients, average mean LV perfusion/unit mass increased significantly less in the group with >50% coronary lesions (Table I). A myocardial blood flow response index was calculated by dividing the increment in myocardial perfusion x 10^3 by the increase in the DP. The mean LV myocardial blood flow response index was significantly reduced in the patients with radiographically significant coronary lesions. Regional myocardial blood flow responses were also different in the two groups (Table II). The increment in average regional perfusion which occurred distal to >50% lesions in response to pacing was significantly less than the flow response elsewhere in the same ventricles. Hence there was a significant difference in the flow response indices in the two areas of myocardium in the group of patients with >50% lesions.

CONCLUSION

Differences in mean LV and regional myocardial blood flow have been found in these studies of patients with radiographically significant coronary artery disease both at rest and during pacing. It must be emphasized, however, that the method used to measure regional myocardial blood flow with ^{133}xenon and a scintillation camera in these studies is still under development. Some of its limitations and the problems currently under investigation are discussed in detail in other reports (3,6). The focus of the present studies was to obtain perfusion data (in the LAO projection) at rest and during right atrial pacing in groups of patients with similar coronary arteriographic lesions, and to make inferences only from statistically significant bodies of data. As the methodology improves, it is our belief that the study of individual patients will be optimized by making multiple measurements of regional myocardial perfusion with radioisotopes in multiple projections at rest and also during an intervention which increases myocardial oxygen consumption. Despite these current methodological limitations, the present data provide evidence for the hypothesis that angina pectoris results in a significant number of patients with coronary artery disease when an obstructive coronary lesion restricts the total or regional myocardial blood flow response to an increased rate of myocardial oxygen consumption.

This work was supported by Grants HL 14148 and HL 14236 from the U.S.P.H.S.

REFERENCES

1. Cannon, P.J., Haft, J.I. and Johnson, P.M. Visual assessment of regional myocardial perfusion using radioactive xenon and scintillation photography. Circulation 40: 277. 1969
2. Cannon, P.J., Dell, R.B., and Dwyer, E.M., Jr. Regional myocardial perfusion in man. J. Clin. Invest. 49: 16a, 1970.
3. Cannon, P.J., Dell, R.B. and Dwyer, E.M., Jr. Measurement of regional myocardial perfusion in man with ^{133}xenon and a scintillation camera. J. Clin. Invest. 51 964. 1972.
4. Judkins, M.P. Selective coronary arteriography. I. A percutaneous transfemoral technicque. Radiology. 89: 815. 1967.
5. Abrams, H.L., Editor. Angiography. Little Brown and Co. 2nd Edition. 1: 421. 1967
6. Cannon,P.J., Sciacca, R.R., Fowler, D.L., Weiss, M.B., Schmidt, D.H. and Casarella, W.J. Regional myocardial blood flow in man: description and critique of the method using ^{133}xenon and a scintillation camera. In press. Am. J. of Cardiol.
7. Kety, S.S. I. Blood-tissue exchange methods. Theory of blood-tissue exchange and its applicaton to measurement of blood flow. Methods Med. Res. 8: 223. 1960.
8. Conn, H.L., Jr. Equilibrium distribution of radioxenon in tissue: xenon-hemoglobin association curve. J. Appl. Physiol. 16: 1065. 1961

9. Herd, J.A., Hollenberg, M., Thorburn, G.D., Kopald, H.H. and Barger, A.C. Myocardial blood flow determined with Krypton^{85} in unanesthetized dogs. Am. J. Physiol. 203: 122. 1962
10. Ross, R.S., Ueda, K., Lichtlen, P.R. and Rees, J.R. Measurement of myocardial blood flow in animals and man by selective injection of radioactive inert gas into the coronary arteries. Circ. Res. 15: 28. 1964.
11. Bassingthwaighte, J.B., Strandell, T. and Donald, D.E. Estimation of coronary blood flow by washout of diffusible indicators. Circ. Res. 23: 259. 1968.
12. Shaw, D.J., Pitt, A. and Friesinger, G.C. Autoradiographic study of the ^{133}xenon disappearance method for measurement of myocardial blood flow. Cardiovasc. Res. 6: 268. 1971.
13. Steel, R.G.D. and Torrie, J.H. Principles and procedures of statistics. McGraw-Hill Book Co., Inc. New York, 1960.
14. Cannon, P.J., Schmidt, D.H., Weiss, M.B., Fowler, D.L., Sciacca, R.R., Ellis, K. and Casarella, W.J. The relationship between regional myocardial perfusion at rest and arteriographic lesions in patients with coronary atherosclerosis. In press. J. Clin. Invest.
15. Cannon, P.J., Dell, R.B. and Dwyer, E.M., Jr. Regional myocardial perfusion rates in patients with coronary artery disease. J. Clin. Invest. 51: 978.
16. Casarella, W.J., Weiss, M.B., Sciacca, R.R., Fowler, D.L. and Cannon, P.J. Myocardial blood flow in patients with left anterior descending disease. Submitted, 48th Scientific Sessions of the American Heart Assoc. Anaheim, Calif. 1975.
17. Klocke, F.J., Bunnell, I.L., Green, D.G., Wittenberg, S.M. and Visco, J.P. Average coronary blood flow per unit weight of left ventricle in patients with and without coronary artery disease. Circulation 50: 547. 1974.
18. Weiss, M.B., Ellis, K., Sciacca, R.R., Schmidt, D.H. and Cannon, P.J. Myocardial blood flow in congestive and hypertrophic cardiomyopathy: relationship to peak wall stress and mean velocity of circumferential fiber shortening. Submitted for publication.
19. Schmidt, D.H., Weiss, M.B., Casarella , W.J., Fowler, D.L., Sciacca, R.R. and Cannon, P.J. Regional myocardial perfusion during atrial pacing in patients with coronary artery disease. Submitted for publication.
20. Katz, I.N., and Feinberg, H. The relation of cardiac effort to myocardial oxygen consumption and coronary flow. Circulation 6: 656. 1954.

(5)

DISCUSSION (CURRENT INVESTIGATIONS IN MYOCARDIAL PERFUSION)

Discussion on Paper of Dr. Bloor

In discussion Dr. Klassen questioned Dr. Bloor's use of the word Model 4 "aortic stenosis". He asked whether the stenotic lesion was introduced below the take-off of the coronary arteries or above it as in coarctation. Dr. Bloor replied that the latter was the case and that the lesion more closely simulated a coarctation than aortic stenosis.

Dr. Cornhill asked Dr. Bloor what was the accuracy of the electromagnetic flow meter when placed on the left main coronary artery, the anterior descending or the circumflex branches because of possible asymmetry of the flow profile immediately distal to a bifurcation. Dr. Bloor replied that he was not aware of this problem. Calibration of the flow meters after long periods of chronic implantation was within an accuracy of $\pm$ 5%.

Discussion on Dr. Klassen's Paper

Dr. Cannon asked Dr. Klassen whether the frequency of fluctuation of flow in small areas of myocardium, which Dr. Klassen had described, was greater in deep or superficial layers of the left ventricular wall. Dr. Klassen replied that he had not analysed his data to determine this point.

Dr. Roberts said that it is accepted that the endocardium is normally maximally vaso-dilated and that this is the mechanism by which flow is maintained homogeneous in the inner layer of the left ventricle. "I take it that you find this not to be true." Dr. Klassen replied that this was correct. The state of water regulation of the myocardium does not effect the distribution of blood across the wall, according to his experiments.

Dr. Mitchell then asked whether Dr. Klassen could explain, in the light of this finding, how the blood is distributed homogeneously in the left ventricle. Dr. Klassen stated that he could not yet give the full explanation, but the data had shown why one might expect subendocardial layers to become selectively under-perfused in conditions such as coronary artery narrowing or aortic stenosis because of the changes in the ratio of ventricular systolic and coronary artery diastolic pressures.

Dr. Chesebro asked whether the distribution of microspheres was sensitive to the relationship of the instant of injection to the period of the cardiac cycle in which they were injected. Dr. Klassen said he did not know this. He made injections in his studies which had a duration of at least 4 cardiac cycles so the timing of injection would not be important to his results.

A questioner asked how Dr. Klassen could explain the well documented gradient in oxygen tension which was observed across the left ventricular wall of the dog heart. Dr. Klassen replied that he was not sure that this difference was really accurate and that in spite of some PO_2 electrode results there was contrary evidence as well.

<u>Discussion on Dr. Maseri's Paper</u>

Dr. McGregor asked how the "tail of the washout curve" was defined in these studies. Dr. Maseri explained that the washout curve was followed down to 10% of peak concentration. The "tail" was then arbitrarily defined as the last 60 seconds before this point.

Dr. Roberts asked how Maseri could deduce a reduction in flow in "ischemia" areas during the induction of angina by pacing from the increased half time of washout. Such a result might also have occurred if the voluble distribution of indicator were increased as a consequence of vasodilatation and the flow were maintained constant because of the narrowed coronary artery. Dr. Maseri replied that you could tell that there was a true reduction in flow because when injections of indicator were made during angina it was apparent that there was a reduced input of indicator to these areas.

Another questioner asked whether, in the light of Klocke's work which showed that it might take up to 20 minutes to equilibrate indicator in the slow flow areas, Doctor Maseri's analysis would not, therefore, under-estimate slow flow. Maseri agreed. The reduced flow which he had been able to demonstrate was an under-estimate.

McGregor asked Dr. Maseri about the extraordinary reduction in flow which was demonstrated by him in patients while experiencing angina. Did he have any views whether this might be due to coronary steal, coronary spasm, or some other mechanism. Maseri replied that he did not know. He pointed out that in each of these patients with angina it was probable that the left ventricular end-diastolic pressure was considerably elevated. This might well result in a major reduction in flow in the subendocardial layers such that the injected indicator was trapped there for a long time.

Roberts asked Dr. Maseri if there were any difference in flow measurements between those patients with angina at rest with elevation of ST segments and those with depression. Maseri replied that he was not aware of any difference. Furthermore he had seen in the same patient sequential elevation and subsequent depression of ST segments in consecutive attacks of angina.

McGregor asked Dr. Maseri whether he had any special technique for precipitating coronary spasm at the time of study since the size of his series of studied patients must be the largest in the World. Maseri replied that the secret was waiting. They chose patients with frequent attacks of angina at rest and made observations when spontaneous angina occurred. He had tried to produce coronary spasm with noradrenalin, with epinephrine without effect. Furthermore he had not been able to confirm that atropine protected from spontaneous spasm. He had not tried ergotamine.

A questioner asked Dr. Maseri how he could account for angina of effort occurring in patients whose angina at rest was precipitated primarily by spasm. Maseri replied that in only 20% of the cases of angina at rest which he had studied was the vessel completely normal. In a further 25% there was single vessel disease, in another 25% there was two-vessel disease and 30% of these subjects actually had three-vessel disease. He stressed that in no patient had he ever encountered an increase in blood pressure or heart rate preceding the onset of electrocardiographic changes. This included a series of patients he had studied during sleep with recording of the EEG. He found no correlation between REM sleep and the occurrence of angina.

In conclusion Maseri stressed that one should be certain to exclude coronary spasm as the principle cause of angina before allowing patients to be subjected to surgery. In 3 patients he had studied surgery had been carried out independently and post-operatively angina persisted in spite of the proven patency of the bypass grafts.

Discussion of Dr. Cannon's Paper

Dr. Sniderman asked Dr. Cannon how it was possible that his data failed to show a reduction in flow in areas of muscle distal to coronary narrowing up to 90%. Cannon pointed out that this result was quite consistent with the animal experimental work in which it had been shown that slow occlusion of the coronary branch in the dog did not result in reduction in resting flow until the vessel was narrowed by more than 90% in spite of the fact that the vessel was quite unable to take part in reactive hyperemia.

(1)

TISSUE CULTURE IN THE STUDY OF ATHEROSCLEROSIS

George H. Rothblat, Ph.D.

Member, The Wistar Institute

36th and Spruce Streets, Philadelphia, PA, U.S.A.

The surge of interest in the use of cell culture systems to study atherosclerosis is perhaps best evidenced by the presence at this meeting of two workshop sessions specifically devoted to reports and discussions of cell culture systems. Among the factors that have contributed to this sudden interest in cell culture are a realization of the distinct limitations of other experimental systems (e.g., whole animals, organ perfusion, tissue slices); standardization of techniques and materials which has taken the "black magic" out of cell culture methodology; and the development of techniques making it possible to obtain and maintain differentiated cells such as vascular cells that are highly relevant to the atherosclerotic process.

Basic to an intelligent assessment of the suitability of a particular cell system is a thorough understanding of both the advantages and limitations of the techniques of cell culture. Although the technique is relatively new to many investigators in the field of lipid metabolism and atherosclerosis, cells have been maintained routinely in culture for many years and a vast amount of information is available. An overview of the literature, however, will show a number of fundamental considerations that must be kept in mind by the researcher contemplating tissue culture as a model system to study the mechanisms involved in atherosclerosis.

I. PROBLEMS AND PITFALLS

A. Model Systems

Questions relevant to the use of tissue culture cells in the study of atherosclerosis are similar to those asked of other experimental systems. For example, just as the question can be raised as to the proper animal model for the study of atherosclerosis similar questions are pertinent to the choice of cell models for such studies. This may be particularly true for those investigators interested in studying fundamental aspects of metabolism and cell regulation, and a cell model system that is readily available and easily maintained can greatly facilitate such investigations.

It is interesting to note that there are relatively few examples of fundamental biochemical pathways and metabolic regulatory mechanisms that are highly specific to one particular cell type. In terms of lipid metabolism, the available information would actually suggest that a variety of cells in culture, including smooth muscle, endothelial and fibroblast cells, all share common metabolic pathways and that differences are quantitative rather than qualitative. If the knowledge gained from investigations on tissue culture is to be profitably applied to the atherosclerotic process, various cell systems must be compared to determine which phenomena are relevant to atherosclerosis and which are antifacts of the cell culture system itself. It should always be kept in mind that the cell in culture is operating as an individual, without the restraints and controls normally imposed upon it by the multiple interactions *in vivo*.

B. Experimental Conditions

Just as careful consideration should be given to the type of cell used, so also should consideration be given to the conditions under which the experiments are conducted. For example, should a study utilize confluent or nonconfluent cultures? Since metabolism of rapidly proliferating cells may be considerably different from that of quiescent cells in a confluent culture,which condition, if either, most closely approximates the conditions of the cells *in vivo*. Even in the supposedly quiescent confluent culture considerable cell division may be present. Cells are continually dying and being replaced, multi-layering occurs with some cells, and extensive cell division can be triggered by manipulations of the culture medium. Again, it is difficult to define the ideal system. What is essential is an appreciation for the characteristics of the particular system to be used and the consistent reporting of the specific conditions of the experiments.

C. Cellular Aging

Another fundamental aspect of cells in culture is that of cellular aging, or cellular senescence. This phenomenon is being extensively investigated and is of particular importance to any investigator conducting experiments utilizing diploid cells. Such populations have a finite life span and at different points in this life span they exhibit changes in various metabolic parameters. Specific diploid cell types have been isolated; for example, the mutant fibroblasts from Type II hyperlipemic individuals. Undoubtedly, other similarly specific cells will be isolated and distributed. For valid comparisons between data from different laboratories it is essential that investigators be aware of the process of "aging in vitro" and accurately monitor and report the age of the culture at the time experimental measurements are taken. Simplified techniques to assess culture age are available: one of the most recent techniques utilized thymidine-labeling of the cell nuclei and can be performed with relative ease (1).

A related aspect of the same problem is the use of primary cells as opposed to cultures maintained in continual passage. Some investigators feel that only cells obtained from the primary outgrowth can serve as valid experimental material whereas others utilize cells that have undergone five, ten, or perhaps fifteen population doublings. In most instances the cut off point seems entirely arbitrary. To date, the information basic to establishing guidelines has yet to be determined. For example, what changes, if any, occur as this cell migrates out of an explant? What changes continue to occur as this cell is passed in culture? It is probable that many parameters are stable and persist throughout the life span of a culture. Thus, for some experiments it may not be necessary to discard cultures after an arbitrary period of time. The acquisition of metabolic data obtained throughout the life span of a cell in culture may provide information that will aid in understanding the phenomenon of cellular senescence which in itself could be highly relevant to atherosclerosis.

D. Experimental Variation

One of the major advantages of the use of cell culture is the ability to produce a cell system under uniform and controlled conditions, however, reliance on a single set of determinations is no more justified when using tissue culture cells than when dealing with whole animals. Biological variations are encountered in tissue culture experiments similar to those occurring between whole animals of the same species. The statistical significance of results in both, therefore, is dependent upon the numbers of experimental determinations. Cells in culture exhibit considerable day-to-day variation in the quantitative cellular responses to specific stimuli or experimental manipulations. Such variation is readily observed using cloned transformed cell populations, and it is to be expected that it might even be greater in experiments using primary diploid cells. In addition, reliance on morphological criteria to define and quantitate metabolic changes is often misleading. Gross cellular appearance is variable and is easily influenced by subtle differences in growth conditions. For example, one often observes in cells large quantities of lipid present as lipid inclusions. In most instances these lipid inclusions are composed of triglycerides, the formation of which can be elicited by a variety of manipulations (2,3). In a few instances, however, such lipid inclusions may be composed of esterified cholesterol (4). Thus, the appearance of lipid inclusions in cells often gives no specific information on the type of lipid being accumulated or the metabolic processes that preceded this accumulation.

II. THE FUTURE

The enthusiasm generated for the use of tissue culture cells in the study of atherosclerosis will entice many new investigators to initiate cell culture studies. The successful use of cells from Type II hypercholesteremic individuals will certainly stimulate the search for other genetic variants that can be used for the study of lipid metabolism. A closely related area that deserves investigation is that of clonal variation. The variability that is often encountered in early passage cellular material may, in part, be attributed to clonal variation. Sophisticated techniques and equipment are available for the isolation and maintenance of cloned populations. Evidence for clonal variation, particularly if observed in aortic medial cells, could help to explain the focal development of lesions in atherosclerosis.

Another potentially useful area for investigation would be the development of cell culture systems that could be used as screening systems. Two different approaches could be taken. The first would develop cell culture as a technique for screening physiologically active compounds that could be useful in the treatment of atherosclerosis. Enough information is currently available on the mechanisms involved in cellular cholesterol metabolism to permit the _in vitro_ testing of compounds that might influence sterol synthesis and/or sterol flux. A second approach would be the use of cell culture to screen for various hyperlipoproteinemias by using either the patients sera or cells. Evidence has accumulated indicating the presence of specific serum lipoprotein receptor sites on the cell surface (5). If this is the case, cells in culture may provide a sensitive recognition system for specific abnormal or modified human lipoproteins. The use of the individual's skin fibroblasts to diagnose familial hypercholesterolemia is already experimentally feasible (6). In the future such systems could be expanded into clinically useful screening techniques.

Finally, rewarding results might be obtained by the use of cell cultures in "multifactor" experiments. All experiments to date have used single populations of cell types. Investigators might consider the use of mixed cell populations or two cell types growing in justaposition. Thus, tissue culture could be used to study the interaction between cell types under easily controlled conditions. A broader approach can also be taken for the study of cellular metabolism. It is now possible to quantitatively and qualitatively manipulate the phospholipid, fatty acid and sterol composition of cells (7,8,9). By combining such techniques one might obtain information on the possible coordinated metabolism of sterols, glycerides and phospholipids in mammalian cells, and to assess the relationship between cellular lipid metabolism, membrane synthesis and cell growth. Integrated information of this type would be highly relevant, not only to atherosclerosis but to a variety of other pathological conditions that affect man.

It is hoped that the workshop sessions on the use of cell culture systems will aid in the understanding of this uniquely multifaceted tool as research continues into the puzzling phenomenon of atherosclerosis.

REFERENCES

1. Cristofalo, V.J., and Sharf, B.B., Exp. Cell Res. 76: 419, 1973.
2. Mackenzie, C.G., Mackenzie, J.B., and Reiss, O.K., IN: "Lipid Metabolism in Tissue Culture Cells", Wistar Monograph, No. 6, Wistar Institute Press, Philadelphia, Pennsylvania, (1967), p. 63.
3. Schneeberger, E.E., Lynch, R.D., and Geyer, R.P., Exp. Cell Res. 69: 193, 1971.
4. Rothblat, G.H., Lipids 9: 526, 1974.
5. Brown, M.S., Brannan, P.G., Bohmfalf, H.A., Brunschede, G.Y., Dana, S.E., Helgeson, J., and Goldstein, J.L., J. Cell. Physiol. 85: 425, 1975.
6. Khachadurian, A.K., Lipson, M., and Kawahara, F.S., Atherosclerosis 21: 235, 1975.
7. Wisnieski, B.J., Williams, R.E., and Fox, F., Proc. Nat. Acad. Sci. 10: 3669, 1973.
8. Glaser, M., Ferguson, K.A., and Vagelos, P.R., Proc. Nat. Acad. Sci. 10: 4072, 1974.
9. Kandutsch, A.A., and Chen, H.W., J. Cell. Physiol. 85: 415, 1975.

Supported in part by UHPHS grant HL-09103 and Established Investigatorship of the American Heart Association.

(2)

ELECTRON MICROSCOPIC TECHNIQUES IN THE STUDY OF CULTURED VASCULAR CELLS

C. Richard Minick, M.D., Eric A. Jaffe, M.D., Ralph L. Nachman, M.D., and Carl G. Becker, M.D.
From the Departments of Pathology and Medicine, The New York Hospital-Cornell Medical Center, 1300 York Avenue, New York, N.Y., U.S.A.

Culture of cells derived from blood vessel walls has provided new information concerning the biology of normal blood vessels and new insight into the pathogenesis of vascular disease (1,2,4,6,7,8, 11-17). Electron microscopy has helped establish the identity of the cells grown in culture and contributed significantly to our understanding of their normal and abnormal biology. The purpose of this communication is to report on techniques used in our laboratory for preparation of cultured cells derived from blood vessels for scanning and transmission electron microscopy. Preparation of human endothelial cells will be emphasized since most of our experience is with endothelium. However, vascular smooth muscle cells may be prepared similarly.

Human endothelial cells and vascular smooth muscle cells are obtained from umbilical veins by an adaption of a technique of Maruyama (10) as described previously by us (6). According to this technique, collagenase is utilized to digest the basement membrane that binds endothelial cells to the vessel wall. A longer digestion may be utilized to digest extracellular protein surrounding subjacent smooth muscle cells. Unattached endothelial or smooth muscle cells may then be flushed from the lumen of the vein with cord buffer (0.14 M NaCl, 0.004 M KCl, 0.001 M phosphate pH 7.4, 0.011 M glucose). Briefly, human umbilical veins, obtained while maintaining aseptic surgical technique, are placed immediately in cord buffer and perfused with 100 ml of this buffer. The lumen of the vein is then filled with 10 ml of a 0.2% collagenase solution and the umbilical cord containing collagenase is incubated at 37°C for 15 minutes. Collagenase solution containing endothelial cells is flushed from the cord by perfusion with 30 cc of cord buffer. Cells are collected in medium 199 with 10% fetal calf serum, washed several times and grown on cover slips, in flask, or in plastic petri dishes in tissue culture medium 199 with 20% fetal calf serum in 5% CO_2 at 37° C.

Cultured vascular cells to be examined by scanning electron microscopy are grown on glass cover slips in the bottom of plastic petri dishes. Cover slips are removed and the attached cells are fixed in 1% glutaraldehyde in 0.15 M phosphate buffer for 1 hour. Cover slips bearing fixed cells are then rinsed in several changes of buffer, and then distilled water. They are dehydrated first in a series of graded alcohols followed by a graded series of amyl acetate and alcohol, and then critical point dried in CO_2 at a temperature of 39-41° C and a pressure of 1300 lbs/inch^2. After drying, small 2x2 mm fragments of tissue-coated cover slips are glued onto polished aluminum stubs, coated uniformly in vacuo with about 200 Å thickness of gold and viewed immediately with a scanning electron microscope.

Scanning electron microscopy is used in observing the growth characteristics of various cultured cells, surface characteristics of cells and junctions between cells (Figs. 1,2). Endothelial cells in culture are homogeneous and are large (30x50 μ), very flat cells that grow in a monolayer, have distinct cell boundaries and a prominent nuclear bulge. They have prominent blebs and pits on their surfaces most often seen around the nucleus or near the edge of the cell and prominent overlaping or interdigitating cell junctions (Fig. 1). In contrast, cultured fibroblasts are spindle shaped and grow in parallel arrays, with different junctions and processes (Fig. 2).

Scanning electron microscopy is also used to study the interaction of blood elements such as platelets with endothelial cells. Platelets adhere to the surface of endothelial cells and their processes in preference to the glass surface of the cover slips (Fig.3). In the future, scanning electron microscopy may be used in studying other functions of vascular cells such as phagocytosis. In addition, more recently developed techniques such as the labeling of proteins or antibodies with methylmethacrylate latex spheres (9) and antibodies with viruses (3) may be used in the characterization of surfaces of endothelial cells and vascular smooth muscle.

Cultured vascular cells to be examined by transmission electron microscopy are grown on cover slips, in flasks or on Falcon plastic dishes. In some instances cells are processed by a modification of a method used by Ross (12). Briefly, cells are grown on the bottom of plastic culture dishes that have been carbon coated in a vacuum evaporator and sterilized in ethylene oxide. After rinsing with several changes of cord buffer, cultured cells are fixed in the dishes at room temperature with slight agitation in solutions containing equal volumes of Karnovsky's fixative (5) and fresh culture medium. Fixed cells are then washed with fresh culture medium, post fixed in osmium tetroxide at room temperature and prestained with uranyl ace-

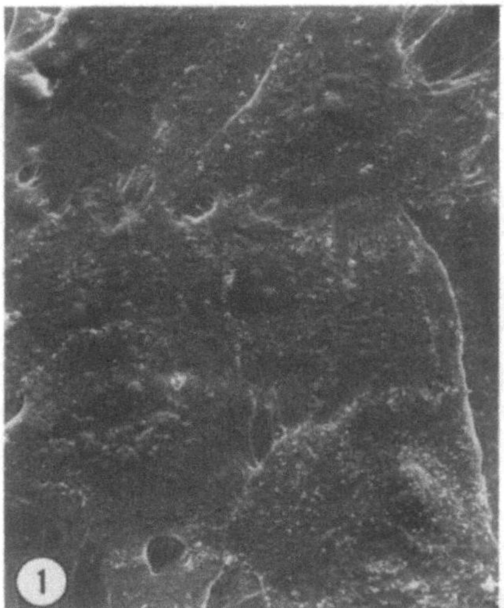

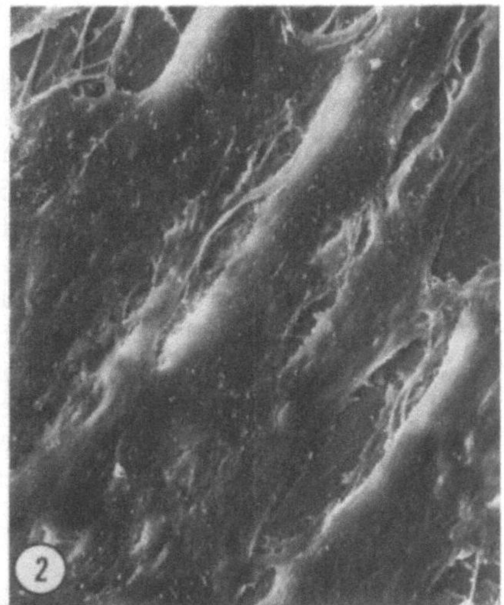

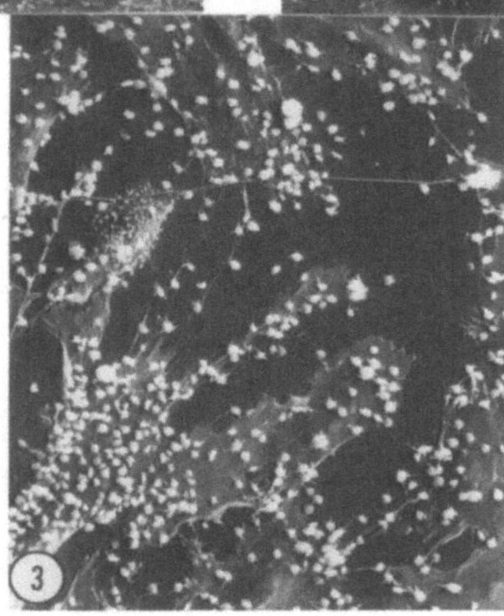

Fig. 1. Scanning electron photomicrograph of cultured endothelial cells. Cells grow in a monolayer and are large, flat and polygonal. They are closely apposed and prominent cellular interdigitations are present. (X 724)

Fig. 2. Scanning electron photomicrograph of cultured skin fibroblasts In contrast to endothelial cells, these cells are spindle shaped and grow in parallel arrays. (X 892)

Fig. 3. Scanning electron photomicrograph of cultured endothelial cells and attached platelets. Platelet rich plasma was added to culture dish 30 minutes prior to fixation. Note platelets are attached to endothelial cell surface and processes and only occasionally to glass. (X 428) tate from 2 hours to overnight. Cells in culture dishes are then infiltrated with Epon by standard techniques. Prior to polymerization Epon filled Beem capsules are inverted over the cells in the bottom of the culture dishes. After polymerization, the capsules with the cells on the surface are twisted free from the dishes with a large surgical clamp. Cells are easily identified on the face of the Epon block. Areas of Epon containing cells are then cut out and reembedded in a flat mold with Epon. Cells may be oriented so that they are cut en face or blocks may be rotated 90° and cut on edge to obtain cross sections of cells. Ultrathin sections are cut and picked up on 200 mesh uncoated copper grids and restained with uranyl acetate followed by lead citrate. Grids are then lightly carbon coated and viewed with a Philips 301 electron microscope.

Cultured vascular cells are also prepared for transmission microscopy as a pellet by detaching them from petri dishes with 0.01% EDTA or 0.1% collagenase in cord buffer. They are then washed in buffer, centrifuged at 500g and the pellet is fixed in half strength Karnovsky's fixative for 20 minutes. The pellet on bottom is then

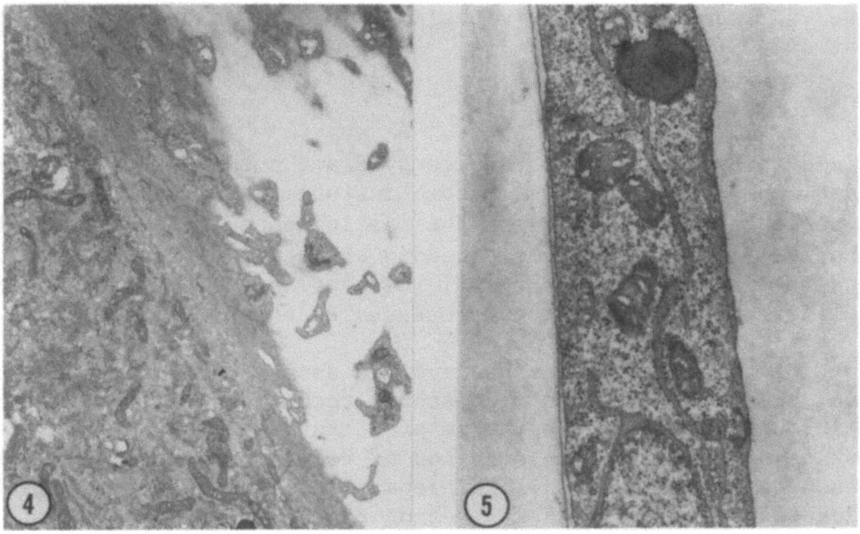

Fig. 4. Transmission electron photomicrograph of cultured endothelial cell prepared en face. Note bundles of fine filaments and dense bodies near edge of cell. Cell membrane is poorly defined. Basement membrane if present is not well defined. (X 8,152)

Fig. 5. Endothelial cell reoriented and cut in cross section. Note distribution of rough surfaced endoplasmic reticulum, clusters of free ribosomes and mitochondria. Folds are not present in nucleus. Condensations of fine filaments are present along upper surface of cell, Basement membrane material accumulates along lower surface against surace of the dish. (X 22,440)

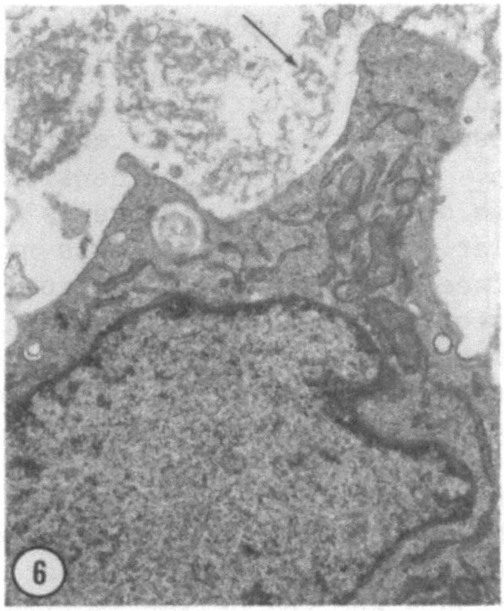

Fig. 6. Transmission electron photomicrograph of cultured endothelial cell prepared in cell pellet. Cell has irregular shape and nucleus is folded. Basement membrane material is distributed along edge of cell (arrow). (X 11,960)

post fixed in osmium, dehydrated, removed and cut into small fragments and embedded in Epon. In some instances only parts of the cells are loosened with EDTA and the remaining cells and extracellular material in which they are embedded are scraped from the bottom of the dish with a rubber spatula. These cells and the surrounding extracellular material are then processed as above (Fig. 6).

Each of these techniques has evolved as a result of a particular need. Scanning electron microscopic techniques are particularly useful in observing growth patterns of cultured cells, surface characteristics of cells, and interaction of cells with other blood elements such as platelets. En face preparations, viewed by transmission microscopy are useful for studying fine filaments and microvesicles as well as lipid droplets in cells, but are not very useful when better definitions of cell membranes are needed (Fig. 4). Examining sections of cells on edge offers a better view of growth characteristics, e.g. whether cells pile or not, cell junctions, and allows more accurate assessment of the quantity and location of intracellular structures such as fine filaments, vesicles, and in the case of endothelial cells, organelles such as Weibel-Palade bodies. This technique is also useful in locating extracellular structures such as basement membrane produced by endothelial cells and assessing the orientation of this material to the cells. For example, in the case of endothelial cells, basement membrane appears to accumulate on the side of cells that face the surface of the culture dish (Fig. 5). This technique should also be useful in studying the effect of vasoactive amines such as angiotensin, on cells in culture, correlating observations made with scanning electron microscopy such as the interaction of platelets with cultured cells, and for immunohistochemical techniques at the ultrastructural level. Preparation of cells as pellets allows examination of relatively large quantities of cells in cross section. These techniques have proven useful in attempting to quantify the proportion of cells in any plane of section containing particular structures such as Weibel-Palade bodies and obtaining larger concentrations of extracellular products such as basement membrane.

In summary, observation by electron microscopy of cultured cells derived from blood vessels has served to establish the identity of cells grown in culture and has contributed to our understanding of their normal and abnormal biology. A variety of preparative techniques are available; the choice of the best techniques depends upon the goals of the experiment. Application of new techniques holds promise for new information about the biology of these cells and further insight into their role in vascular disease.

References

1. Fisher-Dzoga K, Jones RM, Vesselinovitch D and Wissler RW: (1973) Ultrastructural and immunohistochemical studies of primary cultures of aortic medial cells. Exp Mol Pathol, 18:162.

2. Gimbrone MA Jr, Cotran RS and Folkman J: (1974) Human vascular endothelial cells in culture. J Cell Biol, 60:673.

3. Hammerling U, Polliak A, Lampen N, Sabety M and deHarven E: (1975) Scanning electron microscopy of tobacco mosaic virus-labeled lymphocyte surface antigens. J Exp Med, 141:518.

4. Haudenschild CC, Cotran RS, Gimbrone MA Jr and Folkman J: (1975) Fine structure of vascular endothelium in culture. J Ultrastruc Res, 50:22.

5. Karnovsky MJ: (1965) A formaldehyde-glutaraldehyde fixative of high osmolality for use in electron microscopy. J Cell Biol, 27:137A.

6. Jaffe EA, Nachman RL, Becker CG and Minick CR: (1973) Culture of human endothelial cells derived from umbilical veins; Identification by morphologic and immunologic criteria. J Clin Invest, 52:2745.

7. Jaffe EA, Hoyer LW and Nachman RL: (1973) Synthesis of antihemophilic factor antigen by cultured human endothelial cells. J Clin Invest, 52:2757.

8. Koide R, Pollak OJ and Burns DA: (1963) Further observations of aortic cell cultures from untreated and cholesterol-fed rabbits. J Atheroscle Res, 3:32.

9. Molday RS, Dreyer WJ, Rembaum A and Yin SPS: (1974) Latex spheres as markers for studies of cell surface receptors by scanning electron microscopy. Nature, 249:81.

10. Maruyama Y: (1963) The human endothelial cell culture. Z Zelforsch Mikrosk Anat, 60:69.

11. Robertson AL Jr: (1967) Transport of plasma lipoproteins and ultrastructure of human arterial intimacytes in tissue culture, In Lipid Metabolism in Tissue Culture Cells, Rothblat and Kritchevsky, eds. Wistar Institute Press, Philadelphia. Symp Mono 6, 115-128.

12. Ross R: (1971) The smooth muscle cell. II. Growth of smooth muscle in culture and formation of elastic fibers. J Cell Biol, 50:172.

13. Ross R and Glomset JA: (1973) Atherosclerosis and the arterial smooth muscle cell. Science, 180:1332.

14. Ross, R, Glomset JA, Kariga B and Harker L: (1974) A platelet dependent serum factor that stimulates the proliferation of arterial smooth muscle cells in vitro. Proc Nat Acad Sci USA, 71:1207.

15. Rothblat GH, Buchko MK and Kritchevsky D: (1968) Cholesterol uptake by L51784 tissue culture cells: studies with delipidized serum. Biochem Biophys Acta, 164:327.

16. Slater PM and Sloan JM: (1975) The porcine endothelial cell in tissue culture. Atherosclerosis, 21:259.

17. Smith SC, Straut RG, Dunlop WR and Smith EC: (1965) Fatty acid composition of cultured aortic cells from white Carneau and Show Racer pigeons. J Atheroscle Res, 5:379.

(3)

TECHNIQUES FOR CULTURING ARTERIAL ENDOTHELIAL CELLS

Dr. Eva Csonka

2nd Department of Pathology of Semmelweis
Medical University
Budapest, Hungary

Lazzarini (3) was one of the first to make use of the methods of tissue culture in the study of the nature of cells of blood vessels. His pioneer work was continued and extended by Pollack and his group (5). Like any other new approach this also had been vigorously discussed until recently. At the present time a large amount of evidence has been made available from the works of Jaffe et al. (2), Lewis et al. (4), Gimbrone et al. (1) and Slater et al. (6). Thus at present it seems hardly possible to argue against the use of studying the morphology and biology of vessel-wall-cells grown *in vitro*.

We have reported on the successful establishment of pure mini-pig aortic endothelial cell cultures in 1973 at the European Congress of Pathology in Budapest. Our main methodical aim was to cause the least possible damage to the endothelial cells during their isolation. Therefore, we omitted treatment of the dissected aortic specimen with any type of enzyme and made use of the principle of obtaining "Häutchen" preparations. About 0.5 - 1.0 square mm pieces of the aorta were gently pressed with their endothelial faces against the glass onto the surface of a Petri-dish or a tissue culture bottle. Care was taken to ensure tight contact of cells and glass over the total surface and all excess fluid was carefully removed. Firm attachment was ensured by a 15 minutes incubation at 37°C without any medium added. The initial growth medium consisted of 5 parts of 5% lactalbumin hydrolysate, 10 parts of calf serum, 45 parts of HBS and 40 parts of Parker's No. 199 medium. After 2 to 3 days of incubation at 37°C in 5% CO_2 atmosphere the fluid was removed and the aortic fragments were stripped off. Attachment of smaller or greater groups of endothelial cells was easily observed by light microscopy. On further incubation the initial cell islands

Fig.1.
Electronmicrographs of endothelial cells in 5th passage
4 days old monolayer culture.

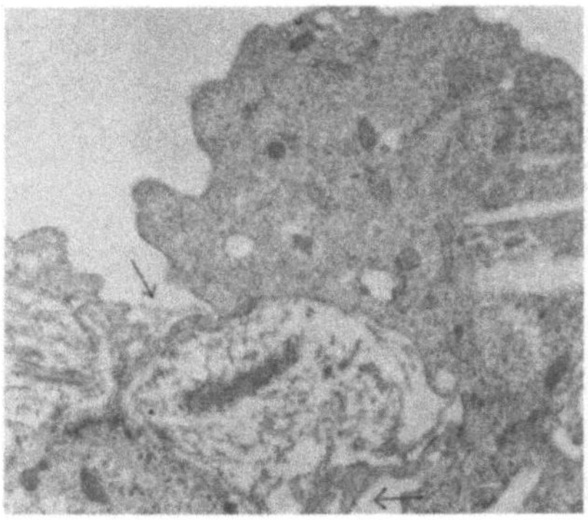

a.Organelle rich cells,
interendothelial junctions
/arrows/. x 12,000.

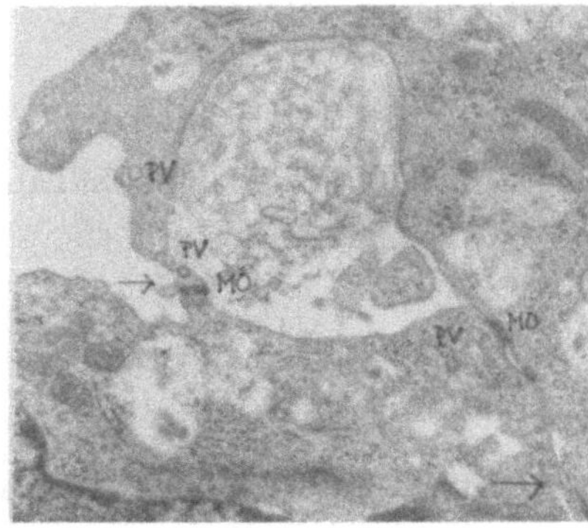

b.Endothelial junctions/arrow/
macula occludens/MO/,pino-
cytotic vesicles /PV/.x18,000.

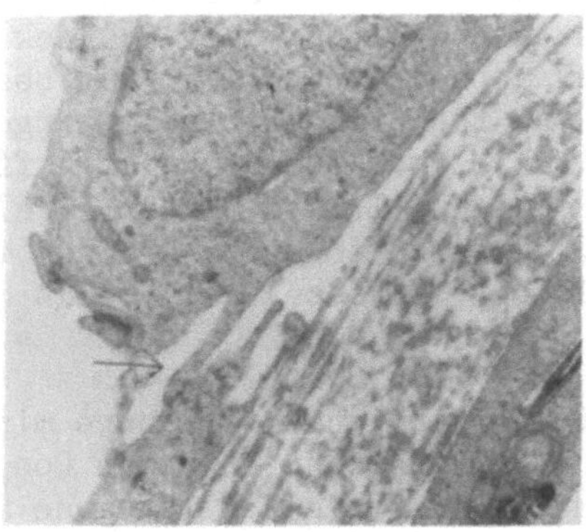

c.Interendothelial junction
/arrow/. x 15,000.

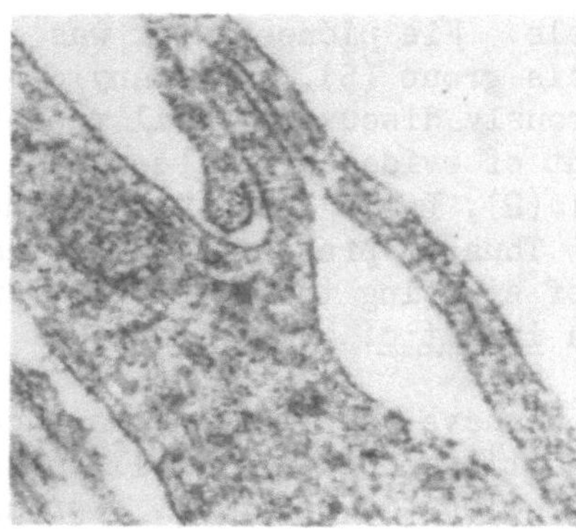

d.Interdigitation.
x 72,000.

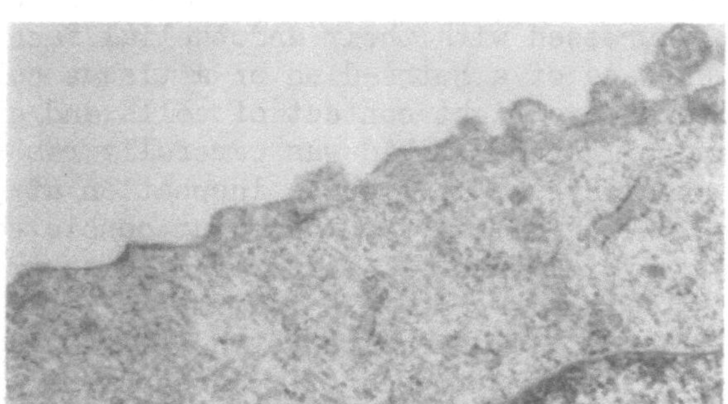

e.Undulant surface,microfilaments,free ribosomes.x36,000.

Fig.2.
Scanning electronmicrographs of endothel.cells in 4th passage,7 days old monolayer culture,at different magnifications.Cell borders,villous cell surface and intercellular junctions,at the lower magnification; crater like holes are seen.

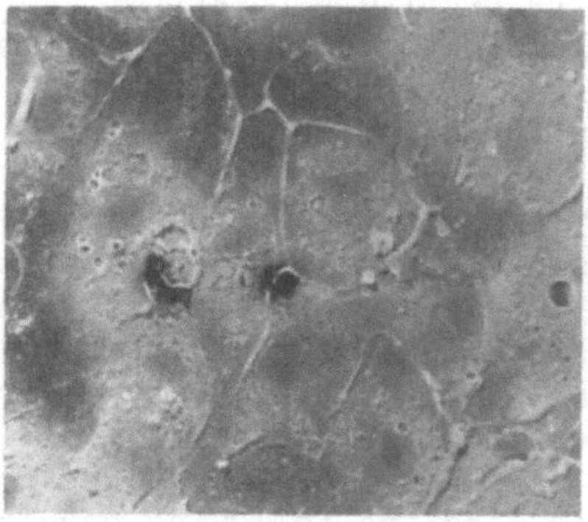

a. x 500

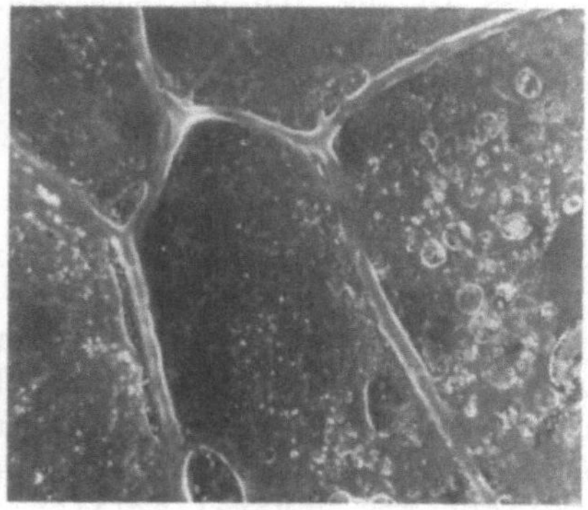

b. x 2000

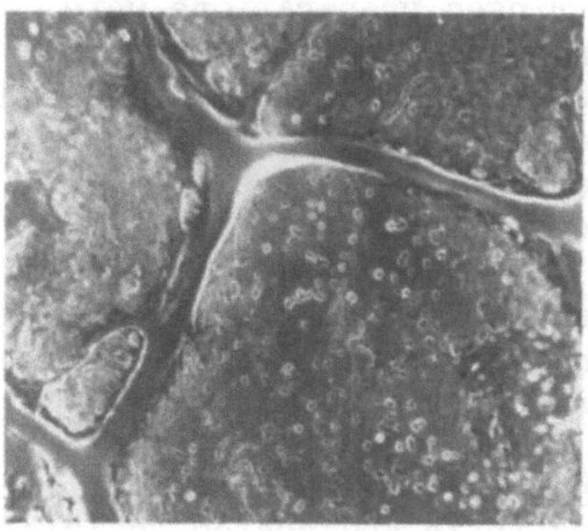

c. x 5000

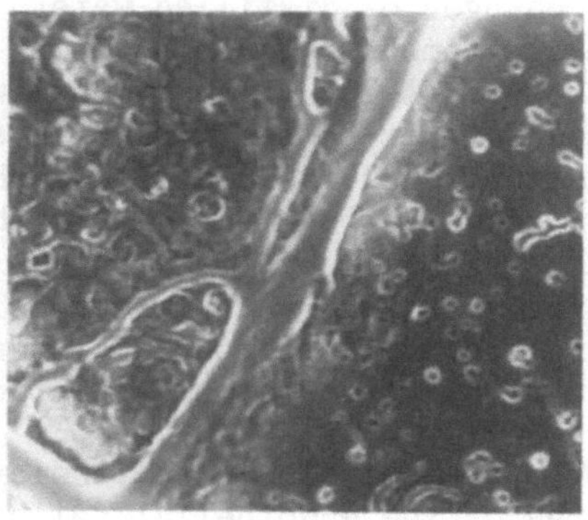

d. x 10,000

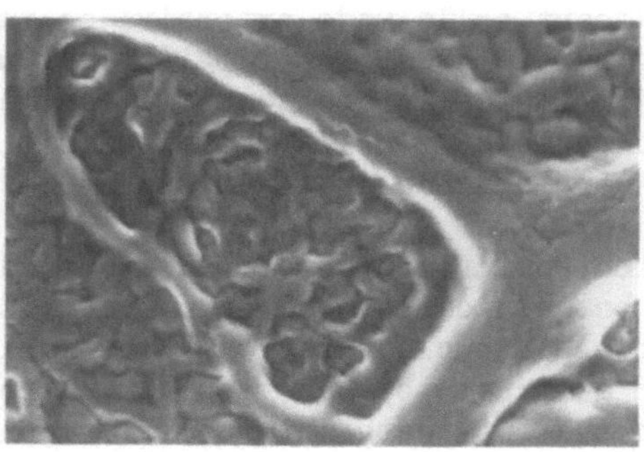

e. x 20,000

developed into a confluent monolayer in 7-21 days.

During the last 2.5 years several endothelium cultures were started and obtained. Out of them a single one maintained its diploid character through 18 passages.

At present we are in possession of 5 different endothelial cell lines in the 5th to 14th passage, respectively. Part of our cell lines has been preserved in fluid nitrogen. According to our experience viability is best preserved if cells are frozen in the presence of 5 percent dimethylsulfoxide.

The cells were identified by light and electronmicroscopy. For light microscopy the cells were grown on coverslips and stained with haematoxylin and eosin. The electronmicroscopic studies were made by both transmission and scanning techniques. The cells grew readily on araldit so they could be easily embedded and cut. For scanning electronmicroscopy coverslip cultures were prepared. Since fixation with glutaraldehyde and osmium tetroxide yielded poor preparations and several artifacts we applied the following process. Coverslip cultures were very briefly (1 second each) dipped into three changes of distilled water. The rinsed preparations were immediately mounted onto scanning stubs and dried in the vacuum evaporator. A 10^{-3} Hg mm vacuum was established in 10 minutes and reduced further to 10^{-6} Hg mm in another 10 minutes. As soon as the latter level was stabilized the preparations were coated with a 50 Å thick carbon and a 250 Å thick copper coat.

The light microscopic morphology shows flat polygonal cells growing orderly in compact islands. The very characteristic close and intricate intercellular contacts are conspicuous.

The transmission electronmicrographs showed the characteristic features of the endothelial cells, pinocytotic and coated vesicles, rough surfaced endoplasmic reticulum, free ribosomes. The cells were rich in mitochondria. Microtubules and microfilaments were also found. The adjacent cells made extensive contacts with one another forming marginal folds or interdigitating junctions. The membranes of adjoining cells are sometime separated by wide spaces. In older cultures some cells contained lipid inclusions, exhibiting amorphous or lamellar internal structures.

The scanning electromicrographs of cultured endothelial cells show close contacts between cells, and numerous pits on the cell surface, mostly in the perinuclear region. The nuclei show a flattened surface in contrast to the cytoplasmic area. At higher magnification the intricate intercellular junctions are evident.

Some preliminary studies have shown that cultured endothelial cells took up added exogenous cholesterol in contrast to various established laboratory cell lines including HeLa. Concentration dependent changes in scanning electronmicroscopic morphology of the cells were also observed within the range of 10^{-4} to 10^{-10} M final concentrations of added cholesterol.

REFERENCES

1. Gimbrone, M.A. Jr., Cotran, R.S., and Folkman, J., J. Cell Biol. 60: 673-684, 1974.
2. Jaffe, E.A., Nachman, R.L., Becker, C.G., and Minick, C.R., J. Clin. Invest. 52: 2745-2756, 1973.
3. Lazzarini, A.A. Jr., Studies of the effect of lipoid emulsion on arterial intimal cells in tissue culture in relation to atherosclerosis. Thesis, The Graduate School of Cornell University. 106 p., 1959.
4. Lewis, L.J., Hoak, J.C., Maca, R.D., Fry, G.L., Science 181: 453-454, 1973.
5. Pollak, O.J., Koide, R., and Burns, D.A., Fed. Proc. 21: 2765, 1962.
6. Slater, D.N., and Sloan, J.M., Atherosclerosis 21: 259-272, 1975.

(4)

CULTURED HUMAN FIBROBLASTS IN THE STUDY OF ATHEROSCLEROSIS

Joel Avigan

National Heart and Lung Institute
National Institutes of Health
Bethesda, Maryland, U.S.A.

Deranged lipoprotein metabolism as well as abnormally high rates of cholesterol synthesis have been implicated as likely causes of hypercholesterolemia and atherosclerosis. Metabolism and biological transport of specific serum lipoproteins and their lipid components and the environmental factors leading to the excessive intracellular accumulation of the latter have been studied in various mammalian cells, in culture, including the easily grown and maintained human skin fibroblasts. Progress in this field has been summarized and reviewed by a number of authors (e.g., 1,2,3).

In an earlier study, Bailey demonstrated that growing mouse fibroblasts adapted to a serum-free medium synthesized less cholesterol when serum lipids were added to the above medium (4). It was subsequently found in human skin fibroblasts by the present author that not only in growing cells but also in confluent stationary cell cultures, cholesterol synthesis readily responded to the presence or absence of lipids in the medium in a manner that could be interpreted as a negative feedback control of this process (5,6). The use of contact inhibited cultures allows the study of cell metabolism in a stable system similar to the one encountered in most tissues *in vivo*.

The incidence of human atherosclerosis is greatly increased in several types of hyperlipoproteinemia, most notably in familial hypercholesterolemia (or type II hyperlipoproteinemia) (7). Extensive studies by Goldstein, Brown and coworkers have importantly contributed to the understanding of normal metabolism of low density lipoprotein (LDL) and of the biochemical basis of the disease (see reference 8 for a recent summary). The above authors have shown that LDL is bound to the fibroblast surface by a high affinity receptor

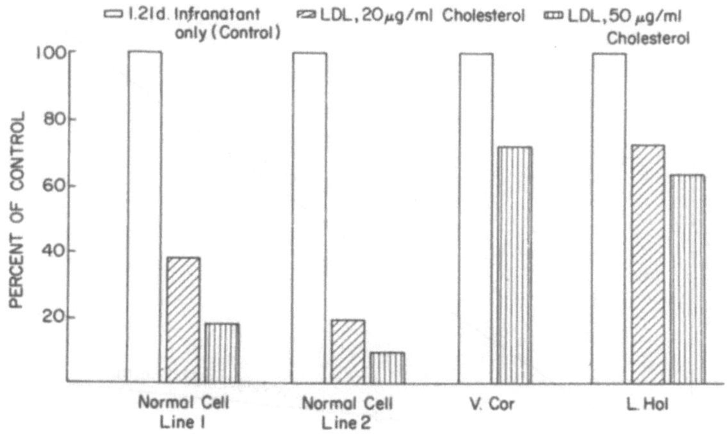

FIGURE 1. The effect of LDL on HMGCoA reductase in human skin fibroblasts. Cells were grown to confluency in 75 cm^2 Falcon flasks and in Eagle's minimum essential medium containing 10% calf serum. The cell cultures were then incubated for 24 hr in Eagle's medium without glucose, containing 5% human serum d 1.21 infranate. Finally the cells were incubated for 8 hr in a medium with 5% d 1.21 infranate without or with LDL at two concentrations, as indicated. The HMGCoA reductase was assayed as described elsewhere (9). V. Cor. and L. Hol. are cell lines derived from two patients with homozygous type II hyperlipoproteinemia that were studied at the N.I.H.

and that such binding precedes specific uptake of LDL and its breakdown. These processes affect the cellular cholesterol metabolism by depressing the enzyme hydroxymethyl coenzyme A reductase (HMGCoA reductase), which is controlling cholesterol synthesis in mammalian tissues, and by activating the esterification rate of free cholesterol. It has been further shown that fibroblasts from patients with a homozygous form of familial hypercholesterolemia do not bind LDL through the high affinity mechanism and consequently are not subject to the above metabolic effects.

In our studies on fibroblasts from several patients with a homozygous form of type II hyperlipoproteinemia, a diminished but significant feedback inhibition of cholesterol synthesis and of HMGCoA reductase has been found (9). It is shown in Fig. 1 that following an incubation with LDL (50 μg/ml of cholesterol), the enzyme was inhibited in the two normal cell lines by 82 and 91%, while in the two mutant cell lines the inhibition was 19 and 37%. Khachadurian and Kawahara (10) and Breslow *et al.* (11) have also

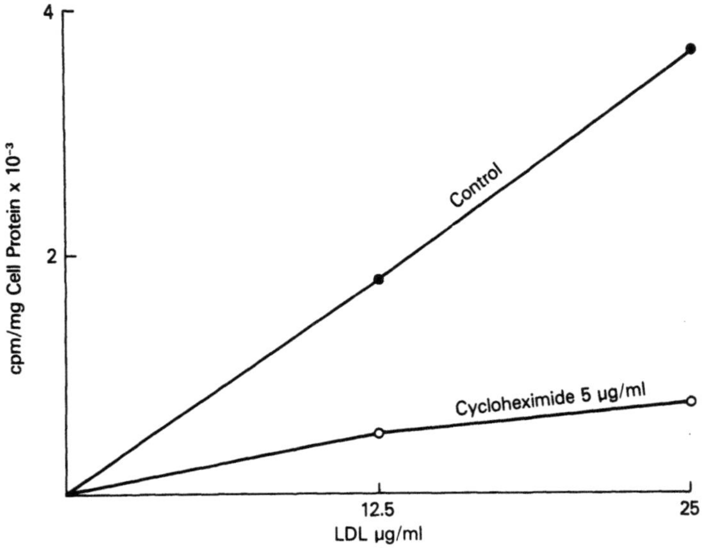

FIGURE 2. The effect of cycloheximide on LDL binding. Normal skin fibroblasts were grown to confluency in 100 mm petri dishes in Eagle's minimum essential medium containing 10% calf serum and were then incubated for 24 hr in Eagle's medium containing 5% solvent extracted serum (6) with or without cycloheximide. Finally the cells were incubated at 4° for 3 hr with Eagle's medium containing 5% solvent extracted serum and ^{125}I-LDL at two concentrations. The cells were washed exhaustively (13) and the bound radioactivity was assayed.

reported similar inhibitory effects in type II homozygous cell lines. Goldstein *et al.* (12) have recently suggested the existence of two different mutations affecting LDL binding, one producing "receptor negative" and the other "receptor defective" cells. There remains a likely possibility that a variety of mutations will eventually be found to be correlated with different degrees of abnormalities of cholesterol metabolism.

The role of the specific receptor of LDL in the regulation of cholesterol synthesis and esterification suggests the potential importance of the formation and metabolic turnover of the receptor molecule itself. Binding of LDL to normal human fibroblasts was greatly reduced following an overnight incubation with cycloheximide (Fig. 2). Furthermore, cells inhibited by cycloheximide recovered slowly the original binding capacity after removal of the inhibitor (Fig. 3). These data suggest that the maintenance of

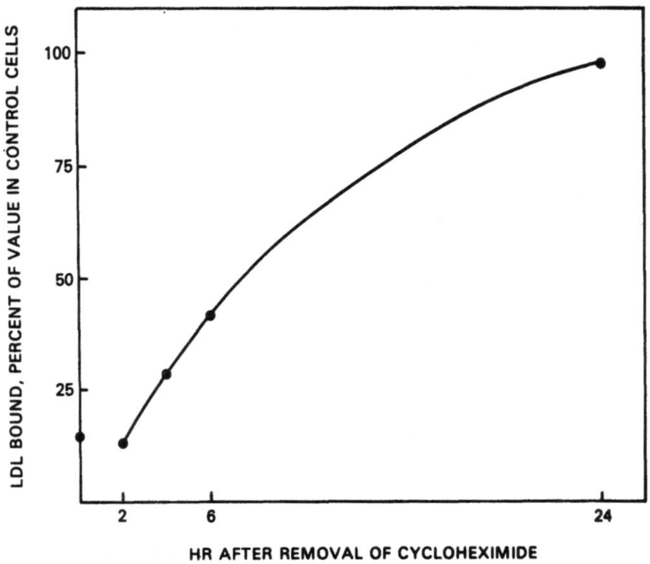

FIGURE 3. Recovery of LDL binding capacity after removal of cycloheximide. Normal skin fibroblasts were grown and incubated with a medium containing cycloheximide, 5 μg/ml as for Fig. 2. Medium was then replaced with one of the same composition, but without cycloheximide, and after incubation of the cells for the indicated times the binding of ^{125}I-LDL was assayed.

binding sites depends on uninterrupted protein synthesis. Changes in concentration of the receptor may conceivably represent a distinct mechanism for the regulation of LDL metabolism and of cholesterol synthesis.

Since the triglyceride-rich very low density lipoproteins (VLDL) have an affinity for the same receptor as LDL (13), receptor defect or deficiency could possibly produce abnormalities in triglyceride metabolism in some of the affected cell lines. The results in Fig. 4 showing considerably lower uptake of labeled triglycerides from VLDL by type II homozygous cells than by normal fibroblasts suggest such a possibility.

In spite of its metabolic limitations, the fibroblast cell has been successfully used as a model system in the study of LDL transport and degradation and of lipid synthesis, especially that

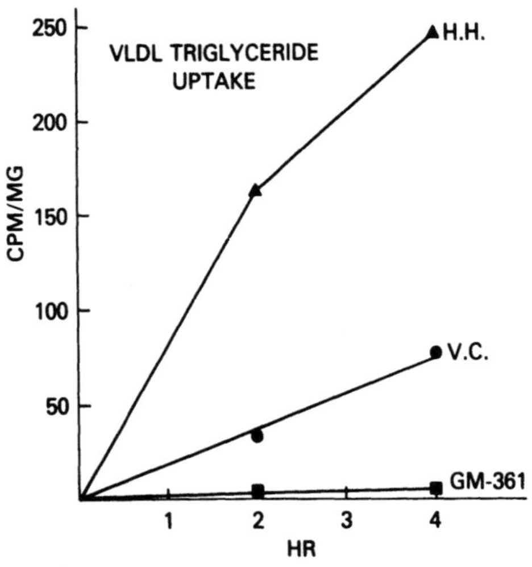

FIGURE 4. Uptake of 1-^{14}C-tripalmitin from VLDL by skin fibroblasts. Cells were grown as for Fig. 1 and incubated for 24 hr in Eagle's medium containing 5% solvent extracted serum. 1-^{14}C-tripalmitin, 28 mC/mmole, was purified by TLC and dissolved in a small volume of acetone. The above solution was injected into a VLDL solution (1 mg protein/ml) dialyzed against saline and filtered through an 0.2 μ filter. Cell cultures grown on petri dishes were incubated for the indicated time periods with 5 ml Eagle's medium containing 0.2% serum albumin and 20 μg/ml VLDL containing 8000 cpm of 1-^{14}C-tripalmitin. Cells were washed, solvent extracted and the radioactivity in the extract was assayed. Data presented per mg cell protein. H.H. - normal cell line; V.C. - cells from a homozygous type II patient studied at the N.I.H.; GM-361 - cells from a homozygous type II patient previously studied by Goldstein, Brown, and coworkers.

of cholesterol which helped to promote the understanding of the biochemical basis of familial hypercholesterolemia. It is to be expected that numerous other metabolic problems important in the study of atherosclerosis will also be approached in the future in this experimental system.

ACKNOWLEDGEMENT. The author thanks Dr. Jan L. Breslow, Dr. Howard R. Sloan, Dr. Arthur E. Greene and the Institute for Medical Research, Camden, N.J. for the fibroblast cell lines used in this study.

REFERENCES

1. Rothblat, G.H. (1972) In Growth, Nutrition and Metabolism of Cells in Culture, Eds. G. H. Rothblat and V. J. Cristofalo, Academic Press, New York, vol. 1, p 297.

2. Bailey, J. M. (1973) In Atherosclerosis: Initiating Factors, Ciba Foundation Symposium 12 (new series), Elsevier, Amsterdam, p 63.

3. Howard, B. V., and Howard, W. J. (1974) Adv. Lipid Res. 12: 51.

4. Bailey, J. M. (1966) Biochim. Biophys. Acta 125: 226.

5. Avigan, J., Williams, C. D., and Blass, J. P. (1970) Biochim. Biophys. Acta 218: 381.

6. Williams, C. D., and Avigan, J. (1972) Biochim. Biophys. Acta 260: 413.

7. Fredrickson, D. S., and Levy, R. I. (1972) In Metabolic Basis of Inherited Disease, Eds. Stanbury, J. B., and Fredrickson, D. S., McGraw-Hill, New York, p 545.

8. Brown, M. S., and Goldstein, J. L. (1975) Adv. Intern. Med. 20: 273.

9. Avigan, J., Bhathena, S. J., and Schreiner, M. E. (1975) J. Lipid Res. 16: 151.

10. Khachadurian, A. K., and Kawahara, F. S. (1974) J. Lab. Clin. Med. 83: 7.

11. Breslow, J. L., Lux, S. E., Spaulding, D. R., and Sloan, H. R. (1974) Ped. Res. 8: 387A.

12. Goldstein, J. L., Dana, S. E., Brunschede, G. Y., and Brown, M. S. (1975) Proc. Nat. Acad. Sci. USA 72: 1092.

13. Brown, M. S., and Goldstein, J. L. (1974) Proc. Nat. Acad. Sci. USA 71: 788.

(5)

CULTURED HUMAN ENDOTHELIAL CELLS AND ATHEROSCLEROSIS

L.J. Lewis, M.J. Welsh and J.C. Hoak

University of Iowa College of Medicine

Iowa City, Iowa, U.S.A.

Until recently our knowledge of the endothelium and its cellular components has been incomplete. However, with present day methods for the culture and replication of these important cells, not only has our knowledge increased but the relationship to atherosclerosis is becoming more apparent[1].

For the major portion of this presentation, we shall limit ourselves to the discussion of the endocytic action of human endothelial cells isolated from umbilical veins. Blumenthal[2] contends that all the hypotheses concerning atherosclerosis are closely and inescapably concerned with the reactions of the endothelium. This relationship is due to endothelial permeability, its endocytic responses to large molecules and its role in microthrombosis and healing. Although it has been demonstrated that blood cells are able to migrate across the endothelial barrier and that this migration may be due to an intracellular process, the significance of endothelial endocytosis in the protection of the organism or in the pathogenesis of disease is not entirely clear. The data presented here may offer some insight concerning how lipids can be exchanged between the blood and the intima. It would seem reasonable that this interchange must be through the endothelium or a defect in the cell itself. It would also seem within reason to consider the transport of macromolecules through the spaces between these cells.

Ideally, the study of endocytosis in cell cultures is by the use of microorganisms. The bacterial organisms utilized in this study were *S. Aureus*, *E. Coli* and *N Gonnorrhea*. In order that an *in vivo* environment would be simulated, the bacteria were suspended in physiological saline and opsonized with fresh human serum. A representative of both DNA and RNA viruses was included by the use of influenza A and vaccinia viruses. Both bacterial and viral agents were inoculated into the endothelial cell culture and incubated at 37°C for varying periods of time. Although the preparations showed the organisms to be both extracellular as well as intracellular, it was difficult to determine whether those appearing to be intracellular might only be adhering to the cell surface. To evaluate this possibility, after incubation of the cells with bacteria, the fluorescent antibiotic tetracycline was added to the cultures and examined by phase and fluorescent microscopy (Fig. 1). The vacuolar membrane surrounding the phagocytized bacteria was relatively impermeable to tetracycline in the intact cell. This impermeability of the phagocytic vacuole to tetracycline prevented its uptake by those bacteria located within the vacuoles. Thus, the intracellular bacteria did not fluoresce and were inapparent. If the endothelial cells were dried or lyzed after the incubation period was completed, the vacuolar membrane was disrupted and the tetracycline was able to gain access to any bacteria that were intracelluar (Fig. 2).

In order to delineate extracelluar bacteria and the cell surface by transmission electron microscopy, it was necessary to coat them with an electron dense material. For this, we added the dye ruthenium red to the osmium tetroxide fixative. The dye does not penetrate to the interior of the cell but coats the extraneous glycocalyx layer that is associated with the outer layer of the plasma membrane.

Two bacterial particles which were completely intracellular as demonstrated by the inability of the ruthenium red to penetrate the cellular membrane can be seen in Fig. 3. Note the bacterial surface is not coated with the dye. When the bacteria were attached to the endothelial cell membrane and were not intracellular, then both cell and bacterial surfaces were coated with the dye (Fig. 4).

What were the fates of the phagocytized bacteria and the endothelial cells after they had been involved in phagocytosis? When bacterial cultures were incubated in culture medium containing cells and in culture medium devoid of cells, the following results were observed when colony counts were made 1-3 hours post-incubation to determine the number of viable cells. The colony counts from the supernatant fluid of the endothelial cell containing fluid were much lower than those from the media devoid of cells due to the phagocytosis of the bacteria. Those cells which had phagocytized bacteria were then scraped from the slide to which they were attached into physiological saline and a colony count was performed on that fluid. A comparison of the number of bacteria

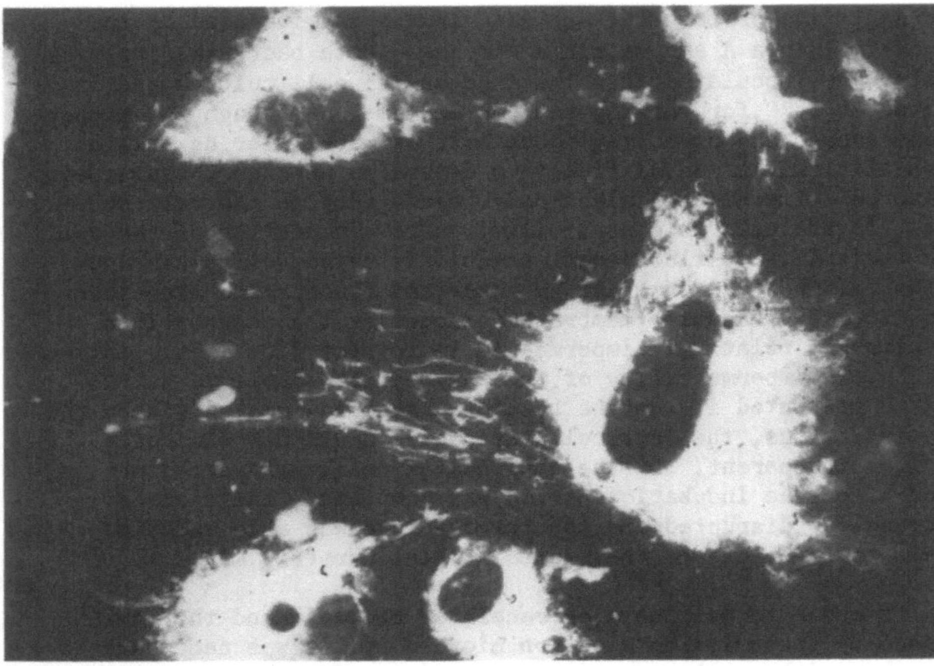

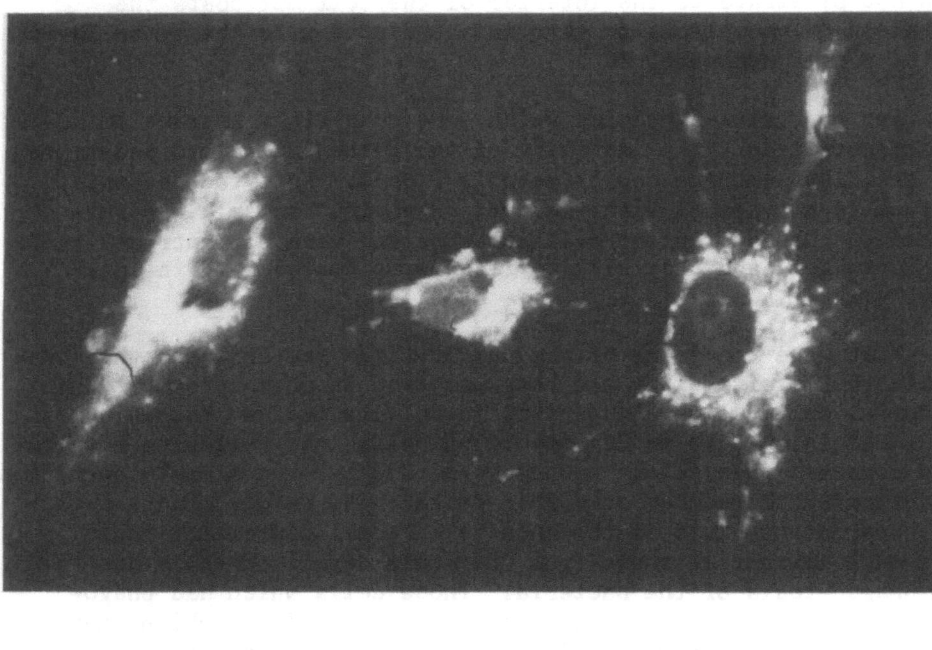

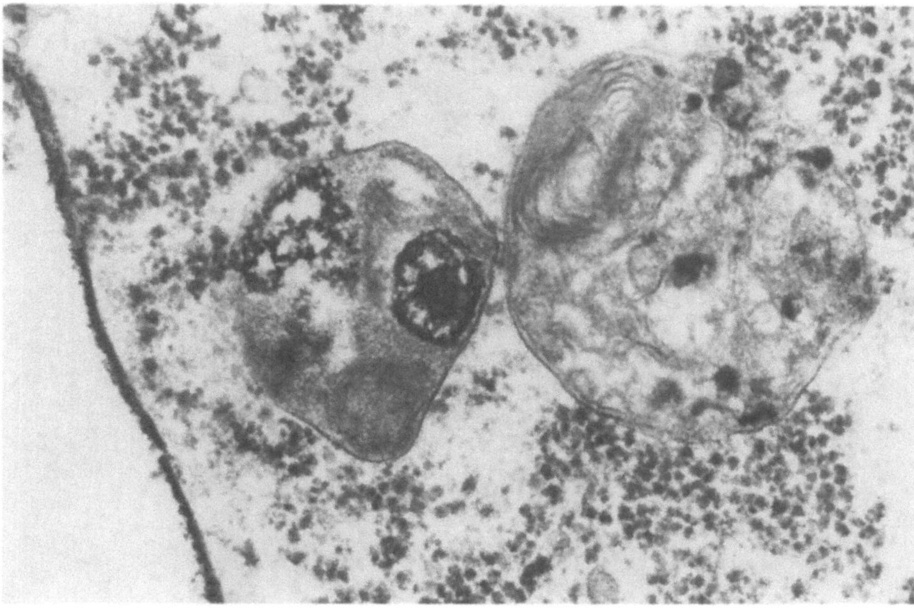

Fig. 3; x79,880

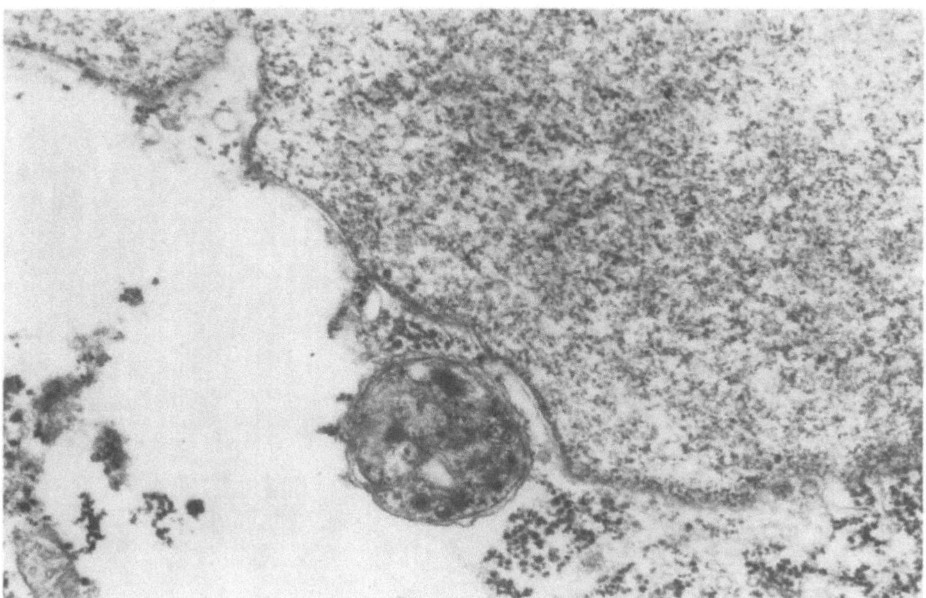

Fig. 4; x41,000

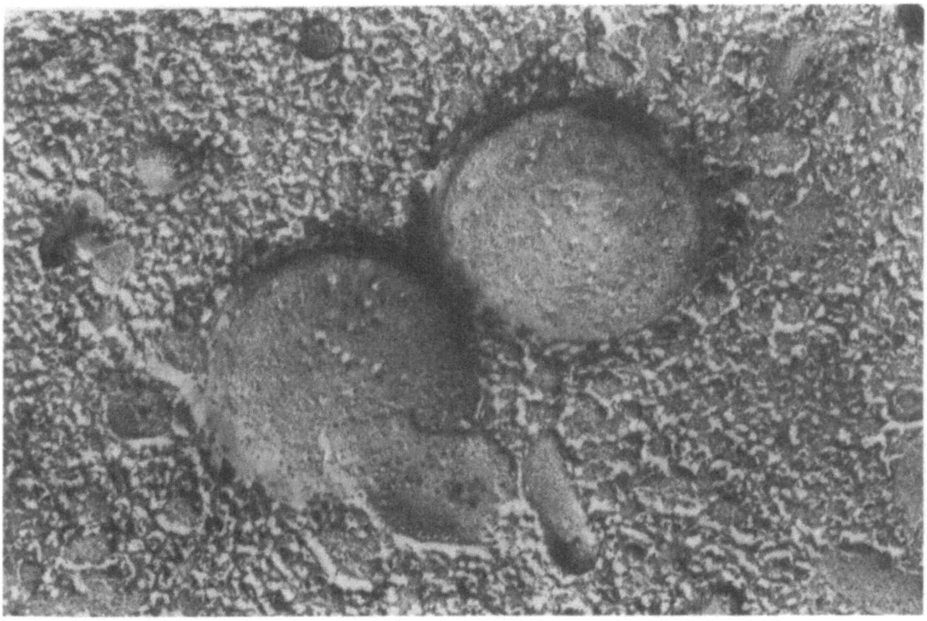

Fig. 5; x120,840

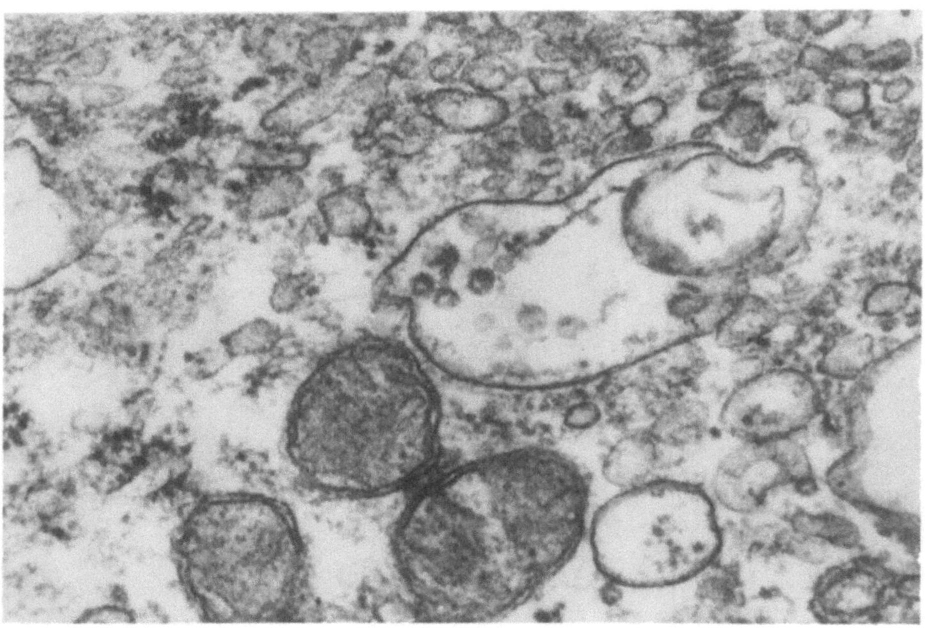

Fig.6; x120,600

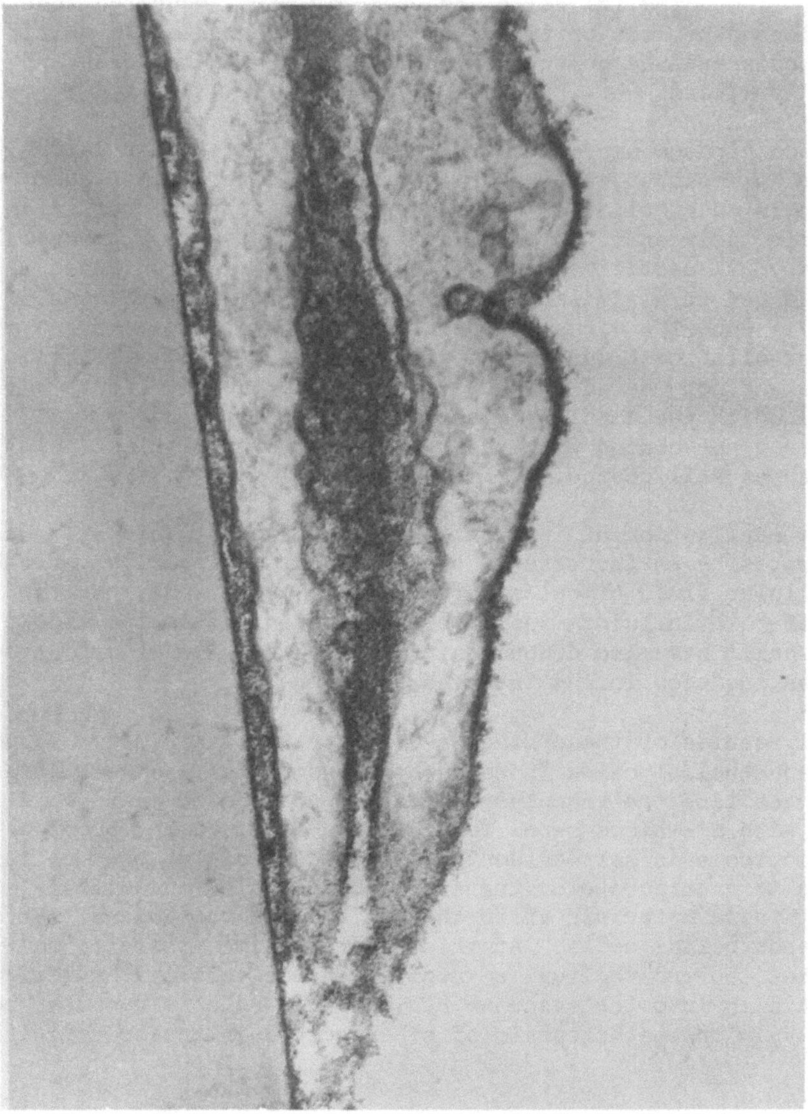

Fig. 7; x120,600

remaining viable after having been phagocytized and the total number of bacteria taken up indicated that many bacteria lost their viability after phagocytosis by the endothelial cells. However, if endothelial cells and bacteria were incubated together for prolonged periods of time, the bacteria continued to multiply in the media and the cultures were overgorwn with bacteria and eventually killed.

Since viruses can only survive and replicate in an intracellular environment, it was of interest to determine whether cultured human endothelial cells would phagocytize viral particles and permit their entry into the cellular cytoplasm. Extracellular vaccinia viral particles were coated with the electron dense ruthenium red in a similar manner as the bacterial particles (Fig. 5). Once the virus had been phagocytosed, the membrane of the endothelial cell was coated with the dye but the intracellular particle was not coated (Fig. 6). A phagocytosed influenza virus (Fig. 7) which was completely enclosed within its phagocytic vacuole was not coated with the dye while the endothelial cell membrane was well coated.

The replication of influenza virus in endothelial cells was demonstrated by an increase in the hemagglutination titer of the extracellular fluid of cells infected with this virus. Multiplication of both influenza and vaccinia viruses within the endothelial cells was also demonstrated by the increase of cytopathology which was produced in the infected cells.

The results of these studies demonstrate the ability of human venous endothelial cells in culture to endocytize. Since these cells which line the vascular system are so located as to come in contact with all blood-borne foreign materials, their opportunity for endocytosis is self-evident. Palade[3] speculated that cells are able to incorporate or transfer substances by endocytosis and that these materials enter the vesicles on the luminal surface of the endothelial cells. At this point in time, there is no doubt that the endothelium is involved in the exchange of fluid and particles into the vascular bed, and its role in vascular permeability in the pathogenesis of atherosclerosis appears significant.

REFERENCES

1. Lewis, L.J., et al.: Science 181:453-454, 1973.

2. Blumenthal, H.T.: Cowdry's Atherosclerosis. Charles C. Thomas, p. 91, 1967.

3. Palade, G.E.: Circulation 24:368, 1961.

(6)

DISCUSSION (TISSUE CULTURE I)

Dr. Pollak, U.S.A. - Is the pinocytotic ability of endothelial cells confined to young cells or does this ability persist in older cultures?

Dr. Lewis, U.S.A. - We have observed pinocytosis in endothelial cells ranging from primary to seventh passage cultures.

Dr. Robertson, U.S.A. - In regard to some of the points that have been made in the presentations concerning the care that should be taken in the interpretation of results, we are currently studying the effect of topographical differences on the cells obtained from the aorta. Our data would suggest that in the human aorta there are regional differences in the endothelial cells both in the dynamics of their response to different concentrations of vasoactive agents and in generation time and turnover rates. Distinct differences seem to exist between endothelial cells taken from different regions of the same aortic segment.

Dr. Rothblat, U.S.A. - I think it would be fruitful for the participants to discuss their views on the possibility of clonal variation in the cells that grow out from explants. For example, in aortic medial cell cultures may only a small population of the cells have the ability to accumulate esterified cholesterol, whereas the majority of the population does not? An example of mixed populations might also be found in the studies that Dr. Avigan has reported today. Intermediate levels of response of HMG-CoA reductase activity are observed in the familial hypercholesteremic fibroblasts exposed to LDL. Could this intermediate response be a reflection of a mixed population of fibroblasts, some of which have a full complement of LDL receptors while others are completely lacking receptors? The extent of the response would then be a function of the relative proportion of two populations in such a mixed culture.

Dr. Federoff, Canada - This is a complex problem. In any culture one can encounter tremendous cell to cell variation. In many experiments one studies the entire population and obtains the average figures for the individual cells in that population. We have recently been studying the development of neurons and although these neurons have morphologically appeared very normal when we investigate them metabolically we encounter marked variation. In any single culture neurons which may have identical morphological characteristics exhibit markedly different biochemical reactions.

Dr. Benditt, U.S.A. - One of the fundamental questions of cell culture is whether cells breed true. There has been a great deal of discussion in the atherosclerosis literature concerning multi-potential cells or cells that change from one type to another. Cells in culture breed true. In our laboratory the endothelial cells that we have carried through nine generations have maintained their endothelial characteristics. In addition, the smooth muscle cells in culture also maintain their smooth muscle properties. However, there can be variations within a population. Dr. George Martin in our laboratory has cloned fibroblasts and then measured the longevity of each cell. He has observed distinct differences among the individual cells. It seems to be entirely possible that there is a great deal of heterogeneity in some cultures and it whould be possible to design experiments to detect the heterogeneity of a particular factor under examination.

Dr. Poole, England - We have been growing arterial smooth muscle cells from rabbit aorta for about three years. We have observed, as have others, that after about two or three months most cultures will exhibit a gradual decrease in the rate of multiplication with the culture eventually dying. However, we obtained one culture of rabbit aortic smooth muscle cells that was growing extremely well after 11 months in culture. A karyological analysis of these cells revealed distinct differences in the chromosome pattern when compared to those obtained from normal cells. We have also observed a similar phenomenon in fibroblasts obtained from the aorta. After a number of months in culture, cell growth temporarily slowed and after this period a new phase of rapid cell growth was observed. These cultures also exhibit chromosome abnormalities.

Dr. Rothblat, U.S.A. - I would like to ask the Drs. Stein why they have chosen approximately the seventh passage as the cutoff for the use of their smooth muscle cells?

Dr. Olga Stein, Israel - In our earlier studies we found we obtained reproducible results with material up to passage seven. This was the passage level that we had achieved at the time we published our results.

Dr. Daoud, U.S.A. - Do endothelial cells synthesize anything else other than basement membrane? Do they make collagen and elastic tissue?

Dr. Becker, U.S.A. - They make material that seems different from basement membrane material. We don't see pure collagen.

Dr. Rothblat, U.S.A. - Is there a polarity to endothelial cells? Is there a consistent top and bottom when you have them in culture?

Dr. Minick, U.S.A. - With regard to basement membrane formation there certainly seems to be a definite polarity. Basement membrane formation is always on the bottom side.

Dr. Pollak, U.S.A. - Would someone comment on the problems involved in growing cells from atherosclerotic tissues?

Dr. Lewis, U.S.A. - We have tried it and it is very difficult to get cells to grow.

Dr. Benditt, U.S.A. - We have cultured the plaque area and the area directly adjacent to it. We found that although cells grow out, they grow with great difficulty. Cells from the plaque have a finite life-span having the same life-span, or slightly less, than the cells that come from the adjacent uninvolved area. In culture you can't tell them apart by their morphology. Part of the difficulty of growing cells from the plaque is that there are far fewer cells in this material than in normal aorta.

Dr. Fisher-Dzoga, U.S.A. - We have had the same experience in that it is more difficult to establish cultures from the atherosclerotic material than from normal aorta. It would seem that they grow slower. There are fewer explants that get outgrowth and it takes longer to establish a culture.

Dr. Pollak, U.S.A. - Perhaps Dr. Avigan would comment on the nature of the LDL binding sites on the fibroblasts.

Dr. Avigan, U.S.A. - At the moment very little is specifically known about the composition of the specific LDL binding sites. From some recent studies that we have conducted, we have found the binding is affected by the ionic concentration. Hypertonic salt concentrations will weaken the specific binding.

Dr. Jagannathan, U.S.A. - Dr. Minick, do you find lysosomes in endothelial cells?

Dr. Minick, U.S.A. - There are structures like lysosomes in these cells. We have not, as yet, done any histochemical or biochemical studies.

CHAPTER 12
CONNECTIVE TISSUES IN ATHEROSCLEROTIC LESIONS

(1)

INTRODUCTION

Robert H. More, M.D.

Institute of Pathology, McGill University

Montreal, P.Q., Canada

Without encroaching on anything the invited speakers have to say, I wish to take this opportunity to make a few remarks. The organizing committee must have considered the role of connective tissue in atherosclerosis as a currently important topic. This is a significant change from views that dominated very active groups investigating this disease in the late 1950's. For instnace, I recall demonstrating at an international meeting that the material having an acidophilic property in an H & E stain of a section of atherosclerotic lesion was protein and not lipid. At the same time the abundance of this material and the relative absence of lipid was emphasized. In the discussion, our revered late colleague, Dr. Russell Holman, jumped to his feet and in his own inimitable style said "No fat, no atherosclerosis". In retrospect he may be right because it would be misleading to suggest that lipid is not a major component of the atherosclerotic lesion. However, times do change and if he were still with us he might paraphrase his previous remarks with the comment, "No connective tissue, no serious disease". This I believe may reflect the current opinion and is a very major shift from the thinking of the past few decades. The importance of connective tissues in the clinically serious lesion may be illustrated in the next few slides. In the classical atherosclerotic plaque the atheroma forms a prominent component of the lesion but it is overlain with a connective tissue plaque producing a very small eccentric lumen. However, some equally advanced lesions have no visibly demonstrable lipid and histologically are composed of connective tissues. Biochemical studies have shown that such lesions still contain a significant amount of lipid, but this is clearly not present in a visibly demonstrable form, and in morphologic terms this lesion is almost totally formed by various components of connective tissues. Many leading investigators of atherosclerosis now realize that much of the advanced atherosclerosis of man is represented by this type of lesion which had previously been ignored in many pathogenic studies of this disease. That connective tissue is a very major component of advanced atherosclerosis in general is no longer in dispute. However, we know very little about the mechanisms responsible for this major accumulation of connective tissue. This panel has brought together the foremost experts in the field of metabolism of connective tissue. Presumably, the organizers of the symposium believe that if we understand the normal production of connective tissue this may lead to an understanding of those factors that contribute to the production of an abnormal quantity of connective tissue in disease and this information may provide a basis for controlling the production of connective tissue in the atherosclerotic lesion.

(2)

SECRETION AND ASSEMBLY OF COLLAGEN - PRESENT STATUS

Jürgen Rauterberg

Institut für Arterioskleroseforschung

44 Münster, Westring 3 , W.-Germany

INTRODUCTION

Collagen and elastin are the essential structural proteins of the arterial wall; the first one is being responsible for tensile strength, the other one for elasticity.

Our knowledge on collagen - its structure and biosynthesis - has remarkably increased during the last years; it has become obvious that its structure is more variable and its synthesis a more complex process than it had been imagined only few years ago.

Figure 1 shows a scheme of collagen structure on several structural levels : (For reviews see Kühn, 1969 ; Traub and Piez, 1971)

Within the poly-peptide chains glycine occupies each third position - often followed by proline and then hydroxyproline. Each chain is wound into a left-handed helix, three of them are linked together in a right-handed supercoiled triple helix. The resulting rod-like molecule is 300 nm in length and 0,15 nm in diameter. Only short regions at both ends do not belong to the triple-helical structure; they play an important role in intermolecular crosslinking.

The collagen fibril is formed by side to side association of molecules with a stagger of 66,8 nm. All molecules are arranged in the same direction. This stagger comprises more than a fifth and less than a quarter of the molecule; therefore there remains a gap of roughly 30 nm between tail and head

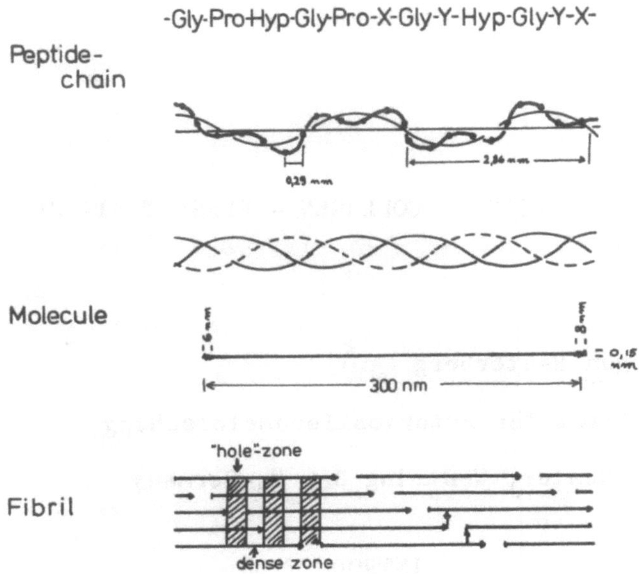

Figure 1: Scheme of collagen structure

of molecules laying in a row. Due to this gap there is a periodic change of dense and less dense periods along the fibril which can be visualized in the electron microscope as light and dark bands after applying the negative staining technique.

The fibril is the functional unit of collagen in the tissue and fibril formation and stabilization by crosslinks marks the final point in biosynthesis of collagen.

It is a typical feature of this protein that the way from chain synthesis to the final product comprises a lot of additional steps. This complexity of the biosynthetic way is related to one of the most essential properties of collagen : its enormous variability and adaptability to numerous possibilities for regulation which are able to influence the properties of the final product.

INTRACELLULAR BIOSYNTHETIC STEPS

Figure 2 comprises the intracellular steps. The synthesis of polypeptide chains takes place at the ribosomes attached to the membranes of the endoplasmatic reticulum; it follows the common rules of protein biosynthesis.

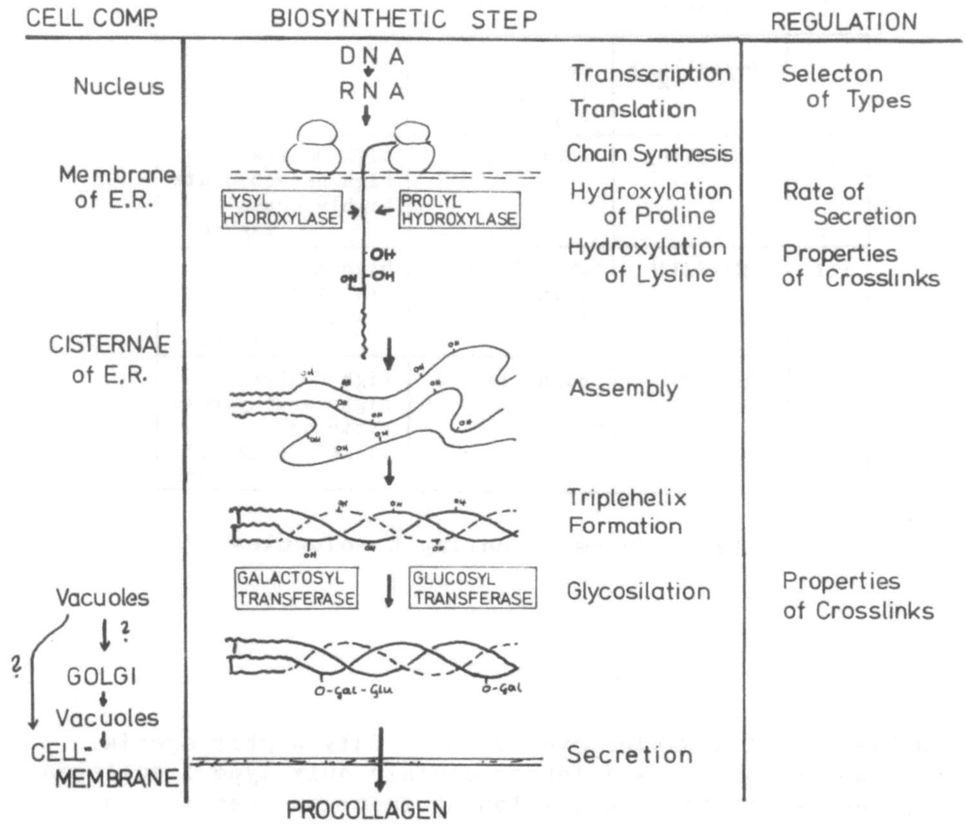

Figure 2: Intracellular steps in collagen biosynthesis

It has been known for a few years only that gene expression is an important factor in regulating the properties of the final product. Each cell contains the genetic information for the polypeptide chains of several types of collagen.

Table 1 comprises the types of collagen which are known so far and describes their chain composition. Only the type I molecule is composed of different polypeptide chains : 2 α1 and 1 α2 chain. The molecules of all other types are composed of three identical chains.

Type I and III are the most widespread distributed types of collagen in mammals and birds; they mostly occur together, type III minor in quantity to type I. (Epstein, 1974 ; Chung

Type	Chain Composition	Tissue	Characteristics
I	$[\alpha 1(I)]_2 \alpha 2$	bone tendon skin	
II	$[\alpha 1(II)]_3$	cartilage	high HO-lys high carbohydrate highly cross-linked
III	$[\alpha 1(III)]_3$	arterial wall skin leiomyoma	high Hyp cysteine highly cross-linked
IV	$[\alpha 1(IV)]_3$	basal lamina	high HO-lys high carbohydrate cysteine linked to globular protein

Table 1: Types of collagen molecules

and Miller, 1974 ; Rauterberg, 1975). Only highly specialized tissues as bone and tendon contain only type I collagen. All tissues which have an enveloping function seem to contain type III collagen; among them the arterial wall has the highest amount of type III, about 40 % of total collagen (Rauterberg, 1975).

Type II collagen is the specific cartilage collagen. Cartilage-bone transition is accompanied by a complete change from type II to type I collagen (For review see Miller, 1973).

The amino acid sequences of polypeptide chains of collagen types are homologous (Butler et al.,1974 ; Fietzek and Rauterberg, 1975) - that means that they have been developed from an unique ancestor chain during evolution.

Figure 3 shows a short piece of sequence of $\alpha 1$ chain from type I, II and III, taken from the central region of the chains.

It should be pointed out that in spite of various exchanges there are only few exchanges which alter the distribution of charges along the chain.

	1 10
α1(I) CB 3	Gly-Phe-Hyp-Gly-Pro-Lys-Gly-Ala-Ala-Gly-Glu-Hyp-Gly-Lys-Ala-Gly-Glu-Arg
α1(II) CB 8	Gly-Phe-Hyp-Gly-Pro-Hyl-Gly-Ala-Asn-Gly-Glu-Hyp-Gly-Lys-Ala-Gly-Glu-Hyl
α1(III)CB 4	Gly-Phe-Hyp-Gly-Pro-Lys-Gly-Asn-Asp-Gly-Ala-Hyp-Gly-Lys-Asn-Gly-Glu-Arg
	20 30
I	-Gly-Val-Hyp-Gly-Pro-Hyp-Gly-Ala-Val-Gly-Pro-Ala-Gly-Lys-Asp-Gly-Glu
II	-Gly-Leu-Hyp-Gly-Ala-Hyp-Gly-Leu-Arg-Gly-Leu-Hyp-Gly-Lys-Asp-Gly-Glu
III	-Gly-Gly-Hyp-Gly-Gly-Hyp-Gly-Pro-Gln-Gly-Pro-Ala-Gly-Lys-Asn-Gly-Glu

Figure 3: Amino acid sequences of homologous regions of α1 type I, II and III

This charge pattern is expressed to a certain degree in the electron microscopic appearance of long spacing segments - arteficial aggregates of molecules ordered exactly parallel and in register. Figure 4 shows the comparison of segments of type I and type III collagen. Except of a few characteristic differences the cross striation patterns are very similar (Rauterberg and v. Bassewitz, 1975). Probably the charge pattern must be an important prerequisite for the function of collagen and is kept very constant during evolution.

Type I

Type III

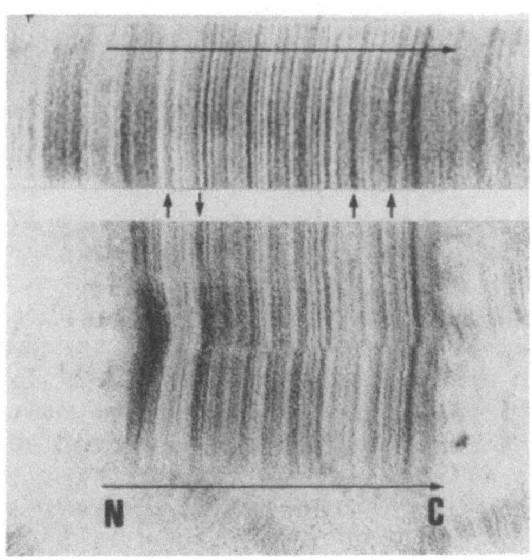

Figure 4: Long spacing segments of type I and type III collagen. Both from calf aorta

In vitro experiments with chondrocytes have shown that the extracellular matrix may be able to determine which type of collagen the cell will produce. These cells switch from type II to type I production if culture conditions are changed (Müller et.al., 1975). That means : Gene expression in collagen synthesis may be regulated by extracellular factors.

Some hereditary diseases indicate the importance of correct selection of collagen types :

Osteogenesis imperfecta patients produce too much type III collagen (Penttinen et.al., 1975). Bone which normally contains only type I is most affected. In Ehlers-Danlos type IV no type III collagen is synthesized. The arterial wall, which normally contains the highest proportion of type III is most severly affected (Pope et.al., 1975).

While the polypeptide chains are still in statu nascendi and attached to ribosomes, selected proline and lysine residues are already modified to hydroxyproline and hydroxylysine, respectively (Miller and Udenfriend, 1970 ; Lazarides et.al., 1971). Two different enzymes are involved : Prolylhydroxylase (peptidyl proline hydroxylase, PPH) and lysylhydroxylase (peptidyl lysine hydroxylase, PLH); both reactions require the same cofactors : α-Ketoglutarate, molecular oxygen, Fe^{++} and a reducing agent, normally ascorbic acid (For review see Grant and Prockop, 1972). Both enzymes are membrane bound (Diegelman et.al., 1973 ; Harwood et.al., 1974) and prolylhydroxylase was shown immunohistochemically to be localized in the cisternae of the endoplasmic reticulum (Olsen et.al., 1973 ; Adnani et.al., 1974).

Hydroxylation of prolyl residues is essential for the formation of the triple-helical structure; without hydroxylation the triple helix is not stable at 37 ^{o} (Jiminez et. al., 1973 ; Jiminez et.al., 1974 ; Berg and Prockop, 1973).

The prolyl hydroxylase probably plays an essential role in regulating the amount of collagen to be released into the extracellular space (Nigra et.al., 1972). Since collagen can only be released as triple-helical molecule inhibition of this enzyme immediatly stops collagen secretion. Underhydroxylated collagen accumulates within the cells and is finally digested by intracellular proteolysis.

Fibroblasts in rapidly deviding cell cultures do not produce collagen. It could be shown, however, that unhydroxylated polypeptide chains accumulate within the cells. As soon as they become confluent there is an increase in the activity of prolyl hydroxylase and the cells start to secret collagen

(Gribble et.al., 1969).

Prolyl hydroxylase probably is synthesized in an inactive precursor form (McGee and Udenfriend, 1972). Therefore only activation of this enzyme is needed to start collagen secretion immediately.

Hydroxylation of lysine takes place at the same time. The inhibition of this enzyme has no influence on the secretion of collagen. Hydroxylation of lysine, however, is an important prerequisite for intermolecular crosslinking. This became obvious by the discovery of a hereditary disease, hydroxylysine deficiency; patients show normal fibril formation but connective tissue disturbances typical for crosslink malfunction (Pinell et.al., 1972).

The polypeptide chains finally released from ribosomes are about 30 % longer than chains from mature collagen. These so called pro-αchains (for review see : Grant and Prockop, 1972 ; Schofield and Prockop, 1974 ; Bornstein, 1974) have an extension of more than 200 amino acid residues at their N-terminal site. Recently evidences were reported also for an additional C-terminal extension in pro-αchains (Tanzer et.al., 1974).

The chain extension of pro-αchains has at least two functions : (1) It serves as "registration peptide" which regulates correct alignment of αchains prior to triple helix formation. (2) After triple helix formation it retains solubility of the procollagen molecule and prevents fibril formation within the cell.

Assembly of these chain extensions even occurs when hydroxylation and therefore triple helix formation are inhibited. In case of type I collagen still the correct stoechiometry of 2 α1 and 1 α2 is observed (Fessler and Fessler, 1974). The assembly of registration peptides is stabilized by interchain disulfide bridges (Dehm et.al., 1972 ; Monson and Bornstein, 1973 ; Sherr et.al., 1973).

Glycosilation of some hydroxylysine residues is the last intracellular modification of procollagen. Two enzymes are involved : A Galactosyl transferase links galactose to hydroxylysine. Glucose is linked to the already covalently bound galactose by a Glucosyl transferase.

There is still some controversy about the question, by which way procollagen molecules are released by the cell. Three different possibilities are discussed which are outlined in figure 5 :

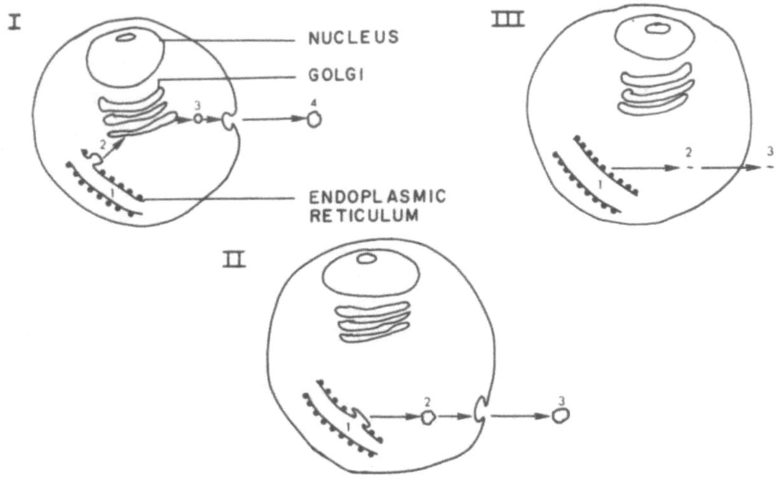

Figure 5: Current theories of collagen transport within cells (From: Miller and Matukas, 1974)

I. Procollagen is transported from the endoplasmic reticulum to the Golgi apparatus and then in vacuoles from the Golgi apparatus to cell membrane. Collagen again is released by exocytosis.

II. Vacuoles, which contain procollagen are formed by the endoplasmic reticulum, transported to the cell membrane and released by exocytosis.

III. Procollagen molecules are released into the cytoplasm, and directly transported across the cell membrane.

There is some strong evidence against theory III: Collagen secretion can be inhibited by microtubule disrupting agents as colchicine and vinblastin; the microtubule system, however, plays an important role in transport of vacuoles within the cell (Dehm and Prockop, 1972 ; Diegelman and Peterkofski, 1972 ; Ehrlich and Bornstein, 1972).

Experiments using ferritin coupled antibodies against procollagen have added further evidence for a transport within vacuoles. But they led to controversial results concerning the involvement of the Golgi apparatus. Electronmicroscopic autoradiography after ^{3}H-proline incorporation can be interpreted in favour of theory I (Weinstock and Leblond, 1974).

III. Extracellular steps

Figure 6 comprises the extracellular steps of collagen synthesis.

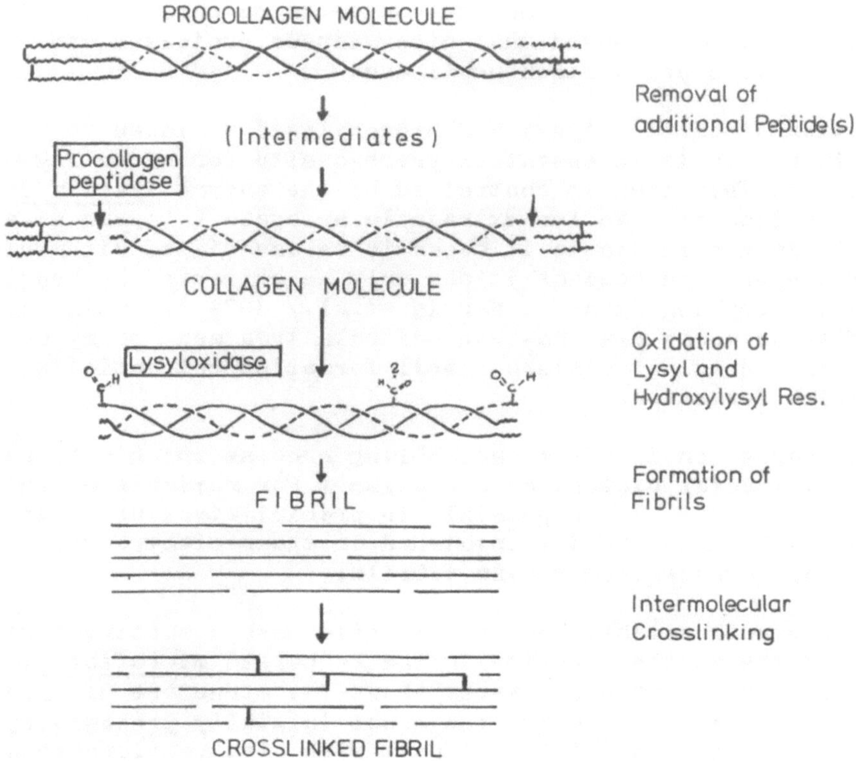

Figure 6 : Extracellular steps of collagen synthesis

Essential for fibril formation is the cleavage of the molecular extension of procollagen. One enzyme has been identified to control this process : Procollagen peptidase, an endopeptidase which acts at neutral pH. There is some evidence, however, that procollagen-collagen conversion occurs in several steps, and the possibility that more than one enzyme is involved cannot be excluded.

In dermatosparaxis, a heriditary disease of cattle, procollagen peptidase is inactive (Lenaers et.al., 1971). Fibril formation is disturbed severely and the skin of these animals is extremely fragile. Procollagen which can be extracted from the skin of these animals, however, is already shortened at its N-terminal extension; instead of pro-αchains so called p-αchains are isolated after denaturation. On the other hand about 50 % of skin collagen of these animals and an even higher percentage in other tissues are converted to normal collagen and it has to be assumed that other tissue proteases can partly replace procollagen peptidase.

Oxidation of certain lysyl and hydroxylysyl residues to aldehyde functions is an essential prerequesite for crosslink formation. This step is controlled by the enzyme lysyloxidase which is localized in the extracellular space (Layman et.al., 1972). In aortic tissue it seems to be associated with some insoluble protein because it can only be extracted by hydrogen bond breaking agents (Harris et.al., 1974). Inhibition of this enzyme by ß-amino-propionitrile treatment or by copper deficiency does not disturb fibril formation but inhibits crosslink formation.

Fibril formation is a self assembling process which does not need any special biological mechanism (For review see Traub and Piez, 1971). It is possible to precipitate fibrils in vitro which cannot be distinguished in their electronmicroscopic appearance from tissue fibrils.

It is now well established that fibrils have a substructure and that the smallest entity is the so called microfibril. There is still some controversy about the structure of this microfibril. Figure 7 shows the model initially proposed by Smith which is believed to fit best with electronmicroscopic and X-ray data. It is a five stranded helical arrangement of molecules (Smith, 1968 ; Miller and Parry, 1973).

The substructure model of collagen fibrils implies the necessity of two nucleation steps :
The first : Five molecules have to form the first helical turn of the microfibril. After that linear growth can be promoted by association of single molecules.
The second : Several microfibrils have to form a fibril nucleus which grows in diameter by association of further microfibrils.

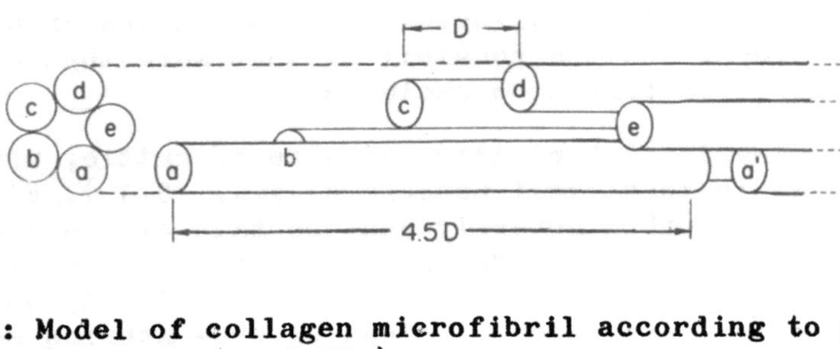

Figure 7 : Model of collagen microfibril according to Smith (from Piez, 1975)

Thus two separate nucleation steps and growth phases determine growth of fibrils in length and in diameter. This is considered to be an important point of regulation of fibril growth in tissue (Piez, 1975).

Intermolecular crosslinking is the last step in collagen biosynthesis. Experimental lathyrism and some hereditary crosslink disorders show how essential crosslinking is for function of collagen in tissue (For review see Bailey and Robins, 1973).

Figure 8 gives a short scheme of crosslink foramtion :

Lysyl and hydroxylysyl residues, mainly within the non-helical regions at both ends of molecules, are transformed to aldehydes. These aldehydes either react with further aldehydes in an aldol condensation or with unchanged lysines or hydroxylysines to form aldimin bonds. The aldol condensation products can further react to form polyfunctional crosslinks.

Characteristic differences have been found in chemical nature, quantity and localization of crosslinks in collagens of different tissues. As mentioned before, some of the intracellular steps of biosynthesis are believed to determine crosslink formation within the fibril. The molecules which are released from the cell are already programmed to form the tissue specific type of crosslinking.

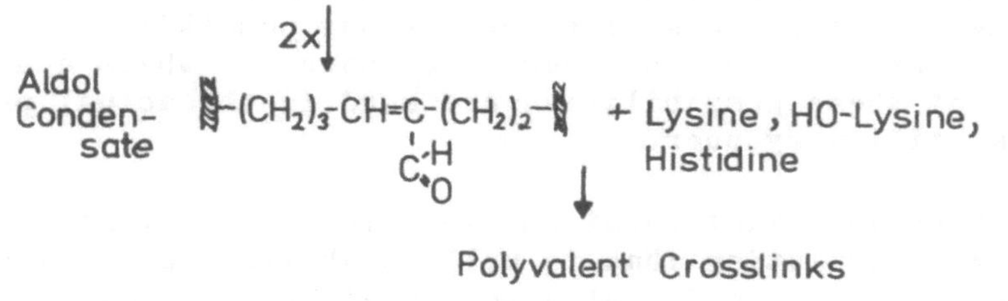

Figure 8 : Scheme of formation of intermolecular crosslinks in collagen fibrils

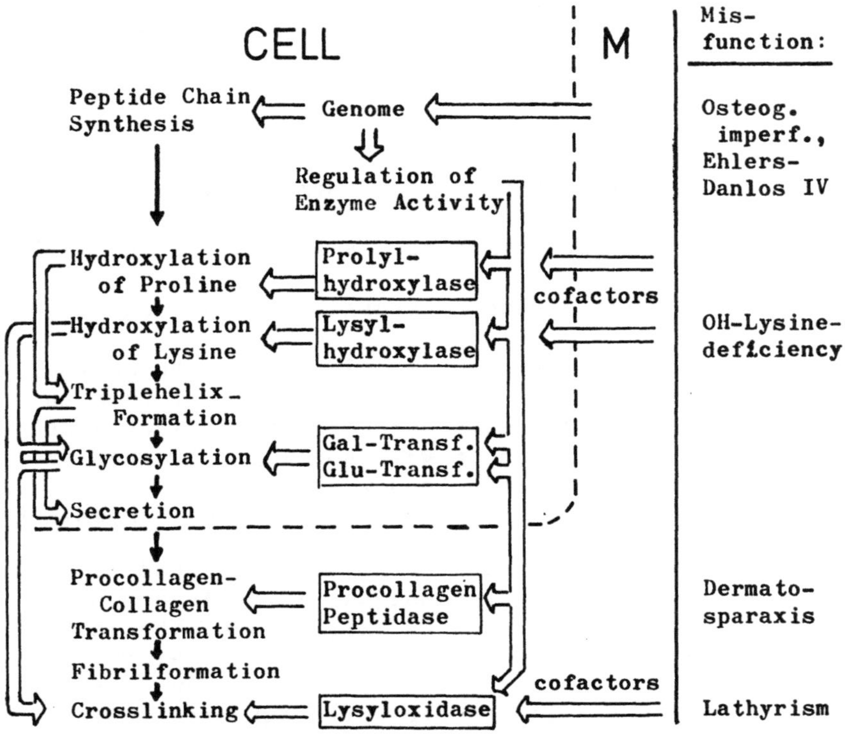

Figure 9 : Possibilities of biological regulation during collagen biosynthesis

IV. Conclusion

The intention of figure 9 is to show once more that formation of collagen is a process offering various possibilities of biological regulation. The knowledge, however, which and to what extent these possibilities are used in the actual process, is still very poor.

Another very important question, too, is at this moment more subject to speculation than to well established knowledge : Which functional role do collagen fibrils play in macromolecular organisation of extracellular matrix? Perhaps some steps of biosynthesis whose functional meaning are unclear so far will be better understood if we have a more detailed knowledge about interaction of macromolecules in the extracellular space.

References

Al-Adnani, M.S., Patrick, R.S., McGee, J.O'D. (1974)
J. Cell Sci. 16, 639

Bailey, A.J., Robins, S.P. (1973)
Front. Matrix Biol. Vol. 1, pp 130-156 (Karger,Basel)

Berg, R.A., Prockop, D.J. (1973)
Biochem. Biophys. Res. Commun. 52, 115

Bornstein, P. (1974)
Annu. Rev. Biochem. 43, 567

Butler, W.T., Miller, E.J., Finch, J.E., Inagami, T. (1974)
Biochem. Biophys. Res. Commun. 57, 190

Chung, E., Miller, E.J. (1974)
Science 183, 1200

Dehm, P., Jiminez, S.A., Olsen, B.R., Prockop, D.J. (1972)
Proc. Nat. Acad. Sci. USA 69, 60

Dehm, P., Prockop, D.J. (1972)
Bioch. Bioph. A. 264, 375

Diegelman, R.F., Bernstein, L., Peterkofsky, B. (1973)
J. Biol. Chem. 248, 6514

Diegelman, R.F., Peterkofsky, B. (1972)
Proc. Nat. Acad. Sci. USA 69, 892

Ehrlich, H.P., Bornstein, P. (1972)
Nature New Biol. 238, 257

Epstein, E.H. (1974)
J. Biol. Chem. 249, 3225

Fessler, L.I., Fessler, J.H. (1974)
J. Biol. Chem. 249, 7637

Fietzek, P.P., Rauterberg, J. (1975)
FEBS-Letters 49, 365-368

Grant, M.E., Prockop, D.J. (1972)
New Engl. J. Med. 286, 194, 242, 286 (three parts)

Gribble, J.T., Comstock, J.P., Udenfriend, S. (1969)
Arch. Bioch. Bioph. 129, 308

Harris, E.D., Gonnerman, W.A., Savage, J.E., O'Dell, B.L. (1974)
Bioch. Biophys. A. <u>341</u>, 332

Harwood, R., Grant, M.E., Jackson, D.S. (1974)
Biochem. J. <u>144</u>, 123

Jiminez, S., Harsch, M., Rosenbloom, J. (1973)
Bioch. Bioph. Res. Commun. <u>52</u>, 106

Jiminez, S., Harsch, M., Murphy, L., Rosenbloom, J. (1974)
J. Biol. Chem. <u>249</u>, 4480-4486

Kühn, K. (1969)
Essays Biochem. <u>5</u>, 60

Layman, D.L., Narayan, A.S., Martin, G.R. (1972)
Arch. Bioch. Bioph. <u>149</u>, 97

Lazarides, E.L., Lukens, L.N., Infante, A.A. (1971)
J. Mol. Biol. <u>58</u>, 831

Lenaers, A., Ansay, M., Nusgens, B.V., Lapière, C.M. (1971)
Eur. J. Bioch. <u>23</u>, 533

McGee, J.O'D., Langness, U., Udenfriend, S. (1971)
Proc. Nat. Acad. Sci. USA <u>68</u>, 1585

Miller, A., Parry, D.A.D. (1973)
J. Mol. Biol. <u>75</u>, 441

Miller, E.J. (1973)
Clin. Orthop. <u>92</u>, 260

Miller, E.J., Matukas, V.J. (1974)
Fed. Proc. 33, 1197

Miller, R.L., Udenfriend, S. (1970)
Arch. Bioch. Bioph. <u>139</u>, 104

Monson, J.M., Bornstein, P. (1973)
Proc. Nat. Acad. Sci. USA <u>70</u>, 3521

Müller, P.K., Lemmen, C., Gay, S., von der Mark, K., Kühn, K.
In: Extracellular Matrix Influences on Gene Expression,
H.C. Slavkin, R.C. Greulich, ed.
Acad. Press New York, pp 293-302 (1975)

Nigra, T.P., Friedland, M., Martin, G.R. (1972)
J. Inv. Derm. <u>59</u>, 44

Olsen, B.R., Berg, R.A., Kishida, Y., Prockop, D.J. (1973)
Science 182, 825

Penttinen, R.P., Lichtenstein, J.R., Martin, G.R., McKusick, V.A. (1975)
Proc. Nat. Acad. Sci. USA 72, 586

Piez, K.A. (1975)
In: Extracellular Matrix Influence on Gene Expression, H.C. Slavkin, R.C. Greulich, ed.
Acad. Press New York, pp 95-100

Pinell, S.R., Krane, S.M., Kenzora, J.E., Glimcher, M.J. (1972)
New Engl. J. Med. 286, 1013

Pope, F.M., Martin, G.R., Lichtenstein, J.R., Penttinen, R., Gerson, B., Rowe, D.W., McKusick, V.A. (1975)
Proc. Nat. Acad. Sci. USA 72, 1314

Rauterberg, J, (1975)
in preparation

Rauterberg, J., von Bassewitz, D.B. (1975)
Hoppe Seylers Z. Phys. Chem. 356, 95-100

Schofield, J.D., Prockop, D.J. (1973)
Clin. Orthop. 97, 175

Sherr, C.J., Taubman, M.B., Goldberg, B. (1973)
J. Biol. Chem. 248, 7033

Smith, J.W. (1968)
Nature 219, 157

Tanzer, M.L., Church, R.L., Yaeger, J.A., Wamper, D.E., Park, E.-D. (1974)
Proc. Nat. Acad. Sci. USA 71, 3009

Traub, W., Piez, K.A. (1971)
Adv. Protein chemistry 25, 243-352

Weinstock, M., Leblond, C.P. (1974)
J. Cell. Biol. 60, 92

(3)

AORTIC PROTOCOLLAGEN PROLINE HYDROXYLASE

K. GRASEDYCK and J. LINDNER

I. Med. Clinic and Pathological
Institute University of Hamburg
Hamburg, Germany

Hydroxyproline and hydroxylysine are not utilized for collagen synthesis by smooth muscle cells as well as by fibro-, chondro-, osteoblasts and other collagen synthesizing cells. First, the peptide chain containing proline and lysine is synthesized. The hydroxylation of these amino acids begins during the assembly and is continued after the release of the polypeptide. Protocollagen proline hydroxylase (PPH) and protocollagen lysine hydroxylase (PLH) are involved in this hydroxylation process. Figure 1 demonstrates the role of these two enzymes although their activity levels do not run parallel to the total collagen synthesis. Therefore they are regarded as key enzymes although their activity levels do not run parallel to the total collagen synthesis in any case. The above subject was discussed in some detail elsewhere (GRASEDYCK et al., 1974).

LANGNER and FULLER (1973) described a sixfold increase of the PPH- activity in rabbit aortic lesions induced by toxic doses of epinephrine and L-thyroxine. We wish to show that such results are at least in part age-dependent.

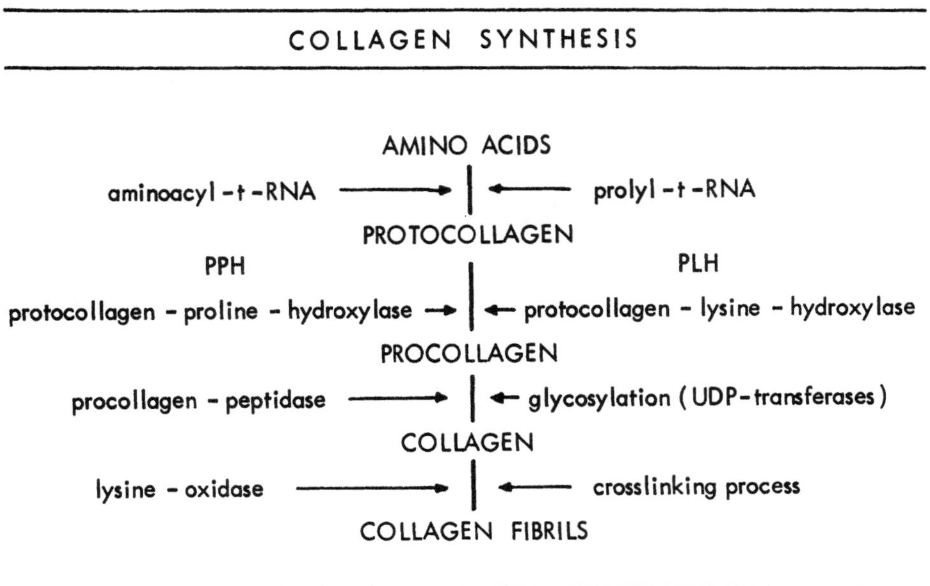

Fig.1: The main steps in collagen synthesis

The decrease of the arterial glycosaminoglycan metabolism with age is indicated by the decrease of ^{35} S-sulfate incorporation as routine indicator method for the synthesis of sulfated GAG. The specific activities and synthesis rates of the several GAG fractions that are typical for arterial connective tissues show identical age-dependent changes. The DNA concentration, a parameter for the muscle cell content, declines with age, too. Smooth muscle cells account for more than 90% of the total cell content of the rat aorta. Related to the DNA content there is a continuous decrease of the aorta GAG synthesis from a newborn to a three-year old (senile) female rat , as demonstrated in this case again by assays of the ^{35} S-sulfate incorporation rates (Fig. 2). We could not show sex-dependent differences in this advanced age of rats.

The PPH activity of rat aortas was assayed by the method of HUTTON et al. (1966). ^{3}H-water liberated from ^{3}H-proline-labeled protocollagen of chick embryos during the hydroxylation process was distilled and its radio-activity was measured in a liquid scintillation counter (TRI-CARB).

Aortas of 4-week-old rats showed the highest PPH activity and almost three times higher than those of 4-month-old rats, i.e., of rats at the end of maturation. The activity was five times higher than that of 25 months old (senile) rats of the same strain and sex. Identical results have been obtained when dry weight or N-content were used as parameters.

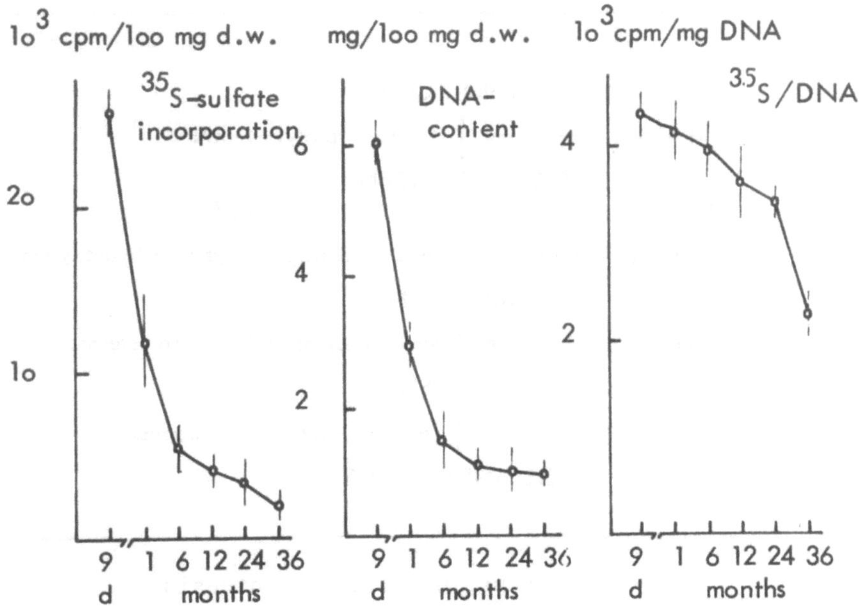

Fig. 2: ^{35}S-sulfate incorporation rates and DNA content in rat aortas of different age

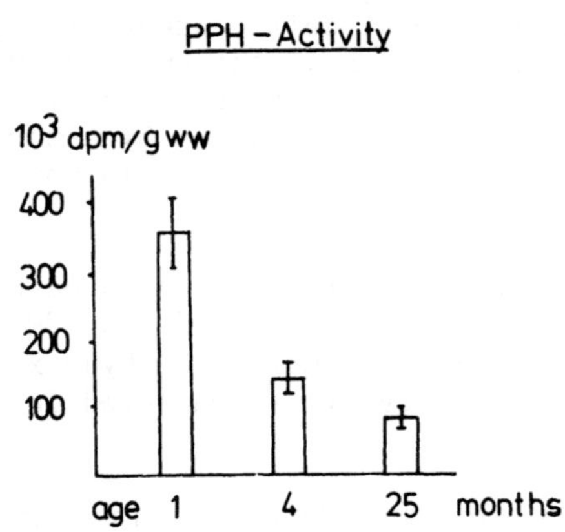

Fig. 3: Rat aorta PPH activity in relation to age

The measure of the PPH activity may be used as indicator method for the collagen synthesis. It is not identical with collagen synthesis, but it represents a main step in the synthesis and it is better accessible than other parameters because only very small tissue samples are needed (GRASEDYCK et al., 1974) for determinations.

The same proline residues of the protocollagen molecule are hydroxylated by this enzyme (PPH) in vitro as in vivo. Therefore, many investigations of the disturbed vascular connective tissue metabolism are possible by this PPH activity assays; using small human biopsy material of the various atherosclerotic stages one may compare their PPH values with unchanged parts of the same arteries.

As mentioned above the PPH activity may be elevated in early atherosclerotic lesions as well as that of the specific activity of hydroxyproline and the collagen turnover rates. In investigations of progressive atherosclerotic lesions age-dependent alterations must be considered. The latter may be caused by the diminution of the cell content in the aging arterial tissue or in progressive atherosclerotic lesions (LINDNER, 1972).

References:

GRASEDYCK, K., M. HELLE, J. LINDNER, K. LANGNESS: Kriterien der Aktivität einer pathologischen Bindegewebsvermehrung bei chronischen Lebererkrankungen. Verh. Dtsch. Ges. Inn. Med. 80, 503-506 (1974).

HUTTON, J.J., A.L. TAPPEL, S. UDENFRIEND: A rapid assay for collagen proline hydroxylase. Anal. Biochem. 16, 384-394 (1966).

LANGNER, R.O., G.C. FULLER: Collagen synthesis in thoracic aortas of rabbits with epinephrine-thyroxine induced arteriosclerosis. Atherosclerosis 17, 463-469 (1973).

LINDNER, J.: Regressive und progressive arterielle Reaktionen bei Atherosklerose: 5.Veränderungen im extrazellulären Kompartment. Verh.Dtsch.Ges.Inn.Med. 78, 1166-1176 (1972).

(4)

PATHOPHYSIOLOGY OF THE INTERCELLULAR MATRIX AS A WHOLE

L. ROBERT and A.M. ROBERT

Laboratoire de Biochimie du Tissu Conjonctif
Fac. Méd., Univ. Paris-Val de Marne, 6 rue du Gl Sarrail
94000 Créteil, France

Arterial wall contains cellular elements and intercellular matrix. The relative importance of the matrix elements varies from the basement membrane in capillaries to a relatively abundant and complex "matrix" in larger arteries of the "elastic" type. This contains all four major classes of the intercellular matrix macromolecules (IMM) : Collagen, Elastin, Proteoglycans and Structural Glycoproteins. The relative proportion of these macromolecules varies also from artery to artery and even in the same artery according to its anatomical location. The differentiation of the cellular elements of the arterial wall during morphogenesis appears to imply the definition of a "program" of biosynthesis of these IMM-s, this program being different according to the anatomical location and the functional role of the artery. This "program" of IMM-biosynthesis changes also with age and appears to be modified in pathological conditions. The study of arterial wall connective tissues "as a whole" is conditioned by the understanding of the mechanisms underlying the "program" of biosynthesis of the IMM-s as well as the mechanisms of their degradation.

Methods used for the study of arterial wall connective tissues "as a whole"

In order to study arterial wall connective tissue "as a whole" several procedures can be used :

a) The analytical approach consists in serial extractions ("chemical dissection") of the arteries. The extracts can be

----

Abbreviations used : IMM : intercellular matrix macromolecules ; SGP : structural glycoproteins ; MF : microfibrils.

analysed for proteins and carbohydrates by the usual analytical procedures (1). Comparative tables may thus be obtained showing compositional differences between normal and sclerotic arteries.

b) A special case of the analytical approach is the thermogravimetric procedure developped by Bihari-Varga and al (2), enabling the qualitative and quantitative analysis of small tissue samples without any previous treatment. This method yielded some interesting results on the macromolecular composition of normal and pathological arterial wall (3, 4, 5).

c) Incorporation of radioactive tracers in normal or pathological aortas was also used for the in vitro study of the "biosynthetic program" in normal and pathological arteries (6).

d) Morphological procedures are particularly apt to reveal modification in the ultrastructural pattern of the IMM-s such as collagen, elastin, structural glycoprotein-microfibrils and even proteoglycans (7).

Recent advances in arterial wall connective tissue biochemistry

Analytical data

Although analytical data were available on separate, more or less purified arterial wall components, the relative proportion of most if not all IMM-s were only recently determined in normal and arteriosclerotic human and animal aortas (8). These studies revealed significant differences between the normal and pathological composition such as increase in salt soluble and stroma-bound (structural) glycoproteins with increasing degree of atheromatosis as determined in the macroscopically lesion-free parts of the human aorta (1). The SGP-MF component of "plaque-elastin" with respect to normal elastin increases and its degree of crosslinking (desmosin content) decreases (9). These findings may be considered as the biochemical equivalent of the often described rarefaction, lysis and disappearance of elastic lamellae.

Changes were also observed in the IMM-composition of the arterial wall with age using both chemical (10) and physicochemical procedures (2, 3, 4, 5). The thermogravimetric method suggested qualitative differences between the modifications of the composition of the arterial wall with age and in arteriosclerosis. The increase of the SGP-MF to elastin ratio and the decrease of the proportion of "highly crosslinked" elastin were observed in aging human aortas also. The regression curve obtained with these parameters as a function of age enabled the authors to calculate a fictive "age" for the pathological aortas. This calculated age of some arteriosclerotic aortas varied from 60 to 120 years for individuals of a chronological age of approximately 40 to 70 years (9).

Studies with radioactive tracers

Both short incubation periods (6) and culture studies (10) were performed on whole aortas or on medias stripped of the other layers. A modification of the incorporation pattern of ^{14}C-lysine in the IMM-s was observed in the aortas of rabbits immunised with K-elastin or fed cholesterol (6). Organ culture studies performed with aortas of newborn, young and adult rabbits showed a regular decrease of the total biosynthetic capacity, expressed as ^{14}C-lysine or ^{3}H-glucosamine incorporated in the IMM-s (expressed as dpm/mg DNA or dpm/g fresh weight) (10). No such global decrease could be demonstrated in cell cultures derived from newborn or adult rabbit aorta explants (11). Cell cultures, although very useful for several purposes, cannot be used therefore to characterise the overall "biosynthetic program" of the normal or sclerotic arterial wall. Some only of the regulatory mechanisms responsible for the synchronised biosynthesis of the IMM-s of the arterial wall manifest themselves in cell cultures, others do not and appear to depend on an "informational feedback loop" between intercellular matrix and cells (11). These results may be of significance in understanding the "vicious circles" that underly the progressive nature of the disease as observed in humans.

Immunological studies

Immunological techniques were used in several laboratories to analyse the role of immunefactors in atherosclerosis (12). Aorta extracts contain many immunologically distinct fractions. Insoluble, stroma components such as SGP and elastin were also shown to be immunogenic and able to initiate a sclerotic process when used in Freund's adjuvant to immunise rabbits (13). Recent studies in Gero's laboratory indicated the existence of specific arterial and venous components as well as the appearance of "autoantibodies" to some of these components extractable from the venous wall by a 1M $CaCl_2$-tris-citrate buffer (CTC buffer) (14). These and other data indicate that some of the matrix components may possess organ as well as species specificity and might be involved in blood vessel wall pathology as targets of auto-immune processes.

Lipid-IMM-interaction

It could be shown recently that lipoproteins interact with smooth muscle cells in culture as well as with aorta organ cultures by altering the metabolic behaviour of the cells (15). This interaction may alter the "biosynthetic program" of the smooth muscle cells. This is shown by the modified incorporation pattern of ^{14}C-lysine and ^{3}H-glucosamine observed in rabbit aorta organ cultures in the presence of hyperlipemic human sera (11).

Another important aspect of lipid-IMM-interactions is the fact that a significant fraction of the "structurally bound lipids" (non extractable with organic solvents without the previous hydrolysis of connective tissue elements) is strongly "associated" with elastin (16). A "hydrophobic stacking" mechanism was proposed for this type of interaction. It was shown recently that the fatty acid composition of the elastin-bound lipid fraction changes with the severity of the atherosclerotic lesion. In the macroscopically intact parts of arteriosclerotic aortas the proportion of longer fatty acid chains ($C > 18$) increases and "odd" chains with known toxicity appear (17).

References

1 - J. Ouzilou, A.M. Robert, L. Robert, H. Bouissou and M.T. Pieraggi., Paroi Artérielle, 1, 105-116 (1973)

2 - M. Bihari-Varga and S. Gerö., in "Protides of the Biological Fluids", ed. H. Peeters (Pergamon Press) 22, 319-322 (1975)

3 - M. Bihari-Varga, J. Feher, M. Varsanyi, S. Gerö, Acta Med. Acad. Sci. Hung. 29, 217-229 (1972)

4 - J. Fehér, M. Bihari-Varga, M. Varsanyi and S. Gerö, Brit. J. Exp. Path. 53, 509-517 (1972)

5 - M. Bihari-Varga, C. Sepulchre and E. Moczar, J. Thermal Analysis 7, 675-683 (1975)

6 - L. Robert, S. Junqua, A.M. Robert, M. Moczar and B. Robert, in "Biology of Fibroblast" ed E. Kulonen and J. Pikkarainen (Acad. Press, London/New-York) pp 637-652 (1973)

7 - H. Jellinek, "Arterial Lesions and Arteriosclerosis" (Plenum Press, London/New York) 1974

8 - L. Robert, A. Kadar and B. Robert., in "Arterial Mesenchyme and Arteriosclerosis" eds W.D. Wagner and T.B. Clarkson (Plenum Press, New-York/London) 43, 85-124 (1974)

9 - Y. Moschetto, M. De Backer, O. Pizieux, H. Bouissou, M.T. Pieraggi and M. Julian, Paroi Artérielle 2, 161-178 (1974)

10 - J. Ouzilou, Y. Courtois, M. Moczar and L. Robert, C.R. Acad. Sc. Paris 280, 209-212 (1975)

11 - M. Moczar, J. Ouzilou, Y. Courtois and L. Robert, in preparation

12 - J. Renais, P. Hadjiisky and L. Scebat, in "Arterial Mesenchyme and Arteriosclerosis" ed. W.D. Wagner and T.B. Clarkson (Plenum Press, New-York/London) 43, 335-354 (1974)

13 - A.M. Robert, Y. Grosgogeat, V. Reverdy, B. Robert and L. Robert, Atherosclerosis 13, 427-449 (1971)

14 - S. Gerö, J. Székely, E. Szondy, A. Zobbagy, A. Orosz and E. Seregélyi, Experientia 29, 1024 (1973)

15 - K. Fisher-Dzoga, R. Chen and R.W. Wissler, in "Arterial Mesenchyme and Arteriosclerosis" ed. W.D. Wagner and T.B. Clarkson (Plenum Press, London/New-York) 43, 299-314 (1974)

16 - B. Jacotot, J.L. Beaumont, G. Monnier, M. Szigeti, B. Robert and L. Robert, Nutr. Metabol. 15, 46-58 (1973)

17 - M. Claire, B. Jacotot, L. Robert and J.L. Beaumont, in "Protides of the Biological Fluids" ed. H. Peeters (Pergamon Press, Oxford/New York) 22, 167-170 (1975)

(5)

MORPHOLOGY OF COLLAGEN AND ELASTIN FIBERS IN ATHEROSCLEROTIC LESIONS

Seymour Glagov, M.D.

Professor of Pathology, University of Chicago

950 E. 59th Street, Chicago, Illinois, U.S.A.

Although there has been no systematic study of the morphology of collagen and elastin fibers in atherosclerotic plaques, most of the detailed descriptions and many of the published photographs of both human and experimental lesions include information concerning the structure, distribution and relative proportions of these elements. A general qualitative overview and some semi-quantitative statements can therefore be formulated. Precise spatial reconstructions of elastin and collagen distribution in plaques from published data are hampered by two serious limitations. First, the sections have usually been taken from the most complex portions of plaques. The disrupted central portion of an advanced or complicated atheroma may not be the best site for observation of the architectural details which might help to unravel plaque morphogenesis. A second limitation is the usual failure to reproduce the *in vivo* configuration of arteries and plaques during fixation. Statements concerning the orientation of plaque and artery wall fibers can not be made readily from undistended material.

It is the purpose of this communication to make a tentative, brief synthesis of the findings gleaned from the considerable descriptive literature and to point out some of the morphogenetic and possible functional implications of these findings. In keeping with my assignment, I shall confine my attention to collagen and elastin fibers and refer, only in passing, to the other extracellular fibrillar or fibrous elements often closely associated with them. The published observations will be complemented by data drawn from our own extensive collection of human and other mammalian arteries fixed while distended at physiologic pressures.

FEATURES OF ARTERIAL FIBERS

I should like, first to describe briefly, the normal appearance of medial and intimal fibers. Smooth muscle cells of the media are associated with a fairly well defined basal lamina (BL). By usual preparation techniques, this structure consists of a relatively clear inner zone next to the cell membrane, a poorly defined midzonal fibrillar network and an outermost dense or compact zone. Fine discrete fibrils, probably collagen, are often embedded in the BL and also occur between the cell membrane and the BL. In the intima, the BL beneath the endothelial cells is essentially similar, but is neither as continuous nor as regularly structured as that of the medial smooth muscle. In addition to the fibrils of the BL, there is in both the media and the intima, a fine, evenly spaced reticular or locular network which, because of its uniform morphology and its staining qualities is considered to represent the mucopolysaccharide matrix. Such material is especially abundant in young arteries, and appears to be increased in the intima when this layer is undergoing abnormal thickening. In the media, collagen fibrils, separate from those which lie near cells in and around the basal lamina, show a range of diameters and generally group to form fibers of varying size. In the intima, collagen fibers are also present but are relatively sparse and not usually arranged in fiber bundles. Elastin in the media occurs as an interconnected network of bars and plates, in very close association with the smooth muscle cells and on both sides of smooth muscle cells. Elastin is seen in two main morphologic forms. One type consists of an aggregate of fine microfibrils of uniform diameter among which an amorphous material accumulates to form irregularly circumscribed islands. In ligamentum nuchae, as well as in growing arteries, this configuration is the morphologic counterpart of the active new formation of elastin. These islands later coalesce to form interconnecting plates and fibers of mature elastin. In the mature form, microfibrils are absent or few and the edge of the elastin fiber has a fairly regular and sharp outline. It stains uniformly, especially in the interior. Fine fibrils, oriented in the long axis of the elastin bar or plate, are embedded in the material. Often the outermost edge of the elastin stains deeply with phosphotungstic acid, in contrast to the poorly stained interior. The newly forming elastin also stains intensely.

The intima is limited on its medial side by the internal elastin lamina (IEL), which in most arteries, is the thickest and most continuous of the elastin plates of the media. Where the IEL is well formed and continuous, the normal overlying intima is nearly completely devoid of elastin islands or plates. Yet, the subendothelial side of the IEL is usually much more irregular than the medial side, and the associated projections, especially in growing animals, may give the appearance of separate intimal elastin islands. These foci are however, uniformly aligned and close to the IEL and can often be shown on sequential sections to be transected projections arising from the IEL. In young animals however, separate intimal elastin islands, soon to merge with the main IEL, are regularly found. In carefully distended specimens, there is a very close association between the IEL and its microfibrils and the endothelial BL. In undistended specimens, the separation of endothelial cells from the IEL leaves a subendothelial "space" between the BL of the endothelium and the IEL; the small elastin islands may then be seen close to the IEL and not to the basal lamina which remains with the endothelial cell.

As concerns the finer infrastructural detail or staining properties of the fibrous elements, there have been no reported consistent differences between intima and media; differences in staining properties and fiber size seem to be related to age of the material rather than to location.

INTIMAL THICKENING

Much has been written concerning the relationship between the diffuse intimal thickening seen in arteries and the formation of atherosclerotic plaques. These processes have been shown to be parallel in time and localization, and morphogenetic links have been established between them. Though advanced plaques are preceded by focally increased intimal thickening and cell accumulation, intimal thickening, per se, does not necessarily or inexorably lead to fibroatheromatous plaque formation. A survey of collagen and elastin morphology in lesions does not as yet provide any decisive insight into the events which may trigger the focal conversion of intimal thickening into plaque formation, but does provide some suggestive indications which may be worthy of deeper exploration.

The earliest intimal change, already evident during development and growth is the so-called splitting, reduplication or fragmentation of the IEL. This consists of the appearance, next to the thick and more or less continuous original IEL, of a thinner, less continuous and less orderly segment of elastin. The process, though focal, occurs at multiple sites around the circumference of the vessel and is also noted in vessels which rarely become atherosclerotic. Close examination reveals that nearly all of these new segments are on the intimal side of the main IEL and are nearly always associated with the presence of smooth muscle cells in the intima between the old IEL and the new segment. Electron micrographs often show the overlying endothelium and its BL closely applied to the new elastin segment in much the same manner as the endothelium is applied to the adjacent IEL where a new elastin segment is not present. Collagen fibers are also in evidence between the IEL and the new elastin segment and between the new segment and the endothelium but in about the same proportions to other elements as is usual for the intima. As the number of cells and the size of this musculoelastic layer increases, new layers as defined by new elastin segments can be discerned. The smooth muscle cells are often arranged in a fairly uniform pattern, each cell surrounded by small islands of newly forming elastin; most often collagen fibers lie between and among adjacent rows of the pericellular elastin islands and the proportion of collagen to elastin tends to be about the same as in the underlying media. There is a tendency toward confluence of these elastin islands, most markedly immediately under the endothelium so that they tend to merge into a more or less continuous subendothelial layer. The underlying IEL is not greatly changed and I have not found convincing evidence, qualitative or quantitative that would support the contention that the old IEL has split or fragmented. The transitions, at least in small thickenings with uniform morphology, suggest instead that there is neoformation of elastin by intimal cells, whatever their provenance, and that there is some reconstruction or imitation of normal intimal and medial structure in the thickened intima.

When relatively limited, and equal to or less then the thickness of the media, accumulations are orderly and more or less uniformly concentric. When intimal thickening develops some degree of eccentricity, layering may be accentuated, but is often less uniform in structure. At these points, thickness may exceed that of the media and the focus tends to take on features of an atherosclerotic plaque. Thus, the layers of elastin and collagen fibers are more variable in thickness and complexity, the cells may be greatly reduced in number or accumulate lipid, and foci of necrosis and disruption appear. Sometimes a series of elastin rich layers can be distinguished beneath the endothelium and has been characterized as an "elastic-hyperplastic" zone. Often, striking contrasts in the connective tissue morphology of adjacent intimal layers, especially in aortas, suggest that the fibroelastic thickening process has been episodic. The intimal thickenings thus far described are not necessarily associated with obvious atrophy of the underlying media, but a decrease in prominence of the IEL with a marked increase in the number of its gaps does tend to occur with moderate to marked increases in thickness of the intima. These findings suggest that non-atheromatous concentric intimal thickening is to some degree a general reactive and mechanically functional state of the arterial wall. Many of the focal changes, described in man and animals as "atherosclerosis" or "arteriosclerosis," are similar to one or another of the manifestations of concentric intimal thickening. The intimal pads and cushions which occur at specific sites in association with ostia, branchings or presumed zones of flow channeling or elevated tension are somewhat different in fibrous architecture. These excrescences tend to be very sharply demarcated and tend also to be highly cellular. Immediately beneath these foci, the IEL is almost always virtually absent and the IEL on either side seems to branch into an intercellular elastin network.

ATHEROSCLEROTIC PLAQUES

Human and experimental eccentric or discrete lesions which contain demonstrable lipid, either intracellular or extracellular, show some distinctive features in their fiber organization. Early changes in the IEL such as swelling or alteration in staining properties with or without associated smooth muscle cell accumulation in the intima have been described even before lipid is demonstrable. It is difficult to know if these sites are really foci of future discrete lipid containing lesions. In early lesions which clearly include numbers of lipid containing cells, accumulations of redundant and disorganized layers of BL-like material have been shown. Also, small islands of newly forming elastin, as seen in other intimal thickenings are also present. An overall impression is gained from descriptions and pictures that the quantity of elastin in such lesions is roughly proportional to the recognizability of the altered cells as smooth muscle. In some animal lesions, the cells containing lipid vacuoles are arranged in a very orderly manner with each cell framed by elastin. In others, lesions are so crowded with lipid filled foam cells that extracellular space is virtually absent and extracellular materials are difficult to evaluate. Yet, foci of increased fine reticular material, accumulating disorganized strips of BL-like material, isolated pericellular elastin islands and collagen fibrils and fibers are described as more or less constant features in these lesions.

With increased cell alteration and disruption, as well as necrosis and disorganization in the central portions of the lesion, especially in the well described human lesions, collagen accumulation becomes an increasingly predominant feature. Fibrils and fibers are intermingled with cells, debris, and other fibrillar material and tend to fill the degenerating zone as the cells decrease in relative number. In addition to collagen, other types of fibrillar or reticular material are also described in such areas. Where structure is relatively loose and cells are sparse but more or less intact or viable, a delicate reticular network is seen. This configuration is not unlike that seen in young arteries and probably represents glycosaminoglycan ground substance material. There is also a more amorphous granular material which tends to accumulate where cells are sparse and disrupted. Fibrin has also been demonstrated in athersclerotic lesions. Elastin formation is not marked in degenerated areas so that the ratio of collagen relative to elastin is much greater than that of normal intima or media or of the more uniform and orderly non-atheromatous or pre-atheromatous intimal thickening. The atheromatous centers of well developed atherosclerotic plaques show much collagen and only small or fragmented islands of elastin. The more peripheral, structured portions of the lesions, where cells are numerous, have more of the features of smooth muscle, and contain less lipid, tend to contain more elastin.

The fibrous cap of an advanced, discrete atheroma is usually a compact, relatively acellular and layered fibrocellular structure with circumferential bars of elastin and bands of collagen. Its thickness and structure is remarkably uniform in any given plaque and it merges with the adjacent non-atheromatous intimal thickening, whose thickness is often very nearly equal to that of the fibrous cap. In very advanced lesions, both human and experimental, which, because of the blandness of their atheromatous interiors and the absence of hemorrhage or thrombosis, may be considered to be quiescent or stabilized, the fibrous cap may contain even denser or more compact layers of collagen and elastin and fewer cells. It is not clear whether this evolution favors the preferential accumulation of collagen or elastin. Though most descriptions describe a predominently collagenized cap, elastin is often abundant and forms structured layers of lamellae. The combination ("diad" or "parite") of atheromatous center and fibrous cap may occur repeatedly in the same segment of an artery, providing an image of an atheroma which has formed in a fibrous cap of a previous atheroma and suggesting that the fibrous cap, like the native wall, is susceptible to atherosclerosis. This finding underlines the episodic nature of the disease and the morphologic features which suggest repair, functional modelling and regression.

The media beneath an advanced plaque is often thinned and may be disrupted. Atrophy, replacement by collagen, relative disappearance of cells and closer approximation of remaining fibers have all been described. A fibrocellular zone, comparable in thickness to the adjacent intimal thickening and to the fibrous cap is often seen between the media and the lesions. Its collagen and elastin content and organization may resemble that of the diffuse intimal thickening in the same artery but it is usually not as well organized as the fibrous cap. Its configuration and transition to the adjacent thickened intima tends repeatedly to suggest that plaques originate from a focal disturbance in an intimal thickening. In atheromatous plaques which are necrotic, the disruption may extend into the media for variable distances, including both underlying intimal and medial collagen and elastin into the atheromatous debris. This direct necrotizing involvement of the media can penetrate quite deeply, and in large and older lesions the subjacent media may be absent or reduced to a thin fibrous band. This data, taken together with the structural features and dimensions of the fibrous cap provide an overall architectural picture suggestive of a continuous artery "wall" formed by the fibrous cap and the adjacent and opposite intact media with its intimal thickening. The atheroma with its atrophic underlying old media thus appears to be sequestered. This concept is emphasized when lesions are studied from vessels which have been fixed while distended and stained for connective tissue fibers. Lumens are then seen to be regularly round or ovoid and the atheroma is, at least topographically, "extrinsic."

PERSPECTIVES

There have not as yet been any special morphologic attributes in plaque collagen or elastin fibers which could, per se, help to assess the disease process. Current preoccupation with the proliferative and fibrogenic response of arterial tissue has generated much new quantitative chemical data concerning collagen and elastin content of vessels and plaques, but morphometric or steriological quantitative studies relating the precise appearance and distribution of extracellular fibers to the natural history and consequences of atherosclerosis have not as yet been undertaken. The individual pattern of connective tissue elaboration in specific portions of the plaque and at specific phases in the disease process could be as important as the total collagen or elastin content of the plaque measured chemically. A collagenous fibrous cap, for example, could be potentially more life threatening than an elastotic cap because of its relative mechanical non-compliance and because of its greater tendency to induce platelet aggregation should its endothelium somehow be disrupted as flow rate is accelerated by luminal narrowing. The fibrous proteins are easily stained differentially, accentuating structural and topographical details. Authors have in the past utilized qualitative data to support various theories of plaque origin and evolution. Quantitative morphometric and steriological studies correlating plaque fibrous composition with clinical features of atherosclerotic disease could conceivably provide further illumination. (Work supported in part by Grant HL 17648 SCOR-IHD of the National Institutes of Health, USPHS)

(6)

BIOCHEMISTRY OF COLLAGEN AND ELASTIC FIBERS IN ATHEROSCLEROTIC LESIONS

Dieter M. Kramsch, M.D. and Carl Franzblau, Ph.D.

Boston University Medical Center

Boston, Massachusetts, U.S.A.

The importance of collagen and elastic fiber alterations in atherosclerosis has long been recognized by morphologists while biochemical evaluation has lagged behind. However, there now is a fair body of biochemical data available which permit some conclusions.

It has been shown (1) that in man the collagen content of lesions increases with increasing severity of atherosclerosis from minimal in fatty streaks and gelatenous lesions to substantial in fibrous plaques with maximal increases in calcified fibrous plaques. Advancing age does not appear to influence the collagen content of lesions (1). Little is known about factors that might enhance the collagen and elastin content of lesions in man. Although a great number of morphologic studies in experimental animals indicate that such factors as dietary cholesterol, butter, peanut oil, hypertension, immune reactions and various mechanical and chemical injuries to the arterial wall or just its endothelial layer may increase arterial connective tissue, few biochemical studies have been reported to validate these microscopic observations. They pertain exclusively to dietary fats and cholesterol (Tables I and II).

The turnover rate of arterial collagen in adults normally is slow; the half-life of normal mature elastin is considered to approximate the life span of the animal (2). In experimental atherosclerosis, however, the turnover of collagen appears to be accelerated early, with the synthesis outweighing degradation (3-5), leading to a net increase in the content of insoluble collagen in advanced lesions (3). No exact data on the turnover rate of elastin in atherosclerosis are available. However, an increased *in vivo* synthesis of arterial elastin has been demonstrated by our

TABLE I. CONTENTS IN AORTIC CONNECTIVE TISSUE PROTEIN OF NORMAL RABBITS AND RABBITS ON ATHEROGENIC REGIMEN WITH AND WITHOUT DRUGS

Experimental Groups	Collagen	"Elastin"	Authors
(Absolute amounts in mg/whole aorta with adventitia; average)			
Control Diet	29.2	36.7	Wartman et al.(1967)
Atherogenic Diet without Drugs	43.5	44.0	J. Atheroscler. Res.
Atherogenic Diet + MgEDTA[a]	32.8	38.8	7: 331.
(% of dry defatted intima-media of whole aorta; mean $\pm$ S.D.)			
Control Diet	12.5 ± 2.4	41.1 ± 3.2	Hollander et al.
Atherogenic Diet[b] without Drugs	20.4 ± 1.8^c	53.8 ± 2.0^c	(1974). Circ. Res.
Atherogenic Diet + Colchicine	11.7 ± 3.5	40.6 ± 2.8	34: Suppl. I: 131.
Atherogenic Diet + Penicillamine	13.1 ± 2.1	42.1 ± 3.1	
(absolute amounts in mg/intima-media of whole aorta; mean $\pm$ S.D.)			
Control Diet	11.9 ± 1.5	65.8 ± 3.8	Kramsch and Chan
Atherogenic Diet[b] without Drugs	18.7 ± 2.3^c	92.7 ± 4.3^c	(1975). Presented.
Atherogenic Diet + EHDP[d]	14.3 ± 1.7^e	81.4 ± 3.2^c	Fed. Proc. 34: 235.
Atherogenic Diet + Colcemid	12.6 ± 1.2	68.9 ± 2.1^e	
Atherogenic Diet + Colcemid & EHDP	12.4 ± 1.4	63.0 ± 3.9	

[a]Magnesium salt of EDTA. [b]Peanut oil and cholesterol, 8 weeks. [c]$p < 0.01$ from control values. [d]Ethane-hydroxy-diphosphonate. [e]$p < 0.05$ from control values.

TABLE II. CONTENTS IN ARTERIAL CONNECTIVE TISSUE PROTEINS IN MONKEYS ON CONTROL –, ATHEROGENIC – AND REGRESSION DIETS (Means without SE of the originals).

(Absolute amounts in mg/intima-media of length-defined artery)

Experimental Groups	Coronary		Pulmonary		Thor. Aorta		Abd. Aorta		Authors
	Coll.	Elast.	Coll.	Elast.	Coll.	Elast.	Coll.	Elast.	
Normal	6.10	1.21	13.42	5.81	7.79	15.32	8.98	7.89	Wolinsky et al. (1975) Circ. Res. 36: 553.
Atherosclerotic[a]	7.09[b]	1.49	12.89	5.24	13.91[c]	19.64[c]	12.16[c]	8.44	

(Absolute amounts in mg/cm length of artery as intima-media)

Experimental Groups	Aorta		Carotid		Subclav.		Femoral		Authors
	Coll.	Elast.	Coll.	Elast.	Coll.	Elast.	Coll.	Elast.	
Normal	3.04	6.06	1.51	2.32	1.03	2.14	1.26	0.93	Armstrong and Megan (1975) Circ. Res. 36: 256.
Atherosclerotic[d]	5.83	9.43	4.27	4.16	3.46	4.30	3.53	2.44	
Regression 1	5.19	5.47[f]	4.13	4.04	4.28	3.60[f]	2.82	1.69[f]	
Regression 2	5.07	3.68[f]	4.10	2.84[f]	4.25	2.88[f]	3.02	1.44[f]	
Regression 3	4.89[e]	4.23[f]	2.86[e]	3.22[f]	3.49[e]	3.41[f]	1.80[e]	1.06[f]	

[a]High cholesterol diet for 6-8 months. [b]$p < 0.05$ from control values. [c]$p < 0.01$ from control values. [d]High cholesterol diet for 17 months - followed (Regression 1) by cholesterol-free diet for 60 days, (Regression 2) 200 days and (Regression 3) 20 months. [e]$p < 0.05$ from atherosclerotic group. [f]$p < 0.01$ from atherosclerotic groups.

laboratory in recent studies in rabbits which revealed a markedly increased uptake of intravenously injected radioactive lysine into the lysine - and desmosine residues of elastin from atherosclerotic lesions. It is possible that the doubling of elastica in lesions may result from new formation of elastic tissue (reduplication). On the other hand, the doubling of lesion elastica also may be caused by degradation (splitting). Recent evidence (6) revealed that naturally occurring hydrophobic ligands, such as free fatty acids and bile salts, bind to elastin in vitro, thereby increasing elastolysis by elastase more than 5-fold with linoleic acid being the most effective fatty acid. An increasing content of free fatty acids has been observed in lesion elastin with increasing severity of atherosclerosis (7) which could play a role in stimulating elastica degradation in vivo. Presumably, both processes, degradation and de novo synthesis of elastin also occur simultaneously in atherosclerosis.

The cells responsible for the synthesis of collagen and elastin in arteries appear to be the smooth muscle cells. Tissue cultures of these cells produce cross-linked collagen, the microfibrillar glycoprotein associated with elastin (8), and as recently demonstrated in the laboratory of Franzblau, they also produce cross-linked elastin containing the desmosines. A sensitive method for detecting early increases in collagen synthesis is the determination of increased activity of prolyl hydroxylase, an enzyme which hydroxylates proline to hydroxyproline (9). It is as yet, not definitely known whether the newly synthetized collagen of lesions has the composition characteristic of normal arterial collagen which consists essentially of 3 α 1 (III) chains (type III). However, there is preliminary evidence (10) that in atherosclerotic intima, type I collagen (α 1 $(I)_2$ α 2) may predominate.

Collagen already normally has a marked affinity for lipids which may be structural components of the protein (11). In atherosclerosis, this association appears to be increased with about 8% (12) to 10% (13) of the total cholesterol of human fibrous plaques being contained in the insoluble plaque collagen. Furthermore, collagen from human plaques, but not from adjacent normal intima, appears to have antigenic properties which could represent autoantigenicity (13). Immunoglobulin G (IgG) and A (IgA) as well as complement were extractable with the acid soluble tissue-bound collagen fractions as well as by collagenase. A small amount of the collagen-bound IgG appeared to be synthetized locally in plaques. These studies also indicated that about 16% of the glycosaminoglycans of plaques are firmly bound to the insoluble plaque collagen. Association of glycoproteins with collagen have been postulated (14). Finally, in later stages of atherosclerosis, collagen also may calcify.

The alkali-insoluble elastin of atherosclerotic aortae of rabbits and monkeys (15) as well as of man (15-18) contained markedly increased amounts of polar amino acids, especially in isolated plaques where the abnormality increased with increasing severity of the disease (16). The amino acid composition of normal elastin from normal arteries or normal areas of diseased arteries was essentially similar in adult experimental animals and man. The compositional abnormalities of elastic fiber protein in atherosclerosis may be the result of a close binding of one or more other proteins to the original elastin, such as the microfibrillar glycoprotein normally associated with elastin (19) or the likewise normally closely associated mucopolysaccharide proteins (20-22); they also may include anti-elastin immunoglobulins (23,24) as well as elastase or lysyl oxidase, both of which are known to bind to elastin (25,26). A small protein of these secondary proteins bound to elastin from plaques appears to be collagen (18,15). It is of interest, however, that newly synthetized alkali-insoluble elastin at certain stages of arterial smooth muscle cell cultures was found by Franzblau also to be rich in polar amino acids, reminiscent of the abnormal elastic fiber protein from lesions.

Normal arterial elastin as well as elastin from plaques appears to be a protein-lipid complex (15,16,27,28) with the lipids presumably bound by hydrophobic stacking to hydrophobic sites of the elastin molecule (29). While the lipid moiety of normal arterial elastin was small, it increased progressively (mainly ester cholesterol) with increasing severity of atherosclerosis in the abnormal elastic fiber protein from plaques in man (16) as well as in atherosclerotic rabbits and monkeys (15). In uncomplicated human lesions (fatty streaks and fibrous plaques), about 30% of the total cholesterol was contained in the abnormal elastic fiber protein (16). As indicated by in vitro studies, the prerequisite for the increased binding of lipids appears to be the markedly altered amino acid composition of the plaque "elastin" protein and the mechanism of binding appears to be a transfer, predominantly of ester cholesterol, from serum or arterial LDL and VLDL but not from HDL or chylomicrons to the abnormal protein (12). In vivo binding of radioactive cholesterol to arterial elastin also was demonstrated in man (16) and rats (30,27).

Calcium may play an important role in the binding of other proteins to arterial elastin in lesions, either through calcium bridges or simply by incrustation of the whole elastic fiber, including the associated proteins, with calcium minerals (18). It has been demonstrated that after thorough demineralization of plaque tissue with EDTA, alkali-isolated elastin, even from calcified plaques of old individuals, had the same amino acid composition as normal elastin from young individuals whereas without demineralization, plaque "elastin" was abnormal (18). In recent studies in our laboratory, the calcium mineral content of the abnormal "elastin" preparation of lesions was shown to increase drastically with increasing severity of atherosclerosis regardless of age. In contrast, the calcium mineral content of elastin from normal aortic intima increased with age only in small increments with minor increases in polar amino acids and insignificant changes in lipid content. The principal target tissue for calcification of arteries in atherosclerosis and aging appears to be the elastica (18,31-34). Mineralization of aortic elastica in preference over collagen also has been demonstrated in vitro (35). The main constituents of the minerals associated with elastins, isolated from normal aorta as well as from plaques, have been shown to be calcium and phosphorus (17,32) which appeared to be present - at least at later stages - in the form of appatite crystals as indicated by x-ray diffraction and electron microscopy (32,33,36). As possible nucleation sites for calcium mineralization of elastic tissue have been proposed the polar matrix proteins associated with elastin (18), the glycosaminoglycans bound to these structural proteins (33, 37) or neutral peptide groups of the elastin itself (38).

TABLE III. CONTENTS IN AORTIC CONNECTIVE TISSUE PROTEINS IN RABBITS ON ATHEROGENIC AND REGRESSION REGIMEN

(Absolute amounts in mg/intima-media of whole aorta; Mean ± S.D.)

Type of Diets	Collagen	"Elastin"
Atherogenic[a]	18.7 ± 2.3	92.7 ± 4.3
Atherogenic, then Control[b] without Drugs	23.7 ± 3.4	124.0 ± 11.5
Atherogenic, then Control + EHDP	16.8 ± 2.1[c]	103.9 ± 12.6
Atherogenic, then Control + Colcemid	14.3 ± 3.3[d]	78.4 ± 4.9[d]
Athero., then Control + EHDP & Colcemid	12.4 ± 1.7[d]	80.0 ± 5.3[d]

[a]Peanut oil + cholesterol, 8 weeks. [b]Normal chow, 8 weeks. [c]$p < 0.05$ from atherogenic values. [d]$p < 0.01$ from atherogenic values.

Alterations of collagen and elastin in atherosclerosis were inhibited partially by MgEDTA and EHDP, substantially by Colcemid and completely suppressed by colchicine, penicillamine and EHDP combined with Colcemid (Table I). Combined EHDP and Colcemid treatment also prevented all alterations of the amino acid -, lipid-and calcium mineral composition of elastin. Partial but significant regression of pre-established connective tissue alterations by diet was achieved in monkeys with the regression for arterial elastin being greater than for collagen (Table II). Regression studies in our laboratory (Table III) confirmed that in rabbits neither collagen nor elastin changes regressed by diet alone but increased further instead. Regression diet combined with drug treatment resulted in rabbits in partial regression of the accumulations of collagen and elastin with MgEDTA (5), of collagen alone with EHDP (Table III) and of both collagen and elastin with Colcemid. Combined treatment with Colcemid and EHDP resulted in complete regression of the alteration of collagen but not of elastin which still revealed marked increases in polar amino acids, cholesterol, and calcium minerals. As indicated by these studies, changes occurring in calcified plaque elastica may be the hardest to reverse once they have been initiated.

REFERENCES

1. Smith, E.B. (1974). Adv. Exp. Med. Biol. 43, 125.
2. Slack, H.G.B. (1954). Nature 174, 512.
3. Lindner, J.P. (1974). In: Atherosclerosis III. Third International Symposium. Schettler, G., and Weizel, A., eds. Springer-Verlag, New York, p. 218.
4. McCullagh, K.G., and Page, I.H. (1974). Ibid, p. 239.
5. Wartman, A., Lampe, T.L., McCann, D.S., and Boyle, A.J. (1967). J. Atheroscler. Res. 7, 331.
6. Jordan, R.E., Hewitt, N., Lewis, W., Kagan, H., and Franzblau, C. (1974). Biochemistry 13, 3497.
7. Jacotot, B. (1974). In: Atherosclerosis III. Third International Symposium. Schettler, G., and Weizel, A., eds. Springer-Verlag, New York, p. 207.
8. Ross, R., and Glomset, A. (1973). Science 180, 1332.
9. Fuller, G.C., and Langner, R.O. (1970). Science 168, 987.
10. McCullagh, K.G. (1975). Presented at the Arterial Wall Workshop, Winston-Salem, N.C., U.S.A.
11. Nikkari, T., and Heikkinnen, E. (1966). Acta Chem. Scand. 22, 3047.
12. Kramsch, D.M., and Hollander, W. (1973). J. Clin. Invest. 52, 236.
13. Hollander, W., Colombo, M.A., Kramsch, D.M., and Kirkpatrick, B. (1974). Adv. Cardiol. 13, 192.
14. Jackson, D.S., and Bentley, J.P. (1968). In: Treatise on Collagen, Vol. IIA. Gould, B.S., ed. Academic Press, New York, p. 189.
15. Kramsch, D.M., Franzblau, C., and Hollander, W. (1974). Adv. Exp. Med. Biol. 43, 193.
16. Kramsch, D.M., Franzblau, C. and Hollander, W. (1971). J. Clin. Invest. 50, 1666.
17. Yu, S.Y. (1971). Lab. Invest. 25, 121.

18. Keeley, F.W., and Partridge, S.M. (1974). Atherosclerosis 19, 287.
19. Ross, R., and Bornstein, P. (1969). J. Cell Biol. 40, 366.
20. Gotte, L., Menegheli, V., and Castellani, A. (1965). In: Structure and Function of Connective and Skeletal Tissue. Fitton-Jackson, S., Harkness, R.D., and Tristram, G.R., eds. Butterworths, London, p. 93.
21. John, R., and Thomas, J. (1972). Biochem. J. 127, 261.
22. Moczar, M., and Robert, L. (1970). Atherosclerosis 11, 7.
23. Mandl, I., Keller, S., and Levi, M. (1970). In: Chemistry and Molecular Biology of the Intercellular Matrix. Balasz, E., ed. Academic Press, New York, 1, 657.
24. Robert, A.M., Grosgogeat, Y., Reverdy, V., Robert, B., and Robert, L. (1971). Atherosclerosis 13, 427.
25. Gertler, A. (1971). Eur. J. Biochem. 20, 541.
26. Kagan, H.M., Hewitt, N.A., Salcedo, L.L., and Franzblau, C. (1974). Biochim. Biophys. Acta 365, 223.
27. Szigeti, M., Monnier, G., Jacotot, B., and Robert, L. (1972). Conn. Tissue Res. 1, 145.
28. Robert, L., Robert, B., and Robert, A.M. (1972). Exp. Ann. Biochim. Med. 31, 111.
29. Jacotot, B., Beaumont, J.L., Monnier, G., Szigeti, M., Robert, B., and Robert L. (1973). Nutr. Metabol. 15, 46.
30. Jacotot, B., Monnier, G., and Beaumont, J.L. (1971). Clin. Chim. Acta 33, 95.
31. Lansing, A.I., Alex, M., and Rosenthal, T.B. (1950). J. Geront. 5, 112.
32. Yu, S.Y., and Blumenthal, H.T. (1963). J. Geront. 18, 119.
33. Weissman, G., and Weissmann, S. (1960). J. Clin. Invest. 39, 1657.
34. Haust, D., and Geer, J.C. (1970). Amer. J. Pathol. 60, 329.
35. Bladen, H.A., and Martin, G.R. (1962). Fifth International Congress on Electron Microscopy. Academic Press, New York, p. QQ-5.
36. Serafini-Fracassini, A. (1963). J. Atheroscler. Res. 3, 178.
37. Yu, S.Y., and Blumenthal, H.T. (1963). J. Geront. 18, 127.
38. Urry, D.W., Cunningham, W.D., and Ohniski, T. (1973). Biochim. Biophys. Acta 292, 853.

(7)

GLYCOSAMINOGLYCANS IN ATHEROSCLEROTIC LESIONS

J. Lindner

Department of Pathology, University of Hamburg

Hamburg, Germany

The increase of metachromasia and of metachromatic material in atherosclerotic lesions was first described by Virchow (1856), first chemically analysed and identified as "chondroitin sulfate" by Mörner (1895) and demonstrated by ever improving stains in the past 65 years. However the best histochemical methods can neither quantify nor specify the several acid glycosaminoglycans (GAG) respectively mucopolysaccharides (MPS) (review: Lindner, 1969, 1974; Velican, 1974). The increased intensities of GAG stains may depend on increased GAG content (or concentration) in the vascular wall, but also on alterations of the chemical composition, the pattern, polymerisation and sulfation range of the GAG, furthermore on the macromolecular structure, organisation and interactions of the proteoglycans especially in the case of decomposition, degradation and decrease of the binding of proteoglycans and GAG to proteins, lipoproteins, phospholipids and other macromolecules (see below). In that case more anionic groups of the GAG become available for reactions with cationic stains (Lindner et al., 1967; Lindner, 1969). The increased intensity of GAG stains is correlated sometimes with increased GAG breakdown, localized histochemically, for example by indicator enzymes like β-glucuronidase, with enhanced activities quantified by biochemical analysis (especially in early lesions), like hexosaminidase and other key enzymes of GAG degradation (Buddecke and Kresse, 1969; Platt, 1969; Lindner, 1974). The increased intensity of GAG stains is often correlated with the enhanced ^{35}S-sulfate incorporation localized in autoradiographs - in and around smooth muscle cells, especially quantified by measurements of the incorporation rates with or without fractionation of sulfated (and nonsulfated) GAG fractions, by assays of their specific activites and half life times, using a TRI-CARB scintillation counter, for assays of double labelled materials (for GAG fractionations or parallel assays of GAG and other structured macromolecules like collagen) using the TRI-CARB sample oxidizer (306/Packard). The increased ^{35}S-sulfate incorporation is proof of enhanced acid GAG synthesis and correlated with increased specific activities and with enhanced turnover rates of sulfated GAG (Lindner et al., 1967; Hauss et al., 1968; Lindner, 1969). These anabolic processes of GAG metabolism are enhanced more in earlier than in progressive atherosclerotic lesions, are higher in the intima than in the media, and highest in fresh oedema plaques in every age group, running parallel to the content of serum components (see below) and decreasing with aging; the above statements are based on the observations of the author and other investigators. The correlation between enhanced GAG synthesis and the increased concentration of serum proteins (including lipoproteins and fibrinogen), analysed and identified by quantitative biochemical, immunological and immunochemical methods, seems to be very important for the atherogenesis: the morphologic equivalent, the well known arterial fresh oedematous plaques, i.e., the vascular oedema, are the first unspecific histologic reactions of the disturbed GAG metabolism after injury to the arterial wall by several unspecific and more specific (atherogenic) factors. Potential atherosclerotic lesions begin with alterations which can be shown 1. only by biochemical methods and can be followed 2. by morphologically demonstrable reactions and alterations (Lindner et al., 1967). The GAG metabolism of the arterial wall shows the first, immediate and most sensitive reaction to any irritation, influence, injury, etc. (Lindner, 1969). It seems that the initial part of this first reaction of the disturbed GAG metabolism is an enhanced catabolism, (with a significant increase of the activities of the responsible GAG resp. proteoglycan degrading enzymes); this is followed immediately by an increased synthesis of GAG. First, their concentration can be reduced and then enhanced resp. regulated at a steady state (changing physiological equilibrium). Later on - in progressive lesions after some repetitions of injuries resp. atherosclerotic events - both processes are reduced, finally the catabolic more than the anabolic one. The total content of GAG can be enhanced, reduced or corresponding to unchanged arterial parts of the same age (related to the dry weight, the DNA-content, etc.) (Lindner, 1974, 1975). As vascular alterations in aging can be (in addition) combined with atherosclerotic alterations it is shown, that synthesis, breakdown, total content and turnover of GAG mainly decrease and their biological half life times increase with arterial aging - related to dry weight or DNA resp. cell content (Lindner, 1975). This typical arterial GAG pattern is largely unchanged in human aging - as far as we know (that means the relation of chondroitin-4-sulfate (C-4-S), hyaluronic acid (HA), heparan sulfate (HS), dermatan sulfate (DS) = 50:29:12:9). The highest turnover rate is found for HA, decreasing in the order DS, HS and CS (Kresse and Buddecke, 1976). This normal metabolic heterogeneity changes in the increased GAG metabolism in early and (less) in progressive atherosclerotic lesions - until to the enhanced total content of acid GAG in the early lesions, to some similarities of progressive lesions with aging, etc. Also the keratan sulfate content increases with this metabolic heterogeneity and with the hybridisation of the proteoglycans in vascular aging. The results about alterations of the GAG patterns in the several atherosclerosis stages are differently and insufficiently analysed, especially because they are (in addition) combined with aging and different in the several arterial layers. Thus, in this summarizing report, one can say only that synthesis, degradation, total content and turnover of these vascular GAG increase in early and decrease in progressive atherosclerotic lesions, whereas the half life times of these GAG are shortened resp. retarded in these phases. The regulation and control mechanisms of the arterial GAG metabolism are manyfold and have been only partly clarified. The arterial smooth muscle cells are responsible for these GAG metabolic processes (as for the metabolism of collagenand elastin) in physiological as well as in pathological conditions. In that case of enhanced metabolism the smooth muscle cells show an increase of the common cytological equivalents (ribosomes, rough ER, Golgi apparatus, secretory vacuoles, mitochondria) and a decrease of their characteristics (myofilaments, dense bodies, basement membranes, pinocytosic vesicles). These cells become modified smooth muscle cells (Haust et al., 1960; Lindner et al., 1967; Wissler, 1968; Lindner, 1969, 1974, 1975). Their first reaction to any injury is the increased GAG turnover (esp. synthesis), followed by an enchanced collagen turnover, whereas elastin is degraded but not resynthesized after severe injuries. The GAG metabolism has the key position in atherogenesis (Lindner et al., 1967; Hauss et al., 1968; Lindner, 1969, 1974). The GAG are responsible for important functions of arteries: exchange, transport, filtration (sieve effect), binding, etc., of water, ions, electrolytes as well as of micro-and macromolecular substances of the smooth muscle cell metabolism (the so-called "trapping" of serum proteins and lipoproteins included), primary interactions of various GAG. resp. proteoglycans (esp. HA is responsible for the proteoglycan aggregates: Hardingham and Muir, 1974), secondary and tertiary interactions and formations of proteoglycan aggregates with collagen, elastin, noncollagen proteins, lipoproteins, glycoproteins, etc., finally producing long-range ordered structures and networks, which can be demonstrated by special electron-, polarisation-, and later on also by light microscopic methods, and are responsible for the physiological function, homeostasis and biorheology of arteries (Lindner, 1969, 1974, 1975; Velican, 1974). Thus, there results a hierarchical order of structures which is disturbed and changed reversibly at the beginning, and more irreversible in the further development of atheroslcerosis. These processes develop with and without primary and secondary actions of the smooth muscle cells (Hauss et al., 1968;

Lindner, 1969, 1974, 1975; Velican, 1974). It requires much more clarification of the relationship of this macromolecular structure of the so-called (but not) amorphous ground substance of arterial walls to their function under the range of physiological and pathological conditions, especially in atherosclerosis (always regarding the differences depending on sex, age, localisation, etc., also). In summary it appears that the GAG metabolism (synthesis, breakdown, turnover rates) 1. is increased in atherosclerosis: a) in early lesions (of any age group), b) at the same time (but less) in morphologically unchanged vessel parts (= the whole arterial system is diseased) (review: Hauss et al., 1968; Lindner, 1969, 1974), and c) partly also in other connective tissues (=unspecific coreaction; atherosclerosis is a generalized connective tissue disease, at first demonstrable by the increased GAG metabolism: Hauss et al., 1968; Lindner, 1969); 2. is correlated - as primary process - to the secondary disturbed resp. diseased collagen-, elastin-, lipid-, coagulation-metabolism, and 3. is therefore at first responsible for the intimal and following medial hyperplasia resp. hypertrophy as well as for the further lesions and stages of the whole disease: atherosclerosis !

References

Buddecke, E., Kresse, H.: Angiologica 6, 89 (1969).
Hardingham, T.E. and Muir, H.: Biochem. J. 139, 565 (1974).
Hauss, W.H., Junge-Hülsing, G. and Gerlach, K.: Die unspezifische Mesenchymreaktion. Thieme: Stuttgart 1968.
Haust, M.D., More, R.H. and Movat, H.Z.: Am. J. Path. 37, 377, (1960).
Kresse, H., and Buddecke, E.: Hoppe-Seylers Z. physiol. Chem. 351 151 (1970).
Lindner, J., Gries, G., Freytag, G. and Kind, J.: Verh. dtsch. Ges. Path. 51, 228 (1967).
Lindner, J.: The histochemistry of atherosclerosis. In: Schettler, F.G. and Boyd, G.S.: Atherosclerosis, p. 73. Elsevier: Amsterdam 1969.
Lindner, J.: Histochemie der Arterienwand. In: Heberer, G., Rau, G. and Schoop, W.: Angiologie, 2.Ed., p. 103. Thieme: Stuttgart 1974.
Lindner, J.: Verh. dtsch. Ges. Path. 59, 181 (1975).
Mörner, K.T.: Z. physiol. Chem. 20, 357 (1895).
Platt, D.: Med. Klin. 64, 1261 (1969).
Velican, C.: Macromolecular changes in atherosclerosis. In: Graumann, W. and Neumann, K.: Handbuch der Histochemie, Vol. VIII/2. Fischer: Stuttgart 1974.
Virchow, R.: Phlogose und Thrombose im Gefäß-system. In: Ges. Abh. Wiss. Med., p. 458. Hirsch: Berlin 1856.
Wissler, R.W.: J. Atheroscler. Res. 8, 201 (1968).

(8)
THE MODE OF CALCIFICATION IN ATHEROSCLEROTIC LESIONS

Wladimir W. Meyer

Institute of Pathology, University of Mainz

65 Mainz 1, Langenbeckstrasse 1, West Germany

Calcific deposits in atherosclerotic plaques are usually considered to be an end stage of advanced atheroma formation. Postmortem studies of coronary arteries showed that pronounced atherosclerotic calcifications are strongly associated with stenosis of the involved segments and ischemic myocardial lesions (Eggen et al. 1965; McCarthy and Palmer 1974). A close correlation has also been found between calcific lesions detected by fluoroscopy or cinefluorography and clinical coronary artery disease (Oliver et al. 1964; Wartburton et al. 1968). Therefore, arterial calcification detected during life may be of important prognostic significance. Moreover, larger calcific plaques may influence the further development of atherosclerotic lesions and be, therefore, of a considerable pathogenetic interest.

POSSIBLE LOCAL FACTORS OF ATHEROSCLEROTIC CALCIFICATION

It is the present consensus of opinion that calcific deposits represent a secondary phenomenon of some focal degenerative changes associated with progressive lipid deposition, for instance, necrosis or hemorrhage. However, extensive areas of the atheromatous necrosis and hemorrhagic infiltration are often seen without any sign of calcification. On the other hand, in numerous atherosclerotic plaques showing pronounced calcification the necrosis and hemorrhage cannot be identified and the exact cause of calcific deposits, i.e., the nature of changes which precede and result in massive incrustation remains obscure. Blankenhorn (1964) estimated that precipitating cause of calcification is evident in only 2o per cent of all atherosclerotic plaques containing calcific deposits.

The electron microscopic studies of Yu and Blumenthal (1963) and Yu (1974) showed that calcium crystallites initially appear between the elastic fibers or membranes, on their surface or in their outer layer as well as in collagen. X-ray diffraction analyses identified the calcific deposits in the arterial wall as apatite. (Serafini-Fracassani, 1963; Yu,1974). This finding accords with chemical analyses showing a Ca/P-relation in apatite (Yu,1974). No definite ultrastructural changes in elastin were evident prior to calcification. However, some findings seem to support the concept that acid mucopolysaccharide which cover the elastic laminae and fibers may be involved in the calcifying process (Yu, 1974). In a departure from "Kalkfänger" hypothesis which suggested the binding of calcium by acid radicals formed within the tissue Urry (1971, 1974) proposed that neutral sites in the protein matrix could function as sites for the selective binding of calcium ion in the initial step leading to calcification.

Different amino acid composition of the elastin formed in the atherosclerotic lesions as compared with normal elastin has often been discussed as a factor increasing the affinity for calcium of diseased or aging arterial wall (Yu and Blumenthal, 1963; Kramsch et al., 1971; Keely and Partridge, 1974). Yu (1974) showed that after injections of ^{45}Ca, the isotope uptake in vivo by aortic elastin is greater in epinephrine injected animals than in normal controls pointing to some undefined biochemical changes of elastin occuring in treated animals. Blankenhorn (1964) suggested that some general metabolic factors may favor both calcific deposits in atherosclerotic lesions and so-called diffuse medial calcification which has been known since the classical studies of Faber (1912) and Blumenthal et al. (1944).

Thus, the biochemical mechanisms involved in the initiation of calcium deposition are still not exactly known, and the morphological substrates preceding deposition of calcium in atherosclerotic plaques remain to be elucidated. Even the natural history of calcification in the individual arterial provinces is still not known in all details.

PATTERNS OF PRIMARY AND SECONDARY CALCIFICATIONS

A dual simultaneous staining of calcific and lipid deposits (Meyer, 1974) shows that in several arterial provinces, atherosclerosis and atherosclerotic calcifications are regularly preceded by another kind of calcification which appears in a seemingly unchanged arterial wall and is initially confined to distinct normal preformed structures. For this reason, on gross examination with the von Kossa reaction these primary calcifications often have peculiar regular patterns which are closely related to some normal structural features. For example gaps in the internal elastic membrane that otherwise are imperceptible grossly become clearly outlined along the arterial luminal surface by pairs of black-stained calcific bands. (Meyer and Stelzig 1967, 1969A, 1969B, Meyer, 1971). In contrast, the atherosclerotic, secondary calcifications are not bound to differentiated normal structures and, therefore, appear irregularly distributed along the arterial wall. In earlier stages, the microradiographs suggest a simultaneous multifocal development of the grain-like deposits in circular areas of the thickened intima (Figure 1).

ASSOCIATION OF PRIMARY CALCIFICATIONS WITH ATHEROSCLEROTIC LESIONS

In several arterial segments not only secondary, i.e., atherosclerotic calcific deposits, but also primary calcifications regularly appear at the predilection sites of atherosclerotic lesions. In the thoracic descending aorta, for instance, primary calcification of the media, seen grossly as a grayish staining after the von Kossa reaction predominantly develops in the dorsal aortic wall which also represents the predilection site of fatty streaking (Fig. 2A and 2B). Microscopically, the calcific and lipid deposits show a different histotopographic distribution, the calcification being predominantly localized in the internal layer of the media, whereas the lipid deposits are initially confined to the thickened intima (Figure 3).

A similar relationship is often present in the trunk of the common carotid artery. A grayish strip of "diffuse" calcification can be seen after the gross von Kossa reaction along the antero-medial wall of this artery (Figure 4A). It has a triangular shape and extends over appoximately the same area as do the lipid deposits that regularly early develop in this artery (Figure 4B) (Meyer and Noll, 1974). However, like in the aorta, the histotopographic distribution of both lesions is different. The granular and lamellar calcifications predominantly appear in the inner media whereas the lipids initially accumulate in the thickened intima. Since the calcific deposits develop not only in the media immediately subjacent to lipid deposits, but also often extend far beyond the

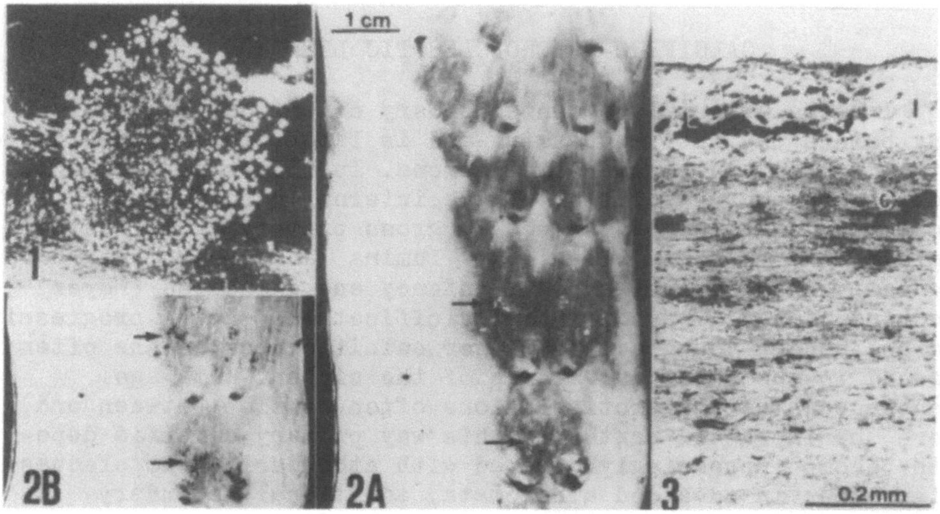

Fig. 1. Microradiograph of the femoral artery from a 58-year-old man showing grain-like calcific deposits in a circular area of an atherosclerotic lesion.
Fig. 2A. Pronounced medial calcification of the dorsal aortic wall seen as grayish staining after the von Kossa reaction. Small lipid deposits (arrows) are confined to the same area. Thoracic aorta from a 37-year-old man.
Fig. 2B. The lower part of the same aortic segment after subsequent gross lipid staining with Fettrot 7B. The small lipid deposits are now seen as black scattered lesions (arrows).
Fig. 3. Microscopic section of the aorta shown in Fig. 2B. The lipid deposits (L) are confined to the thickened intima (I), whereas the calcifications (C) are predominantly localized in the inner half of the media. Von Kossa reaction and Fettrot 7B stain.

areas of fatty streaking, medial calcification cannot be regarded as the consequence of intimal lipidosis. Nor can lipid deposition be interpreted as the sequel to calcification, even in the portions of the arterial wall where calcific deposits appear earlier than fatty streaking. At least in the initial stages, both lesions probably represent independent processes. However, their appearance at the same sites strongly suggests that a common factor, e.g., a higher hemodynamic load may be involved which might induce the development of both calcific and lipid deposits.

PRIMARY AND SECONDARY CALCIFICATIONS IN THE ADVANCED CALCIFERO-ATHEROSCLEROTIC LESIONS

In some arterial segments primary calcification develops long before the fatty streaking and is later closely associated with advanced atherosclerotic lesions. In the carotid siphon, i.e., in the curved portion of the internal carotid artery located at the base of the scull, gross primary calcifications limited to the internal elastic lamina and inner media have regularly been demonstrated in infancy and childhood (Meyer and Lind, 1972). These primary calcifications show a progressive course, and in young adults larger calcific plaques are often present in the upper curvatures of the siphon. With age, pronounced atherosclerotic lesions often develop between and above the incrusted parts. In this way primary calcific deposits become increasingly covered with atherosclerotic plaques (Figure 5). In advanced atheromata, additional secondary deposition of calcium may develop in the disintegrating intima. Then compound lesions appear in the siphon which are characterized by close association and overlapping of calcific in-

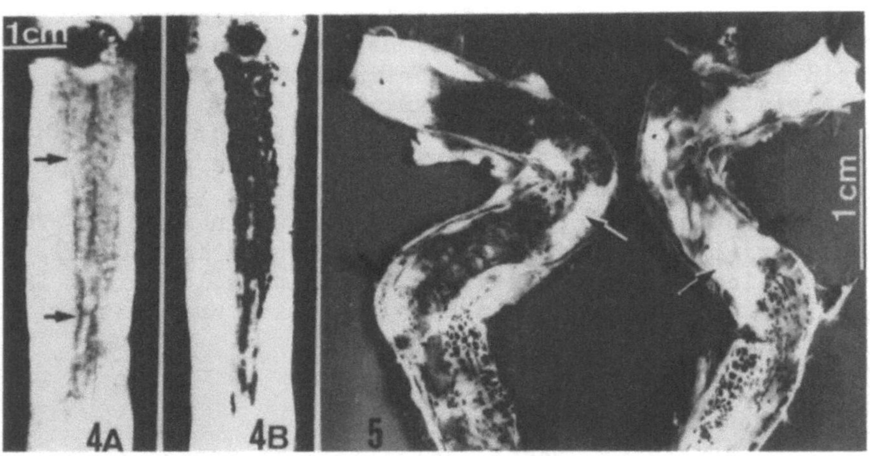

Fig. 4A. and 4B. 4A.- A grayish strip of medial calcification (arrows) is seen after the von Kossa reaction at the anteromedial wall of the common carotid artery from a 36-year-old man. It extends over appoximately the same area as do the lipid deposits seen in Figure 4B after subsequent gross lipid staining. Fig. 5. Extensive primary calcifications (black) are seen in both halfs of the longitudinally opened carotid siphon from a 32-year-old man who died after myocardial infarction. In many areas the primary calcific deposits are covered by advanced atherosclerotic plaques (arrows). Von Kossa reaction.

crustations, lipidosis and atherosclerosis. Similar compound calcifero-atherosclerotic lesions regularly occur at the carotid bifurcation.

Additional pathogenetic factors may arise from the co-existence and interaction of the initially independent lipidosis and calcinosis, and influence the further progression of these complex arterial lesions. Combining cholesterol feeding of rabbits with hypervitaminosis D, Hass et al. (1961) observed rapid and selective accumulation of lipids in the proliferating intima overlying the medial calcific deposits. With the permutation of the vitamin D - induced medial calcification and cholesterol-induced atherosclerosis not only synergistic but also antagonistic relations between both lesions became apparent (Harrison, 1933; Hass et al., 1961). Similar relations between calcific plaques and lipidosis may also be present in human arteries. In Mönckeberg's sclerosis, grooves that are formed above the calcific deposits often become filled with proliferating intima which may then level the deformation. Hemodynamic factors are probably involved in this activation of the intimal mesenchyme. In cases of diabetes, the proliferated intima accumulates large amounts of lipid and may, therefore, become the starting point for later atherosclerotic lesions. In contrast, above the large calcific plaques that appear in the atherosclerotic lesions and extend near the lumen, there is often only a thin layer of lipid infiltrated intima. The spreading calcific incrustation obviously results in extinction of the intimal cell population and, moreover, acts as a barrier preventing immigration of muscular cells from the deeper parts of the arterial wall.

SUMMARY

In several arterial provinces, atherosclerosis and atherosclerotic calcifications are preceded by primary calcifications which develop in a seemingly unchanged arterial wall and often show regular gross patterns. In contrast, secondary calcifications which appear in the atherosclerotic lesions are irregularly distributed along the thickened atherosclerotic intima. At the predilection sites of atherosclerotic lesions, pronounced primary calcifications often precede the fatty streaking representing an independent pathological process. The deformation of the arterial wall resulting from calcific plaques may favor the activation of intimal mesenchyme and contribute to increased accumulation of lipid above and around calcific deposits. The exact nature of structural and biochemical changes which precede and result in primary and secondary arterial calcification still remains obscure.

REFERENCES

BLANKENHORN, P.H., J.Atheroscler. Res. 4: 313, 1964.
BLUMENTHAL, H.T. et al., Am. J. Path. 2o: 665, 1944.
EGGEN, D.A. et al., Circulation, 32: 948, 1965.
FABER, A., Die Arteriosklerose. Jena, G. FISCHER, 1912.
HARRISON, C.U., J.Path. Bact. 36: 447, 1933.
HASS, G. M. et al., Am. J. Path. 38: 289, 1961.
HASS, G. M., In: Cowdry's Arteriosclerosis, ed. H.T.BLUMENTHAL. Ch.C. THOMAS, Springfield, Ill., 1967, p.p. 698.
KEELY, F.W. and PARTRIDGE, S.M., Atherosclerosis, 19: 287, 1974.
KRAMSCH, D.M., FRANZBLAU, C. and HOLLANDER, W., J.Clin.Invest. 5o: 1666, 1971.
McCARTHY, I.H . and PALMER, F.J., Brit.Heart J., 36: 499, 1974.
MEYER, W.W., Comment in: The Artery and the Process of Arteriosclerosis, S. WOLF, ed., Plenum Press, New-York-London, 1971, p.p. 15-21 and 36-42.
MEYER, W.W., IXth. Intern. Congress of Angiology, Florence, April 1974 (in press).
MEYER, W.W. and LIND, J., Arch. Dis. Childh. 47: 355, 1972.
MEYER, W.W. and NOLL, M., Artery 1: 31, 1974.
MEYER, W.W. and STELZIG, H.H., Virchows Archiv 342: 361, 1967.
MEYER, W.W. and STELZIG, H.H., Angiology, 2o: 424, 1969 A.
MEYER, W.W. and STELZIG, H.H., Calc.Tiss. Res. 3: 266, 1969 B.
OLIVER, M.F. et al., LANCET, 1: 1964, p.891.
SERAFINI-FRACASSINI, A., J. Atheroscl. Res. 3: 178, 1963.
WARTBURTON, R.K. et al., Radiology 91: 1o9 1968.
URRY, D.W., Proc. Nat. Acad. Sci. USA. 68: 81o, 1971.
URRY, D.W., Perspectives in Biol.Med., 18: 68, 1974
YU, S.Y., In: Arterial Mesenchyme and Arteriosclerosis. Ed. W.D. WAGNER and Th.B. CLARKSON, 425, Plenum Press, New York and London, 1974, p.p. 4o3.
YU, S.Y. and BLUMENTHAL, H.T., J. Geront. 18: 127, 1963.

(9)

ROLE OF ARTERIAL LIPOPROTEINS IN THE FORMATION OF THE FIBROUS PLAQUE

W. Hollander

Boston University Medical Center

Boston, U. S. A.

Previous studies from our laboratory (1, 2) have indicated that the lipoproteins contained in the human atherosclerotic plaque are extractable into saline and have biochemical properties which are similar to those of the serum lipoproteins except for very low density lipoproteins (VLDL). The major lipid component of arterial VLDL appears to be cholesterol ester as opposed to triglycerides for serum VLDL. It also was found that the saline extractable content of VLDL and LDL (low density lipoproteins) in atherosclerotic vessels was much higher than that of the normal intima and increased with increasing severity of atherosclerosis (Table 1). On the other hand, the high density lipoprotein (HDL) content of the arterial intima was small and did not appear to change with the progression of atherosclerosis. Of the total lipids contained in the diseased intima about 35 to 40% appeared to be extractable into saline (1.65 M NaCl) and recoverable as lipoproteins.

Recent studies from our laboratory suggest that the arterial lipids which are not extractable by saline may be bound as lipoproteins to the acid mucopolysaccharides (AMPS) and fibrous proteins contained in the plaque (3). Most of the lipids bound in the human intima appear releasable by enzymatic digestion of the tissue and recoverable as lipoproteins following separation by differential density ultracentrifugation. It is estimated from the initial findings that of the total lipoproteins isolated from the plaque about 35 to 45% is extractable into 1.65 M NaCl; 15 to 20% of the lipoproteins appear to be released following collagenase digestion and another 20 to 25% following elastase treatment. The final treatment with chondroitinase A, B and C appears to release about 15% of the lipoproteins recovered from the arterial wall.

Table 1

CONCENTRATION OF SALINE EXTRACTABLE LIPOPROTEINS ISOLATED FROM THE HUMAN ATHEROSCLEROTIC INTIMA

mg/gdt

	VLDL (d < 1.006)	LDL (d 1.006-1.063)	HDL (d 1.063-1.210)
Normal intima	7.2 ± 2.1	9.4 ± 2.3	7.0 ± 1.7
Athero-sclerotic intima	37.5 ± 5.3	44.2 ± 6.8	7.1 ± 2.4

Chemical analyses of the ultracentrifugally isolated arterial lipoprotein fractions have shown that they contain small amounts of AMPS and calcium in addition to having a characteristic protein and lipid composition (Table 2). The LDL and VLDL preparations also appear to react immunochemically with LDL antisera. Further studies are being conducted to characterize completely the protein, lipid and AMPS compostion of the isolated lipoprotein fractions.

The close association of AMPS with the arterial lipoproteins also has been demonstrated by electrophoresis. The electrophoretic behavior of LDL released from the plaque by elastase treatment of the tissue is illustrated in figure 1. When LDL was released from the plaque by enzymatic treatment and then isolated in the ultra-

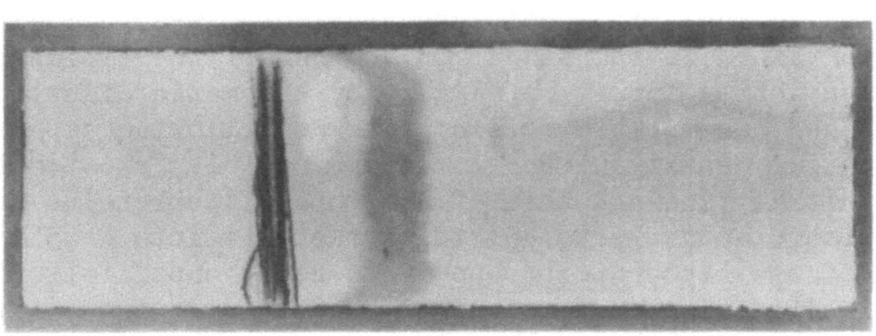

Figure 1

Table 2

COMPOSITION OF ARTERIAL LDL FROM A FIBROUS PLAQUE

	Protein mg/gdt	Cholesterol mg/gdt	AMPS (Uronic Acid) µg/gdt	Calcium µg/gdt
Saline Extractable	8.0	18.6	237	202
Collagenase Releasable LDL	3.3	7.1	182	184
Elastase Releasable LDL	4.2	9.2	195	201
Chondroitinase Releasable LDL	2.8	6.0	-	-

centrifuge and electrophoresed on cellulose acetate at pH 8.6 it showed a migrating beta band which stained for lipid and protein and a non-migrating band which stained not only for lipid and protein but also for AMPS with alcian blue (figure 1). This non-migrating band is also present in arterial VLDL and could represent an aggregated complex of lipoprotein and AMPS. Some of the highly concentrated lipoprotein preparations also showed migrating as well as non-migrating AMPS bands. However when these preparations were electrophoresed at pH 3.2 which is optimum for AMPS, the AMPS did not migrate but remained at the origin along with the lipoproteins. These findings suggest that the interaction of lipoproteins and AMPS in the arteries may be influenced by pH.

The electrophoretic and chemical behavior of the enzymatically released lipoproteins appear to be similar to that of the saline extractable lipoproteins. These lipoproteins appear to contain aggregated and non-aggregated lipoproteins as revealed by their electron microscopic appearance as well as by their electrophoretic, immunochemical, chromatographic and ultracentrifugal behavior (4). When saline-extractable arterial LDL was examined by gel filtration on Biogel A-150, it gave two peaks. Fraction 1 appeared to contain aggregated lipoprotein with an apparent molecular weight of over 30 million while fraction 2 contained non-aggregated lipoprotein with properties resembling those of serum LDL. The protein, lipid and apoprotein composition of both fractions appeared about the same. However small amounts of AMPS and calcium were detectable in fraction 1 but were not found in fraction 2. Arterial VLDL which appeared to be almost completely aggregated also contained small quantities of AMPS and calcium similar to those shown for arterial LDL in table 2. These studies suggest that the aggregation of arterial LDL and VLDL may involve an interaction with AMPS and calcium. They also are consistent with the earlier work of Srinivasan and co-workers who have extracted atherosclerotic lesions with 0.15 M NaCl and have reported the presence of lipoprotein-AMPS complexes in the ultracentrifugally isolated fractions (5).

Studies have been initiated to determine the role of the apolipoproteins in the formation of lipoprotein-AMPS complexes. In these studies serum lipoproteins (LDL and VLDL) were precipitated with heparin (2 mg/ml) and Mn^{2+} (2.7 mg/ml). Following delipidation with alcohol-ether and solubilization with 100 mm SDS the complexes were analyzed by Sephadex G-150 chromatography (figure 2). Three fractions were isolated from the column and had elution volumes corresponding to apoB, apoA and apoC. The first fraction (SF-1) was immunochemically identified as apoB whereas the identity of the other 2 fractions (SF-2, SF-3) were not established. Large amounts of heparin eluted with the apoB fraction with negligible amounts being eluted with the other fractions. These findings suggest that apoB may be the major apoprotein with which AMPS interact.

The lipoproteins contained in the arteries, including those that are closely associated with the AMPS and fibrous proteins, appear to be derived at least in part from the synthesis of lipoproteins in the arterial wall (1, 6). In Table 3 is shown the incorporation of ^{14}C-acetate and ^{3}H-leucine into lipoproteins isolated from the human atherosclerotic plaque following treatment with saline, collagenase, elastase and chondroitinase A, B and C. Both the protein and lipid components of the ultracentrifugally isolated lipoproteins were radioactively labeled following incubation of the intima with the labeled substrates. The distribution of radioactivity appeared to be similar to that of the lipoproteins contained in the intima with the saline extractable lipoproteins containing the greatest amount of radioactivity.

Figure 3 illustrates the incorporation of ^{3}H-leucine into apoB and C of saline extractable VLDL following acrylamine electrophoresis in 10% gels of the chromatographically separated apoproteins. ApoB showed a characteristic single band which appeared to contain more than 90% of the ^{3}H-radioactivity. ApoC showed 4 characteristic peptide bands all of which appeared to contain ^{3}H radioactivity.

Table 3

THE INCORPORATION OF ^{14}C-ACETATE AND ^{3}H-LEUCINE INTO VLDL, LDL AND HDL ISOLATED FROM THE HUMAN ATHEROSCLEROTIC PLAQUE FOLLOWING TREATMENT WITH SALINE, COLLAGENASE, ELASTASE AND CHONDROITINASE A, B AND C.

CPM/gdt x 100

	Saline		Collagenase		Elastase		Chondroitinase	
	Protein	Lipid	Protein	Lipid	Protein	Lipid	Protein	Lipid
VLDL ($d<1.006$)	76±12	107±19	32±6	25±5	22±4	32±6	19±4	21±5
LDL (d 1.063-1.006)	199±24	243±32	23±5	24±4	51±9	33±6	22±5	27±6
HDL (d 1.210-1.063)	54±10	81±14	26±6	26±6	54±10	38±8	17±3	28±5

Work in progress also indicates that the lipoproteins which move from plasma into the arterial wall have a distribution which is much like that of the newly synthesized lipoproteins (7). In these studies, the distribution of ^{125}I-radio-activity in the atherosclerotic aorta of the cynomolgus monkey was determined at 24 hours following the intravenous administration of ^{125}I-labeled serum LDL. Approximately 55% of the radioactivity in the arterial wall was extractable into saline (1.65 M NaCl) with 30% being isolated as LDL and 25% as degraded apoprotein. Of the 45% of the labeled LDL which was not saline extractable almost all was released following sequential treatment of the arterial tissue with collagenase, elastase and chondroitinase.

SUMMARY

The lipids contained in the atherosclerotic plaque appear to accumulate in the lesion as low density and very low density lipoproteins. Studies on the extractability of arterial lipoproteins with saline and specific enzymes (collagenase, elastase, chondroitinase) suggest that the plaque may contain at least 3 different

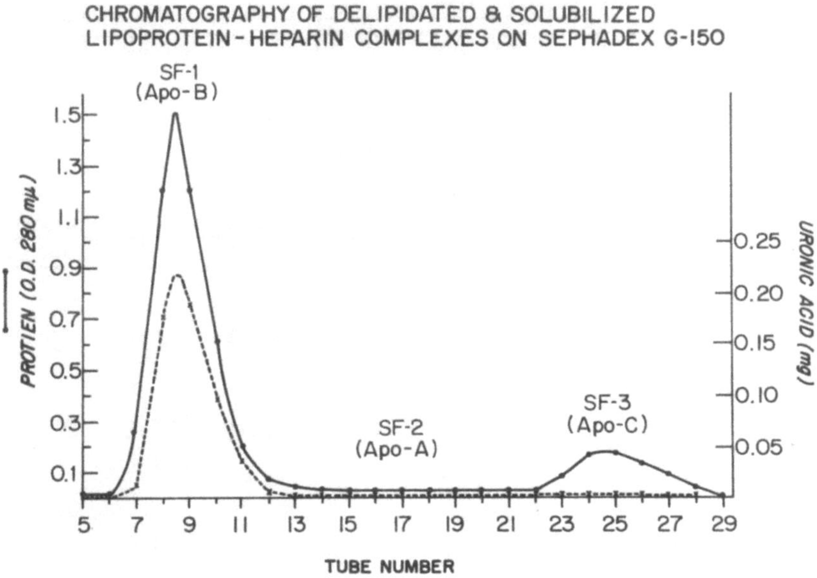

Figure 2

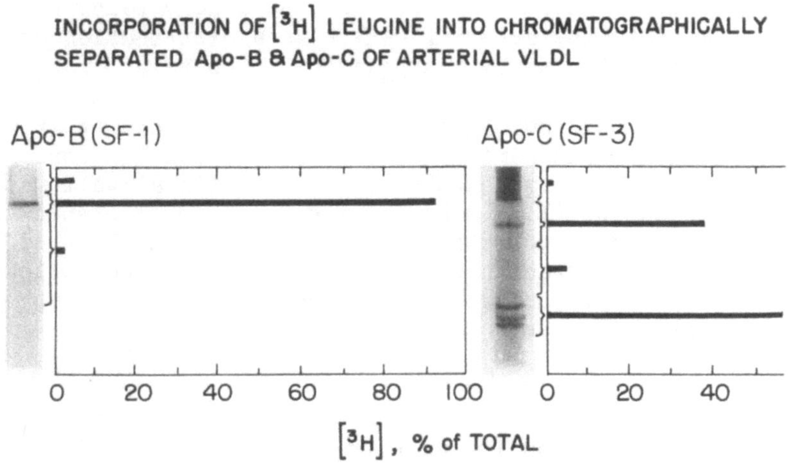

Figure 3

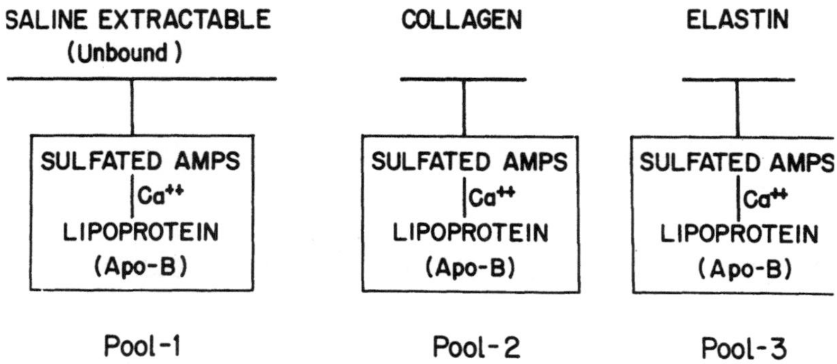

Fig. 4. Lipoprotein distribution in the atherosclerotic plaque.

pools of lipoprotein with each pool consisting of a lipoprotein-acid-mucopolysaccharide calcium complex (figure 4). These pools include a saline extractable or an unbound lipoprotein pool and pools of lipoprotein bound to collagen or elastin. The data reviewed also suggest that the lipoprotein pools may be derived from newly synthesized lipoprotein in the arteries as well as from the plasma lipoproteins which enter the arterial wall. The interaction of LDL and VLDL with AMPS and calcium together with the binding of these complexes to the connective tissue proteins could provide an explanation for the accumulation of lipids, lipoproteins and calcium in the fibrous plaque. The interaction of these macromolecules also could operate as an important determinant of the morphological appearance of the plaque. This interpretation is consistent with histochemical and immunofluorescent studies of atherosclerotic vessels which indicate a close association of lipids and lipoproteins (LDL, apoLDL) with the AMPS and with the elastic and collagen fibers contained in the plaque (8, 9, 10).

REFERENCES

1. Hollander, W. Exper. Mol. Pathol. 7: 248, 1968.
2. Hollander, W. et al. Progr. Biochem. Pharmacol. 4: 270, 1967.
3. Hollander, W. and Paddock. Atherosclerosis, III International Symposium, Springer-Verlag, 1974.
4. Hollander, W. et al. Fed. Proc. 31: 219, 1972.
5. Srinivasan et al. Atherosclerosis 16: 95, 1972.
6. Hollander, W. et al. Proc. III International Symposium, p. 354. Springer-Verlag, New York.
7. Paddock et al. Circulation 50: III-269, 1974.
8. Curran and Crane. J. Pathol. Bact. 84: 405, 1962
9. Walton and Williamson. J Atheroscler. Res. 8: 599, 1968.
10. Hoff et al. Arch. Pathol. 99: 253, 1975.

(10)

DISCUSSION (CONNECTIVE TISSUES IN ATHEROSCLEROTIC LESIONS)

Discussion following Dr. Rauterberg's presentation:

An unidentified Discussor: What is the possible role of prolyl hydroxylase for the regulation of collagen synthesis?
Dr. Rauterberg: In my presentation I referred to experiments with fibroblast cultures; Gribble, Comstock and Udenfriend showed that prolyl hydroxylase is not found during the growth period. During this phase cells make underhydroxylated polypeptide chains which cannot be secreted. When cells become confluent, active PPH appears and collagen secretion starts. It is not clear whether this result applies in some way to the in vivo regulation of collagen secretion.
An unidentified Discussor: What physiological meaning have the carbohydrates which are attached to the collagen molecule?
Dr. Rauterberg: There is no exact knowledge about this. The existence of hydroxylysine deficient collagen in patients with a hereditary collagen disease shows that carbohydrate residues are not, as people believed for a long time, necessary for secretion of collagen from the cell. The occurrence of carbohydrates in some crosslinking compounds may suggest that they determine in some way the properties of crosslinking in collagen.

Discussion following Dr. Robert's presentation:

Dr. Adams (London): What is the type of association between lipids and elastin as lipid stains react with elastic fibers?
Dr. Robert: This can be interpreted as a result of the hydrophobic association of lipids with elastin. There is also an association of proteoglycans with lipoproteins in the intima.
Dr. Zempleny (Los Angeles): What is the role of arterial elastase

in the degradation of elastic tissue?
Dr. Robert: No doubt the discovery of this new elastase in arterial wall by the Creteil team proves the possibility of a locally determined destruction of elastic fibers during the atherosclerotic process and also raises the question of the regulation of the biosynthesis of this enzyme as a function of age and arteriosclerosis.
Dr. Constantinides (Vancouver) discussed the relation between the composition of the arterial wall and the different atherogenic factors and insisted on the importance of acidic mucopolysaccharides. This subject was studied recently by several teams. The role of acid mucopolysaccharides of the intima in the fixation of lipids and lipoproteins was confirmed recently by the New Orleans team of Dr. Berenson, and supports the original hypothesis of GERO and BIHARI-VARGA from Budapest who first demonstrated the complex formation between glycosaminoglycans and lipoproteins as an essential factor in atherogenesis.
Dr. Daria Haust (London) discussed the mechanism of elastogenesis on the basis of recent electron microscopic observations; there is evidence that the micro-fibrillar-structural glycoprotein components and tropoelastin play an important and distinct role during the morphogenetic process of elastogenesis.
Dr. Robert: The observations of Dr. Haust also confirm the importance of the regulation of the relative rate of biosynthesis of these two macromolecular components of intercellular matrix of the vessel wall which was discussed in my presentation.
Dr. Daoud and Dr. Wissler (United States) agreed that correlative studies by both organ culture and cell culture are necessary for the comprehension of the regulatory processes responsible for the biosynthesis of intercellular matrix macromolecules.
Dr. E. Smith (Aberdeen) discussed the compositional aspects of the arterial wall on the basis of her observations made by microtechniques performed on human arterial intima.
Dr. Robert: There appears to be a general consensus on the importance of further efforts to understand the regulation of the biosynthesis and catabolism of intercellular matrix macromolecules as related to the age and arteriosclerosis.

Discussion following Dr. Kramsch's presentation:

Dr. Serge Renaud asked whether in the studies on primary prevention and regression of pre-established atherosclerosis in rabbits the various substances, particularly connective tissue, of the arterial intima and media were expressed per gramm dry tissue or as absolute amounts per intima-media of whole aorta. He pointed out that this distinction was important, since frequently cell proteins, collagen and elastin as well as other arterial wall components increase and decrease in proportion during progression and regression of atherosclerosis, so that on a per gramm dry tissue basis no changes may be discovered as this type of measurement only reflects concentrations

of a particular material but not its actual amounts in a given tissue.
Dr. Kramsch: I agree completely on the importance of this distinction, and our results were expressed in absolute amounts per intima-media of the aorta in rabbits of about equal body weight and age.
Dr. Bjorkerud (Sweden) asked whether the drugs that were used to effect primary prevention and regression of pre-established rabbit atherosclerosis had any side effects endangering the general health of the animals.
Dr. Kramsch: Both drugs used, when given in too large doses, are known to cause serious side effects in men. Ethane-hydroxy-diphosphonate (EHDP) in high doses can cause osteomalacia and Colcemid in high doses can cause agranulocytosis. However, our animals were given doses that in men have not shown any serious side effects (EHDP treatment in myositis ossificans and Colcemid as an anti-tumour agent) and we did not discover any such side effects in our animals, including monkeys.
An unidentified Discussor: Do you believe that focal arterial calcification, especially of the internal elastica, precedes lipid accumulation in a lesion?
Dr. Kramsch: I am not prepared to make such a statement since it would be guesswork on my part; however, Dr. Meyer of Mainz, West-Germany, who is a noted specialist in arterial calcification and its relationship to atherosclerosis, knows much more about this subject than I do and will perhaps talk about it in his presentation.

CHAPTER 13
RECOMMENDATIONS TO THE PUBLIC FOR PREVENTION OF ATHEROSCLEROSIS

(1)

CHOICE OF OBJECTIVES IN ATHEROSCLEROSIS PREVENTION

David Hewitt

Department of Preventive Medicine and Biostatistics

University of Toronto, Toronto, Canada

What is the true value of any recommendation that an expert group, such as yourselves, can make?

Clearly, one limit to the value of such recommendations is set by the theoretical efficacy of the action recommended - and I shall return to this for the second of my two points - but a more confining, and therefore, more critical limit is set by the likelihood that the recommendation will in fact be followed.

Doctors are said to be aware of this limitation as it applies to the recommendations they offer their own patients, and considerable effort is now directed to the study, along scientific lines, of factors that affect "patient compliance". But recommendations addressed to the general public will run into a "compliance" problem that is right off the scale of difficulty encountered within the doctor-patient relationship. Members of the general public are not, and should not be thought of as if they were patients: they have not put themselves into the role of clienthood or dependency on a doctor to tell them how they should order their lives. Certainly they do not have a special concern about the prevention of atherosclerosis, or about any other medically perceived long-term threat to their well-being. They are not disposed to follow even the best intentioned advice from authority unless to do so is convenient, agreeable and rewarding in the short term.

Therefore, the best type of recommendation would be one that could be accepted by an entirely passive public. Recommendations that depend for their effect on having people (other than sick or anxious patients) change their lifestyle are of doubtful value, especially if the first step to be taken in modifying behavior is the deliberate arousal of anxieties about sickness and death. I know that there is widespread enthusiasm for health education and for "motivating" people to adopt better lifestyles: these may be heroic aspirations and yet poor policy.

To make the point more concretely, I ask you to consider a parallel between the task of preventing atherosclerosis and that of preventing venereal disease, bearing in mind that Gluttony as well as Lust has traditionally been listed among the seven deadly sins. An important cause of venereal disease is promiscuous behavior; so whoever preaches continence can claim to be serving a public health purpose but, in order to succeed, he must persuade people that a continent life is good and rewarding in itself. Now it also happens to be the case that some of the people with the lowest apparent risks of atherosclerotic disease are those who have adopted dietary self-restraint for religious or aesthetic reasons (1,2). This does not make it necessary, or even appropriate, for health professionals to join some crusade against the "unhealthy lifestyles" that go with either type of sinful indulgence. A ship's doctor may listen respectfully while members of the crew are told how they ought to behave in port, but will make it his job as a doctor to ensure that prophylactics are distributed. In keeping with this professional style, our preferred and proper objective should be to build some safety factors into existing, freely chosen behavior patterns. As a single, very homely example, you might consider recommending fiscal or other measures to increase the share of the soft drinks market taken up by low calorie products.

The first test of a good recommendation is, then, that it entail a minimum of disturbance to, and a minimum of active participation by, individual members of the general public. An ideal recommendation would be one on the model of the historic recommendations to fluoridate drinking water. Nothing was then required or expected of members of the general public, who were assured of substantial benefit in the form of reduced caries risk even while continuing to eat "too much" candy, neglecting their toothbrush, and staying away from the dentist. I leave it to you to judge whether there are any actions of the fluoridation type yet in view that could be effective against atherosclerosis - or its complications. One possibility of which I have been made aware through some connection with the underlying research is that supplementation of magnesium intake might benefit broad segments of our population, and possibly the whole of it. However, I don't seek to debate the merits of any specific proposal, only to argue that a certain type of recommendation is much more valuable than other types of equivalent theoretical efficacy. There could be no better way to show that we are serious about preventing atherosclerotic disease than by working to develop measures that would benefit the public health directly and unconditionally. At the same time we should be very wary of recommendations that would operate indirectly, via behavior modification, a part of whose appeal may be that, under the guise of preventive care, they promise to inflate still further the demand for services of physicians, dietitians or other health professionals.

My second point has to do with the amount of benefit that may reasonably be expected to result from particular preventive measures. In order to secure initial support for action on your recommendations you will have to state the objectives of your prevention programme in quantitative terms, that is, to select target levels of mortality, morbidity, or average fitness. Even more important, these target levels will be needed for evaluating the outcome of action taken on your recommendations, for it is mandatory that your recommendations be coupled with a definite proposal for judging their effectiveness.

For lack of much experience in experimental modification of risk factors, these target figures will have to be set on the basis of interferences drawn from observational data, including vital statistics and sources such as the Framingham study and the "Seven Countries" study of Keys and his colleagues. Without presuming to state what I think the actual target figures should be, I would like to say two things about the way in which they are to be formulated. First, you should have as little as possible to do with soft or debatable endpoints such as episodes of sickness, ECG changes or physical performance, but should try for a sharp focus on mortality. Second, the mortality measures used should be death rates from all causes, rather than from arteriosclerotic disease alone. The reasons for this latter stipulation are that the component of mortality attributable to arteriosclerotic disease cannot be dissected out cleanly from the general aggregate of deaths, and that the preventive actions proposed are likely to have effects - hopefully but not necessarily beneficial - on the risk of dying from other diseases. Prevention of atherosclerosis is not, for the general public, an end in itself; postponement of death may be.

Most discussion of the potential benefit from action against atherosclerosis risk factors has been within the narrower framework of avoiding heart attacks. I would like to refer to the contribution on these lines recently made by Whyte (3), who concluded in part:

> "that if 100 men who are non-smokers, with normal blood pressure and electrocardiogram, lower their plasma-cholesterol from 310 to 260 mg per 100 ml starting at 35 years of age, 6 could potentially benefit by avoiding a coronary incident, 94 would be likely to follow the regimen without apparent benefit, and 8 of these would have an attack within 20 years despite adherence to the regimen."

Statements in this form express the objectives of a cholesterol lowering programme with some precision, and can certainly be useful in sorting out priorities as between lowering lipid levels, discouragement of smoking and control of blood pressure. However, I believe that the statement quoted may give too rosy an impression of the prospects, partly because of an assumption underlying the calculation, and partly because, as Whyte clearly stated in his paper, women have less to hope for from lipid lowering than men do, and men past early adult life have less to hope for than do younger males. This distribution of expected benefit would also be a feature of the formulation which I have suggested is preferable, in terms of all causes death rates. The particular objective we should set for an atherosclerosis prevention programme is a net reduction in deaths (however certified) of men in their forties and fifties.

The likelihood that benefits from controlled fat intake (or whatever dietary reform you decide to recommend) will be restricted to one sex is regrettable in itself, but may be scientifically opportune, because it opens up the intriguing possibility of conducting an informative experiment without the need for an untreated control group. The pattern we should look for was, I suggest, discernible in the results of the Finnish hospital experiment reported three years ago by Miettinen et al (4). When certain institutions were placed on a low saturated, high polyunsaturated fat diet, the mortality of the male residents decreased, but that of the female residents did not. A net reduction of 12% in the mortality of males from all causes came about through an apparent 39% drop in cardiovascular deaths accompanied by a 14% increase in deaths from other causes.

In summary, I have made two suggestions concerning choice of objectives in atherosclerosis prevention:

1. Top priority in research and action should be given to the development of preventive strategies not requiring active participation by individual members of the general population.

2. Outcome should be assessed in terms of a net reduction in the death rate from all causes, expected to have its main expression in middle aged men.

REFERENCES

1. Sacks, F.M., Rosner, B., Kass, E.H.: Blood pressure in vegetarians. Am. J. Epidemiol. 100:390-398, 1974.
2. Sacks, F.M., Castelli, W.P., Donner, A., Kass, E.H.: Plasma lipids in vegetarians and controls. N. Engl. J. Med. 292: 1148-1151, 1975.
3. Whyte, H.M.: Potential effect on coronary heart disease morbidity of lowering the blood cholesterol. Lancet (i):906-910, 1975.

4. Miettinen, M., Turpeinen, O., Karvonen, M.J., Elosuo, R., Paavilainen, E.: Effect of cholesterol-lowering diet on mortality from coronary heart disease and other causes. A twelve year clinical trial in men and women. Lancet (ii):835-838, 1972.

(2)

NATIONAL VIEWS: AUSTRALIA

Malcolm Whyte

Department of Clinical Science, The John Curtin School of Medical Research,
The Australian National University, Canberra, Australia

RECOMMENDATIONS OF THE ACADEMY OF SCIENCE

The most recent set of recommendations for preventing atherosclerosis was publicly promulgated this year by The Australian Academy of Science.[1] Its Working Group comprised "not experts in the cardiological field, but biologists, all of whom have had some experience in evaluating scientific evidence." It reviewed the extensive literature on the subject, consulted many experts working in the cardiological and biochemical fields and tendered a report as "a judicious assessment of some aspects of the present status of one of the most important health problems in Australia", commenting that "the field is rapidly developing and the recommendations may need to be changed in the future". Their task "was focused on diet in relation to coronary heart disease, largely because of the many factors that may be involved in the growing epidemic of the present century, and diet may perhaps be more readily managed than most other environmental factors".

In common with all reviewers of the situation, they recognized the magnitude of the coronary and atherosclerotic problems in our community, the multifactorial causes, the importance of genetic influences and of diseases such as hypertension and diabetes, variation among individuals in susceptibility and in response to dietary and other changes, and the associations which have been repeatedly demonstrated between diet, hyperlipidaemia and atherosclerotic diseases. They noted, of course, the lack of proof of any causal relationship between lipids and these diseases and the somewhat equivocal results of dietary trials aimed at prevention. Passing recommendations were made about reducing cigarette smoking and encouraging programs of moderate exercise for sedentary workers and they suggested numerous lines of research work which should be promoted but their main advice to the public concerned diet.

Dietary recommendations were to restrict the caloric intake, reduce the consumption of cholesterol to less than 350 mg. per day and of fat to about 35% of calories with roughly equal amounts of saturated, monounsaturated and polyunsaturated fats, and to reduce the intake of refined carbohydrates and alcohol. They recommended that "such dietary changes could reasonably be adopted by the entire population" and that more extensive changes for people at high risk should be decided by physicians taking account of lipid status and other risk factors. They concluded that widespread use of "polyunsaturated" foods by the general community was justified in that "it was virtually certain that they would produce no untoward effects". They emphasized that true prevention "may necessitate changes of the kind outlined (reduction in caloric intake and a decrease in the consumption of cholesterol and saturated fatty acids) in the diet of the whole Australian population, including and especially in children and adolescents" and recognized that "such a program would require a major re-orientation of many food-producing and food-processing industries in Australia, and would need to be introduced by a program of education of the community, including food producers, in dietary matters". Some of their recommendations were aimed in these directions.

We can well imagine that a dietary prescription such as this would not be received with signs of great rejoicing, nor would it be followed at all assiduously by any substantial proportion of a population comprised largely of affluent, self-satisfied people who are obese and indolent, who love bacon and eggs and all manner of meats and dairy products, who are addicted to sweetness and who boast of their beer drinking! Not that I would dare publicly to describe Australians in these terms, any more than I would make sweeping generalisations like this about North Americans. But those are the recommendations and Australians, like so many others in this modern world, have been subjected in recent years to such a bombardment through the news media that they are by no means unaware of the topics mentioned - heart disease, cholesterol, polyunsaturates, obesity and so on. But what has the impact been? The Academy of Science Report received scant attention and will have had a negligible effect on the population as a whole. They have heard it all before, there is still no proof and there are persisting uncertainties, controversy and confusion which bolster up the natural inclination to carry on as usual.

However, the Report is likely to be more effective in professional and governmental circles where its support for the probable causal role of lipids in atherosclerosis and for the advisability of changes in diet as a precautionary measure will be taken seriously. The results could well become evident in the promotion of research and education in human nutrition, in changes in legislation which will loosen restrictions on the availability of polyunsaturated fat products and impose demands on the labelling of foodstuffs and on food standards, in encouraging industry to develop different types and qualities of food products and in the composition of diets provided on a mass scale especially in government-controlled organisations.

RECOMMENDATIONS BY THE HEART FOUNDATION

It is true that Australians have heard it all, or nearly all of it, before. The recommendations put forward in the Academy of Science Report were virtually the same as have been widely promulgated by the National Heart Foundation of Australia[2], except that the Academy emphasized that the dietary changes should be advised for the entire population rather than for selected subjects alone. The National Heart Foundation's Position Statement put forward the usual generally accepted points about the high toll of coronary heart disease, its relationship to the level of blood fats, the responsiveness of blood fats to changes in the diet and the general prescription for lowering the blood levels of cholesterol and triglyceride. They recommended that the diet should be changed in these ways when the blood cholesterol level is higher than 250 mg./100 ml. or when the triglyceride level exceeds 160 mg./100 ml. or when other risk factors are also present. As with the Academy's report, it looked especially towards youth, advocating dietary education along the lines suggested and claims that the diet is safe (though reference was made to the possibility of predisposing to gallstone formation).

More specifcally, the Heart Foundation's dietary advice referred to the adjustment of caloric intake to achieve "ideal" body weight; fat consumption to provide 30-35% of all calories with a reduction of saturated fats, a moderate increase of polyunsaturated fats and a P/S ratio of 1.0 to 1.5; a reduction in dietary cholesterol to less than 300 mg. per day; and restriction of refined carbohydrates and alcohol.

These are the two main sets of recommendations which have been put forward nationally, the general public and the doctors being more exposed to and cognizant of statements from the Heart Foundation than from the Academy of Science. As you would expect, there has been prominent support from industries which have a commercial interest in promoting the use of polyunsaturated oils and counterblasts from the dairying industry.

COMMENTS BY GOVERNMENT

Governmental bodies have refrained, as might be expected, from committing themselves to any strong and clear edicts and recommendations in this field. However, they have made pronouncements from time to time, seemingly based on Heart Foundation reviews, and not always expressed as carefully as might be expected or as warranted by the evidence. In 1967, the statement was made[3] that "The National Health and Medical Research Council supports the conclusions concerning the relationship of dietary fats to coronary heart disease which have been reached by the National Heart Foundation after careful consideration of all the available evidence" but no particular precautionary measures, dietary or otherwise, were advocated. The most recent comments were made in 1972[4] when "Council supported the view that dietary influences are inter alia, important in the cause of coronary heart disease", "Council agreed that in people who are overweight it is important for them to reduce their total calorie intake", and "in addition, when the level of blood cholesterol is significantly raised, current evidence indicates that this should be lowered by weight reduction in people who are overweight, by avoiding the consumption of cholesterol-rich foods and by consuming a diet in which the fats present are predominantly of the polyunsaturated type".

The Council has also recommended that no measures should be taken which would in any way prevent individuals from obtaining the type of fat they wish or have been advised to eat (being mindful of current legislation which restricts the production of polyunsaturated margarine) and they formulated standards for the composition and labelling of polyunsaturated margarine, fats and oils. It was recommended that the P/S ratio should be not less than 2:1.

For the most part, laws have not been enacted along these lines as the Australian Government has no powers of enforcement in these matters for which legislative prerogative remains with individual States.

These then are the main sets of recommendations and statements on this subject which have been put before the public in Australia. The basis for them in all instances has been a review of the literature which is universally available and there is little, if anything, which has been uniquely derived from Australia itself. That the magnitude and nature of the problems of atherosclerosis in Australia are similar to those in other affluent western populations are shown by national mortality statistics, the results of cross-sectional and prospective population studies in Busselton, Western Australia, and the findings of the acute myocardial infarction register which was carried out for one year in Perth, Western Australia. No controlled clinical intervention trials have been carried out to date. There is nearing completion, a 5-year secondary intervention trial, mainly concerned with dietary changes and there is under way a massive multicentred single-blind study of the effect of blood pressure reduction in mild hypertension. Two notable features of the Australian experience which are similar to what have been observed elsewhere are the decline in mortality due to cerebrovascular disease over the last two decades and a more recent down-turn in mortality attributed to coronary heart disease. Perhaps better treatment of hypertension and earlier, more intensive, care of coronary attacks have contributed to this but no clearly supportable claims can be made for any specific therapeutic manoeuvres or for any sizeable proportion of the population having adopted the preventive measures which have been recommended.

FACILITATION BY THE FOOD INDUSTRY

The more specifically Australian contribution to this scene has been the development of polyunsaturated ruminant foods, that is, a contribution towards how dietary changes may be implemented rather than anything pertinent to the rationale for recommending dietary or other measures which might help to prevent atherosclerosis. The story of these relatively new products is now well known. Linoleic acid-enriched milk and meat fats can be produced in ruminants by feeding them vegetable seed oils protected against the hydrogenating action of micro-organisms in the rumen by coating the oil droplets with formalin-treated casein[5] and consumption of these products - meat, milk, butter, cheese, yoghurt, cream, ice-cream - can effectively and predictably contribute to the lowering of blood lipids.[6-8] The linoleic acid content of the food is usually of the order of 20% of the total fatty acids and their cholesterol content is unchanged. So far they have been released onto the market in only one city in our country - cheese and a variety of yoghurts and meats - and it is too soon to assess their popularity. Prices are higher than for ordinary products, some of the promotional material is questionable and production and marketing are hindered by legislative restrictions and opposing commercial interests.

The extent to which these products are likely to affect the plasma cholesterol concentration as compared with the effects of normal products is shown in the table. The estimates were derived[9] by applying predictive formulae to the amounts of cholesterol and fatty acids contributed by the items of food to an average daily diet. It can be seen that cholesterol promotion by these products is about 40% to 60% less than for ordinary products. They can be regarded as useful additions to the range of foodstuffs from which some lipid-lowering dieters might choose their menu, allowing them to enjoy, at least on occasions, some of their familiar and favourite dishes but they do not obviate the need for more radical

ITEM	PORTION	Plasma Cholesterol Contribution (mg./100 ml)		
		Ordinary Products	Poly Products	Difference
Meat:				
Beef & Lamb: Aver.	2 servings (200g) p.d.	20.3	12.6	7.7
" " "	1 serving (100g) p.d.	10.1	6.3	3.8
" " : Lean	1 serving (100g) p.d.	6.4	3.7	2.7
Butter	1 1/2 tbsp (30g) p.d.	11.6	6.7	4.9
Dripping	" " " " "	8.9	3.5	5.4
Cheese:				
Cheddar	1 cube (1 1/4":40g)p.d.	6.1	3.8	2.3
Cream	1 1/2 tbsp (30g) p.d.	6.3	2.9	3.4
Ice Cream	1 scoop (32g) p.d.	1.8	1.0	0.8
Milk: Whole	1/2 pint (300 ml) p.d.	5.0	2.9	2.1

TABLE I: The extent to which polyunsaturated ruminant meat and other products will predictably affect the plasma cholesterol concentration as compared with the effects of ordinary products.

dietary changes if recommended targets are to be achieved, such as reduced fat intake, drastic restriction of cholesterol consumption and a dietary P/S ratio above 1.0.

SUMMARY

The Australian scene in this area would seem to show the same features, and haze, as are found in many other countries. There is general recognition of atherosclerotic problems, of the common risk factors and of the need for prevention. Learned and informed bodies such as The Australian Academy of Science and The National Heart Foundation of Australia have made recommendations along familiar lines, involving especially dietary changes, as preventive measures. The basis for these recommendations has been a general review of the subject and does not include anything uniquely Australian. The admission of uncertainty about causes and prevention, awareness of controversy, confusion, ignorance and a natural reluctance to change habits no doubt contribute to popular disregard for the recommendations at the present time.

REFERENCES

1. Australian Academy of Science, Canberra. Report No. 18, 1975.

2. National Heart Foundation of Australia, Med. J. Aust., 1974, 1, 575,616, 663.

3. Australian Government, Canberra. 64th Report, National Health and Medical Research Council, 1967.

4. Australian Government, Canberra. 74th Report, National Health and Medical Research Council, 1972.

5. Cook, L.J., Scott, T.W., Ferguson, K.A., McDonald, I.W. Nature, 1970, 228, 178.

6. Nestel, P.J., Havenstein, N., Whyte, H.M., Scott, T.J., Cook, L.J. New Eng. J. Med., 1973, 288, 279.

7. Nestel, P.J., Havenstein, N., Scott, T.W., Cook, L.J. Aust. N.Z.J. Med., 1974, 4, 497.

8. Nestel, P.J., Havenstein, N., Homma, Y., Scott, T.W., Cook, L.J. Metabolism, 1975, 24, 189.

9. Whyte, H.M., Havenstein, N. Unpublished.

(3)

PREVENTION PROGRAMS IN CANADA

L. Horlick, M.D.

Department of Medicine, University of Saskatchewan

Saskatoon, Saskatchewan, Canada

I would like to begin by quoting from a recent statement by the Hon. Marc Lalonde, Minister of National Health and Welfare (Published as "A new perspective on the health of Canadians" 1974).[1]
"Good health is the bedrock on which social progress is built.
....The Governments of the Provinces and of Canada have long recognized that good physical and mental health are necessary for the quality of life to which everyone aspires. Accordingly they have developed a health care system...which substantially removes financial barriers to medical and hospital care.
....At the same time as improvements have been made in health care, in the general standard of living, in public health protection and in medical science, ominous counterforces have been at work to undo progress in raising the health status of Canadians. These counterforces constitute the dark side of economic progress. They include environmental pollution, city living, habits of indolence, abuse of alcohol, tobacco and drugs, and eating patterns which put the pleasing of the senses above the needs of the human body.
For these environmental and behavioural threats to health, the organized health care system can do little more than serve as a catchment net for the victims..."

"The Government of Canada now intends to give to human biology, the environment and lifestyle as much attention as it has to the financing of the health care organization so that all four avenues to improved health are pursued with equal vigor. Its goal will be not only to add years to our life but life to our years, so that all can enjoy the opportunities offered by increased economic and social justice."

The report goes on to make a penetrating analysis of the health problems of Canadians and terminates with a series of "strategies" for the future. These have been divided into -

Health Promotion Strategy

- to inform, influence and assist individuals and organizations to accept more responsibility and become more active in matters affecting health.

Regulatory Strategy

- to use federal regulatory powers to reduce hazards to health, and to encourage and assist provinces to do the same.

Research Strategy

- to discover and apply knowledge needed to solve health problems.

Health Care Efficiency Strategy

- to help the provinces re-organize the system for health care delivery so that cost, accessibility and effectiveness are balanced for all Canadians.

I have chosen to extract the "strategies" relating to Exercise and to Nutrition (Table 1) so that you may see the direction in which Canada is moving. It is fair to say that many of the "strategies" remain mere "paper tigers", but the Federal Government and some of the Provinces are moving to implement others.

Exercise: As an outgrowth of this policy position, the Federal Government has sponsored three major national conferences (The National Conference on Fitness and Health - December 1972, the National Conference on Employee Physical Fitness - December 1974, and the National Conference on Women and Sport - May 1974), and has created three organisms which relate to sport and physical fitness. "Sport Canada" is devoted to the pursuit of excellence in sport, to raising national performance levels and concentrates on developing top competitive athletes for Canada. "Recreation Canada" is more important from our point of view. It functions in a support role encouraging and supporting the provision of opportunities for physical activity, stimulating participation and generally striving to raise the national level of fitness. "Sport Participation Canada" is a "private" company, although the impetus for its founding, and much of its support comes from the Federal Government. It was modelled after some of the European efforts to mobilize both the private and public sectors. It has sponsored the "participaction" program in several Canadian communities. Perhaps its greatest success has been in Saskatoon where a very enthusiastic local committee has sponsored and carried through a sustained media supported campaign for greater citizen physical activity. One device used was to sponsor a competition with Umea, Sweden (a town with similar ecology) to see which community could get more of its citizens out to walk 2 Km on each of three successive days. An amazing 64,195 Saskatonians (49.9% of the population) turned out on the third day to defeat Umea (47.5%). The daily turnouts were 32.5%, 35.9%, and 49.9%. Women and school age children were the largest contributors to the victory. Out of a total female population of 66,000, 52.1% (or 34,410) took part on the final day, whereas only 47.5% of eligible males walked, 74% of boys and 76.9% of girls under 18 participated. Dr. Howard Nixon, Chairman of the "Project Sweden" said, "The whole idea of project Sweden is to transfer to Canada that part of the Swedish mentality which makes them among the fittest people in the world".

Another outgrowth of the National Program has been the development of a simple "home fitness test" pioneered by Dr. Don Bailey of Saskatoon, and which is now being test marketed. Dr. Bailey (with the help of several thousand volunteer Saskatoon citizens) has established standards of fitness based on pulse rate after 3, 6 and 9 minutes of stair climbing. This simple test should permit the average citizen to determine his fitness and motivate him to undertake a fitness program and also evaluate his progress. These programs have had a considerable impact on public awareness and have greatly increased the demands on all existing sports facilities. Its impact in the schools (especially at the elementary level) has been most marked.

The Provincial Governments have also been active in this field - time does not permit me to do more than mention two examples - the first is Action B.C. - which grew out of the B.C. Conference on Health and Physical Activity of November 1973. Action B.C. is sponsored by the Provincial Department of Health and its role is to act as a stimulator or "animateur" of physical fitness programs for B.C. It will help in developing regional programs by providing advice, expertise, training and money. (B.C. stands for British Columbia.)

The Saskatchewan Provincial Government has offered bursaries to Elementary School Boards to send teachers in for upgrading Physical Education skills. Last year a three week course in eight centres was provided for 800 teachers (at a cost of $60-70,000). This year, a further 200 will be trained.

Nutrition: Lalonde's "Perspectives" have listed a number of important "strategies" in this area which I have included in Table 2. Important moves have already been taken with a view to implementing

these strategies.
1. The Nutrition Canada Study has been completed. This extremely ambitious undertaking has provided data on most regions of Canada and on many population samples including native population.

2. The Health Protection Branch of NHW has sponsored an expert committee to examine the relationship between diet and cardiovascular disease and to make recommendations. That committee is in the process of finalizing its recommendations. The committee has looked very carefully at the Swedish model of a broadly based Nutrition Council which would include representatives of all groups interested in this area and would attempt to reach a consensus on practical changes in the Canadian Dietary. The committee has also been concerned over the large number of independent jurisdictions which are involved in decision making about nutrition and which act in an unco-ordinated manner. A set of public recommendations will be issued which represent a "prudent" approach to diet. National Health and Welfare have already begun to take action in this field as well as in the exercise area by issuing attractive pamphlets with the Family Allowance cheques.

Smoking: The importance of smoking as a risk factor for diseases of the heart and lungs is widely recognized. Because the risk largely ceases when smoking stops, this may well be the risk factor with the greatest potential for change. In 1969-70 a standing committee of the House of Commons brought down a report which recommended a "phased" program to completely eliminate all cigarette promotional activity within four years. This was to be coupled to increased educational activities to discourage smoking, and measures making for less hazardous smoking. Unfortunately, the major portions of this legislation have not been implemented. It is clear that tobacco represents a very powerful vested interest and that the Federal and Provincial Governments have not decided to take a firm stand on the issue of either banning its cultivation or promotion. Instead attempts have been made to increase public awareness of the evils of smoking, to reduce the hazards of smoking, and to promote non-smoking movements. One of the most successful activities of the Federal program has been the publishing of "tar-nicotine" reports. These have been instrumental in driving the high tar-nicotine brands off the market. The non-smokers movement has led to the segregation of smokers in public transport (airlines). Research is going on at Canada Agriculture to develop tobacco with less toxic smoke. Attempts have been made to establish co-ordinating councils for agencies opposed to smoking at the Federal and Provincial levels, but except for a few provinces (N.B., Sask.) they have not been successful. An interesting experiment has been the peer group leader program developed in Saskatchewan by Dr. George Piper in 1968. These are grade eight students selected by carefully constructed questionnaires - up to 140 students attend each seminar (5 seminars/year) and consider all aspects of smoking. They then go back to their schools and spread the word. Studies of the schools sending students to the seminars show a measureable decrease of smoking among these school populations, but have not really reversed the trend toward increased smoking by adolescents. Educational programs must start at kindergarten and grade one level, and the approach used in one such program is that tobacco is an addicting drug.

The non-smoking movement is gaining ground. A cross Canada survey by the Canadian Press shows as much as 50% of passenger space on many buses, trains and airplanes reserved for non-smokers. Many hospitals, theatres and sports arenas now limit smoking to a few designated areas and most large department stores have prohibited it. (Air Canada now reserves 50% of its passenger space as "non-smoking".) No cigarettes are sold in vending machines and stores in some hospitals. However, a 1974 report by the Alberta T.B. and Respiratory Disease Association said a significant number of 100 hospitals surveyed provided no protection for non-smoking respiratory patients or patients in general.

So, what does it all add up to - we appear to have reached a plateau in cigarette consumption - smokers are increasing at the rate of 1%/year, while the population growth is 2%/year. Cigarette advertising has been restricted on TV but has expanded in other media. More adolescents and women are smoking and fewer adult males. Educational programs are becoming more sophisticated and will be more successful in the future, but whether smoking can be beaten in this way is dubious. Smoking is a health hazard - as hazardous - or more so than pathogens in food and drinking water. It should be treated the same way.

Hypertension: Another important risk fact - and one that can be prevented - is hypertension. Some 20% of the population are believed to have a genetic predisposition to hypertension - but in many of these environmental factors are important in bringing hypertension out. It is known that children's blood pressure correlates highly with their parents blood pressure but no attempts at primary prevention of hypertension have yet been mounted. Efforts thus far have been directed to secondary prevention through case finding, diagnosis, treatment and follow-up, and some or all of these activities are currently underway in almost all Provinces. The first major screening program in Canada was that initiated by Dr. Don Silverberg in Edmonton in 1972, and it has served as a model for many other studies in this country and elsewhere.[2] An important contribution made by Silverberg has been the incorporation of pharmacists into the follow-up system which measureably improved treatment results. The follow-up of individuals found to be hypertensive still represents a very major problem, largely due to the mobility of most patients and health care personnel, and the poor compliance to

Table 1

EXERCISE

Health Promotion Strategy

1. Activities to promote a more widespread understanding of the importance and causes of CAD, (especially exercise).

2. Continued and expanded marketing programs promoting increased physical activity by Canadians.

3. Enlistment of the support of the Educational System in increasing opportunities for mass physical recreation in primary and secondary schools, community colleges and universities.

4. Promotion and development of simple intensive-use facilities for physical recreation including fitness trails, nature trails, ski trails, etc.

5. Pressure for full community use of existing facilities.

6. Reinforced support for mass sports programs.

7. Encouragement for sports clubs to accept more social responsibility for extending the use of their facilities to others.

8. Support for special programs of physical activity for the aged, the handicapped and the poor.

9. Enlisting the help of women's movements in getting more mass physical recreation programs for females.

10. Enlisting the support of employers and trade unions for exercise programs for sedentary workers.

11. Increase the awareness of health professionals of factors affecting physical fitness.

12. Completion of the development of a home fitness test.

Research Strategy

1. A program for assessing the effect of social and environmental change on health, including calculation of risk factors due to lifestyle.

2. Support for research on physical and mental fitness and for fitness testing.

Table 2

NUTRITION

Health Promotion Strategy

1. The development for the general public of educational programs on nutrition.

2. Enlisting the help of the food and restaurant industries to make known the caloric value and nutritional content of the food they sell.

Regulatory Strategy

1. Regulations for improving the nutritional content of food.
2. Increased control of health hazards due to food, etc.

Research Strategy

Continuing study into the ways and means of informing the Canadian people on changes in behaviour which will reduce self imposed risks.

Health Care Efficiency Strategy

cost - accessibility - effectiveness

1. Support of programs aimed at reducing risk of premature CAD, including weight control, exercise, stress reduction and anti-smoking.

2. Identification, treatment and follow-up of Canadians suffering from high serum cholesterol level (hypercholesterolemia).

Goal Setting Strategy

The extension of national standards of nutrition to include definite recommendations on safe levels of intake for hazardous substances occurring naturally in food.

treatment regimens. In this respect Sackett's group found that intensive indoctrination of hypertensives by an industrial health setting had little effect on treatment outcomes.[3] At the present time there is little or no co-ordination of hypertension programs at a National level. There is a role here for the Department of National Health and Welfare in setting up a national co-ordinating function and I believe that some action is being taken. We need some agreement on how best to carry out case finding and follow-up, and we certainly need much more information on compliance. We need some guidelines on acceptable amounts of sodium in the national diet. Current infant formulas may provide up to 8 mEq Na/Kg/day as compared to 1 mEq for breast milk. The importance of Na as an environmental factor in bringing about the expression of a genetic tendency to hypertension has already been alluded to.

Conclusion: The Provincial and National Heart Foundations have waged an active program of public and professional education against coronary heart disease for nearly 20 years. They have sponsored symposia, distributed literature, used the media widely and have aimed their message at every segment of the population. Much of the current awareness of the importance of risk factors by the health professionals and the public results from their work. Health professionals in this country are well indoctrinated concerning the importance of risk factors and are consciously trying to do something about it. The problem is that neither they, the Heart Associations or the Governments are really able to assess the impact of what they are doing on the population as a whole. There is a feeling abroad that preventive campaigns thus far have not been successful. What is most important is the realization that we are only just beginning to learn what is involved in behaviour modification and that we must monitor our efforts scrupulously if we are to have success in this area.

REFERENCES

1. A new perspective on the health of Canadians. Marc Lalonde, Minister of Health. Ottawa 1974.

2. Silverberg, D.S., Smith, E.S., Juchli, B. et al. Use of shopping centres in screening for hypertension. Can Med Ass J. III, 769, 1974.

3. Sackett, D. A randomized trial of clinical strategies for improving compliance with antihypertensive therapy. Presented in abstract form Jan. 1975, Royal College of Physicians of Canada Annual Meeting.

(4)

DIET AND CORONARY HEART DISEASE - A BRITISH POINT OF VIEW

J. R. A. Mitchell

Department of Medicine

Nottingham University, Nottingham, England

In 1970, the British Government's Department of Health and Social Security set up a Panel to advise it on the relationship between nutrition and vascular disease. In particular, it wished to know whether steps should be taken to modify the national diet and whether there ought to be any modification of the British advertising code which up to that time had not permitted claims to be made that particular foods were of benefit in preventing or treating cardiovascular disease.

The panel had as its Chairman a biochemist, Sir Frank Young, and consisted of eleven members (three physicians with an interest in nutrition, three nutritionists, two cardiovascular physicians, two epidemiologists, and one paediatrician). At the outset we took a series of crucial decisions:

1. That our brief was to establish a link between nutrition and cardiovascular disease. If such a link was proved to exist the mechanisms by which it operated could then be analyzed. If we could not demonstrate an overall link, then however tempting, logical or well-established the theoretical links in this non-existent chain might be, they were irrelevant to our deliberations.

2. That there were no adequate animal models for human atheroma and thrombosis, nor for the heart and brain lesions which these processes produce.

3. That "risk factors" are not causative agents in the way that tuberculosis can only be caused by a specific bacillus. Coronary heart disease can develop in the absence of any of the known risk factors, while individuals with all known risk factors may not

develop the disease at all. Modification of a risk factor need not be beneficial; the crucial test is whether modifying the level of the risk factor confers benefit on the individual or community. Thus, the results of adequately-controlled intervention studies aimed at modification of risk factors were of key importance in our discussions.

4. That we would not necessarily achieve a unanimous view and that where this was so, it should be recorded, so that the areas of agreement and disagreement could be identified.

5. That even in Britain, where the Registrar-General has a unique record of the nation's pattern of death and where war-time needs have led to close monitoring of food consumption, factual information about cardiovascular disease and about diet is not as clear and unequivocal as we would have wished. In the cardiovascular disease field it is not easy to separate true changes in incidence and prevalence from shifts in labelling produced by fashion, by increasing awareness of cardiovascular disease and by new diagnostic tools. In the dietary field, it is easy to measure the total foods moving into consumption in the country as a whole, and to survey the food bought by households. This does not tell you, however, what each individual is eating unless food wastage, meals taken outside the home and the way in which bought food is actually distributed within a family are known.

6. That people eat food and not nutrients; eating forms part of the social culture and eating habits cannot readily be changed. Unlike drugs, food is necessary for day-to-day survival, so dietary modifications cannot be tested against an inert placebo.

After many meetings and draft reports, we were able to agree on certain conclusions:

a. Ischaemic heart disease appears to have many contributory causes, and more than one is likely to be involved in determining the incidence of the disease in a population, or its occurrence in an individual. There is at present no evidence that any one cause has the essential importance for ischaemic heart disease which, for example, the tubercle bacillus has for tuberculosis.

b. Populations which have a high death rate from ischaemic heart disease have certain environmental features in common. In any individual, the liability to develop ischaemic heart disease is the result of an interaction between external risk factors and internal ones.

c. There are many risk factors for ischaemic heart disease only some of which are dietary in nature (a consideration of "diet" can not take account of smoking, physical activity, etc.). No single dietary factor can be regarded as predominant in determining susceptibility to the disease, and any claim to the contrary is not acceptable in the contest of the United Kingdom diet.

d. Recognizable obesity increases the risk of ischaemic heart disease and of other conditions. A substantial reduction of the body weight of overweight people diminishes the greater death rate associated with obesity.

e. Changes in the composition of the diet of an individual can reduce the serum lipids but there is no certainty that such a reduction diminishes the susceptibility to ischaemic heart disease.

f. A rise in the ratio of polyunsaturated to saturated fatty acids in the diet of an individual or of a group of people may be followed by a reduction in the mean serum cholesterol concentration. The panel were not convinced by the available evidence that the incidence of ischaemic heart disease in the United Kingdom, or the death rate from it, would be reduced in consequence of a rise in the ratio of polyunsaturated to saturated fatty acids in the national diet. In the present state of knowledge, any suggestion or claim to that effect, with respect to the nation or to an individual, would be unjustified.

g. Sucrose is a widely available, cheap, palatable and concentrated source of food energy; it can easily be consumed beyond satiety in a way that is unlikely to occur with other sources of food energy. The panel believed a reduction in the incidence of obesity to be desirable, and considered that a continued fall in the intake of sucrose would assist in achieving this aim.

h. There was too little evidence on which to assess the possible importance of indigestible material (fibre) in the food in relation to ischaemic heart disease.

i. Within the United Kingdom and in other countries it has been observed that the softer the local water supply, the higher the death rate from cardiovascular disease. The reason for this relation has yet to be elucidated.

Thus, the panel's agreed conclusions reinforce actions which are common ground among all health-care groups (don't get fat; if you are fat get thin; don't smoke). Several members of the panel could not support any additional conclusions, but the remaining members were able to agree on one further point. They accepted the evidence derived from international comparisons that the death rate from ischaemic heart disease in a population correlates positively with the proportion of the food energy derived from fat, and with the proportion of the food energy derived from the saturated fatty acids in the diet. They recognized that such statistical correlations did not of themselves, establish causal relationships, but in their judgement the fact that in the United Kingdom the consumption of dietary fat and the percentage of the food energy which is derived from fat (animal and vegetable) have both been steadily rising was viewed with concern. These members, therefore, recommended that the amount of fat in the diet should be reduced.

Not only did the "minority" disagree with this conclusion, but they were also unable to agree that the "majority" conclusion could be translated into useful action. Total fat restriction could, of course, be achieved by reducing total calorie intake, while leaving the mix of dietary constituents unchanged; this seemed to say little more than the agreed recommendations about obesity. If on the other hand, fat is to be reduced while the total calorie intake remains unchanged, this must either imply an increase in protein intake (which the Third World and the budget-conscious housewife in a developed country might express views about), or an increase in carbohydrate, which appears to run counter to conclusions (g) above. The "minority" members therefore disagreed with their colleagues on two counts: first, they felt that the recommendation about total fat intake went beyond the evidence available, and second, they did not consider that a simple limitation of total fat intake was practicable in the context of the British National diet.

Our Chairman described us as "intelligent, eloquent, critical, strong-minded protagonists of various views". Many individual members of the panel had had reservations about the overall conclusions and recommendations but had resolved these by agreeing to the "majority" and "minority" reports. Had the opportunity been provided, many of us might have wished to amplify our arguments and to have been identified with them, but we had all agreed to prepare a corporate report. Some of us were therefore surprised to find that one member of the panel had stated his own position in a "note of reservation". Moreover, this note adduced as "evidence" items which the panel had agreed were theoretical speculations, bearing no proven relationship to the matter in hand (e.g. "disturbances in hormonal balance"; "increased blood concentrations of insulin and 11-OH corticosterone"; "stickiness and electrophoretic behavior of blood platelets"). These were "Black Box" items, the box being marked "only to be opened if a link between nutrition and vascular disease is established". It is my personal opinion that if the other members of the panel had been aware that the final report would include Yudkin's note of reservation, they would either have wished to add their own notes of reservation or to have recast the report, since our deliberations had established that incontrovertible facts were rare birds, and that the extent to which each member accepted community action based on incomplete information was a matter of personal judgement.

Perhaps the most important conclusion to emerge from our travail was that the advertising code set by the 1966 British Food Standards Committee should not be changed. Thus, in Britain the position is still "that no claim be permitted that any type of dietary fat affords protection against heart disease or is of benefit to sufferers from this condition". It will be a long time before acceptable evidence from controlled intervention studies emerges to challenge that recommendation.

(5)

NEW ZEALAND PERSPECTIVES

F. B. Shorland

Department of Biochemistry, Victoria University, Wellington, New Zealand, currently Visiting Professor, Department of Food Science and Human Nutrition, Michigan State University, East Lansing, Michigan, U.S.A.

I would like to thank the organizers of the Workshop-Conference for inviting me to give this presentation as the convener of a Committee of the Royal Society of New Zealand (1971) on coronary heart disease (C.H.D.).

NEW ZEALAND REPORTS ON CORONARY HEART DISEASE

In the preface of the report, the President of the Royal Society of New Zealand (R.S.N.Z.) noted with concern that more than one-third of all deaths of males of middle age and over was from C.H.D. It is indeed sad that the President at the conclusion of his term of office died from this cause. That animal fats involving meat and butter, upon which the national economy depends, may provoke the disease was also an important matter. However, the report showed the need to avoid excessive caloric intake as the main requirement for the prevention of the disease.

Unbeknown to our Committee, a Committee was set up by the National Heart Foundation of New Zealand (1971). Their report appeared very shortly after ours with similar recommendations summarized as follows: (a) keep weight down to 'ideal' levels; (b) avoid cigarette smoking; (c) minimize cholesterol intake by reducing consumption of such foods as brains and eggs; (d) recognize and treat diabetes and hypertension; and (e) lower high plasma cholesterol levels by limiting intake of cholesterol and saturated fats and increasing intake of polyunsaturated fats.

Whereas the R.S.N.Z. Committee made no specific recommendations in regard to exercise, the National Heart Foundation Committee advised regular exercise and focused more on diagnostic screening. The R.S.N.Z. Committee was against aggressive attempts to increase the consumption of polyunsaturated fats but recommended that butter fortified with linoleic-rich vegetable oil be made available for medical use.

The R.S.N.Z. Committee attempted to consider all aspects though obviously the literature was too wide to succeed in this target. Nevertheless, it was gratifying to note the comments - doubtless all too flattering - in the Lancet of February 19, 1972, "The result is an excellent and detailed summary of all aspects of coronary heart disease." I propose here to touch upon only a few of the points made in our report and to pass on from there to recent developments. The R.S.N.Z. Committee found the absence of knowledge of the cause of atherosclerosis which underlies C.H.D. and the lack of proof of a causal relationship between serum cholesterol levels and the incidence of C.H.D. disconcerting. Likewise, it was disturbing to find that lowering high serum cholesterol levels gave little protection against the disease. In contrast, clearly manifest increases in incidence of C.H.D. were shown between the following population groups, the first named group in each comparison being at the higher level: (a) populations migrating from areas of low prevalence to those of high prevalence of C.H.D. compared with corresponding non-migrant populations; (b) populations after war compared with corresponding populations subject to wartime stresses; (c) cigarette smokers compared with non-smokers (except in Finland and Japan); and (d) diabetics compared with non-diabetics. From the above and related evidence, it was concluded "that C.H.D. is provoked by environmental factors which may be dietary or non-dietary or both."

In evaluating the effect of diet on C.H.D., the R.S.N.Z. Committee selected those trials on humans in which the criteria of randomization, blind reading of diagnostic data, continuation for 5 or more years and of documentation of noncardiac events were most nearly met. Of these, the replacement of saturated fats by polyunsaturated oils in a primary prevention trial has been shown to reduce significantly ($P < 0.05$) the number of atherosclerotic deaths (Dayton et al., 1969) and also to lower significantly ($P < 0.05$) myocardial reinfarcation (Leren, 1966). However, as Dayton et al.,(1969) point out "total longevity was not favorably affected." It is perhaps for this reason the Committee on Medical Aspects (1974) in Great Britain "cannot recommend an increase intake of polyunsaturated fatty acids in the diet as a measure intended to reduce the risk of the development of ischaemic heart disease." This view contrasts strikingly with that prevalent in the U.S.A. as shown for example, by Blankenhorn (1974). The reduced caloric intake (1500 kcal/day) low fat diet without recourse to polyunsaturated oils applied by Morrison (1960) is the only satisfactory procedure so far demonstrated for prolonging the lives of those afflicted by C.H.D. It is now proposed to consider the role of fats and other lipids in atherosclerosis.

REAPPRAISAL OF THE ROLE OF FATS AND OTHER LIPIDS IN ATHEROSCLEROSIS

Linoleic-rich oils especially in the absence of vitamin E promote exudative diathesis and encephalomalacia in chicks (Dam, 1944); muscular dystrophy in rabbits and guinea pigs (McCay et al., 1938); poor growth in calves, when fed in filled milk (Adams et al., 1959); gallstones in humans (Sturdevant et al., 1973) and possibly cancer in man (Pearce and Dayton, 1971). Corn oil has been shown to be a carcinogen promoter as tested on rats (Carroll and Khor, 1970, 1971). Likewise malonaldehyde, the product of autoxidation of polyunsaturated oils is a carcinogen promoter if not an ultimate carcinogen (Shamberger et al., 1974).

To correct for the elevation of serum cholesterol levels incurred by the intake of saturated fatty acids, requires the ingestion of twice as much linoleic acid (Keys et al., 1957), which could be hazardous and without beneficial effect on female coronary heart mortality (Miettinen et al., 1972). Hegsted et al., (1965) regard the regression equations involving the effects of the dietary lipid components on serum cholesterol levels as descriptive rather than functional. Reiser (1973) has even suggested that the effects of oils and fats in this regard are due to their phytosterol and cholesterol contents. However, this view fails to account for the fact that dietary β-sitosterol lowers cholesterol levels in both serum and tissues (Gerson et al., 1964, 1965) whereas corn oil raises the levels of cholesterol in tissues (Gerson et al., 1961). From our present knowledge of dietary lipids, albeit incomplete, it would seem preferable to reduce the levels of serum cholesterol by restricting cholesterol and saturated fat intake while perhaps increasing that of phytosterols rather than adding high levels of linoleic acid to the diet.

Carroll and Hamilton (1975) have recently shown that plasma cholesterol levels of rabbits are greatly influenced by the nonfatty components. Using a synthetic diet containing 27% protein and 60% dextrose in the absence of fat and cholesterol, animal proteins yielded plasma cholesterol levels several times higher than those found for wheat gluten and soybean protein. The differences in levels were not greatly changed by adding 15% corn oil or butter to the diet. However, substitution of dextrose by potato starch lowered the plasma cholesterol in a casein diet from 200 mg to 100mg/100ml. Wheat was without effect. These results

Table 1. Effect of isonitrogenous substitution of meat by potato on serum lipid levels (mg/100 ml) of men receiving 45% of the caloric intake as lamb perinephric fat* (Ahmad et al., 1975).

	Triglycerides			Cholesterol			Serum urea nitrogen			Urinary pH		
Subjects	D.W.	F.S.	M.A.	D.W.	F.S.	M.A.	D.W.	F.S.	M.A.	D.W.	F.S.	M.A.
At start of experiment	212	92	80	219	267	225	12.0	18.0	12.5	-	-	-
At end of meat diet	136	100	100	234	291	267	8.5	18.0	12.5	5.30	5.83	5.87
At end of potato diet	196	92	92	213	255	222	6.0	8.5	6.5	7.44	7.31	7.31

*The dietary protein expressed as a percentage of the total calories comprised lamb, 4.9; potatoes, 1.1 and bread 1.7. In both the meat and the potato diets the daily intake was made up to approximately 2,500 kcalories by the addition of jam or honey, 2 oranges or apples, lettuce or other greens and beverages. The lamb fat was more than 95% digestible. The meat diet was continued for 7 days before changing to the potato diet which lasted 4 days. Immediately before starting the experiment the subjects had been taking a meat type of diet for at least one week.

are consistent with those shown in Table I in which the isonitrogenous substitution of meat by potatoes was associated with a rapid drop in serum cholesterol levels.

In conclusion, aside from persons at risk I can see no objection to increasing the proportions of potatoes in the diet up to or beyond the level pertaining to the beginning of the century. The increased incidence of C.H.D. in U.S.A. and elsewhere has been accompanied by a misguided craving for first class protein. The intake of protein, which is unnecessarily high, has remained constant in the U.S.A. but its nature has changed from equal parts of plant and animal protein during 1909-1913 to two-thirds animal and one-third vegetable by 1965 (Leveille, 1975). With these changes, the consumption of bread, the protein of which is adequate for humans (Vaghefi et al., 1974) and of potatoes has been halved since the beginning of the century. It is considered that increased intake of potatoes and bread to replace the over-indulgence in first-class proteins might well lead to a decreased incidence of C.H.D. without incurring any health hazard. In addition, it would seem useful to extend the work of Morrison (1960) on dietary restriction as a means of combating C.H.D. Apart from these remarks and caution in the use of polyunsaturated oils I wish to uphold the recommendations of the R.S.N.Z. Committee.

REFERENCES

Adams, R.S., Gullickson, T.W., Gander, J.E. and Sautter, J.H. 1959. J. Dairy Sci., 42:1552.

Ahmad, M., Foy, R.B., Mickelsen, O. and Shorland, F.B. 1975. Unpublished observations. Dept. Food Science and Human Nutrition, Michigan State University, East Lansing, MI 48824.

Blankenhorn, D.H. 1974. Nutrition and the M.D. 1, No. 1.

Carroll, K.K., and Hamilton, R.M.G. 1975. J. Food Sci. 40:18.

Carroll, K.K. and Khor, H.T. 1970. Cancer Res. 30:2260.

Carroll, K.K. and Khor, H.T. 1971. Lipids. 6:415.

Committee on Medical Aspects of Food Policy. 1974. Diet and Coronary Heart Disease. Dept. of Health and Social Security. Her Majesty's Stationery Office, London.

Dam, H. 1944. J. Nutr. 27:193, 28:297.

Dayton, S., Pearce, M.L., Hashimoto, S., Dixon, W.J. and Tomiyasu, U. 1969. Circulation 40, Suppl. 11, 1-63.

Ellis, R. Kimoto, W.I., Bitman, J. and Edmondson, L.F. 1974. J. Am. Oil Chemists' Soc. 51:4.

Gerson, T., Shorland, F.B. and Adams, Y. 1961. Biochem. J. 81:584.

Gerson, T., Shorland, F.B. and Dunkley, G.G. 1964. Biochem. J. 92:385.

Gerson, T., Shorland, F.B. and Dunkley, G.G. 1965. Biochem. J. 96:399.

Hegsted, D.M., McGandy, R.B., Myers, M.L. and Stare, F.J. 1965. Am. J. Clin. Nutr. 17:281.

Keys, A., Anderson, J.T. and Grande, F. 1957. Lancet i:959.

Leren P., 1966. Acta Medica Scand. Suppl. 466.

Leveille, G.A. 1975. J. Anim. Sci. In Press.

Miettinen, M., Turpeinen, O., Karvonen, J.J., Elosuo, R. and Paavilainen, E. 1972. Lancet ii:835.

Morrison, L.M. 1960. J. Am. Med. Assn. 173:884.

National Heart Foundation of New Zealand. 1971. Coronary Heart Disease: A New Zealand Report. National Heart Foundation, Wellington, New Zealand.

Pearce, M.L. and Dayton, S. 1971. Lancet, i:464.

Reiser, R. 1973. Am. J. Clin. Nutr. 26:524.

Royal Society of New Zealand. 1971. Coronary Heart Disease: Report of a Committee. Royal Society of New Zealand, Wellington, New Zealand.

Shamberger, R.J., Andreone, T.L. and Willis, C.E. 1974. J. Cancer Inst. 53:1771.

Sturdevant, R.A.L., Pearce, J.L. and Dayton, S. 1973. New Eng. J. Med. 288:24.

Vaghefi, S.B., Makdani, D.D. and Mickelsen, O. 1974. Am. J. Clin. Nutr. 27:1231.

(6)

THE STATUS IN SWEDEN

Björn Isaksson

Institute of Clinical Nutrition, University of Gothenburg

Sahlgren s Hospital, S-413 45 GOTHENBURG, SWEDEN

The discussion in Sweden as to which external factors may give rise to the development of atherosclerosis is still very lively. We are far from having reached the stage where it is generally accepted that changes in the diet would be of value in the prevention of atherosclerosis. With respect to tobacco, however, the situation is entirely different. Smoking can be measured in units in about the same way as is done with tablets. This immediately makes it easier for physicians to accept the idea that if the dose is changed, this will affect the organism in a negative or positive direction. As to the importance of physical exercise, we are still lacking evidence in Sweden to support the notion that physical exercise may delay the development of atherosclerosis, prevent heart infarction diseases or reduce the blood pressure.

A sufficiently strong public opinion supports the idea to improve our dietary habits, reduce our tobacco consumption and increase our physical exercise, however. Such recommendations have gradually developed out of the activities of individuals, medical societies or idealistic organizations. Today, these recommendations have been given a more official character as they are issued by the Committee on Health Information of the Swedish Board of Social Welfare. Practically all other types of information have been adapted to the official message and this has undoubtedly influenced the product development of the food industry, the advertising of the Swedish Tobacco Monopoly and the activities of the sports organizations.

The recommendations, which most often are made in connection with nationwide campaigns or campaigns aimed at special target groups, usually serve the purpose of being generally health promoting. It is almost a rule, however, that the importance of the campaigns in the prevention of atherosclerosis is given special emphasis.

RECOMMENDATIONS CONCERNING DIET

The background of the recommendations concerning improved dietary habits is, of course, the severely changed dietary habits in our country during this century. Most of these changes have been of a negative character (Fig. 1). Some changes, of course, are positive such as the increase in the consumption of vegetables and fruits, but the drastic decrease in the consumption of bread and potatoes and the simultaneous strong increase in the consumption of fats and sugar are clearly negative. As for milk products, there has been a decrease in the total consumption but an increase in the fat products. As regards the meat product group, lean meat has given way for pork and fat sausages.

These changes, which have resulted in the diet consisting of more than 60 % fats and sugar towards the end of the 60's, have been combined with a gradually decreasing physical activity because of the continuous mechanization of our society. These changes are responsible both for overconsumption and underconsumption diseases in our country (Fig. 2). The risk of undernutrition diseases is caused by the fact that fat- and/or sugar-rich food with their low nutrition density cover so much of the plate that there is not sufficient space for food which - in addition to energy - also contain significant amount of essential nutrients (Fig. 3). An extensive study of the whole situation in low-income groups in Sweden showed a higher percentage of people with wrong food habits than in other social classes.

These data and the failure of earlier activities to improve the dietary habits, together with the enormous and still increasing costs for the medical care of people with different nutrition diseases forced the National Board of Health and Welfare to have its Committee on Health Education to start an active campaign. From the very beginning, it was found desirable to combine the campaign for better nutrition with propaganda for increased physical activity. The organization of the campaign "Diet and Exercise" started in 1968-69 and the purpose was to give the individual more opportunities to improve his health by means of different health policy methods. Its symbol (Fig. 4) is a heart and an arrow, "a heart on the move". The Leadership group (LKM) (Fig. 5) have representatives from national and municipal organisations, agricultural organizations, the labor union movement, certain idealistic organizations, and the food industry. The responsibility to work out a scientific basic material was given to the MEK group. The first report of this group was published in 1971 and a summary of the recommendations is given in Figure 6. We were all rather suprised to learn that this publication was accepted as an official guide with respect to the product development of the industry and to an increasing extent

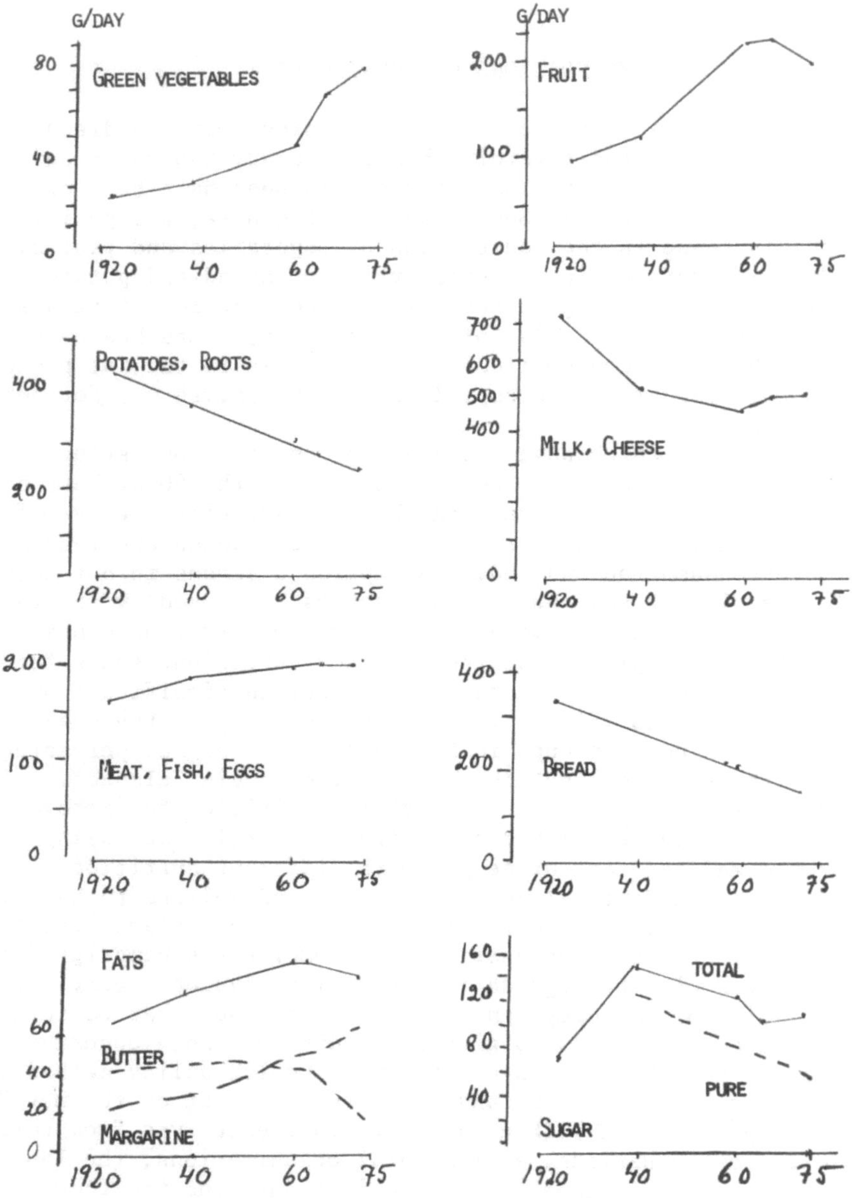

Figure 1. Changes in mean daily consumption, Sweden 1920-1973

	Clinical conditions
Overconsumption	
Energy	obesity
Saturated fat	atherosclerosis ?
Sugar	caries
Underconsumption	
Iron	anemia
Vitamins, other minerals	"suboptimal health"
Fibre	constipation

Figure 2. Malnutrition in industrialized countries

also by other producers and the commercial organizations.

An Effect Measuring Project Group performed a sociological study in 1971 in order to define the knowledge and attitudes of the population with regard to diet and exercise. The diet knowledge did not turn out to be very good: 60 % thought that calcium in milk was harmful for the blood vessels, while 40 % did not know if saturated or polyunsaturated fatty acids were good or bad in that connection and so on, but most people were relatively conscious of the fact that we ought to avoid fat and sweet food.

The project group Institutions made a basic investigation of 225 lunch canteens, which showed that good nutrition was strived for only in a couple of cases. Therefore, several large household conferences were held all over the country, and the project group worked out diet recommendations for employee restaurants, for the old age care institutions, for nursery schools. Furthermore, they produced special information packages to be used in the training of the large household staff.

Another project group called Exercise cooperated with the sports movements whose 200,000 leaders were expected to be able to function as communicators of the dietary principles, at the same time as they should motivate people to increase their physical exercise. The national sports movements have an extensive secretariate which produced and distributed a lot of pamphlets.

Furthermore, it was considered particularly important to establish good relations with the food industry and to gain their support - especially economically - in making the message reach the general public. Therefore, the so-called Coordination Group became perhaps the most important one and included representatives from the food industry and from commerce. The group decided to promote theme activities and the first was called "Begin your day in a better way" - thus, it had been found that most people had an entirely insufficient breakfast meal. Most of the remaining people eat a qualitatively bad breakfast. The food industry promoted its best products in this connection. The shop windows showed complete

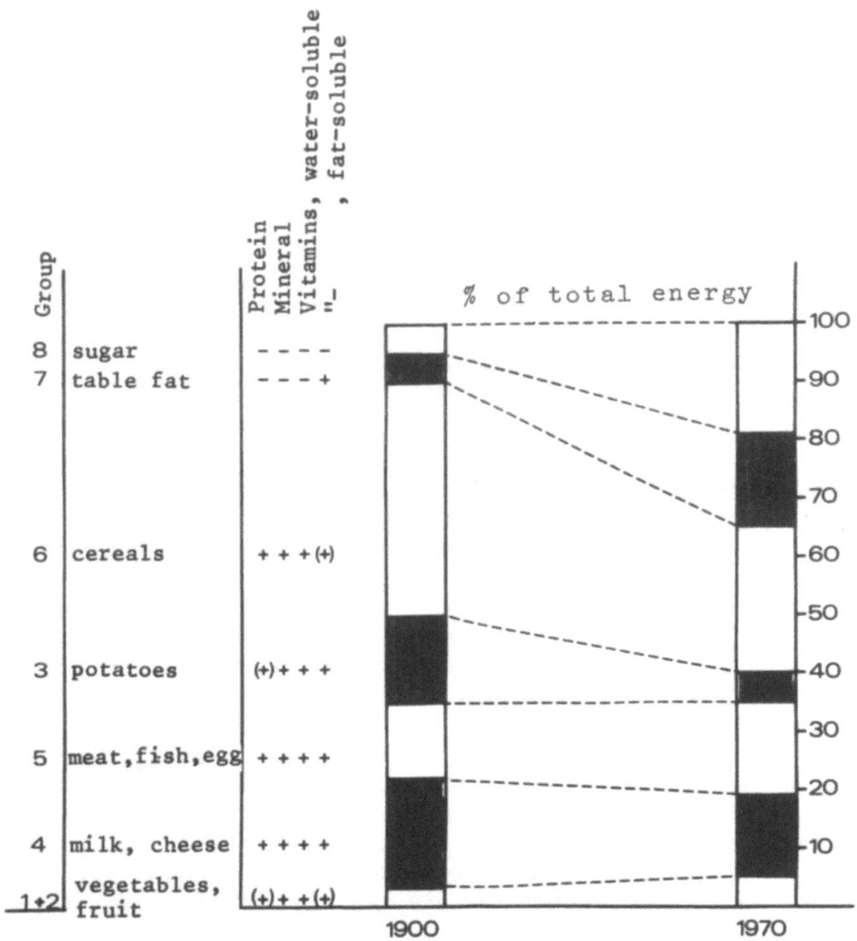

Figure 3. The effect of the changed dietary habits during this century on the caloric and nutrition density.

breakfast meals and centrally produced pamphlets were given to the customers. This campaign had very positive results for all parties involved and has served as a model for future campaigns which, during 1976, will involve all aspects of the diet and which will be aimed at all categories of people in the country. The recommendations are still based on the MEK-rapport which will be published in a revised edition, and on the work of the project group Diet and Expenses. This group was formed because it was a generally held opinion that nutritious food was too expensive - a misconception which was easy to defeat by means of practical exemplifications. In future campaigns, some of the objectives are to correct prejudices and misconceptions in dietary matters and to

Figure 4. The symbol of the Swedish campaign "Diet and Exercise"

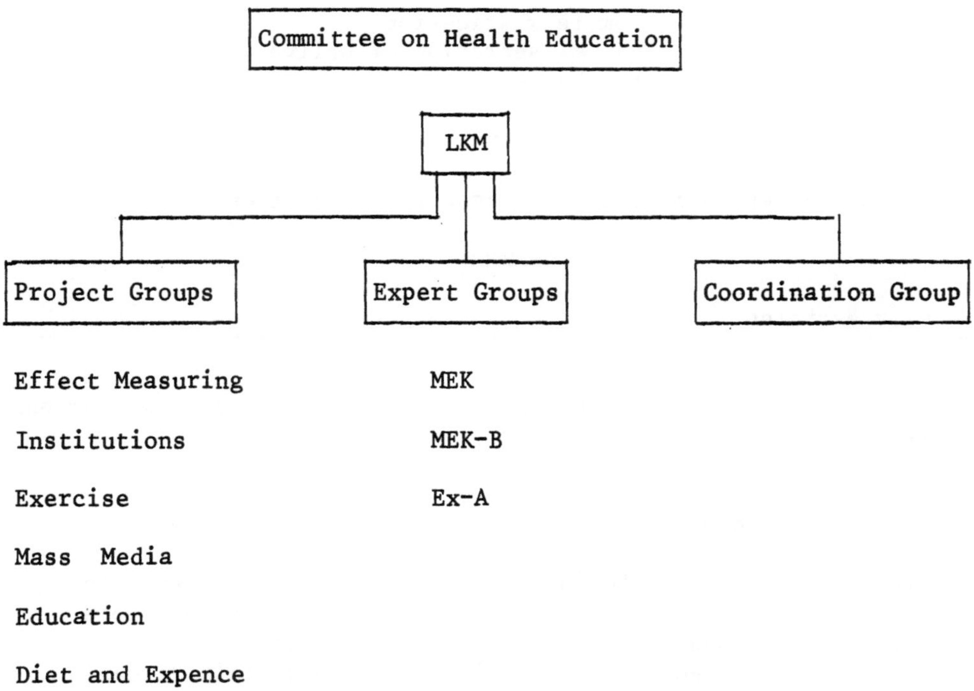

Figure 5. The organisation of the campaign "Diet and Exercise"

Fat ↓ from 42 cal% to <35 cal%

Sugar ↓ 17 cal% to about 10 cal%
Saturated fat ↓, PUFA ↑

Green vegetables ↑, fruit ↑, potatoes ↑, roots ↑, lean milk ↑,
fish ↑, lean meat ↑, poultry ↑, bread ↑, other cereals ↑.

xxxxx

Breakfast:	1/4 of daily energy need.	Most food groups.
Lunch:	1/3 "-	All 7 food groups.
Dinner:	1/3 "-	"-

xxxxx

Dental health: sugar-containing products ↓
regular meals
few snacks
promote mastication
" secretion of saliva
oral hygiene

xxxxx

Institutional meals must fulfil these recommendations

xxxxx

Regular exercise

Figure 6. Summary of the Medical Expert Group (MEK) recommendations 1971.

inform the public where hidden fats and hidden sugar are to be found.

The campaign of the Social Welfare Board has given rise to a great number of local and special target group campaigns. Some activities are aimed at the risk groups. This applies, for instance, to children of parents with high blood lipid values, adults who in connection with physical examinations have been found to have high blood lipid values without clinical symptoms, or persons who have had a heart infarction. In these cases, the treatment has been combined with tests of different types of information channels for the purpose of trying to find the channels which give the best results. Our own studies of patients at risk at the Section for Preventive Cardiology in Gothenburg have given the expected result that individual advice by a dietitian has the best effect, especially in subjects who have the motivation of a previous infarction, while advice only through pamphlets has no effect whatsoever on the blood lipid values. Mention should also be made in this connection of Professor Malmros' "Klostergårds-projekt" where the population of an entire section of a city can buy a great number of special products with a high P/S-quotient, receive both oral and written information, and have their blood lipid values controlled regularly.

RECOMMENDATIONS CONCERNING SMOKING

Sweden does not belong to the high tobacco consumption countries. The average cigarette consumption is only half of that in Canada, but we have tripled our consumption since the middle of the 1940's. Smoking starts in younger and younger people and the number of smokers among the girls increases considerably quicker than among boys. Different anti-smoking campaigns have been carried out and a tobacco research committee was appointed by the Social Welfare Board in 1971. The committee published its report in 1973. The objective of their activities during a 25-year period is to reduce the cigarette consumption to the same relative extent that it had during the 1920's in Sweden. It is proposed that children born in 1975 and later should be subjected to measures which mean that they will encounter environments which are as smoke-free as possible.

RECOMMENDATIONS CONCERNING PHYSICAL EXERCISE

As to the recommendations concerning increased physical activity, the national sports movement has started a campaign "Sweden in trim" with the slogan "sports for everyone". It is made clear, however, that it is not a question of elite sports.

RESULTS

What has been the result of these efforts? Apparently, many persons have improved their breakfast habits and the sale of good breakfast products has increased considerably. The meat has become much leaner, and milk with only 0.5 % fat is available. We can buy butter mixed with polyunsaturated fatty acids and several excellent margarines with 25 % linoleic acid or with only 40 % fat. Convenient food has been given a nutritionally more correct composition and the demand for all these products is increasing. Totally, the fat content of our diet has decreased from an average of 42 % of the total energy at the end of the 1960's to a little less than the present 38 %. We seem to be the only OECD country which shows a decrease in our consumption of fat. The smokers have become more considerate towards non-smokers and many - especially physicians -

have stopped smoking. Probably, we tend to move around a little more although we still can be described as homo sedentarius.

It would be difficult, of course, to prove that these changes are the result of the information campaigns and the preventive measures. It is still too early to form an opinion as to whether the changes have or will result in a reduced number of atherosclerosis cases.

(7)

THE ALTERNATIVE AMERICAN DIET

William E. Connor and Sonja L. Connor

The Department of Medicine,
University of Oregon School of Medicine
Portland, Oregon, U.S.A.

Almost all responsible organizations and individual authorities in the United States firmly suggest that atherosclerosis is a preventable disease. Recommendations to prevent atherosclerosis have centered upon five objectives which are: (1) The abolition of cigarette smoking; (2) the control of high blood pressure; (3) the institution of regular exercise; (4) the lowering of elevated serum cholesterol levels and (5) finally and most importantly, changes in the habitual diet to lower the serum lipid levels. No one disagrees that the public at large should follow the first three recommendations related to smoking, blood pressure and exercise. Nor is there any controversy about the desirability of treating persons with identified hyperlipidemia. Strong differences of opinion are expressed about the wisdom and safety of diet modification for the general public. The Intersociety Commission for Heart Disease Resources and the American Heart Association have both urged dietary change for the public at large in an effort to prevent coronary heart disease and atherosclerosis (1,2). Others have advised caution and delay until the "final proof is in".

The authors of this paper believe that there should be no further delay in advising a national change in the way people eat. The seriousness of the coronary heart disease epidemic, the scientific bases for advocating dietary change, the economic problems associated with the present diet and the nutritional soundness and safety of the proposed changes in eating all suggest that dietary change will lead to an improvement in the health of people in the United States and will produce no adverse results.

Four lines of scientific work have provided evidence about the key role of nutritional factors in the causation of atherosclerosis.

First, worldwide epidemiological studies have related the kind of diet eaten to the plasma cholesterol level and to the incidence of coronary heart disease. Second, animal experiments have established that dietary cholesterol and fat are the only nutrients which induce hypercholesterolemia and atherosclerosis. The third line of evidence relates to human studies which have shown that plasma cholesterol levels are elevated by dietary cholesterol and saturated fat. Fourth, there is evidence that cholesterol is the major chemical constituent of the atherosclerotic artery and that this excessive cholesterol is derived from the plasma cholesterol.

The proposed dietary changes have the propensity of shifting the entire serum cholesterol distribution curve of the population to the left, with lower serum cholesterol levels at all ages. Specifically to be stressed at the onset is that all of the dietary recommendations are feasible. Many individuals in our country and especially throughout the world are already following them. These recommendations have been a part and parcel of the life styles of many population groups historically as well as at the present time. Paramount to these changes is the development and implementation of an "alternative" to the American diet which is based on five criteria:

(1) Such a diet should prevent diseases associated with the usual American diet, primarily coronary heart disease.
(2) The diet must be nutritionally adequate with no undue excesses or deficits.
(3) Any dietary change should be ecologically sound at this time of world food shortages.
(4) Such a diet should be economical for all peoples of the world.
(5) The "alternative diet" should be based in part upon foods eaten by the peoples of past civilizations.

The Alternative Diet: People do not make abrupt changes in their dietary habits. It may take from 2 to 10 years or longer to make permanent changes in one's manner of eating. It is suggested that the changes to the present American diet be approached in a gradual manner, with each phase introducing more changes toward the alternative dietary pattern desired.

Phase I: The aim of the first phase is to reduce the consumption of foods very high in cholesterol and saturated fat. This can be accomplished by deleting egg yolk, butterfat, lard and organ meats from the diet and by using substitute products when possible: margarine for butter, vegetable oils and shortening for lard, skim milk for whole milk and egg whites for whole eggs. In addition, a decrease in the use of table salt is encouraged. This is because dietary salt is related to the occurrence of hypertension which is a risk factor for the development of coronary heart disease (1,3,4).

The majority of recipes which Americans are currently using can be easily altered to meet the criteria for the "alternative diet" through the use of substitute products. Many of the recipes can also be altered to use less fat and salt. In addition, there are many appropriate recipes now being printed in cookbooks, magazines and newspapers.

Phase II: In Phase II some reduction in meat consumption is the goal, with a gradual transition from the American ideal of up to 16 ounces of meat a day to no more than 6 to 8 ounces per day. In addition, we propose the use of less fat and less cheese as well as the use of fewer products containing large amounts of salt, salt being a chief additive of many processed foods. New recipes to replace current recipes which cannot be altered to meet the requirements of the "alternative diet" will be made available. Recipes not easily altered are those using meat as the principal ingredient and recipes using high fat dairy products. Industries will be encouraged to develop recipes and products which meet the specifications of less meat and fat. As more and more new recipes and products become available, people can incorporate these into their lifestyles of food consumption.

Phase III: In Phase III we take an historical approach to the consumption of meat. Man has always eaten meat. What he has not done is to eat meat every day, let alone several times a day. Even today daily meat consumption is only possible for the affluent minority of the world's population. It is not to our advantage, either health-wise or resource-wise, to consume large amounts of meat every day. As President Thomas Jefferson said in a letter to Dr. Utley, "Like my friend the doctor (i.e. Rush), I have lived temperately, eating little animal food, and not as an aliment, so much as a condiment for the vegetables which constitute my principal diet" (5).

It is proposed in Phase III, that meat, fish and poultry be used as condiments rather than aliments. The total of these foods should average no more than three to four ounces per day. Fish and poultry should be emphasized instead of meat. Also in Phase III, the use of low cholesterol cheeses and a decrease in the amount of salt used in cooking is recommended. Certain foods should be saved for special celebrations: Extra meat, regular cheese, chocolate, coconut and "salty" foods. During Phase III, the transition from the American diet to the "alternative diet" will have been completed.

Composition of the "Alternative Diet": The cholesterol content of the American diet and of the three phases of the "alternative diet" is shown in Figure I. The American diet contains approximately 750 mg, cholesterol per day. This is decreased in Phase I to 450 mg in Phase II to 300 mg, and in Phase III to 100 mg per day. The "alternative diet" is adequate in both the quantity and quality of protein required for body needs. In addition, this diet meets

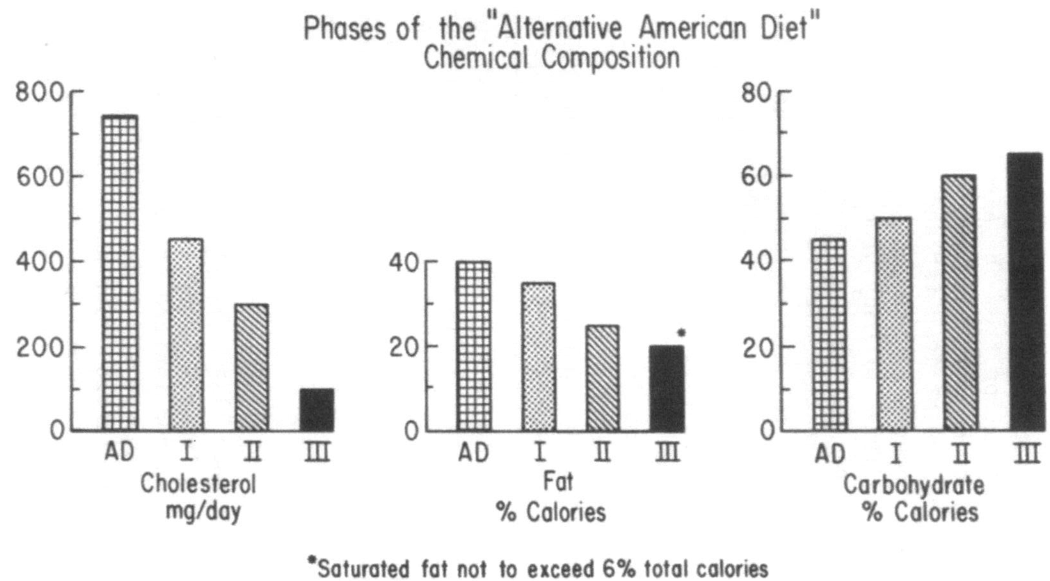

Figure 1: The chemical composition of the 3 phases of the "Alternative American Diet". The symbol "AD" refers to the usual American diet whose composition can then be compared to the phases of the "alternative diet".

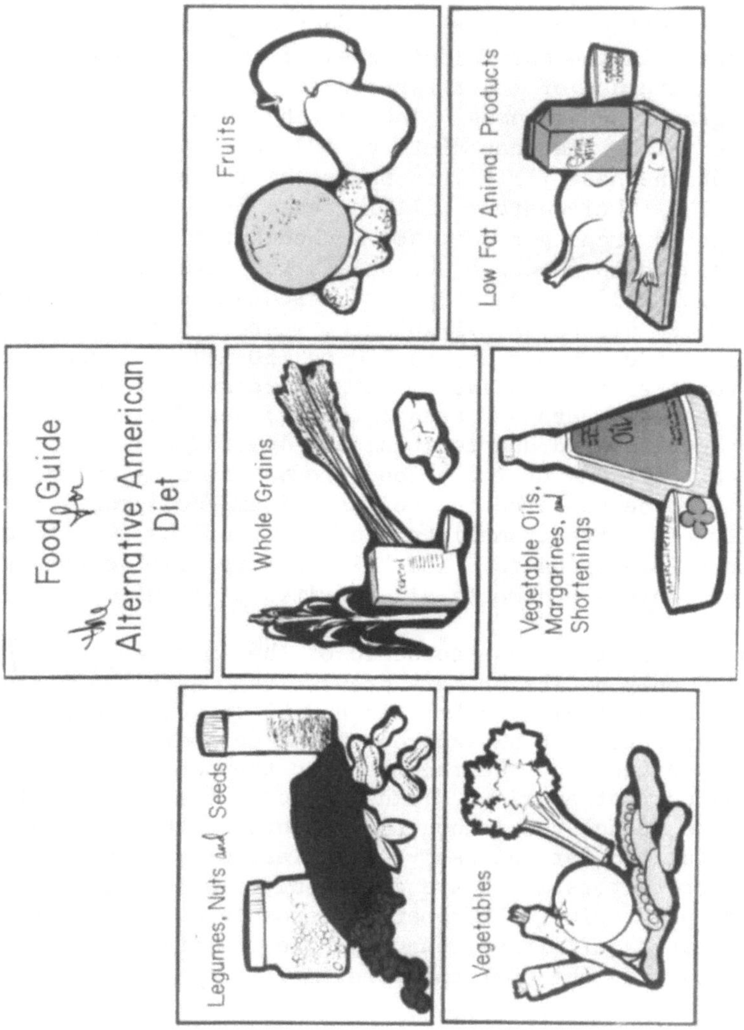

Figure 2: Food Guide for the "Alternative American Diet" with foods categorized into 6 food groups.

the recommended dietary allowances for all other nutrients (6). The fat content decreases from 40% of calories in the American diet to 35% in Phase I, to 25% in Phase II, and to 20% in Phase III. The polyunsaturated fat content is kept at 6 to 7 percent of calories in order to prevent any possible toxic effects of consuming large amounts of a food not eaten previously by any group of people (7,8). In order to have sufficient calories to meet body needs, we propose a gradual increase in the physiologic fuel of the body, carbohydrate, with emphasis on the use of the fiber-containing complex carbohydrates, whole grains and legumes. The carbohydrate increases from 45% of calories in the American diet, to 50% in Phase I, to 60% in Phase II, to 65% in Phase III. This increases the bulk of the diet considerably. The fiber content will increase from 2 to 3 grams per day to 12 to 15 grams per day. Even though the total carbohydrate is increased to 45-65% of calories, the sugar content is decreased from 20 to 10% of calories. The sodium content decreases from 200 to 300 mEq per day to 75-100 mEq, whereas potassium increases from 30 to 70 mEq per day to 120 to 150 mEq. Figure 2 is a food guide for the "alternative diet". There are 6 food groups: Whole grains; legumes, nuts and seeds; fruits; vegetables; vegetable oils, margarines and shortenings; and low fat animal products. Note that only one of the 6 food groups contains animal products. This is to be compared to the Basic Four Food groups (9) which exemplify the current American diet. Two of the four food groups contain animal products. The "alternative diet" offers a wide variety of choices and meets all nutritional requirments (10).

The coronary heart disease epidemic of the American population can be curtailed only by its primary prevention. As already demonstrated, both by past clinical trials and by logic, secondary prevention in patients with already developed coronary heart disease is not very effective. We recommend to the public at large a change in the current American "luxus" diet to the "alternative diet" in order to reduce the pathogenic factors in the diet, namely cholesterol, saturated fat, excessive calories, sugar and salt and to increase other factors which are deficient; complex carbohydrate and fiber. The prevention of coronary atherosclerosis will occur to the extent that a definitive change in the dietary life style is adopted and carried out over the lifetime.

* This study was supported by U.S. Public Health Service Research Grant HL 19,130 from the National Heart and Lung Institute and by the General Clinical Research Centers Program (RR-334) of the Division of Research Resources, National Institutes of Health.

REFERENCES

1. Report of Inter-Society Commission for Heart Disease Resources: Primary Prevention of Atherosclerotic Disease. Atherosclerosis and Epidemiology Study Groups, Inter-Society Commission for Heart Disease Resources. Circ. 42:A-55, 1970.

2. Committee on Nutrition: Diet and Heart Disease. American Heart Association, 1968.

3. Kirkendall, W.M., Page, L. and Langford, H.: Diet and Hypertension in National Nutrition Policy-Study-1974. Hearings before the select committee on nutrition and human needs of the United States Senate. U.S. Government Printing Office, Washington, D.C. 20402. Series 74/NNP-6A:2848.

4. Dahl, L.K., Salt and Hypertension. Am. J. Clin. Nutr. 25:231, 1972.

5. Padover, S.L.: The Writings of Thomas Jefferson. The Heritage Press, New York. 1967.

6. Food and Nutrition Board, National Academy of Sciences. National Research Council, Recommended Dietary Allowances. 8th Ed. Washington D.C.: National Academy of Sciences, 1974.

7. Studevant, R.A.J., Pearce, M.L. and Dayton, S.: Increased Gallstone Prevalence in Men on Serum-Cholesterol Lowering Diets. New Eng. J. Med. 283:1358, 1970.

8. Pearce, J.L., and Dayton, S.: Incidence of Cancer in Men on a Diet High in Polyunsaturated Fat. Lancet 1:464, 1971.

9. A Guide to Good Eating. 3rd Ed. Copyright, National Dairy Council, Chicago, Illinois, 1973.

10. Bickel, J.H., and Connor, S.L. Nutrient content of the "alternative diet". Unpublished observations. The University of Oregon and the University of Iowa.

(8)

RECOMMENDATIONS TO THE PUBLIC FOR PREVENTION OF ATHEROSCLEROSIS FROM SIX WESTERN COUNTRIES - THEIR APPLICATION TO CHILDREN

Shiela C. Mitchell, M.D.
Division of Heart and Vascular Diseases,
National Heart and Lung Institute,
Landow Building, Room C808,
Bethesda, Maryland, U.S.A.

In considering the recommendations for the prevention of atherosclerosis, developed primarily for adults, for application to the younger members of society, specifically those in the first two decades of life, five major facts must be kept in mind. The first of these is that the recommendations must have all the hallmarks necessary for creditability.

If suggestions are made for too much change for too many people too quickly, then, not only will these recommendations, but subsequent ones, lose their creditability with the public to whom they are directed. A data base which is not firm will also imperil creditability. Accordingly, since all the causes of coronary heart disease and atherosclerosis are not known at this time, and any universal recommendations are therefore sure to fail to prevent <u>all</u> coronary disease, the prudent course would appear to be one which focuses upon those at highest, and at documented, risk.

Not only is this prudent but it is likely to be effective since it is the approach most similar to current medical practice. Physicians are accustomed to making as precise a diagnosis as possible; and to recommending as specific therapy, as possible. Accordingly, they will be most comfortable making recommendations for prevention, to youngsters and teenagers who carry established risk factors of premature coronary heart disease.

Limiting the recommendations to individuals or families at high risk also avoids the unfortunate connotations associated with omnipotent pronouncements from "big brother" addressed to all the people.

Recommendations focusing on this group of potential patients have other inherent benefits as well. One of these is that this "targeted" or "focused" philosophy allows for the education of physicians, which can only be compressed so far in time; education which alerts them to the presence of risk factors in children, to the problems of dealing with these, and to the prerequisites of effective, preventive therapy. It also provides time to develop, evaluate, and improve the effectiveness of educational materials for those at high risk, and of grade school or teen age.

In considering the general characteristics of the recommendations to be directed towards children and teenagers, it is imperative to recognize that neither are simply small, nor young, adults. Nor are they a homogeneous group. Preschoolers are not the same as preteens; high achievers are not the same as dropouts. Accordingly, a variety of approaches will be needed in order to motivate adoption of preventive measures and the maintenance of them during the growing as well as the adult years.

Particularly in the young, one must be careful not to make recommendations that can, or may, result in adverse effects. Such effects are often unforeseen and totally unexpected. About the only thing which <u>is</u> certain is that some unexpected results will turn up. A potential "side effect" of a diet high in polyunsaturated fats is the possible atherogenic property of the phytosterols, substances readily absorbed in the intestine and found in many polyunsaturated fatty acids. Another potential "side effect" is seen in animal experiments utilizing hypertensive rats where it has been shown that one strain has extrinsic sympathetic, "salt resistent" hypertension, the other intrinsic, renal, salt sensitive hypertension. Restricting salt in the first group, if this differentiation holds true in man, might have undesirable affects both physiological and psychological. No one likes to be denied a pleasurable activity such as eating a favorite food, only to subsequently discover that the restriction was unnecessary.

All of these considerations presuppose that recommendations are needed for all children who bear the stigmata of high risk for premature coronary heart disease. While there may be little doubt that preventive measures are needed in youngsters, the efficacy of full implementation of these has yet to be established. However, clear epidemiologic proof does exist that some young people notably, young black males, must receive preventive measures in their teens, or perhaps earlier, if they are to be spared crippling strokes or cerebrovascular death in their twenties. Furthermore, the vital statistics in most western countries clearly indicate that a nontrivial number of young adults in their thirties suffer a fatal myocardial infarction. It is difficult to believe that the atheroslcerosis leading to this only began sometime during the third or fourth decade of life.

The data from the Evans County Georgia Study have shown that there is tracking of serum cholesterol levels from age 20 onward. Blood pressure values show a similar tracking in this study, tracking which is evident by age 15. These data have also revealed that the weight/height ratio in the late teens is almost as accurate a predictor of blood pressure, as is that pressure itself, with the obese having the highest blood pressure levels. While more data are needed from other population groups, it would seem unwise to ignore these data, pointing, as they do, to the need for prevention in the high risk child.

From other studies there are emerging data that cigarette smoking is, for some people, a true addiction that is virtually impossible to cure. Here, the only therapy is prevention. Given the ever decreasing age at which young people are beginning to smoke cigarettes regularly, it would seem prudent to expend some energies to encourage more of these youngsters to forego the tobacco habit.

Having decided then that recommendations for prevention of atherosclerosis are needed in children, and that these should be focused upon those at high risk, issues of feasibility come to the fore. One of the first of these is the family, in which the child is one of several people, with needs and desires requiring satisfaction. Since a positive family history is, apparently, one of the strongest risk factors, it makes good sense to direct the recommendations at the entire family.

It is obviously essential that the recommendations be feasible, within the family <u>and</u> for the individual members. If a change in diet is recommended, then the foods to be consumed must be available to the patient and be socially acceptable to him and his peer group. The primary physician, who, in most cases will be dispensing this preventive therapy, needs to know, have the opportunity to learn, or be able to refer his patients to someone who does know about the problems of translating nutrients into foods, and foods into shopping lists, menus, cooking techniques, and social settings. None of this can be learned even by an intelligent patient in one brief visit. So it would seem to be imperative that "diet teachers" be trained and made available to physicians and to their patients. The availability of such paramedical personnel would do much to insure the consistency and efficacy of the advice given. Particularly is this essential for teenagers whose mobility is one of their chief characteristics.

Having developed and implemented recommendations which have all the hallmarks of creditability and feasibility and therefore can be expected to be effective, care needs to be taken that in their implementation these recommendations do no harm. Accordingly, one of the approaches that is not recommended is that of mass screening. All the evidence to date suggests that this is not the most cost effective way to identify youngsters at high risk and it does bear potential for harm if a youngster is mislabelled as coronary prone. Not only may such mislabelling lead to neurosis, but it may haunt the youngster as he seeks employment and as he attempts to acquire life insurance. It may even render him more prone to other illnesses since any and all symptoms may be blamed on his supposed risk factors or their underlying cause.

Adopting the general recommendations made to adults in the hope of preventing premature atherosclerosis in children, lead to the following recommendations;

1. That primary physicians be alerted to, and their active participation enlisted in, this preventive approach to medical therapy. This is relatively easy to do with pediatricians who are already attuned to their preventive role in medicine, but it may require some special preparation for those who treat children but are not pediatricians.

2. That a family history be taken in depth and in detail at the first examination, and that this be updated at each subsequent examination. For children and teenagers it would be ideal to have such an examination each year. However, realistically it might be better to aim at one complete examination every five years.

3. At each physical examination the blood pressure should be carefully taken and recorded upon the youngsters chart, even though "hypertension," at present, can only be identified in adult, or statistical, terms.

4. Youngsters, and their parents, should be made aware as to why height and weight are measured and recorded at each examination. These measurements are fairly routine, yet their prognostic import, particularly the synergism of obesity and hypertension, is not well known to the average patient.

5. Every five years, a random (which is to say non-fasting) serum cholesterol level should be obtained and recorded. In part this is in order that the child may serve as the propositus for identifying the family at high risk and in part because it is becoming increasingly more common for one parent in the home not to be the biological parent of the child. Obviously, for adopted children, neither parent may be the biological progenitor. Using only family history as the index of suspicion would leave these children unidentified.

6. No test result whether blood pressure reading, serum cholesterol, or obesity index should be recorded or reported to the child or his parents as an abnormality until the test has been repeated at least three times and the abnormality found to be consistent.

7. The creation of "diet teachers" is highly recommended both for work with youngsters and adults at high risk of atherosclerosis.

8. That both practicing and research physicians should work closely with the food industry in order to ensure the valid and relevant labelling of foods. The source of the fat is important but equally important is the knowledge of the effect of the manufacturing and processing upon the polyunsaturated ratio of that fat.

9. That practicing and research physicians become working partners with psychologists, sociologists, psychiatrists, and others in the fields of motivation, and adherence, particularly with respect to the social and pyschological implications both of dietary practices, and smoking habits, and of alterations in these areas.

10. That more attention be paid to providing older children and teenagers with valid information about cigarette smoking, offering them alternate expressions of virility and maturity, and providing them with a suitable data base upon which to make a rational choice.

Most of the recommendations here made apply to the medical profession or to paramedical personnel, suggesting activities and approaches they might use with the lay public. Why then are they being made at a session entitled "Recommendations to the Public?"

The reasons for this are five fold. In the first place it is the people who make the social mileau into which the recommendations must fall and wherein they must be effective, if they are to be effective. Secondly, it is lay people who are peers to lay people. Peer pressure is an important part in any preventive therapy.

In the third place it is only people themselves who can decide to take themselves or their children to the doctor for identification of risk factors and for preventive therapy. Not even in a totalitarian society can one order people to be healthy. In a democracy one is foolish even to try to order people to acquire good health habits.

Then too, in the final analysis it is people that underwrite the cost of medical research and medical practice. Accordingly, recommendations made to either of these professional groups are in effect recommendations for the people.

And finally, it is the people who will benefit from the preventive therapy, or suffer disease from the lack of preventive measures, if appropriate recommendations are not made and not made available to them.

(9)

PRACTICAL CONSIDERATIONS REGARDING AVAILABILITY OF FOOD SUPPLIES

Ralph Witty, Ph.D.

Assistant Director of Research, Canada Packers Limited
2211 St. Clair Avenue West
Toronto, Ontario, Canada

The average North American consumes in excess of 100 lbs. of fat per year from all sources. While Canadians consume only slightly less total fat than Americans, there are some substantial differences in the types of fat consumed by the two groups. On the average Canadians consume more butter (11.2 vs 3.6 lbs.) and less salad and cooking oils (7.5 vs 18.6 lbs.) than their U.S. counterparts. Also, because of their lower intake of beef and pork, the Canadian consumption of meat fats is lower. These differences in the types of fat consumed affect the polyunsaturated fatty acid (PUFA) intake in the two countries. The PUFA intake is also affected by the vegetable oils available to the oil processing industries. Soybean oil is by far the major oil produced and used in the U.S.A.; it accounts for about half of the edible oil used. In Canada, canbra oil (rapeseed oil) is the only oil produced in excess of their requirements and canbra and soybean oils share the lead with butter in total use.

It is possible to estimate the average PUFA consumption of Canadians and Americans by applying what we would consider to be normal manufacturing procedures to the different fats and oils used to produce shortening, margarine,and salad and cooking oils. These calculations show the PUFA consumption in the U.S. is 16 lbs. per person per year and 11 lbs. in Canada. This substantial difference is not reflected in the incidence of heart disease.

We can, with our present technology, increase the PUFA intake in both countries. It is well known, for example, that feeding monogastric animals or poultry a diet rich in PUFA will increase the degree of unsaturation in the tissue fats. Recently, Scott et al., have shown that similar changes can be achieved in ruminant tissue fats and milk fat by feeding specially processed unsaturated fats to the animal. The conversion efficiency of dietary fat to tissue fat is only 20 to 40%. In addition to this poor transfer, there is the loss during preparation and cooking, plus the plate loss. It is doubtful if the conversion in the human amounts to more than 10%.

There is a very simple and efficient method of increasing the PUFA content of milk products, that is, to remove all or part of the butter fat, and replace it with a suitable vegetable oil. This procedure is not legal in many states and provinces, but filled-milk products are on the market in some areas.

Many changes in the visible fats are technically feasible, but these changes cannot be made without added costs and without some changes in the oilseed production. It is technically possible to produce margarine with 44% PUFA, shortening with 40% PUFA and salad oils with 60% PUFA. A complete substitution of butter, margarine, shortening, salad and cooking oils for these new products, plus a change in 50% of the milk fat, would increase the average PUFA intake by approximately 10 lbs. per capita per year. These drastic dietary changes would also reduce the intake of monoenoic acids and trans-acids, and increase the amounts of saturated fatty acids slightly. Whether or not these changes would be sufficient to make a significant difference in the health of the population is open for discussion.

There are sufficient supplies of soybean oil in the U.S. market to make the suggested changes in margarine, shortening and milk fat. However, it would not be possible to change the salad oil to the recommended 60% PUFA without a major increase in the production of sunflower, safflower and corn oils.

The Canadian product changes are much more limited by the availability of suitable oils. It would be necessary for Canada to double its oil purchases abroad in order to obtain the quantities of the desired oils. The production of the required quantities of sunflower, safflower or corn oil is virtually impossible under our climatic conditions.

REFERENCES

Scott, T.W., Cook, L.J., Ferguson, U.A., McDonald, J.W., Buchanan, R.A., and Hills, G.L. Aust. Jour. Sci. 32:291, 1970.

(10)

DISCUSSION (RECOMMENDATIONS TO THE PUBLIC FOR PREVENTION OF ATHEROSCLEROSIS)

Dr. Hewitt made two important points in his opening remarks. 1) That any strategy aimed at prevention should be one in which public compliance is not a problem, that is, the strategy should not require the active participation of individual members of the general public. 2) The outcome of any intervention should be assessed in terms of its impact and the net reduction of the death rate from all causes rather than from only the specific health problems for which the intervention is designed. Most of the speakers seemed to accept the evidence that smoking is detrimental to health and contributes to the development of cardiovascular disease. Although the evidence concerning exercise is incomplete, nobody would disagree with the concept that exercise is "good for you". The question of diet does not appear to be settled. Obviously, some believe that reduction of cholesterol intake and an increase in the ratio of polyunsaturated fats to saturated fats in the diet is desirable, particularly for prevention of the development of atherosclerosis and its complications. Others believe that there is not enough evidence at the present time that this would be of much value to the population as a whole. The Swedish experience of a national approach to establish a nutritious diet for adults is interesting in relation to the compliance issue raised by Professor Hewitt. In Sweden, there appears to be general acceptance that reduction of cholesterol and alteration of the fat content in the diet is desirable.

Dr. Connor brought forward a basic point when he pointed out that food requirements for the future will inevitably lead to changes in the composition of diet. He was of the opinion that vegetables will become an increasingly important source of protein for all of us; those of us who usually eat a large amount of meat will eventually find ourselves in the position of most of the people in the world for whom meat is usually a condiment and is eaten in large quantities only at feasts. The point was made that if one believes that diet is important and modification of diet is desirable, some thought should be given to how the diet of children can be modified. Information about this would have to reach each family.

Dr. Mitchell noted that if one examines Dr. Gerry Morris' study on bus drivers and conductors one finds that, although the study has been interpreted as showing that exercise protects individuals against the development and complications of atherosclerosis, detailed examination indicates that the subjects were different before they began driving and conducting. The results observed could be unrelated to exercise but related to the characteristics of the subjects before they took the jobs.

Dr. Whyte raised a question about a man who has been on a high cholesterol diet and is then given a low cholesterol diet. Does this change convert the individual to the same state as an individual who has always been on a low cholesterol diet? It is questionable that convincing people to stop smoking, increase their exercise, and lower their cholesterol levels will change them into the same kind of individuals as those who have never smoked, always exercised and have a low cholesterol level. Dr. Whyte also asked Dr. Mitchell about the approach of the British Committee in bringing forward their recommendations about diet and cardiovascular disease. Although they do not come down in favour of diet changes, they are quite clearly in agreement about the horror of obesity and the desirability of staying thin, or becoming thin. Since Dr. Mitchell is concerned about evidence, what is the evidence that led the Committee to accept the theory that becoming thin would be of benefit? Dr. Whyte was not aware of any prospective studies and wondered if the Committee had some evidence which led them to accept this particular point. In his opinion, there is much less evidence about the harmfulness of obesity than there is about diet and cholesterol. Dr. Mitchell replied that it is easy for a person to tell whether he or she is fat, and there is general acceptance that one should be thin. Life insurance statistics show that people with lower weights are better risks than people who are overweight. Therefore, even though these data are incomplete, there is general acceptance that avoidance of obesity is a good thing. Obviously, the data are poor and we need better evidence.

A speaker from the audience asked Dr. Mitchell if he thought the evidence about overweight and health is better than the evidence that he disregarded about diet and lowering serum cholesterol. Dr. Mitchell replied, "Yes."

Dr. Mishkel asked Dr. Witty whether he has any evidence that the Federal Government of Canada is going to implement any of the changes which he discussed concerning changes in food products or the development of food substitutes. The only thing Dr. Mishkel has noticed in his particular area is that they can now buy "Egg Beaters" (a modified egg product with low cholesterol) and he has seen advertisements for "Egg Beaters" on television. Dr. Mishkel then asked Dr. Witty whether he thinks the government will be prepared to collaborate with physicians, industry and agriculture in setting up a coordinated approach to tackling the problems of nutrition and atherosclerosis. Dr. Witty replied that there has been little change. The government does have a committee of which he is a member, but it has not made much progress in setting up collaborative arrangements. Most of them do not talk to industry.

Dr. Mustard wondered if the discussion could be focussed on the question of the suitability of dietary recommendations.

A speaker from the audience asked if Dr. Connor could indicate to the audience whether any of the Indians in his study were obese, and had elevated blood triglyceride levels. He was interested to know the effect of a 75% carbohydrate diet on these people. Dr. Connor replied that obviously some of the Indians were overweight but not to the same extent as some individuals in his own community. The ones who were overweight tended to be the women who had had a number of children. They did not find any hypertriglyceridemia in the 390 people they surveyed.

Dr.Little asked if we could have some idea of the panel's views on a suitable diet, and dietary change, and what is meant by increasing the polyunsaturated content of the diet in relation to the saturated fat level. It has been suggested that we should perhaps lower the amount of saturated fat to a moderate intake but nobody is prepared to stand up and say what the amount should be. Dr. Hewitt stated that he would like to say something about this since it is one of the areas in which there cannot be unanimity. It should be recognized that there will not be agreement about this. There may have to be a number of solutions and perhaps it might be more appropriate if, in countries like Australia, different approaches to these problems are tried to see if it is possible to learn something.

Dr. Brown remarked that obviously the total fats, and the balance among saturated and polyunsaturated fats and cholesterol are all interdependent factors in a diet. He thinks that any approach to dietary modification has to take into account the interdependence of all these factors.

A speaker from the audience (Johns Hopkins University) questioned if universal application of a diet may not be harmful for certain groups in the population. For example, a dietary modification which might be suitable for one particular group of people may be harmful to others because it causes their triglyceride level to go higher. Is there not a risk of significant side effects, for example, from excess polyunsaturated fats in the diet? Dr. Mustard stated that these questions really raise the point of how confident we can be that dietary recommendations for the public are not going to be harmful to some members of the population. Furthermore, this raises the question about whether the diets which are being recommended will be beneficial to people with vascular disease.

Dr. Horlick felt that the speaker from Johns Hopkins was focussing his attention on individuals in the population with very special requirements. It was recognized long ago, when iodized salt was advocated for everyone to cope with problems of thyroid glands, that any individual who needs special treatment should come under the advice of a physician and be given appropriate therapy. Obviously, a dietary recommendation for the general public may not necessarily apply to every individual. One aspect about which there is uncertainty at this moment is the desirable degree of supplementation with polyunsaturated fats. Investigators who have looked at the various trials in which high levels of polyunsaturates have been used in the diet have arrived at different opinions as to whether or not harm was done. The consensus appears to be that there is no real danger in polyunsaturated fats in the diet. Dr. Isaacson stated that he did not think the recommendations which have been made for Sweden have been a problem for anyone in the population. The recommendation in Sweden is designed to reverse the situation in which people have deviated from what is considered to be the so-called natural diet. They have not stressed the polyunsaturated fatty acids in their diet. They did not think they had sufficient evidence to do so.

A speaker from Baltimore in the audience returned again to Dr. Mitchell's point about the position of the British Advisory Group on the question of the diet, and wondered what kind of evidence Dr. Mitchell would require before he would be prepared to make a recommendation. Dr. Mitchell replied that the question of diet was carefully considered by the Committee but it is evident that it would be of enormous cost to the country if the national diet were to be altered. They were not concerned with the question of what might be done for an individual person who is at risk. He thinks that, in a situation where major change is to be recommended in the diet, with enormous implications in terms of food supplies and cost, particularly in a country like England, one would have to have very convincing proof of its benefits. These decisions cannot be made on the basis of hearsay or half-completed trials. Although he understands the problems in this and knows that Seymour Dayton's study and the one in the Finnish Mental Hospitals were good studies, they just are not sufficient, in his opinion, to form the basis for national recommendations.

A speaker from the floor asked Dr. Mitchell if he thought that we will ever have a good enough study. Dr. Mitchell replied that he did not think so. On the other hand, if one does not know the answer, should one give an answer based on belief? He would prefer to wait since he does not see the harm in waiting. If someone is going to ask the question, "Is there harm in waiting?", he can equally well ask, "What is the benefit in going ahead?". People have to die of something, haven't they? It seems to him that it is what is put on the death certificate that gives concern, rather than the fact that people have died. If there is a 40% death rate from heart attacks, one should show a shift in the total death rate by manoeuvers which are supposed to prevent deaths from heart attacks. For example, if we modified the diet and eliminated deaths from heart attacks, and the actual death rate remained the same, would we really have accomplished anything other than to change the cause of death on the death certificate? We would not have changed the life expectancy statistics of the country. If we were really able to modify this problem, then we should be able to show a change in life expectancy.

Dr. Shorland stated that he had always felt that the experimental evidence from the primary prevention trials with polyunsaturated fatty acids indicated that no benefit was gained. Because of this, he found it difficult to see why we should progressively increase the level of polyunsaturated fats in the diet.

Dr. Mustard summarized the discussion to this point as follows: As far as smoking is concerned, all of you would agree that we should urge that it be stopped or restricted. Do what you can about it. Although the evidence is weak about exercise, all of you seem to think it is a good thing, particularly if it keeps individuals in caloric balance. It is interesting that, although there is no convincing evidence, this is one area in which you will let your beliefs dictate your decision. As far as diet is concerned, your opinions range from Dr. Mitchell's point of view that there is insufficient evidence that diet is important in cardiovascular disease, to those of you who believe that there should be a reduction in the amount of fat in the diet, together with an increase in polyunsaturated fats and reduction of the amount of cholesterol in the diet. Perhaps an interesting point about diet is the decision of Sweden to go ahead and develop a nutritious diet concept for its population. It seemed to him that in Dr. Isaacson's comments he mentioned that they were trying to achieve a balanced diet, which from historical perspectives and good nutrition was more in keeping with what Sweden's people used to eat. An interesting point is that individuals from agriculture and the food industry, health professionals, nutritionists, and others have come together to develop a strategy for the campaign. This suggests that if you are going to introduce dietary recommendations, you need the full cooperation of all the groups that are involved in determining public attitudes and accessibility to food, along with information on the kinds of foods which are available. He wondered whether there were any questions the audience would like to direct to Dr. Isaacson in view of this very radical approach in Sweden.

A speaker form the audience asked how you prevent people from overeating in the Swedish system. Dr. Isaacson replied that it is perhaps not correct to say that they control everything. What they try to do is to get people to understand and they use information and peer pressure to try to help people to cope with such problems as overeating.

Dr. Little asked Dr. Isaacson and the other members of the panel whether they believe that substitute foods are necessary for the programs that are being recommended. Dr. Isaacson then asked what was meant by substitute foods. Dr. Little stated that he would consider substitute foods as special foods such as the ones that Dr. Whyte described in Australia; for example, the specially prepared beef rich in polyunsaturated fat. To this Dr. Isaacson replied that he did not think it necessary to provide "special" foods for the population as a whole. They may be needed for certain types of people, but as far as the general public is concerned, he thinks it best to use foods which are produced within the country.

Dr. Mitchell remarked that he would like to turn to a point raised by Dr. Sheila Mitchell. This concerns the matter of collaborating with other groups to get a message across. It is interesting that people who know how to manipulate behavior did not find it very hard in Britain to get across a campaign about crash helmets for motorcyclists. In this case everyone who rode motorcycles had generally visited a friend in hospital who had smashed himself up on his motorcycle. Then, if you go to another sort of behavioral change where you need to get the person to believe that there is a risk but he does not see anyone involved in it, you have another problem. The medical profession as a whole has promoted scares of one sort or another - sedentary life, coffee, sugar, and so on. If you go into a school now, for instance, and say that not smoking will prevent lung cancer, they say "Oh! What is lung cancer?" They do know, however, all about smoking and peer group acceptance. You know whether you are fat or not and you may worry about if you are, but you certainly do not worry about whether you are going to get coronary artery disease 20 or 30 years from now. So there is a difficult problem with people not being able to understand a risk which is not visible to them. Why should the public believe doctors, because so much of what doctors have said has proven to be nonsense?

Dr. Mustard asked Dr. Isaacson, in the light of Dr. Mitchell's comments whether he might like to give some idea of the effect of the campaign on the Swedish population. Dr. Isaacson replied that they did not have enough figures to give any concrete statement at the present moment. His general impression, however, was that they had produced changes in the dietary habits of the Swedes.

A member of the audience asked if any member of the panel would care to comment on the significance of fibre in the diet in relation to the so-called "consumption diseases" other than atherosclerosis. The public, in particular the younger generation, are very much exposed to unnatural things. A number of people wish to go back to farming and producing their own foods so that they can have natural foods. Dr. Horlick replied that he thinks we need a variety of strategies. One point that Dr. Hewitt made earlier was that any changes which are brought about should be similar to the natural habits and the way we generally behave. He thinks it may be somewhat easier to get people to change if the kind of food they buy resembles the kind of food they ordinarily use. He would prefer to see desirable changes built into foods which people normally accept. In the case of fibre, he believes there is reasonable evidence that diets which are high in fibre are desirable for reasons other than the prevention of atherosclerosis. For example, they are good for intestinal function.

Dr. Mustard noted that Dr. Connor raised a very important question about the ecological balance and food. This applies to Dr. Witty's remarks about the sources of fatty acids and the restrictions if one were to make general changes in the diet along the lines some have recommended. In reply, Dr. Connor stated that the public the world over has been sold a bill of goods about protein. It is not true that animal protein is necessary for human nutrition. Margaret Olsson said many years ago that people who get enough calories from a variety of food stuffs will never suffer from protein malnutrition and he thinks this is true. Dr. Polarin from Beirut pointed this out in an article in Lancet a few months ago. The truth is that a variety of vegetable proteins will produce just as much growth and just as balanced a diet as one rich in animal protein. The only problem one might face is a source of vitamin B_{12}. There is evidence in studies of protein malnutrition that the condition can be managed very well by a mixture of vegetable proteins. Dr. Mitchell felt that this was an important point in a world where we are short of resources. For example, we catch fish, turn the fish into meal, feed it to animals in order to produce meat for us to eat. The same argument holds true with vegetable protein. Obviously this cannot go on. This problem will have to be faced but it should be emphasized that it is not only a question of resources but also of public acceptance.

CHAPTER 14

BIOCHEMISTRY OF ARTERIAL WALL; FACTORS IN MURAL LIPID ACCUMULATION

(1)

INTRODUCTION

D. B. Zilversmit

Division of Nutritional Sciences and Section of Biochemistry, Molecular and Cell Biology, Cornell University, Ithaca, New York, U.S.A.

Although much attention has been directed to the structure and metabolism of plasma lipoproteins, relatively little effort has been given to the study of the arterial wall. Recent reviews on the interaction of serum lipids with the artery have been published by Walton (1) and by Zilversmit (2); a 1972 Ciba Symposium on the mechanisms of early atheromatosis (3) summarizes various aspects of this topic. Much of today's session deals with vascular enzymes, a topic which has been reviewed recently by Zemplényi (4).

One particular enzyme--lipoprotein lipase--has recently drawn our attention, and elsewhere (2, 5). I have summarized the literature, which tends to support the hypothesis that the interaction of triglyceride-rich lipoproteins with arterial lipoprotein lipase may be a key element in the development of arterial lesions. A lipase with the activating and inhibiting properties similar to those of adipose tissue lipoprotein lipase has been found in bovine arteries (6). The specific activity of this enzyme appears to be higher near the endothelial surface than in deeper-lying strata of the arterial wall.

Our discussion today will look more deeply into various metabolic factors that may enhance or diminish the accumulation of plasma lipid and protein constituents in the arterial wall.

REFERENCES:

1. Walton, K.W. (1975) Amer. J. Cardiol. 35:542.

2. Zilversmit, D. B. (1975) Amer. J. Cardiol. 35:559.

3. "Atherogenesis: Initiating Factors" (1973) Ciba Foundation Symposium 12 (new series), Associated Scientific Publishers, Amsterdam.

4. Zemplényi, T. (1974) Med. Clin. N. Amer. 58:293.

5. Zilversmit, D. B. (1973) Circ. Res. 33:633.

6. DiCorleto, P. E., and Zilversmit, D. B. (1975) Proc. Soc. Exptl. Biol. Med. 148:1101.

(2)

EFFECT OF LIPID ACCUMULATION ON ARTERIAL WALL BIOENERGETICS

E. S. Morrison and R. F. Scott

From the Department of Pathology and Special Center for Atherosclerosis Research
Albany Medical College, Albany, New York, U.S.A.

Smooth muscle cell (SMC) proliferation of arterial wall is one of the earliest phenomena observed in atherosclerosis. We have been investigating selected metabolic changes associated with this SMC proliferation process in various experimental models. The rationale is that if we understand the molecular events associated with, and possibly initiating arterial wall SMC proliferation, it may be possible to devise a therapeutic regimen which would inhibit the development of the early atherosclerotic lesion, to such an extent that the advanced lesions associated with high mortality would not appear.

Most of the data to be presented are from swine fed a hypercholesterolemic diet. Depending on the degree of hypercholesterolemia produced, swine receiving such diets begin to develop grossly visible atherosclerotic lesions in the arch and distal abdominal aorta in one to two months; lesions in the coronary arteries take longer to appear.[1] That SMC proliferation is an early event in cholesterol-fed swine was demonstrated biochemically by showing a significant increase in the rate of uptake of tritiated thymidine into aorta long before the development of gross lesions.[2] In a later study we demonstrated a greater rate of entry of arterial SMC into mitoses after the swine were on a high cholesterol diet for only 3 days.[3]

Because the SMC proliferation in early atherosclerosis must be an energy-requiring process, we decided to investigate initially O_2 uptake, by which pathways (glycolysis or oxidative phosphorylation) most ATP is synthesized in the artery wall, and what substrates are used for oxidative phosphorylation. Some of these earlier studies have been reviewed elsewhere,[4] and will be only briefly outlined here. Oxygen uptake in aortic intima-media in proliferative lesions from cholesterol-fed swine, in grossly normal areas of aorta in cholesterol-fed swine and in aorta of normal swine were compared.[5] As might be expected, per mg of DNA, O_2 uptake was significantly elevated in the actively proliferating lesions. However, tissue respiration was also significantly greater in grossly normal intima-media from cholesterol-fed swine than in the aorta of normal swine suggesting that hypercholesterolemia possibly increased oxidative phosphorylation in aorta even before the onset of overt SMC proliferation. Studies of glucose utilization in aortic intima-media strips showed that in normal tissue the majority of glucose metabolized by the artery goes to lactate with very little entering the Krebs cycle and thus being available for oxidative phosphorylation.[6] In addition, very little glucose entered RNA, DNA protein or lipid pools. In atherosclerotic aortic intima-media, the amount of glucose utilization more than doubled, but virtually all of the increased glucose was metabolized via the glycolytic pathway to lactic acid.*

Having determined that glucose was not the substrate accounting for the increased O_2 uptake in atherosclerotic tissue, we investigated the possibility that free fatty acids (FFA) might be utilized for this purpose by the artery.[8] Table I shows the results of a study using U-^{14}C palmitic acid in control and atherosclerotic rabbits. Atherosclerotic tissue not only had a greater endogenous level of FFA, but when incubated in appropriate medium had a much greater uptake of FFA than normal tissue. More importantly, however a great deal more FFA was oxidized to CO_2, and presumably was acting as a substrate for oxidative phosphorylation.

Even on the assumption that the increased amount of FFA was oxidized via the β-oxidative pathway in atherosclerotic aortas, the amount was not sufficient to account for the increased O_2 uptake in this tissue. Among the substances to investigate next as possible substrates for oxidative phosphorylation were amino acids and ketone bodies. We have begun preliminary studies of utilization of amino acids by the Krebs cycle; the initial results suggest that at least some amino acids are oxidized extensively in normal arterial wall.

*This and subsequent studies on arterial wall metabolism were carried out in tissue kept constantly at 37°, with the analyses being done within 10 minutes after the tissue was secured. Pre-cooling of aortic tissue irreversibly damages both glycolysis and tissue respiration.

TABLE I

FREE FATTY ACID UPTAKE, CONTENT AND DEGRADATION IN NORMAL AND ATHEROSCLEROTIC RABBIT INTIMA-MEDIA

	Uptake of FFA* into Intima-Media umoles/g/hr	Endogenous FFA umoles/g wet wt	FFA degraded to CO_2 nmoles/g/hr
Stock (7)	0.129 $\pm$ 0.018	1.031 $\pm$ 0.076	6.1 $\pm$2.6
	$p < 0.001$	$p < 0.001$	$p < 0.001$
Cholesterol (5)	0.314 $\pm$ 0.029	1.731 $\pm$0.076	92.6 $\pm$3.6

*U-^{14}C palmitate.

TABLE II

CALCIUM-STIMULATED RESPIRATION, OXYGEN UPTAKE, Ca^{2+}/O AND RESPIRATORY CONTROL RATIOS

	State 3	State 4	RCR	Ca^{2+}/O
Mash Group (14)	20.9 $\pm$1.68	3.96 $\pm$0.28	5.48 $\pm$0.38	7.01 $\pm$0.19
Cholesterol Group (11)	23.0 $\pm$2.0	5.93 $\pm$0.53	4.15 $\pm$0.36	7.66 $\pm$0.52
		$p < 0.001$	$p < 0.05$	

Substrate: 10 mM Glutamate, Ca^{2+}: 100 nmoles/mg protein -- protein 1-2 mg/ml

State 3: natoms oxygen/mg mitochondrial protein/min -- Ca^{2+} present in medium

State 4: natoms oxygen/mg mitochondrial protein/min -- Ca^{2+} absent in medium

The last subject we would like to discuss is one aspect of the utilization of metabolic energy by atherosclerotic intima-media. ATP is of course utilized for many functions in SMC, but one of the ways it is expended is in maintaining arterial wall compliance. Some idea of the efficiency of contraction in SMC can be gained by examining Ca^{2+} metabolism. Ca^{2+} uptake into various subcellular particles is thought to be, in part at least, energy-dependent. In a preliminary study using normal swine aorta utilizing maximum loading with Ca^{2+}, the uptake of Ca^{2+} into isolated mitochondria was found to be twice as great as in sarcoplasmic reticulum, in contrast to the findings in heart.[9] Mitochondria from normal and atherosclerotic aortas were then compared using methods of both massive loading and light loading (Ca^{2+}-stimulated respiration). With massive Ca^{2+} loading there were significant decreases in uptake in mitochondria from atherosclerotic tissue at 2, 4 and 8 minutes incubation time. The results with light loading of mitochondria with Ca^{2+} are shown in Table II. The findings suggest that even in the earliest phases of atherosclerosis, utilization of metabolic energy to maintain normal Ca^{2+} flux within the cell is abnormal. Whether or not this is reflected in abnormal arterial compliance due to abnormal smooth muscle cell function must await further study.

REFERENCES

1. Florentin, R. A. and Nam, S. C. Dietary-Induced Atherosclerosis in Miniature Swine. I. Gross and light microscopy observations; time of development and morphologic characteristics of lesions. Exp. & Mol. Path., 8: 263-301, 1968.

2. Thomas, W. A., Florentin, R. A., Nam, S. C., Kim, D. N., Jones, R. M., and Lee, K. T. Preproliferative Phase of Atherosclerosis in Swine fed Cholesterol. Arch. Path., 86: 621-643, 1968.

3. Florentin, R. A., Nam, S. C., Lee, K. T., Lee, K. J., and Thomas, W. A. Increased Mitotic Activity in Aortas of Swine After Three Days of Cholesterol Feeding. Arch. Path., 88: 463-469, 1969.

4. Morrison, E. S. and Scott, R. F. Arterial Wall Metabolism in Atherosclerosis. Adv. Cardiol., 13: 127-133, 1974.

5. Scott, R. F., Morrison, E. S., and Kroms, M. Aortic Respiration and Glycolysis in the Preproliferative Phase of Diet-Induced Atherosclerosis in Swine. J. Ather. Res., 9: 5-16, 1968.

6. Morrison, E. S., Scott, R. F., Kroms, M., and Frick, J. Glucose Degradation in Normal and Atherosclerosis Aortic Intima-Media. Athero., 16: 175-184, 1972.

7. Scott, R. F., Morrison, E. S., and Kroms, M. Effect of Cold Shock on Respiration and Glycolysis in Arterial Tissue. Am. J. Physiol., 219: 1363-1365, 1970.

8. Morrison, E. S., Scott, R. F., Kroms, M., and Frick, J. Uptake, Oxidation and Esterification of Free Fatty Acids in Normal and Atherosclerotic Rabbit Aorta. Biochem. Med., 11: 153-164, 1974.

9. Cheney, C. P., Morrison, E. S., Frick, J., and Scott, R. F. Effect of Cholesterol Feeding on Calcium Metabolism in Mitochondria From Swine Vascular Smooth Muscle. Fed. Proc., 34: 347, 1975.

(3)

QUANTITATIVE STUDIES OF THE INTERACTION BETWEEN PLASMA AND TISSUE COMPONENTS IN HUMAN INTIMA

Elspeth B.Smith, K.M.Alexander and I.B.Massie

University of Aberdeen, Department of Chemical Pathology

Foresterhill, Aberdeen, Scotland

It is now apparent that the arterial endothelium does not form an impermeable barrier, and that plasma macromolecules pass across it into the arterial wall in substantial amounts, even in healthy young animals. A large number of plasma proteins have been identified in intima by immunological techniques, and the concentration of low density lipoprotein (LDL) in normal aortic intima of adult humans is highly correlated both with its concentration in the subjects plasma and with blood pressure level. (1,2) Localized areas containing excessive concentrations of plasma proteins have been identified by immunofluorescence (3) and quantitative immunoelectrophoresis (1,2). It is suggested that these "insudation" or "gelatinous" lesions, which are characterised by a loosely structured proliferation of smooth muscle cells and collagen fibres, are the precursors of fibrous plaques.

ACCUMULATION OF INTACT PLASMA MACROMOLECULES

In gelatinous lesions the concentrations of thrombin-clottable fibrinogen and of LDL (4,1) are increased 2-4 fold compared with adjacent normal intima. On a crude basis of total intimal volume the concentration of LDL is about the same in normal intima and plasma, thus in these lesions its overall concentration is much greater than in plasma and the concentration in the extracellular space must be very high; by contrast, the concentration of albumin is much lower in intima than in plasma. (1,2) This could arise by preferential retention of LDL,

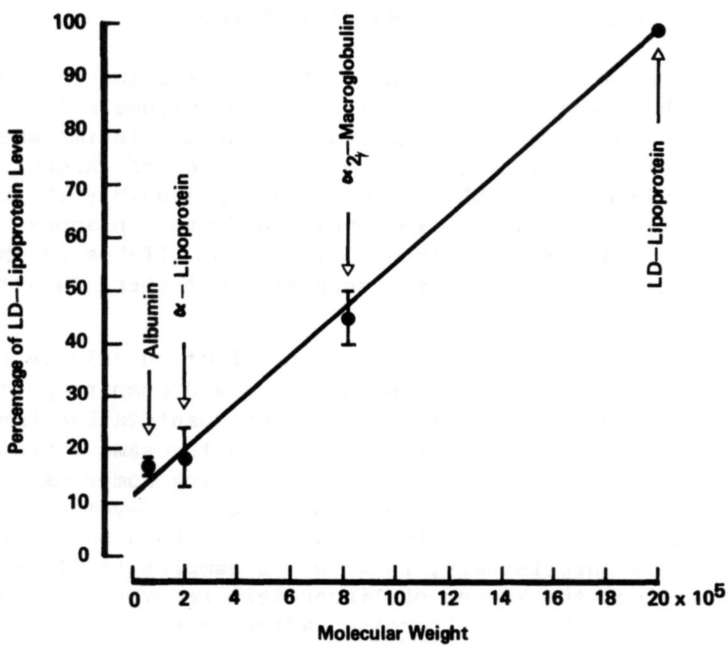

FIGURE 1. The relative retention of plasma proteins in normal intima in relation to molecular weight. The concentration of each protein is calculated as microlitres of the patient's plasma per 100 mg dry tissue, and the relative concentration is expressed as percentage of the LDL level. Points represent mean $\pm$ SEM; 8 samples. (Reproduced from Protides of the Biological Fluids, 22nd Colloquium, 1975) (Reference 7).

possibly through formation of reversible complexes with glycosaminoglycans (GAG) (5), or by molecular sieving through the GAG gel (6); it seems unlikely that the large lipoprotein molecule enters the intima at a faster rate than albumin. We have examined the relative retention of LDL, α_2-macroglobulin, α-lipoprotein and albumin in 8 samples of normal intima (FIG.1) and 5 gelatinous lesions, and found retention to be a linear function of molecular weight (7). This does not support the idea of specific reversible complex formation, but suggests that enrichment of electrophoretically mobile LDL is the result of molecular sieving, and that rate of egress from the intima is an important factor in determining tissue concentration.

"DEPOSITION" OF PLASMA MACROMOLECULES

In gelatinous lesions insoluble "fibrin" and the residual cholesterol that remains in the tissue after immunoelectrophoresis (RC) show only small changes compared with normal intima whereas there are 3-fold increases in the concentrations of thrombin-clottable fibrinogen and LDL (4), which are presumably their soluble precursors. However, in developed fibrous plaques "fibrin" increases 5-fold and RC increases 10 to 30-fold (Table 1) while the soluble fractions decrease, which suggests that there is active deposition from the precursors.

We have attempted to demonstrate an effect on soluble LDL by incubating aliquots of finely minced tissue and comparing the LDL content of incubated and control samples by quantitative immunoelectrophoresis (1) in adjacent positions on the same plate. Some loss of LDL occurred in fatty streaks containing numerous fat-filled cells, and there was marked diminution in developed white fibrous plaques, particularly in the atheroma lipid bottom layer (Table 2). Very surprisingly, in 17 of 23 samples (74%) from gelatinous lesions the amount of lipoprotein recovered on quantitative immunoelectrophoresis increased after incubation (Table 2).

TABLE 1

THE CONCENTRATIONS OF "SOLUBLE" AND "INSOLUBLE" PLASMA DERIVATIVES IN AORTIC INTIMA

	CONCENTRATION: mg/100 mg dry tissue			
	"Fibrin"	Fibrinogen	LDL	RC
NORMAL (9)[1]	2.0	2.2	5.2	3.8
FATTY STREAKS (5)	2.4	2.5	1.2*	25.6*
GELATINOUS LESIONS				
Thickenings (6)	2.9	6.9*	10.5*	2.8
"Heads and tails" of plaques (5)	4.0*	6.2*	13.4*	4.2
FIBROUS PLAQUES				
Edges (12)	9.7*	6.8*	6.0	27.2*
Central cap:				
opaque (9)	2.1	1.4	2.9	11.2
Translucent (6)	6.8*	1.6	4.0	11.2
Underlying atheroma				
lipid: early (6)	1.3	1.0	2.8	37.3*
advanced (9)	10.3*	4.0	3.7	97.8*

[1] Number of samples

*Significantly different from normal intima ($p < 0.02$)

TABLE 2

EFFECT OF INCUBATION ON THE CONCENTRATION OF SOLUBLE LDL IN AORTIC INTIMA

	Time after death: hours	Incubation time: hours	LDL: % of control level
NORMAL (4)	3 - 4½	2½ - 4	78
(3)	9 -12½	3½ - 4	101
FATTY STREAKS (4)	2½ - 5	3 - 3½	60
(4)	7 - 9	4 - 4½	58
WHITE FIBROUS PLAQUES (4)	3 - 8	3 - 4	
Upper cap			55
Lower cap			43
"Atheroma bottom			24
GELATINOUS LESIONS			
Thickenings (5)	2½ - 4½	2 - 5	144
Plaques			
Whole cap			181
Bottom* (3)	2½ - 7	3 - 4	101
Upper cap			124
Lower cap (4)	4 - 7	3 - 4½	94
Bottom*			104

*Contained "early" atheroma lipid, mean RC = 41.7mg/100mg.

This increase was most marked in early thickenings and the upper layers of larger gelatinous plaques. In white fibrous plaques maximum loss of LDL occurred in the bottom atheroma layer, and it is possible that in the bottom layers of larger gelatinous plaques "release" of LDL was masked by rapid degradation.

The apparent increase in LDL on incubation could be an artefact resulting from loss of tissue weight following excessive proteolysis of tissue components. To investigate this, and to obtain a measure of proteolytic activity against other plasma proteins, samples were assayed on double antibody plates in which the mobile components migrated into gels containing anti-α_2-macroglobulin or anti-transferrin before reaching the anti-LDL gel. Whole lesions were analysed in order to obtain enough tissue to examine the time-course of the reaction. Results are shown in Table 3; in white plaques there was some loss of α_2-macroglobulin, but LDL disappeared at a three-times faster rate. In gelatinous lesions LDL first increased, and on longer incubation, decreased rapidly relative to α_2-macroglobulin or transferrin.

TABLE 3

COMPARISON OF THE CHANGE IN CONCENTRATION OF LDL AND OTHER PLASMA PROTEINS ON INCUBATION OF TISSUE SAMPLES

(Samples taken from three aortas $2\frac{1}{2}$, 3 and 3 hours after death)

		Incubation time: hours	LEVEL IN INCUBATED SAMPLE: % OF CONTROL. LDL	α_2-macroglobulin	Transferrin
NORMAL	(3)*	$2\frac{1}{2}$	75	93	-
WHITE FIBROUS PLAQUES	(4)	$2\frac{1}{2}$	76	86	-
	(2)	5	64	83	-
	(2)	8	43	75	-
GELATINOUS LESIONS	(2)	$1\frac{1}{2}$	121	-	100
	(3)	$2\frac{1}{2}$	104	99	-
	(3)	5	84	94	-
	(2)	7	69	-	100
	(3)	8	39	92	-

* Number of Samples.

CONCLUSIONS

Presumably the function of a workshop is to stimulate discussion. We postulate that the gelatinous or insudation lesion is an early stage in fibrous plaque formation. Our findings suggest the following sequence of events:-

(1) Excessive accumulation of plasma macromolecules and proliferation of smooth muscle cells and collagen. Accumulation seems, at least in part, to be controlled by rate of egress and molecular sieving so that the largest molecules - LDL, α_2-macroglobulin and fibrinogen (which has an apparent molecular weight of 10^6 on gel columns) - accumulate most. It is not known if the initiating factor is increased permeability or proliferation leading to decreased egress.

(2) Fibrinogen seems to be converted to fibrin or some other insoluble complex within the intima. The large pool of soluble LDL in the intima is further increased by a "tightly bound" fraction.

(3) LDL is either degraded or irreversibly precipitated in the atheroma lipid pool.

ACKNOWLEDGEMENTS

This work was supported by grants from The British Heart Foundation and The Medical Research Council.

REFERENCES

(1) Smith, E.B., and Slater, R.S. (1972) Lancet i, 463
(2) Smith, E.B. (1974) Advan.Lipid Res. 12,1.
(3) Haust, M.D. (1971) Hum.Pathol. 2, 1.
(4) Smith, E.B., Alexander, K., and Massie, I. (In Press) Atherosclerosis.
(5) Gerö, S., Gergely,J.,Devenyi, T.,Jakab, L. and Virag, S. (1961) J.Atheroscler. Res. 1, 67.
(6) Iverius,P.-H., Atherogenesis: initiating factors. Ciba Foundation Symp., New Series, 12, 185 (1973)
(7) Smith, E.B., and Crothers, D.C. (1974). Protides of the Biological Fluids 22, 315 (H.Peeters, ed.)

(4)

ARTERIAL CHOLESTEROL ESTERASE

David Kritchevsky

The Wistar Institute of Anatomy and Biology

Philadelphia, Pennsylvania, U.S.A.

Windaus (1) first reported that cholesteryl esters accumulated in atherosclerotic aortas. His findings were confirmed and extended by Böttcher (2) and Smith (3). Newman and Zilversmit (4) demonstrated the steady increase in aortic cholesteryl ester with continuing feeding of cholesterol to rabbits and Kritchevsky and Tepper (5) showed that cholesteryl ester increased in rabbit aortas even when the animals were subjected to a cholesterol-free, atherogenic semipurified regimen. Despite the absence of cholesterol, the diet was hypercholesterolemic and hyperbetalipoproteinemic. The Virchow hypothesis that increased aortic lipid levels were due to filtration of serum gained currency when several groups showed that the lipids of serum and aorta were qualitatively similar (6-8). However, they analyzed adult aortas and adult sera. Analysis of infant's aortas shows almost complete absence of cholesteryl ester (9). The work of Dayton and Hashimoto (10,11) and of Smith (3) now leaves little doubt than an appreciable amount of aortic cholesteryl ester arises from synthesis *in situ*.

We have investigated the esterification of cholesterol and hydrolysis of cholesteryl esters by aortic acetone powder preparations (12,13). Both enzymic activities are optimum at acid pH--synthesis at pH 6.1 and hydrolysis at pH 6.6. The fatty acid specificity for esterification activity is: oleic (1.00), linoleic (0.85), linolenic (0.56), arachidonic (0.46), palmitic (0.40) and stearic (0.28). When different sterols were used as substrate for esterification of [1-^{14}C]oleic acid, specificities ranged: cholesterol (1.00), epichoesterol (0.05), cholestanol (0.93), coprostanol (0.25), desmosterol (0.35), β-sitosterol (0.20) and ergosterol (0.21). Hydrolysis of cholesteryl esters (compared to the oleate) showed: oleate (1.00), linoleate (1.28), linolenate (0.86), palmitate (0.83), stearate (0.77) and laurate (0.62). The foregoing data were derived using rat aortic powder but rabbit aortic powder yielded similar results (13). It is evident that there is a disparity between various fatty acids and sterols with regard to esterification, but hydrolyzing activity falls within a narrower range.

The ratio of cholesteryl ester synthesizing (S) to hydrolyzing activity (H) is greater in animal species susceptible to atherosclerosis than that in resistant species (14), and may vary within specific aortic sites (15). The S/H ratio also rises in rabbits shortly (5 days) after establishment of a cholesterol regimen (16).

The influence of hypocholesteremic drugs on the S/H ratio using aortic acetone powders of rabbits was investigated. A number of drugs have shown hypolipidemic activity and several have been shown to affect the course of experimental atherosclerosis. These drugs have been found to increase the free/esterified cholesterol ratio in the aortas of treated rabbits, but whether the changes were a result of lowered lipid levels or of a direct effect on aortic metabolism was not known.

Seven groups of four rabbits each were used in the experiment. One group (B) was maintained on a regimen of commercial laboratory feed. A second group (BC) was fed laboratory ration augmented with 5% corn oil and a third (BCC) was fed ration plus 1% cholesterol and 5% corn oil. Three other groups were fed diet BCC with 0.5% nicotinic acid, 0.3% ethyl p-chlorophenoxyisobutyrate (CPIB) or 1% β-sitosterol added. The last group was fed BCC and given 0.5 mg/day of D-thyroxine by gavage. After 10 days the rabbits were killed, serum total cholesterol levels were determined (17), and the aortas taken for preparation of acetone powders. There were no grossly visible lesions. The esterification of [4-^{14}C]cholesterol and hydrolysis of [4-^{14}C] cholesteryl oleate was assayed using aliquots of each powder. Our findings are summarized in Table I.

Addition of corn oil to the basal diet increased cholesteryl ester synthetase activity and had a slight effect on hydrolase activity with a resultant increase in the S/H ratio. Cholesterol feeding resulted in an almost three-fold increase in S/H activity. This has been previously demonstrated in pigeon (18) and rabbit (16) aorta. The various drug treatments all decreased S/H ratios vis-a-vis the group fed the atherogenic diet. Nicotinic acid exerted the greatest effect, returning the S/H ratio to normal levels. The S/H ratios in the groups fed CPIB, D-thyroxine and β-sitosterol were lower than that observed in the group fed the atherogenic diet by 17, 33, and 44%, respectively.

Regimen	Serum Cholesterol*	Enzymatic Activity**		
		Synthetase (S)	Hydrolase (H)	S/H
Basal (B)	76 ± 7 a	1.00	1.00	1.00
B + 5% Corn Oil (BC)	83 ± 3 b	1.38	0.84	1.64
BC + 1% Cholesterol (BCC)	463 ± 36 abcd	1.10	0.39	2.82
BCC + 0.5% Nicotinic Acid	285 ± 54 abc	0.98	1.04	0.91
BCC + 0.3% CPIB	464 ± 87 ab	1.10	0.47	2.34
BCC + 1% β-sitosterol	366 ± 98 ab	1.68	1.07	1.57
BCC + D-thyroxine (0.5 mg/day)	279 ± 55 abd	1.20	0.64	1.88

*In terms of mg/dl ± the standard error of the mean; values bearing same subscript are significantly different.

**nmoles cholesterol esterified or liberated per hour per mg protein.

Table I. Influence of Hypolipidemic Drugs on Aortic Cholesterol Esterase. (4 Rabbits per Group : Fed 10 days)

These experimental findings are preliminary and will have to be repeated using larger numbers of animals and, possibly, other regimens such as a semipurified, cholesterol-free atherogenic diet. The results indicate, however, that hypolipidemic drugs can influence aortic cholesterol metabolism.

ACKNOWLEDGEMENT

This work was supported, in part, by grants (HL-03299 and HL-13722) and a Research Career Award (HL-00734) from the National Heart and Lung Institute and by the John A. Hartford Foundation.

REFERENCES

1. A. Windaus, Z. Physiol. Chem. 67:174, 1910.
2. C.F.J. Bottcher in "Drugs Affecting Lipid Metabolism". Eds. S. Garattini and R. Paoletti; Elsevier, Amsterdam, 1961, p. 54.
3. E.B. Smith. J. Atheroscler. Res. 5:224, 1965.
4. H.A.I. Newman and D.B. Zilversmit. J. Atheroscler. Res. 4: 261, 1964.
5. D. Kritchevsky and S.A. Tepper. J. Atheroscler. Res. 8:357, 1968.
6. S. Weinhouse and E.F. Hirsch. Arch. Pathol. 29:31, 1940.
7. I.H. Page. Ann. Int. Med. 14:1741, 1941.
8. J.F. Mead and M.L. Gouze. Proc. Soc. Exp. Biol. Med. 106: 4, 1961.
9. N. Tuna and H.K. Mangold, in "Evolution of the Atherosclerotic Plaque". Ed. R.J. Jones; Univ. of Chicago Press, Chicago. 1963, p. 85.
10. S. Dayton and S. Hashimoto. Exp. Molec. Pathol. 13:253, 1970.
11. S. Dayton and S. Hashimoto. Atherosclerosis 12:371, 1970.
12. H.V. Kothari, B.F. Miller and D. Kritchevsky. Biochim. Biophys. Acta 296:446, 1973.
13. H.V. Kothari and D. Kritchevsky. Lipids 10:322, 1975.
14. D. Kritchevsky and H.V. Kothari. Steroids and Lipids Res. 5:23, 1974.
15. D. Kritchevsky and H.V. Kothari. Biochim. Biophys. Acta 326: 489, 1973.
16. D. Kritchevsky, S.A. Tepper, J.C. Genzano and H.V. Kothari. Atherosclerosis 19:459, 1974.
17. S. Pearson, S. Stern and T.H. McGavack. Analyt. Chem. 25: 813, 1953.
18. R.W. St. Clair, H.B. Lofland and T.B. Clarkson. Circulation Res. 27:213, 1970.

(5)

PARTICIPATION OF PHOSPHOLIPIDS IN ARTERIAL METABOLISM OF CHOLESTEROL ESTERS

J. Patelski

Lipid Metabolism Laboratory, Department of Biochemistry

Medical Academy, Poznan, Poland

Enzymes involved in the metabolism of cholesterol esters

The increased concentration of cholesterol esters in the arterial wall attracts attention because this could be due to decreased hydrolysis or increased synthesis in atherosclerosis (3, 6). The following enzymes involved in the metabolism of cholesterol esters have been demonstrated in the arterial wall: cholesterol esterase * (5), along with the enzyme-catalyzed acylation of cholesterol by oleic acid without the addition of ATP and CoA (4, 5); lecithin : cholesterol acyltransferase (1) and acyl-CoA : cholesterol acyltransferase (4).

Phospholipids participate in arterial metabolism of cholesterol esters, as indicated by the presence of the LCAT enzyme and the known effects of injected polyunsaturated (soya) lecithin on enzymes involved in lipid metabolism (3, 6). However, there is relatively little information about the arterial LCAT enzyme as compared with the plasma LCAT enzyme which has been extensively studied in recent years (2). Moreover, the published literature is concerned with the enzyme-catalyzed transfer of an acyl group from

---

* Cholesterol acyltransferase = ACAT = acyl-CoA : cholesterol acyltransferase (EC 2.3.1.26), LCAT = lecithin : cholesterol acyltransferase (EC 2.3.1.43), LLAT = lysolecithin : lysolecithin acyltransferase (EC 2.3.1.), phospholipase A = phosphatide acyl-hydrolase (EC 3.1.1.4), phospholipase B = lysolecithin acyl-hydrolase (EC 3.1.1.5), cholesterol esterase = sterol-ester hydrolase (EC 3.1.1.13), Acid : CoA ligase(AMP) (EC 6.2.1.3).

lecithin to cholesterol (LCAT+) but not with the reverse reaction, i.e. the acyl transfer from cholesterol esters to lysolecithin (LCAT-). Therefore, it seemed to be of interest to study this reaction in both directions as well as other relevant enzyme activities of the aorta, to learn more about arterial synthesis and degradation of cholesterol esters.

Phospholipid-dependent synthesis and hydrolysis of cholesterol esters

Protein extracts of acetone-butanol powders from pig aortas, substrate hydrosols and two-point assay methods of the enzyme activity at optimum experimental conditions, with chemical determinations of the reaction products were used as previously described (5, 6, 8-10).

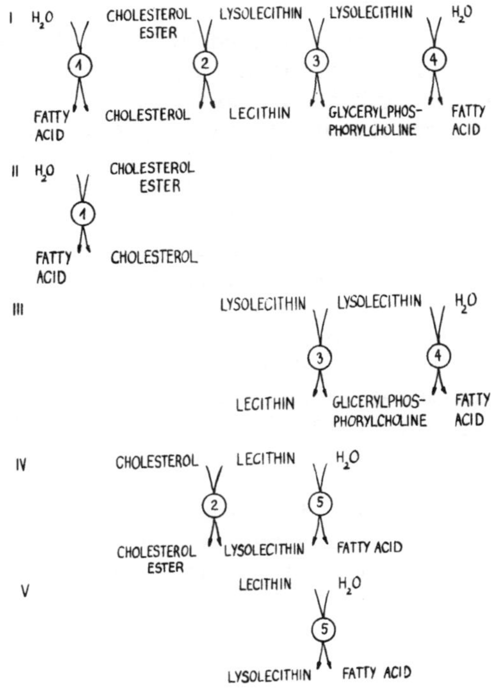

Figure 1. Reaction systems.

1. Cholesterol esterase
2. LCAT
3. LLAT
4. Phospholipase B
5. Phospholipase A

The reaction systems are summarized in Figure 1. It may be seen that other enzymes contribute to the reactions catalyzed by the LCAT enzyme. Lecithin, lysolecithin and cholesterol esters are in part hydrolyzed by the appropriate lipolytic enzymes, and lecithin is synthesized by the lysolecithin : lysolecithin acyltransferase, as indicated also by the appearance of the other reaction products (free fatty acids and glycerylphosphoryl choline). Results obtained for the (control) one-substrate systems have been subtracted from those for the two-substrate systems and expressed in nmoles of free cholesterol (I-II) for LCAT-, and lysolecithin (IV-V) or esterified cholesterol (IV) for LCAT+, per min per mg of protein of the enzyme preparation (mU/mg).

A higher enzyme-catalyzed synthesis of lecithin was found in the one-substrate (lysolecithin) systems (III) than in the two-substrate systems for LCAT when tested at different concentrations of the substrates (I). This is likely to be due to substrate competition for the enzymes, as indicated by a negative correlation between the LCAT and LLAT activities.

Classical product inhibition and also substrate inhibition of LCAT can be demonstrated in vitro. However, it is difficult to distinguish between these two effects because of the other enzymes interfering.

Smaller amounts of cholesterol esters synthesized by the arterial LCAT were found in the presence of polyunsaturated (soya) lecithin, as compared with the results obtained with a more saturated substrate (egg yolk lecithin); the amounts of released lysolecithin were not significantly different (7). It was suggested, therefore, that in the former case, more polyunsaturated cholesterol esters were formed and subsequently underwent preferential hydrolysis, than in the latter case. To check this point, investigations were made on the effect of cholesterol esters with fatty acids of different chain length and saturation on both the cholesterol ester hydrolase and cholesterol ester : lysolecithin acyltransferase activities. The results appeared to confirm the preferential hydrolysis of polyunsaturated cholesterol esters and demonstrated preferential transacylation with lysolecithin of cholesteryl oleate, as compared to other cholesterol esters (9).

The results seem to indicate the relative importance of these two reactions for degradation of cholesterol esters and a particular role of the phospholipid-dependent transacylations with respect to cholesteryl oleate.

Metabolism of cholesteryl oleate

Preferential esterification of cholesterol with oleic acid by ACAT (4, 8) and preferential hydrolysis of other cholesterol esters (8, 9) may favour accumulation of cholesteryl oleate in the arterial wall.

As regards hydrolysis of cholesteryl oleate, three pH optima at 8.6, 7.0 and 8.0 with reaction rates of 6.6 ± 1.04, 4.7 ± 0.91 and 3.3 ± 1.03 mU/mg (Mean $\pm$ standard deviation from N=4,6 and 6 series of estimates) respectively, and one optimum pH 8.0 for the rate of both hydrolysis and transacylation with lysolecithin, amounting to 5.7 ± 1.05 mU/mg (N=4) were found (Figure 2).

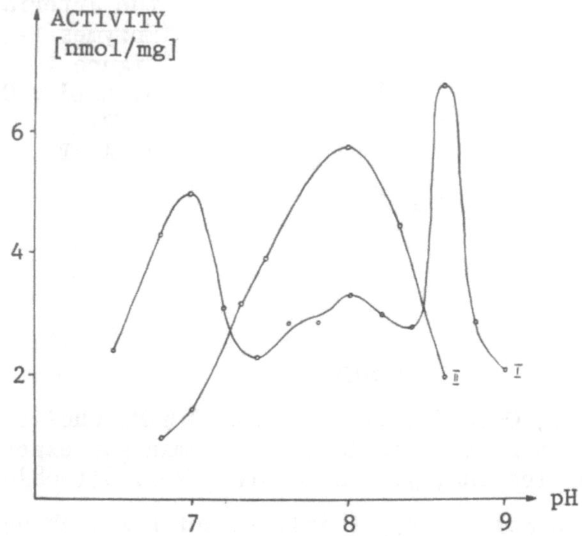

Figure 2. Effect of pH of the reaction mixtures on (I) cholesteryl oleate hydrolase and (II) cholesteryl oleate: lyscolecithin acyltransferase + the hydrolase activities.

The transacylation with lysolecithin seems, therefore, to compensate for the lower degradation of cholesterol oleate by hydrolysis, at less alkaline pH and perhaps at other conditions changed.

Metabolic pathways of phospholipid and cholesterol esters

Considering the data, it is possible to suggest that the phospholipid-mediated acyl exchange in cholesterol esters would render the esters more susceptible to hydrolysis and transportation and thus promote their removal from the arterial wall.

The metabolic pathways of phospholipid and cholesterol esters in the arterial wall are presented in Figure 3.

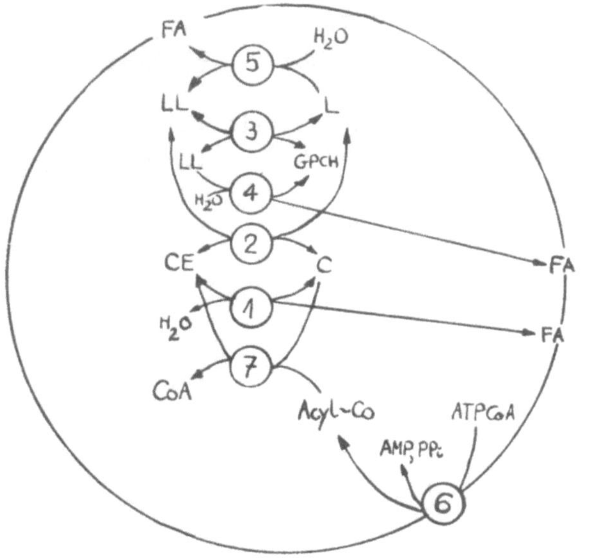

Figure 3. Metabolic pathways of phospholipid and cholesterol esters in the arterial wall. Enzymes 1-5 as in Figure 1.
6. Acid : CoA ligase (AMP)
7. ACAT

REFERENCES

1. Abdulla, Y.H., Orton,C.C., and Adams,C.W.M. Cholesterol esterification by transacylation in human and experimental atheromatous lesions, J. Atherosoler, Res. 8(1968)967.

2. Gjone,E., and Norum,K.R., (Eds), Recent research on lecithin: cholesterol acyltransferase, Scand. J. Clin. Lab.Investig. 33 Suppl. 137(1974).

3. Howard, A.N. and Patelski J., Hydrolysis and synthesis of aortic cholesterol esters in atherosclorotic baboons. Effect of polyunsaturated phosphatidyl choline on enzyme activities, Atherosclerosis, 20(1974)225.

4. Klimińska-Pniewska,B., Enzymatyczna estryfikacja cholesterolu w tętnicy głównej (Enzymatic esterification of cholesterol in the aorta), Pozn. Tow. Przyj.Nauk, Prace Kom. Med.Dośw. 42 (1970)167.

5. Patelski,J., Esteraza cholesterolowa tętnicy głównej (Cholesterol esterase of the aorta), Państwowy Zakład Wydawnictw Lekarskich, Warszawa 1964.

6. Patelski,J., Bowyer,D.E., Howard,A.N., Jennings, I.W., Thorne, C.J.H. and Gresham,G.A., Modification of enzyme activities in experimental atherosclerosis in the rabbit, Atherosclerosis, 12(1970)41.

7. Patelski,J. and Torlińska,T., Lecithin : cholesterol acyltransferase and phospholipase A activities of the aortic wall. In: Samochowiec,L. and Wójcicki,J. (Eds), Proceedings of the 1972 International Symposium on Phospholipids. Internat. Soc. Biochem. Pharmacol. and Polish Pharmacol. Soc., Szczecin 1973,p.91.

8. Patelski,J. Pniewska, B., Pioruńska,M. and Obrębska,M., The arterial acyl-CoA: cholerterol acyltransferase and cholesterol ester hydrolase activities. In vitro effect of substrates with fatty acid of different chain length and saturation, Atherosclerosis, 22 (1975) 287-291.

9. Patelski, J., and Pioruńska,M., Cholesterol ester: lysolecithin acyltransferase activity of the aorta, this book.

10. Patelski, J., Pioruńska, A., and Pioruńska, M., Effect of substrate composition and concentration on the aortic cholesterol ester hydrolase activity, to be published.

(6)

THE SIGNIFICANCE OF 'BOUND' AND 'LABILE' FRACTIONS OF LOW-DENSITY LIPOPROTEIN AND FIBRINOGEN IN THE ARTERIAL WALL

K. W. Walton and H. Bradby

Department of Experimental Pathology

University of Birmingham, England

INTRODUCTION

It is now widely agreed that arteries are not impermeable tubes and that atherosclerosis is not simply a process of passive accretion (like sludge formation) on their inner surfaces. Instead, three different techniques: namely: the use of radioisotopically labelled plasma proteins; the analysis of extracts of arterial tissue by chemical or immunological methods; and immunohistological examination, give essentially similar results which are compatible with the 'insudation' of plasma into the arterial intima (for review of evidence, see Walton, 1975) as the underlying mechanism of atherogenesis.

However, some results suggest that although many, if not all, the proteins present in plasma enter the intimal gel, only the low- and very low-density lipoproteins (hereafter collectively referred to as the total low-density lipoproteins or TLDL in this communication) and fibrinogen, are selectively localised in atherosclerotic lesions (Walton and Williamson, 1968). It has been proposed that entrapment of these proteins occurs because they selectively form complexes (co-acervates) with the sulphated glycosoaminoglycan components of the intimal gel (Amenta and Waters, 1960; Gero et al, 1960).

It has been shown by Smith and Slater (1971) that if arterial intima is finely minced and electrophoresis is carried out from the tissue sample into agarose containing antisera to human plasma proteins the presence of various plasma proteins in the interstitial fluid of the arterial wall can be demonstrated and their concentrations measured. Using this procedure, these authors have shown (a) that the amount of TLDL recoverable from the intima is related to the severity of atherosclerosis and to the level of serum lipids and lipoproteins in life (Smith and Slater, 1973); and (b) that fibrinogen is similarly recoverable from intima and that a proportion of this is clottable with thrombin (Smith, Slater and Hunter, 1973). Nevertheless this technique necessarily only measures that fraction of the plasma proteins which can be mobilised by electrophoresis. Any protein firmly and irreversibly bound to the tissue would probably not be demonstrated and measured by this method. The purpose of the present investigation was to see whether a 'bound' fraction of this kind could be shown to be present in relation to atherosclerotic lesions by combining immunofluorescence with electrophoresis of intimal samples.

MATERIALS AND METHODS

Two-dimensional (crossed) immuno-electrophoresis was carried out by the method of Laurell (1965). One-dimensional electrophoresis into agarose containing antiserum was performed essentially as described by Smith and Slater (1971) except that the intimal sample was used intact and not minced.

Immunofluorescence and conventional histological examinations of intimal samples before and after electrophoretic extraction was performed using the methods, reagents and apparatus described in previous publications (Walton and Williamson, 1968; Walton, Williamson and Johnson, 1970; Walton, 1973). Samples of intima were examined from 16 subjects aged 45-75, coming to routine autopsy.

RESULTS

Using polyvalent antiserum and two-dimensional electrophoresis it was established that a wide range of plasma proteins could be mobilised just as effectively from intact as from minced intima (Fig. 1). Using monospecific antiserum and single-dimensional electrophoresis it was established that quantitation of a given serum protein (e.g. TLDL as in Fig. 2) could similarly be carried out on intact intima (see below). It was found that no further material could be mobilised from the tissue in this latter manner after it had been exposed to electrophoresis for 18 hours.

The intima from early raised fibro-fatty lesions from the aorta and other major arteries was stripped and divided into two portions. Frozen sections were prepared from one portion and these were examined by immunofluorescence, using antisera to TLDL and fibrinogen, or after staining with haematoxylin and eosin, or with haematoxylin,

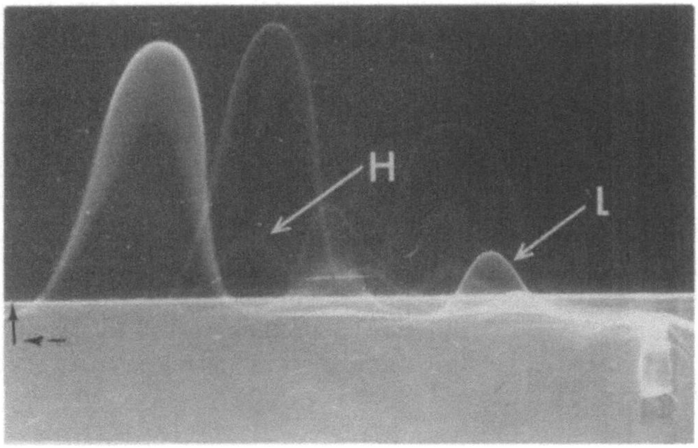

Fig. 1. Two-dimensional electrophoresis of intact aortic intima, from male aged 51, into polyvalent sheep anti-whole human serum. Note many precipitin arcs including high-density (H) and low-density (L) lipoproteins.

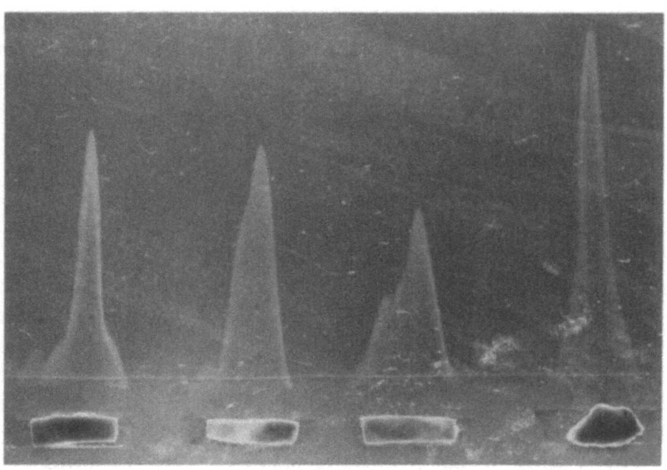

Fig. 2. One-dimensional electrophoresis of 4 pieces of intact aortic intima of male aged 67 against anti-TLDL.

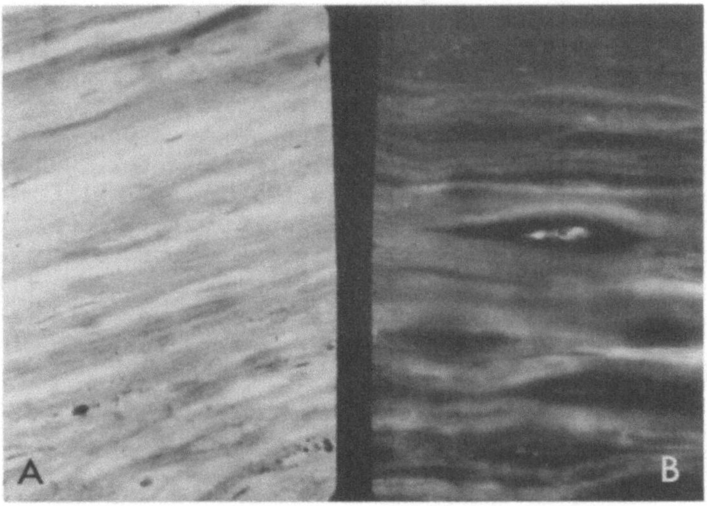

Fig. 3. Corresponding fields from adjacent frozen sections of portion of intima, from fibro-fatty aortic plaque of female aged 75, after one-dimensional electrophoresis of this tissue for 18 hours.

Fig. 3A from section stained with Haematoxylin, Oil red O and Light Green. Note very fine 'perifibrous' lipid on collagen of intima (grey in picture, red in original).

Fig. 3B from section treated with fluorescein-labelled anti-TLDL and examined in U.V. light. Note specific fluorescence (white in picture, green in original) in distribution corresponding to 'perifibrous' lipid as seen in Fig. 3A.

X250.

Oil red O and light green. The other portion of intima from the same lesion was submitted to single-dimensional electrophoresis into agarose containing antiserum for 18 hours. Following this, the portion of tissue was removed, frozen sections prepared, treated as described above and similarly examined.

Comparison by immunofluorescence of the tissue from a given lesion before and after single dimensional electrophoresis establishes: (i) that samples of intima which have not been subjected to electrophoresis show the presence of fibrinogen and of TLDL, especially in areas with atherosclerotic plaques. The distribution of extracellular lipid reactive with Oil red O corresponds closely with that of specific fluorescence for TLDL, suggesting the presence of intact lipoprotein (Walton and Williamson 1968); but (ii) that on examining samples of intima after their submission to electrophoresis until no further plasma components can be extracted, residual fibrinogen (or fibrin) and TLDL are still detectable in the tissue by immunofluorescence and lipid is still present in an identical distribution by conventional staining methods (Fig. 3).

DISCUSSION AND CONCLUSIONS

The findings reported above suggest that both 'labile' and 'bound' fractions of TLDL and fibrinogen are demonstrable in intima in relation to atherosclerotic lesions. It seems likely that electrophoretic mobilisation, like simple saline extraction of intima, yields only the 'labile' fraction. Attempts to measure the 'bound' fraction, at least in terms of lipid (cholesterol) content, by the difference in concentration before and after electrophoresis, have given inconsistent results in our hands. This is probably because the 'bound' fraction is relatively small (near the limits of error of the method of estimation). Nevertheless, if even a small fraction of the total plasma traversing the intima at any one time is irreversibly bound to the tissue, over a life-time this may be of great significance in relation to atherogenesis.

ACKNOWLEDGEMENT

This work was supported by the British Heart Foundation.

REFERENCES

Amenta J. S. and Waters, L. L. (1960) Yale J. Biol. Med., 33, 112.

Gero, S., Gergely J., Devenyi T., Jakab L., Szekely J. and Virag S. (1960) Nature (Lond.) 187, 152.

Laurell C. B. (1965) Analyt. Biochem. 10, 358.

Smith E. B. and Slater R. S. (1971) Biochem. J. 123, 397.

Smith E. B. and Slater R. S. (1973) Nutr. Metab. 15, 17.

Smith E. B., Slater R. S. and Hunter J. A. (1973) Atherosclerosis 18, 479.

Walton K. W. (1973) J. Path. 111, 263.

Walton K. W. (1975) Amer. J. Cardiol. 35, 542.

Walton K. W. and Williamson N. (1968) J. Atheroscler. Res. 8, 599.

Walton K. W., Williamson N. and Johnson A. G. (1970) J. Path. 101, 205.

(7)

SUMMARY

Dr. George S. Boyd

Department of Biochemistry
University of Edinburgh Medical School
Edinburgh, Scotland

Dr. Elspeth Smith and colleagues (University of Aberdeen) investigated quantitative aspects of the interaction of plasma and human intimal components. The theme that plasma macromolecules pass into the arterial wall has been studied as a physiological process. They have identified a number of plasma proteins in arterial intima and have correlated the concentration of LDL in normal aortic intima with the plasma concentration of LDL and with the blood pressure. These insudations or gelatinous lesions are suggested to be precursors of fibrous plaques. It is proposed that the accumulation of these macromolecules may be controlled in part by the rate of egress of these complexes and by molecular sieving so that the largest molecules such as LDL and fibrinogen accumulate to the greatest extent. The fibrinogen may be converted to fibrin and the LDL may be degraded or precipitated in the atheroma lipid pool.

On a similar theme, Walton and associates (Birmingham) have studied the significance of bound and labile fractions of low density lipoproteins and fibrinogen in the arterial wall. They have established that there is present both labile and bound fractions of total low density lipoproteins and also fibrinogen in the intima. The amount of these materials in the vessel is correlated with the degree of atherosclerosis. These authors suggest that even if a small fraction of the total plasma macromolecules traversing the intima at any one time is irreversibly bound to the tissue, then over a life-time this binding can be of great significance in relation to atherogenesis.

Morrison and associates (Albany) have investigated the effect of lipid accumulation on arterial wall bioenergetics, on arterial tissue from pigs, some of whom have been fed a hypercholesterolemic diet. This group has been concerned with smooth muscle cell proliferation in arterial wall and have been studying selected metabolic changes associated with this proliferation process. The oxygen uptake in tissues in which the proliferative lesions were present were significantly elevated. Hypercholesterolemia appears to increase oxidative phosphorylation in aorta even before the onset of overt smooth muscle cell proliferation. Most of the glucose metabolized by arterial tissue appears to go to lactate with very little entering the citric acid cycle. It was shown that atherosclerotic tissue had a greater endogenous concentration and a greater uptake of free fatty acids than had normal arterial tissue. Atherosclerotic tissue oxidized more free fatty acids to CO_2 and arterial tissue used amino acids extensively for oxidative phosphorylation. In the early phases of atherosclerosis there appears to be an abnormal utilization of metabolic energy to maintain the normal calcium flux within the cell.

Kritchevsky (Philadelphia) has investigated the "esterification" of cholesterol to produce cholesterol esters in aortic tissue and the "hydrolysis" of cholesterol esters in arterial tissue. Accordingly, it is possible to work out a synthesis/hydrolysis ratio using rabbit aortic acetone powders. Seven groups of rabbits were used: a control group, a group fed the control diet augmented with 5% corn oil, and a group fed the control diet with 5% corn oil and 1% cholesterol; four other groups were fed this cholesterol diet but also containing nicotinic acid or CPIB or sitosterol or thyroxine for 10 days. The rabbits were then killed, the serum total cholesterol level was determined, and the synthesis/hydrolysis ratio of cholesterol esters determined in portions of the aorta. Corn oil increased cholesterol ester synthetase as did cholesterol feeding. Nicotinic acid had a very marked effect on the synthesis/hydrolysis ratio, bringing this ratio back to normal level in animals on the hypercholesterolemic regimen. CPIB, D-thyroxine and sitosterol also affected this level but to a lower extent than did nicotinic acid.

Patelski (Poznan) has studied the participation of phospholipids in arterial metabolism of cholesterol esters. Attention is drawn to the need to investigate rates of synthesis of cholesterol esters in arterial tissue and simultaneously study rates of hydrolysis of these esters in that tissue. The role of the LCAT enzyme in arterial tissue has been studied with regard to the possibility of this enzyme being involved in both cholesterol ester synthesis and hydrolysis. The possible role of cholesterol ester: lysolecithin acyl transferase activity in the metabolism of cholesterol esters by arterial tissue is emphasized by the author. This reaction may compensate for the lower rate of degradation of cholesterol oleate by the hydrolytic process in arterial tissue. It is suggested that a phospholipid mediated acyl exchange renders cholesterol esters more susceptible to hydrolysis and transportation, thus promoting removal.

(8)

DISCUSSION (BIOCHEMISTRY OF ARTERIAL WALL; FACTORS IN MURAL LIPID ACCUMULATION)

Discussant X: Dr. Walton, did you look at the early fatty lesions for biochemical changes?

Dr. Walton: We have been able to show very low density lipoproteins in the early fatty streaks. In this case the VLDL appears to be an extracellular lipid.

Discussant Y: Dr. Smith, would you care to comment on the role of VLDL in atheromatosis, in view of the very large size of this macromolecule?

Dr. Smith: I have not convinced myself that I have found VLDL in these lipid lesions. There is, however, a large amount of LDL and HDL. If VLDL is present in these lesions, it is not there as intact VLDL.

Dr. Walton: One can show the presence in the lesions of apoprotein C. This would suggest that VLDL is present in the atheromatous lesions.

Dr. Zilversmit: In our studies using the bovine aorta, we have established that there is lipoprotein lipase in the arterial wall near the endothelial surface. We think that chylomicrons and VLDL may be degraded at the surface of the arterial intima and hence as the lipoproteins are rendered smaller in size they may be taken up by the arterial wall.

Dr. Bradford: Is it possible to reconcile some of the differences between the apparently normal intima and the intima with lesions? Do you suggest, Dr. Smith, that there was no preferential binding with respect to LDL?

Dr. Smith: The relative concentrations of the lipoproteins in the vessel wall appear to be the consequence of molecular sieving. There is also a tightly bound fraction of lipoprotein material in the vessel wall.

Dr. Howard: The results reported by Dr. Kritchevsky on effects of nicotinic acid are interesting and seem to fit with the results obtained by Altschul over twenty years ago. It will be remembered that Altschul fed this compound to rabbits and showed a dramatic effect on atherosclerotic lesions. I have one question for Dr. Kritchevsky: did the phospholipid, present in the cholesterol ester hydrolase assay, have any effect on the cholesterol esterase activity?

Dr. Kritchevsky: We tested this and found that apparently the lecithin had nc effect on this enzyme.

Dr. Zemplenyi: I would like to ask Dr. Patelski whether he has considered the possibility of measuring the ATP-dependent and the ATP-independent ester synthesizing systems.

Dr. Patelski: I think that there are only three enzymes involved in the synthesis of cholesterol esters. I should like to mention that in 1964 I found that there appear to be two pH optima for the cholesterol ester hydrolase enzyme system, one at pH 8.6 and the other at pH 8.0. Recently, when we changed the assay method we found a third pH optimum at pH 7.0. Thus, there are many factors which appear to affect the apparent pH optima of these hydrolase enzymes in vitro. For example, so much depends on the physical state of the substrate and enzyme particles and the method of preparation of the substrate and the enzymes.

Dr. Adams: I would like to remind the audience of the possible importance of the cholesterol ester hydrolase enzyme found in lysosomal organelles. As many of us are aware, there is supposed to be a deficiency of cholesterol ester hydrolase activity in vasculature smooth muscle. It has been shown that in atheroma-susceptible animals, there is a deficiency of cholesterol ester hydrolase, an enzyme with a pH optimum at pH 5.5. This same enzyme appears to be deficient in Wohlman's disease, in which there is an accumulation in the lymph nodes of cholesterol esters. It is possible that the smooth muscle cell is poorly equipped to deal with cholesterol esters. It seems that at least the lysosomes in these cells are not too efficient at dealing with the metabolism of cholesterol esters. I think that this is an important concept. We should also pay attention to the possibility that in some lipid storage diseases there may be a deficiency of certain lysosomal enzymes.

Dr. Zemplenyi: I think that someone has shown that in Wohlman's disease there is a high incidence of atherosclerosis.

Dr. Adams: That is very interesting.

Dr. Smith: I would like to ask Dr. Patelski whether the LCAT enzyme present in the arterial wall is associated with the HDL fraction or with some other macromolecules in the wall. Is this LCAT enzyme produced locally?

Dr. Patelski: I am afraid that I cannot answer this question at present.

Dr. Smith: I would like to make a comment on substrates used in these enzyme studies. In the atheromatous lipid, which I assume to be derived from the plasma lipoproteins, it is interesting to note the following. If one calculates the amount of the various lipids in the atheromatous lesions, then a large amount of the plasma phospholipids have been "lost" in the atheromatous lesions. This phospholipid has gone somewhere and if we remember that there is also active synthesis of phospholipids in the vessel wall, then a great deal of the arterial phospholipid must be eliminated from the vessel wall and from the lesion by some mechanism. It is important to try to link up phospholipid metabolism with cholesterol ester metabolism as indicated in Dr. Patelski's paper. I would, however, like to state my concern about all the in vitro assays of the hydrolase and synthetase enzyme systems, because the critical state of the substrate can influence the experimental result.

Dr. Patelski: I agree with these comments.

Dr. Boyd: Dr. Smith, if you state that there is an active removal of phospholipids in the vessel wall and in the atheromatous lesion, then presumably this creates a situation for the deposition of other lipids at that site.

Dr. Smith: That is correct and there must be an enormous amount of phospholipid going somewhere by some, as yet unknown, mechanism.

Dr. Nikkila: I would like to ask Dr. Kritchevsky whether he has any idea on how nicotinic acid acts on these synthetase and hydrolase enzymes described in his paper.

Dr. Kritchevsky: We have not looked into this aspect of the problem. There appear to be so many possibilities for the mechanism by which this compound could affect these enzymes. For example, the effect could be by an allosteric mechanism or by influencing the availability of co-factors. It must be appreciated by all that these enzymic observations made in vitro have been performed using a relatively crude system.

Dr. Beaumont: I am grateful for the studies of Drs. Patelski and Kritchevsky for helping me to understand certain aspects of lipid metabolism. We sometimes see in Type II lipoprotein disorder during the treatment of these subjects with nicotinic acid or with CPIB, there may be no change in the blood cholesterol concentration and yet we see a definite change, a regression, in cutaneous xanthoma lesions. I would like to know whether these experimental findings of Dr. Patelski and Dr. Kritchevsky could explain these clinical observations.

Dr. Kritchevsky: I am not in a position at present to say much more on this topic. We hope to be able to answer questions of this sort at a later date. We are trying to evolve assays for these enzymes, using as substrates the physiological substrate which the enzyme in vivo may encounter.

Discussant Z: There are several points which should be noted in connection with the use of nicotinic acid. There is the low dose of this compound which nutritionists use in the prevention of pellagra. There is the dose which clinicians use in the treatment of certain hyperlipemic states and this is often in the range 50-100 mg/kg body weight. There is then, the high dosage of nicotinic acid which may cause fatty livers. It is possible that Dr. Kritchevsky's observations may have been made at the high dosage range. It has to be appreciated that nicotinic acid behaves in a different fashion at these different dosage ranges.

Dr. Kritchevsky: We have used this drug in these studies at the dose range of 250 mg/kg body weight.

Discussant Z: I would be inclined to try these experiments again at the dose range 50-100 mg/kg body weight, as I suspect that this would produce results different from those reported in the study.

Dr. Zilversmit: In the question of the effect of drugs on tissue cholesterol compared with the effects on plasma cholesterol it is possible that this situation could be like that which is seen in the cholesterol fed rabbit. When rabbits are fed cholesterol and then cholesterol is removed from the diet, the plasma cholesterol concentration does not decline for a long time, presumably because the tissues are emptying their cholesterol into the plasma. I might assume that in the subjects with xanthoma, the same situation might exist. Thus, the xanthoma may disappear but while they are emptying their cholesterol into the plasma, the plasma cholesterol concentration may not change. In some cases it may require several years before the plasma cholesterol concentration decreases.

Dr. Beaumont: I would like to comment on this. In rabbits it takes only a few weeks for the animal to return to fairly normal blood cholesterol levels. In the human subjects to which I refer, the plasma cholesterol concentration is still high after five years of treatment.

Dr. Klimov: I would like to ask Dr. Patelski about the methods for the separation of the enzyme activity which he has described in this paper. How were these enzymes separated from the vascular tissue?

Dr. Patelski: Initially, we attempted to try to purify these different enzymes in arterial tissue but due to difficulties we have not pursued this aspect very far. There are, however, reports of the purification of some of these enzymes from aorta. Particularly, there is a report of the isolation of cholesterol ester hydrolase from aorta.

Dr. Kritchevsky: I would like to comment on data we have on two strains of pigeons. These are the Show Racer pigeon and the White Carneau pigeon. The latter strain are susceptible to spontaneous atherosclerosis and in these birds we have found a higher aortic synthetase to hydrolase ratio than we have observed in the other birds which are less susceptible to atherosclerosis.

Dr. Boyd: I would like to ask Dr. Scott whether he has tried adding cholesterol to the mitochondria isolated from arterial tissue to see whether exogenous cholesterol influences the respiratory control ratio in these mitochondria.

Dr. Scott: We have not tried this. How would we get the cholesterol into the mitochondria?

Dr. Boyd: Using rat adrenal cortical mitochondria and rat corpora luteal mitochondria, we have added cholesterol to these organelles in acetone solution and demonstrated that the exogenous cholesterol is rapidly metabolized by these specialized mitochondria to the hormone precursor pregnenolone.

Dr. Scott: Does the acetone influence the respiration of these mitochondria?

Dr. Boyd: At the concentration of acetone which we employ, this organic solvent has no effect on the respiration of the mitochondria.

Dr. Zilversmit: I would like to ask Dr. Smith how she manages to differentiate in aortic tissue between post-mortem effects and ante-mortem effects.

Dr. Smith: There is, of course, no easy way to differentiate between post-mortem and ante-mortem effects. We have attempted to do this by the use of time sequences. In general, the earliest that we obtain the tissues is about 2½ hrs after death of the subject. In general, the albumin content of the tissue appears to increase with increasing time after death but the differences were not significant.

Dr. Zilversmit: Dr. Smith, in your studies would it not be necessary to take into account the size and the shape of the proteins in such an infiltration concept? For example, the plasma protein fibrinogen is quite different from LDL.

Dr. Smith: I agree, while we do not have plasma samples available from all these subjects, if we assume that the subjects have normal fibrinogen concentration, then the data do in fact suggest that fibrinogen behaves as if it had a molecular weight of about a million!

Discussant A: I have a question for Dr. Walton. In connection with the immunofluorescence studies, in some of the slides you showed areas of the lesion which appear to be positive immunologically for LDL but negative for lipid. And a second question, do you obtain positive evidence for the presence of HDL in these atheromatous lesions?

Dr. Walton: It is possible that there is a greater sensitivity of the immunoreactive tests than for the lipid stain test. There are also other technical reasons for the problems which you have highlighted and are encountered in the demonstration of the specific localization of proteins and lipids. In some cases the tissue must be fixed in alcohol or in acetone to localize the protein. This procedure slightly increases the sensitivity of some tests and it is possible to show the presence of HDL reactive material in these lesions.

Dr. Zemplenyi: Dr. Walton, you showed slides showing the localization of heparin in the vessel wall. You indicated that this substance would localize in the vasa vasorum. Are you sure that the heparin was in the vasa vasorum and not in the vasa lymphatica?

Dr. Walton: There are publications relating to this point. It has been shown that the vasa lymphatica of the arterial wall appears to grow into the vasa vasorum and so it would be almost impossible to give a definitive answer to your question.

Dr. Boyd: In concluding this Workshop, I would like to thank all the speakers and the discussants. I am sure that all will agree that this has been a most stimulating session and that we leave with the impression that we still have a great deal to learn about the mechanism by which lipoproteins enter the vascular tissue. The processes associated with the movement of lipoprotein macromolecules within the vessel wall seem to be similar to many of the techniques used in chemistry and biochemistry for the separation of macromolecules. Thus, the vascular wall behaves in some ways like a molecular sieve in separating large lipoprotein complexes from smaller lipoprotein complexes and from the smaller plasma proteins. It is also possible that the vascular system behaves like an adsorbent in chromatography and there is also the possibility that the vessel wall behaves towards some of these macromolecules like an affinity chromatography adsorbent. No doubt, future studies on the physico-chemical behavior of the vessel wall and of the enzymes contained in the vessel wall will throw light on the underlying pathogenesis of atherosclerosis.

CHAPTER 15
TISSUE CULTURE II

(1)

THE LIPOPROTEINS AND ARTERIAL SMOOTH MUSCLE CELLS: UPTAKE OF VLDL, LDL, HDL

Olga Stein and Yechezkiel Stein

Department of Experimental Medicine and Cancer Research,
Hebrew University-Hadassah Medical School, and
Lipid Research Laboratory, Department of Medicine B,
Hadassah University Hospital, Jerusalem, Israel.

Serum lipoproteins are considered the main source of cholesterol of "peripheral" cells and studies with perfused aorta have shown that human LDL and HDL can cross normal aortic endothelium, most probably via the plasmalemmal vesicles (1). Thus even under normal conditions aortic smooth muscle cells are exposed to some serum lipoproteins, the presence of which is highly augmented under pathological conditions. Recently, Hoff et al. have established the presence of apolipoprotein B in atherosclerotic intima, using a highly purified antibody to human apoLDL (2). However the study of uptake of lipoproteins by aortic smooth muscle cells in the intact artery is not readily feasable and therefore most investigators have turned to the smooth muscle cells in culture to study this problem. In our studies we have used the system developed by Ross (3) and have used cells of a locally bred strain of rats. The cells can be grown for several generations in Falcon flasks and passed into Petri dishes for the individual experiments.

Since the ^{125}I is the common marker used for the study of uptake of lipoprotein-protein it seems important to review briefly some problems one encounters using this method. Even under the optimal conditions for iodination of the protein moiety a certain percent of the label is present in the lipid. This is much more pronounced with rat than with human lipoproteins. However, even in the case of human lipoproteins the percent of lipid label recovered in the cells exceeds that in the labeling medium, a factor which should be taken into account in final calculations. It seems worthwhile to take notice also of the fact that the (4) efficiency of counting

Figure 1

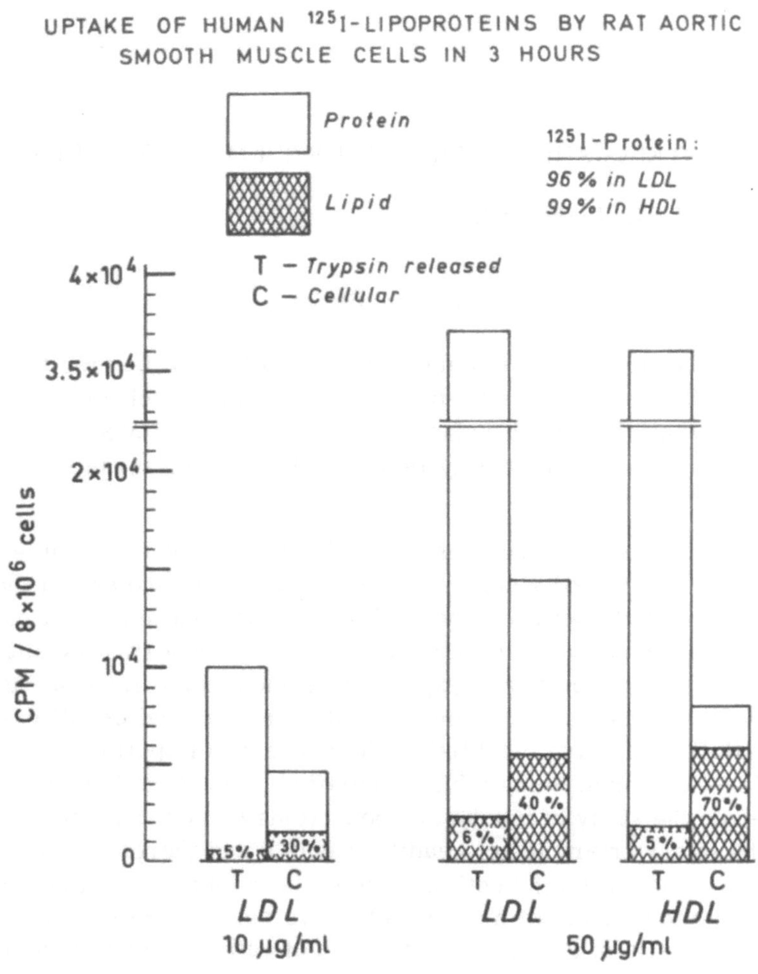

of ^{125}I is highly reduced in the presence of chloroform (a common lipid solvent) and KBr, which is used for separation of lipoprotein classes (5).

The interaction between the cells and lipoproteins proceeds in two stages - binding and uptake, which are related but do not necessarily follow each other. The two stages can be distinguished with the help of trypsinization, which is superimposed on six washes with buffer (6); as seen in Fig. 1 the label removed by trypsin is different from that remaining with the cells. While in the trypsinate the ratio of lipid : protein radioactivity is similar to that in the incubation medium, this is not so for the label remaining with the cells, which is usually enriched in respect to lipid label (7). As another evidence that trypsin can help to distinguish between surface bound and interiorized label are the results performed at 0°, under conditions where no uptake occurs, and under which about 90% of the radioactivity can be removed by trypsin (8). On the other hand, radioautography of cells which had been trypsinized shows that the remaining label is indeed intracellular (6) and that can be verified also by electron microscopic radioautography. Following incubation of rat smooth muscle cells with various homologous lipoproteins the highest uptake is seen with rat LDL and HDL (Fig. 2). That this represents most probably interiorization of entire particles is supported by the findings with labeled apoproteins, as even after exposure to much higher concentration of apoproteins the protein uptake is considerably lower than that following incubation with entire lipoproteins (4). Are there species differences in lipoprotein uptake? Such a comparison was done by Bierman and Albers (9) who have concluded that human aortic cells in culture take up more homologous lipoproteins than do rat aortic cells. We have obtained also similar results with human skin fibroblasts and have wondered whether this is solely due to a species difference. Even though we have grown the human skin fibroblast and the rat smooth muscle cells under the same conditions, there were usually $1 - 1.5 \times 10^{6}$ fibroblasts and $6 - 10 \times 10^{6}$ smooth muscle cells per Petri dish. This prompted a study of the effect of cell density on lipoprotein uptake and the two types of experiments designed are summarized in the next two figures (Figs. 3 and 4).

In the first experiment the same number of cells was present in three Petri dishes of different diameters and therefore the relative cell density was unequal. Concomitantly the lipoprotein uptake per 10^{6} cells was dissimilar and was inversely proportional to the cell density. In the second experiment in which the relative cell density was kept constant the lipoprotein uptake was proportional to the cell number (7). Thus it seems that apart from species differences, variation in cell density has to be considered when comparing lipoprotein uptake in vitro.

The cholesterol transported in the form of an LDL particle is about 60-70% esterified and the ester bond has to be hydrolyzed prior to the utilization of the sterol moiety. This process occurs most probably in the lysosomes, which were shown to be active in the hydrolysis of the protein moiety (4). The presence of secondary lysosomes in smooth muscle cells is not limited to cells in culture as secondary lysosomes can be demonstrated also in the smooth muscle cells of the artery in vivo (10) (Fig. 5). Thus it seems that aortic smooth muscle cells are able to bind and interiorize serum lipoproteins and are equipped with the enzymic

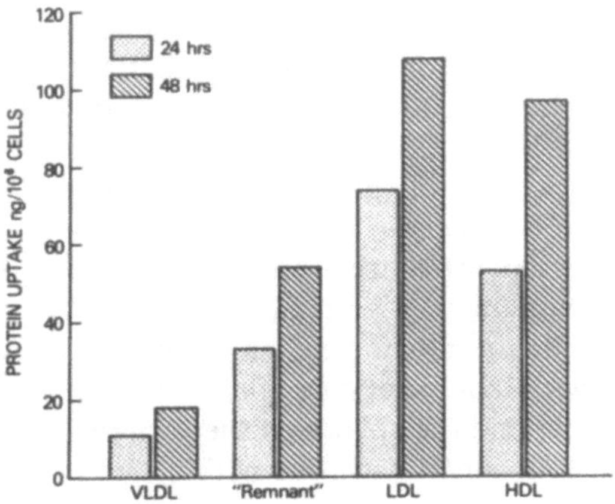

Fig. 2. Uptake of Homologous Lipoproteins by Rat Aortic Smooth Muscle Cells.

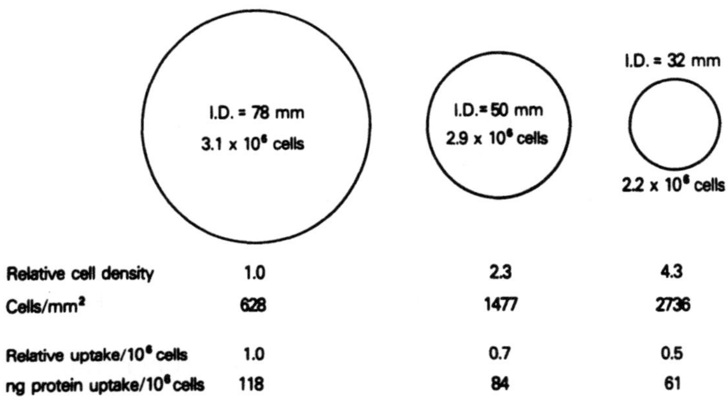

Fig. 3. Relation of Uptake to Cell Number at Varying Cell Density.

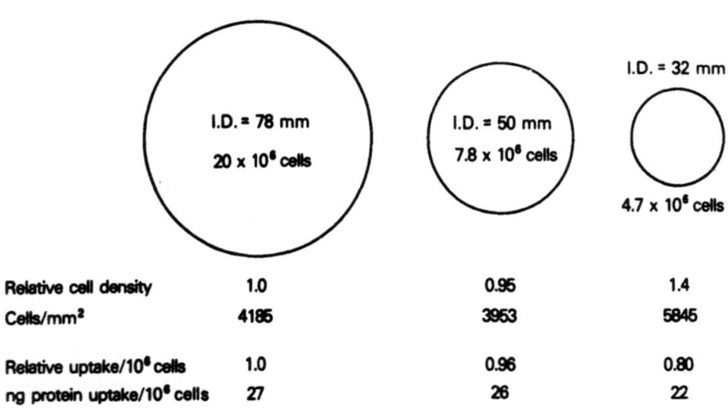

Fig. 4. Relation of Uptake to Cell Number at Equal Cell Density.

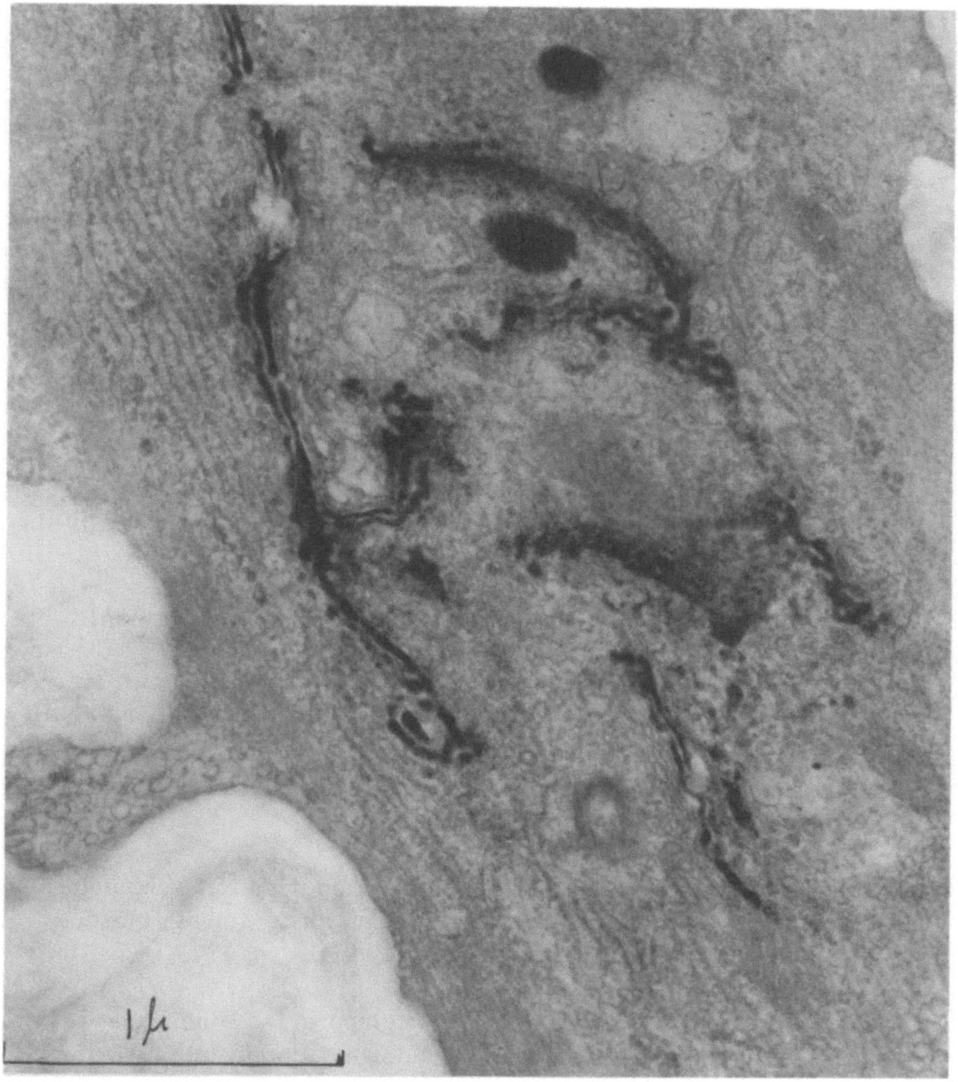

Figure 5. Electron micrograph of aortic media of 3-week-old rat. Tissues stained for acid phosphatase which is represented by the electron opaque product in the secondary lysosomes and in the Golgi apparatus.

apparatus to degrade the protein moiety as well as the cholesterol ester bond. The fate of the cholesterol molecule is different and mechanisms for its removal from cell which regulate the cholesterol content of the cells are under current investigation.

References

1. Stein, O., Stein, Y. and Eisenberg, S.: A radioautographic study of the transport of ^{125}I-labeled serum lipoproteins in rat aorta. Cell & Tissue Res. 138: 223, 1973.

2. Hoff, H. F., Lie, J. T., Titus, J. L., Bayardo, R. J., Jackson, R. L., DeBakey, M. E. and Gotto, A. M.: Lipoproteins in atherosclerotic lesions. Localization by immunofluorescence of apo-low density lipoproteins in human atherosclerotic arteries from normal and hyperlipoproteinemics. Arch. Pathol. 99: 253, 1975

3. Ross, R.: Smooth muscle cell: II. Growth of smooth muscle in culture and formation of elastic fibers. J. Cell Biol. 50: 172, 1971.

4. Stein, O. and Stein, Y. : Comparative uptake of rat and human serum low density lipoproteins by rat aortic smooth muscle cells in culture. Circulation Res. 36: 436, 1975.

5. Eisenberg, S., Stein, O. and Stein, Y.: Radioiodinated lipoproteins: absorption of ^{125}I radioactivity by high density solutions. J. Lipid Res. In press, 1975.

6. Bierman, E. L., Stein, O. and Stein, Y.: Lipoprotein uptake and metabolism by rat aortic smooth muscle cells in tissue culture. Circulation Res. 35: 136, 1974.

7. Stein, O. and Stein, Y: Surface binding and interiorization of homologous and heterologous serum lipoproteins by rat aortic smooth muscle cells in culture. Biochim. Biophys. Acta, In press, 1975.

8. Stein, O., Weinstein, D. B., Stein, Y. and Steinberg, D. Binding, internalization and degradation of low density lipoprotein by normal human fibroblasts and by fibroblasts from a new case of homozygous familial hypercholesterolemia. In press, 1975.

9. Bierman, E. L. and Albers, J. J.: Lipoprotein uptake by cultured human arterial smooth muscle cells. Biochim. Biophys. Acta 388: 198, 1975.

10. Stein, O., Sanger, L., Zajicek, G. and Stein, Y.: Acid phosphatase in aortic smooth muscle cells studied by electron microscopic cytochemistry. Paroi Arterielle 1: 187, 1973.

(2)

LIPOPROTEINS AND ARTERIAL SMOOTH MUSCLE CELLS: REGULATION OF CELLULAR METABOLISM BY SWINE LIPOPROTEINS.

Robert W. Mahley, M.D.

Comparative Atherosclerosis and Arterial Metabolism Section, NHLI
Bethesda, Maryland, U.S.A.

The purpose of this paper is to review our findings related to the regulation of cellular metabolism in cultured smooth muscle cells and fibroblasts by control and cholesterol-induced lipoproteins and to speculate on possible mechanisms. Miniature swine fed diets composed of 15% lard and 1% cholesterol develop a hypercholesterolemia of ≈500 mg% and accelerated atherosclerosis (1). The atherogenic hypercholesterolemia is characterized by marked changes in the types of plasma lipoproteins as revealed by paper electrophoretograms of various ultracentrifugal density fractions (Fig. 1). Control swine have lipoproteins equivalent to human VLDL, LDL and HDL with respect to physical and chemical properties. Following cholesterol feeding there are three primary alterations in the lipoprotein pattern: 1) the presence of B-VLDL, as in human Type III disease, in the d<1.006; 2) an increase in LDL; 3) the appearance of a unique lipoprotein referred to as HDL_c (c indicating cholesterol induced). HDL_c have α-mobility, lack the B apoprotein, and are related to HDL with respect to the presence of apo-A-I.

The occurence of HDL_c as a major cholesterol-transporting lipoprotein similar to LDL in many respects, but differing in apoprotein content, offered a unique opportunity to test the importance of various physicochemical properties of lipoproteins to the regulation of cellular metabolism. As shown in Figure 2, LDL and HDL_c are both cholesterol rich (50-60% of the total composition) and are similar in size (mean diameter ∿190 Å). By comparison, HDL_2 are rich in protein and phospholipid and have a particle size of 60 to 100 Å, with a mean of ∿85 Å (similar to human HDL). The apoprotein pattern on Tris-urea polyacrylamide gel electrophoresis is shown in Figure 2. The B apoprotein is a major protein component of LDL. In addition, the cholesterol-induced LDL contain a variable

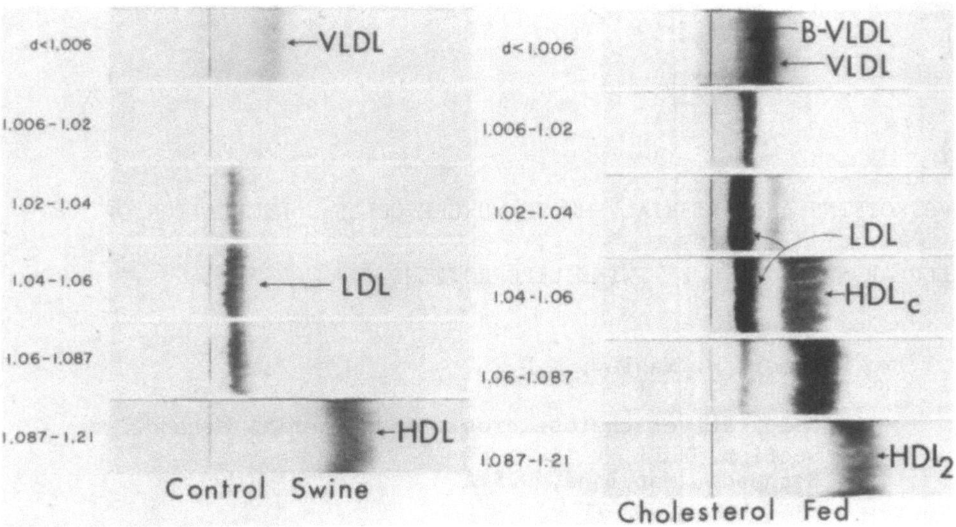

Figure 1. Paper electrophoretograms of ultracentrifugal density fractions (reproduced with permission (1)).

amount of other peptides. A major difference between LDL and HDL_c is that HDL_c lack any detectable B apoprotein. HDL_c contain the arginine-rich, A-I and C apoproteins. HDL_2 of the swine have as their primary protein apo-A-I and little, if any, of the arginine-rich apoprotein (1).

	Triglyceride	T. Cholesterol	Phospholipid	Protein	Size (Å)
d<1.006	40.0	38.1	14.2	7.7	240-800
LDL	0.5	59.7	21.7	18.0	160-240
HDL_c	0.5	50.0	29.3	20.3	140-240
HDL_2	0.5	24.2	34.3	41.0	60-100

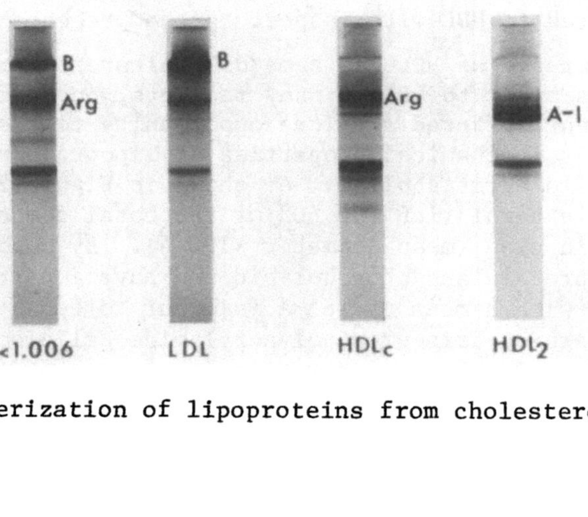

Figure 2. Characterization of lipoproteins from cholesterol fed swine.

Since the accelerated swine atherosclerosis induced by cholesterol feeding is characterized by smooth muscle cell (SMC) proliferation and cellular lipid accumulation, we undertook to determine the effects of the various classes of swine lipoproteins on SMC growth and cholesterol metabolism. SMC from the inner media of the swine thoracic aorta were derived and maintained by procedures described by Ross (3). The studies were performed in collaboration with Dr. B. G. Brown (4). Cells were grown in limiting media containing 1.5% swine serum for 4 days prior to the addition of the lipoproteins to the media. At a concentration of 10 mg/dl of lipoprotein cholesterol, LDL from control and hypercholesterolemic swine increased the growth rate 6.1-fold compared to cells grown in the limiting media. However, the HDL_c and HDL_2 from the hypercholesterolemic swine had significantly less growth-promoting effect at the same cholesterol concentration (∿3-fold increase in rate). The typical 85 Å HDL from control animals give results similar to those obtained with HDL_2 and HDL_c from the hypercholesterolemic animals. VLDL or the d<1.006 fraction from controls and hypercholesterolemic animals were equally as stimulating as LDL (∿7-fold). The observation that HDL_c stimulated growth less than LDL may be of importance in eventually determining the mechanism of cell growth regulation by lipoproteins.

With respect to lipid metabolism, we undertook to determine the effects of swine lipoproteins on regulation of cholesterol metabolism in SMC. This work was performed in collaboration with Drs. G. Assmann and B. G. Brown (5). We were able to demonstrate that both swine LDL and HDL_c at equal cholesterol concentration caused a similar and nearly complete suppression of 3-hydroxy-3-methylglutaryl coenzyme A reductase activity. HMG-CoA reductase has been shown to be the rate-limiting enzyme for de novo cholesterol synthesis in several different cell lines. As shown in Figure 3, when the

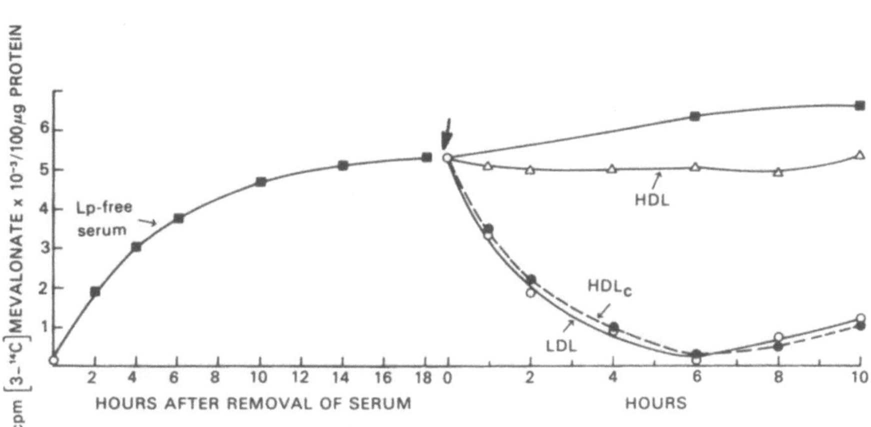

Figure 3. Regulation of HMG-CoA reductase (modified from 5).

cellular growth media containing serum was replaced by lipoprotein-free serum, a marked increase in HMG-CoA reductase activity was observed which reached a maximum at 18 hr. At this point, the addition of LDL or HDL_c containing 100 mg/ml of lipoprotein cholesterol resulted in almost complete inhibition of reductase activity within 6 hr. VLDL or d<1.006 fraction from control or cholesterol-fed swine likewise suppressed reductase activity. On the other hand, swine HDL_2 had much less effect (Fig.3). These data in SMC suggested that HDL_c, a lipoprotein lacking the B apoprotein, could regulate cellular cholesterol metabolism in a manner similar to LDL, whereas the typical 85 Å HDL_2 had little effect on reductase activity.

In order to determine if swine LDL and HDL_c interact with the same or a different cell surface receptor and if they regulate cholesterol synthesis by similar mechanisms, we undertook studies with the swine lipoproteins using the lines of cultured human fibroblasts established by Drs. Goldstein and Brown. This work was performed in collaboration with Drs. T. P. Bersot, M. S. Brown and J. L. Goldstein (6). The ability of the swine lipoproteins to compete with iodinated human LDL for binding and uptake at 37°C was determined in fibroblasts cultured under standard conditions (7). On day 6 the growth medium was replaced by 2 ml of a medium containing lipoprotein-deficient serum plus 23 μg/ml of iodinated LDL and varying amounts of unlabeled human LDL or swine LDL, HDL_c, or HDL_2. As presented in Figure 4A, swine LDL and HDL_c were as effective as human LDL in competing with human iodinated LDL for binding and uptake. Swine HDL_2 were much less effective in displacing the iodinated LDL from its binding site, as has been shown for human HDL.

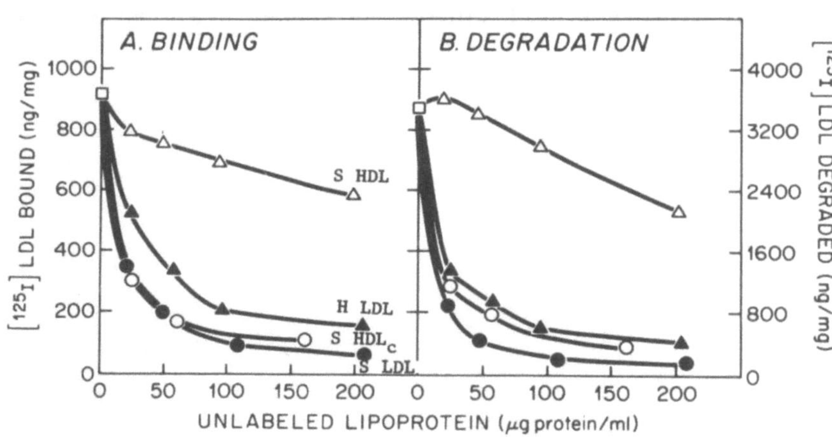

Figure 4. Competitive inhibition of binding and degradation of ^{125}I-human (H)-LDL by swine (S) lipoproteins (modified from 6).

Proteolytic degradation of iodinated human LDL by fibroblasts has been shown by Goldstein and Brown to require the binding of LDL to its receptor (8). In Figure 4B, human LDL and swine LDL and HDL_c are shown to competitively inhibit the degradation of iodinated LDL. This is further evidence which suggests that HDL_c interact with the cell and are bound, taken up, and degraded in a manner similar to LDL.

With respect to HMG-CoA reductase activity, swine and human LDL at comparable levels in the media caused nearly identical suppression of reductase activity in normal human fibroblasts. The HDL_c also suppressed reductase activity in human fibroblasts, as was shown in the swine smooth muscle cells. Swine HDL_2 had less effect on reductase activity even at high lipoprotein levels. Regulation of HMG-CoA reductase activity in fibroblasts from patients with the so-called receptor negative form of homozygous Type II disease by the swine lipoproteins has been studied. Swine LDL and HDL_c do not significantly suppress HMG-CoA reductase activity in these cells as has been shown for human LDL (6).

Extension of these data to another species, the dog, allowed further comparison of the parameters of lipoprotein structure essential for recognition by cell receptors and for cholesterol uptake. Free and esterified cholesterol content of SMC from dog aorta was determined by gas chromatography after a 24-hr incubation with various canine plasma lipoproteins (Table I). After incubation with lipoprotein-deficient plasma the cellular free cholesterol was 19 and the esterified 4 μg/mg cell protein. The typical dog HDL_2 at a concentration of 500 μg/mg cholesterol did not significantly alter the sterol level in the cells. However, dog LDL and HDL_c at the same cholesterol concentration resulted in a marked elevation to comparable levels (Table I). The LDL and HDL_c of the dog have a similar composition and size but differ in apoprotein content (2) as has been shown in the swine.

Table I. Cholesterol Content* of Canine Smooth Muscle Cells

	Control			Hypercholesterolemic	
	Free	Esterified		Free	Esterified
LDL	78	22	VLDL	72	37
HDL_1	74	26	LDL	80	41
HDL_2	21	3	HDL_c	73	35
d>1.21	19	4			

* μg sterol/mg cell protein

SUMMARY

Cell Growth. Ross and Glomset (9) and Dzoga et al (10) have shown that lipoproteins can effect SMC growth in culture, although the mechanism remains obscure. Despite the observation that HDL_c are taken up by cells and regulate cholesterol metabolism in a manner similar to LDL, HDL_c do not have a similar growth-promoting effect. The LDL have a greater growth-promoting effect than HDL_c. HDL_c and

LDL have similar chemical composition and particle size but have a different apoprotein content, which may be of importance with respect to cell growth. LDL contain primarily the B apoprotein, whereas HDL_c lack apo-B and contain the A-I and arginine-rich apoproteins. HDL_2, which contain primarily apo-A-I, have growth-promoting effects similar to HDL_c. A possibility, as we have suggested previously (4), is that cell growth may be stimulated by the presence of apo-B as occurs with VLDL and LDL or, conversely, that cell growth may be inhibited by the presence of apo-A-I in HDL_c and HDL_2.

Cholesterol Metabolism. LDL and HDL_c suppress HMG-CoA reductase activity in both SMC and fibroblasts, whereas HDL_2 do not. In addition, LDL and HDL_c compete for binding, uptake and degradation (unlike HDL_2). Thus HDL_c, a lipoprotein devoid of apo-B, can interact with the cell surface receptor, deliver cholesterol to the cell and regulate cholesterol synthesis. The nature of the cell surface receptor which interacts with both LDL and HDL_c, but not HDL_2, is open to discussion.

We speculate that lipoproteins which exert regulatory control and are taken up by cultured cells may have at least two parameters in common: first, they are >120 Å in size, as described in this paper and previously by the Steins (11), and, second, they contain the B apoprotein and/or the arginine-rich apoprotein or a structural sequence common to both apoproteins. Rat HDL, the only high density lipoproteins demonstrated to be taken up by cultured cells, have a larger mean particle size than HDL of man or swine (11). In addition, rat HDL contain more of the arginine-rich apoprotein (∿10-15% of the total protein; unpublished observation) than is present in either human HDL or swine HDL. Distinguishing among the specificity of apoprotein content, particle size or other physical properties as the initiating event for internalization of the lipoproteins and regulation of cholesterol synthesis awaits further data.

References

1. Mahley, R.W., Weisgraber, K.H., Innerarity, T., Brewer, H.B.,Jr., and Assmann, G. Biochemistry 14:2817, 1975.
2. Mahley, R.W., Weisgraber, K.H., Innerarity, T. Circ. Res. 35:722, 1974.
3. Ross, R. J. Cell Biol. 50:172, 1971.
4. Brown, B.G., Mahley, R.W., and Assmann, G. Submitted.
5. Assmann, G., Brown, G., and Mahley, R.W. Biochemistry In Press.
6. Bersot, T.P., Mahley, R.W., Brown, M.S.,and Goldstein,J.L. In preparation.
7. Brown, M.S., Dana, S.E., and Goldstein, J.L. J. Biol. Chem. 249: 789, 1974.
8. Goldstein, J.L., and Brown, M.S. J. Biol. Chem. 249:4143, 1974.
9. Ross, R., and Glomset, J.A. Science 180:1332, 1973.
10. Dzoga, K., Wissler, R.W., and Vesselinovitch, D. Circ. 44: Suppl. II-6, 1971.
11. Stein, O. and Stein Y. Circ. Res. 36:436, 1975.

(3)

THE LIPOPROTEINS AND ARTERIAL SMOOTH MUSCLE CELLS: CELLULAR PROLIFERATION AND MORPHOLOGY

K. Fischer-Dzoga, R. W. Wissler and A. M. Scanu

University of Chicago, Depts. of Pathology, Medicine and Biochemistry
Chicago, Illinois, U.S.A.

We have been using primary cultures of aortic media as an *in vitro* model to study the response of these arterial smooth muscle cells to lipoproteins, and in particular to study their differential responses, if any, to lipoproteins from hyperlipemic serum compared to lipoproteins from normal serum.

The cultures are obtained by placing small round explants of arterial media in plastic culture flasks, and allowing them to attach to the bottom of the flask. In a few days outgrowth can be observed forming a cell colony around the explant. Eighty to ninety percent of the explants show outgrowth, and once the cell colony is well established the original explant can be removed. The diameter or surface area of the culture can be measured as an indication of proliferation. Eagle's Basal Media supplemented with serum is adequate for satisfactory growth. All our efforts to culture these cells in serum-free media have failed, even when using media enriched in known growth-promoting factors. Nor have we been able to obtain satisfactory growth in lipid-free media, e.g. using the >1.21 protein residue instead of whole serum. Only a few cells grow out when cultures are grown under these conditions.

According to morphological and immunohistochemical criteria, these cells appear to be smooth muscle cells (1). They retain their ability to produce mucopolysaccharides, collagen and elastin (1, 2). This can be demonstrated chemically or by special stains: cultures stained with a Gomori-Trichrome stain for collagen show large amounts of the stainable material at the site of multilayers, and to a lesser degree throughout the culture, even in areas of monolayers when cell density is high. High magnification frequently reveals the formation of new fibers, apparently oriented at right angles to the longitudinal axis of the cells. The presence of mucopolysaccharides can be visualized using Alcian blue for staining. Extracellular pools of the blue material can be seen throughout the culture, but are usually most evident in areas of high cell density. Other cultures have been stained with aldehyde fuchsin for elastin. The purple elastin fibers form a distinct pattern with dense fibers along the multilayers and fine fibers throughout the culture.

With 100% normal serum as the media supplement, these cells show a very reproducible growth pattern. The cell colonies grow to about 15 mm in diameter before reaching a relatively stationary phase with little mitotic activity and a very slow increase in culture size (Fig. 1). This phase is reached after 6 to 8 weeks, and without changing the culture conditions such cultures can be kept for a long period of time without showing much evidence of necrosis.

The substitution of the normal serum in the medium by hyperlipemic serum during this phase triggers the cells into a second phase of proliferation: pulse labeling with ^{3}H-thymidine and subsequent autoradiography indicate an increased mitotic activity within 24 to 36 hours, accompanied by an increase in culture size, measurable after a few days (3, 4). When the lipoprotein fractions of the hyperlipemic serum are added separately, the low density lipoprotein (LDL) fraction can be identified as the one largely responsible for this increase in proliferation. Table 1 gives the results of a representative experiment. It shows that the cultures receiving the whole hyperlipemic serum, as well as the group receiving its LDL fraction, undergo a remarkable increase in size during a 10-day experimental period, paralleled by an increase in

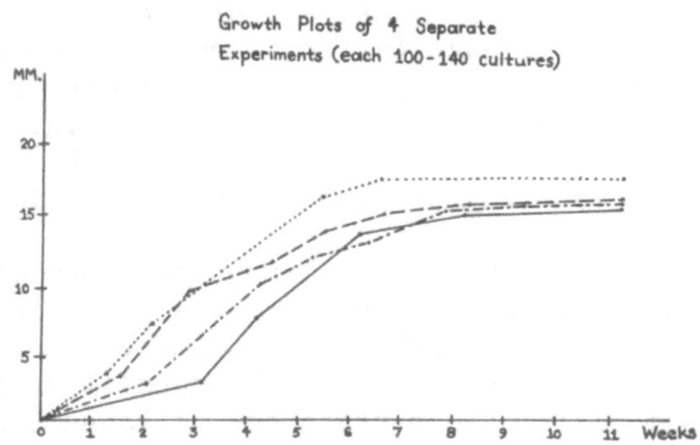

Fig. 1. Growth curves of primary cultures of aortic media in Basal Eagle's Medium supplemented with 10% normal serum.

ADDITION TO CULTURE MEDIUM	AVERAGE GROWTH INCREASE mm^2	% OF CELLS LABELED WITH H^3 THYMIDINE
5% Normal monkey serum	14.9 ± 13.3	6.2% ± 1.5
5% Hyperlipemic monkey serum	81.9 ± 21.9	39.5% ± 5.0
5% Serum VLDL	18.9 ± 5.9	6.5% ± 1.6
5% Serum LDL	79.2 ± 17.5	39.4% ± 8.1
5% Serum HDL	24.5 ± 12.5	4.9% ± 0.7
Serum protein	12.8 ± 4.5	3.8% ± 1.0

Table 1. Effect of hyperlipemic serum and its lipoprotein fractions on incorporation of ^3H-thymidine and on surface area of primary aortic smooth muscle cell cultures.

labeled nuclei. The other lipoprotein fractions, as well as the LDL from normal serum, have no effect. Recently we have tried to narrow down the fractions further in order to identify more exactly the responsible lipoprotein. Lipoprotein fractions were isolated by sequential ultracentrifugation and the following density cuts were used:

LDL_1	= d 1.006-1.019 g/ml
LDL_2	= d 1.019-1.063 g/ml
Narrow Cut (N. C.)	= d 1.02-1.05 g/ml
Bottom Fraction (B. F.)	> 1.21 g/ml

LDL_1 and LDL_2 were used in two experiments, and in two additional experiments we used what we call the "narrow cut" fraction (1.02-1.05 g/ml) which gives a homogenous fraction as judged by agarose electrophoresis and density gradient ultracentrifugation, and contains only apoprotein B by immunological criteria.

Fig. 2 summarizes the results obtained in these experiments. Whole hyperlipemic serum and normal serum were included as positive and negative controls in each experiment. For comparison the results are expressed in percent of growth increase, with the increase from hyperlipemic serum set at 100%. It is evident that the proliferative activity is in the LDL_2 fraction, while the LDL_1 fraction has no effect. The narrow cut fraction is also active in inducing proliferation, although somewhat less than LDL_2. Comparable fractions of normal serum have no effect, even when given in concentrations approaching cholesterol levels of the fractions from hyperlipemic serum (5).

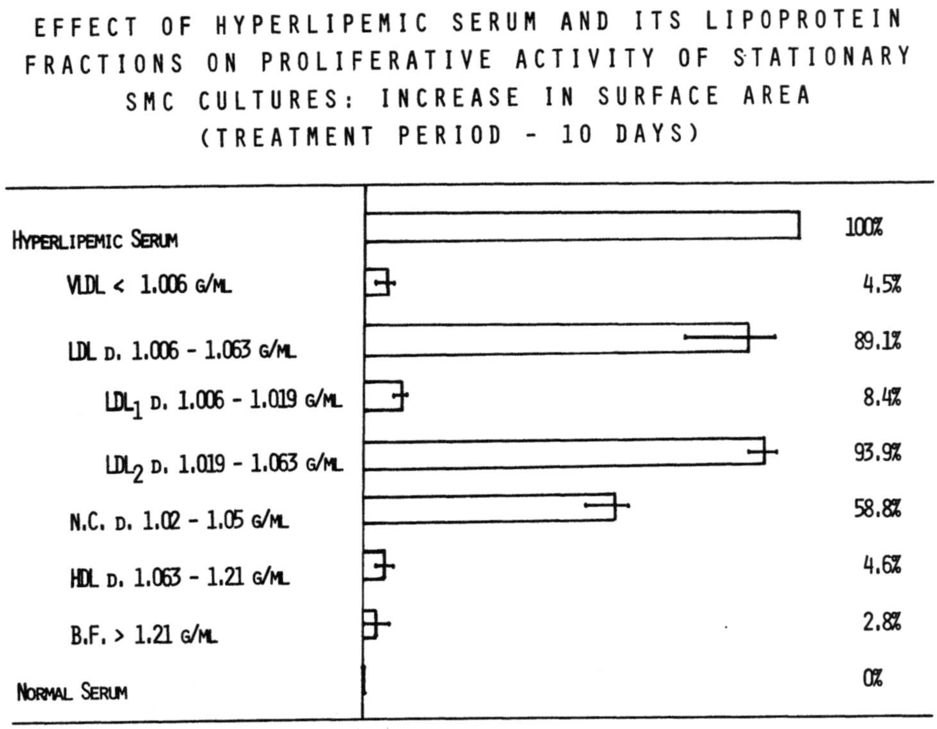

Fig. 2. Relative increase in surface area of primary aortic smooth muscle cell cultures caused by the addition of hyperlipemic serum and its lipoprotein fractions to the culture medium.

When the cultures are grown in media which has been supplemented with 10% hyperlipemic serum from the time of explantation, they frequently show outgrowth somewhat sooner. Outgrowth is usually present in over 90% of the explants--a higher percentage than in normal serum-supplemented media. Furthermore, the average culture size is often (but not always) larger, although on the whole the average growth curve is similar to that of the control cultures in normal serum. There is, however, quite a difference between the normal and hyperlipemic groups in the distribution of size of individual cultures at 8 weeks. The bell-shaped curve shown in Fig. 3, with 70% or more of the cultures within a relatively narrow range, is typical for cultures grown in normal serum-supplemented media, although it may be shifted slightly to the right or left. On the other hand, the size distribution curve of a group of cultures in hyperlipemic serum looks quite different. These cultures show a much wider distribution in size--in this particular case there are two bell-shaped curves, one with cultures much larger and the other with smaller cultures than are usually found in the normal serum group.

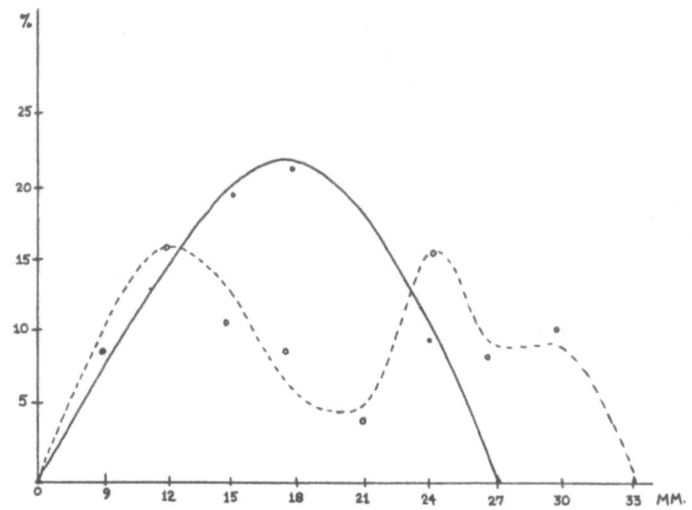

Fig. 3. Size distribution of aortic medial cultures grown in Eagle's Basal medium supplemented with either normal (•——) or hyperlipemic (o------) serum.

One interesting finding is that there are often multiple colonies per flask in the hyperlipemic serum group. These new colonies apparently form even after the explant is removed. We have noted before that at least some cells must migrate, since single cells can often be observed away from the periphery of the culture. In the presence of hyperlipemic serum this might take place at an increased rate, with migrating cells apparently able to form new colonies more readily than in media supplemented with normolipemic serum.

Not only the size but also the morphology of the cultures in hyperlipemic serum show much more variation than their controls in normal serum. When the cells are grown in hyperlipemic serum from the beginning, the cultures tend to form multilayers more rapidly and frequently. However, these cultures reveal areas with apparently healthy cells right next to areas of incipient cell degeneration at a relatively early stage. Staining for collagen or elastin is often less positive than in comparable cultures grown in normal serum. The reason that there is less extracellular material made by the culture in hyperlipemic serum is not that there are less cells to produce it. In fact, these cultures regularly exhibit more cells per field than comparable cultures in normal serum (6).

All these findings indicate that cultures grown in hyperlipemic serum from the time of explanting tend to grow faster. However, just as in the early human plaque, there are signs of simultaneous cell degeneration at a relatively early stage, resulting in a wide variation in morphology and culture size.

On the other hand, cultures media-supplemented with 10% normal serum show a reproducible growth pattern, with a prolonged stationary phase during which they can be stimulated to enter another phase of proliferation, thus making them an ideal model for studying the effects of a given atherogenic stimulus.

Acknowledgements: This research was made possible by USPHS HL15062 (SCOR).

REFERENCES

1. Fischer-Dzoga, K., Jones, R.M., Vesselinovitch, D. and Wissler, R.W.: Ultrastructural and immunohistochemical studies of primary cultures of aortic medial cells. Exp. Mol. Path. 18: 102, 1973.

2. Jarmolych, J., Daoud, A.S., Landau, J., Fritz, K.E. and McElvene, E.: Aortic medial explants: Cell proliferation and production of mucopolysaccharides, collagen and elastic tissue. Exp. Mol. Path. 9:171, 1968.

3. Fischer-Dzoga, K., Chen, R. and Wissler, R.W.: Effects of serum lipoproteins on the morphology, growth and metabolism of arterial smooth muscle cells. In: Arterial Mesenchyme and Arteriosclerosis, p. 299. Wagner, W.D. and Clarkson, T.B., eds. Plenum, New York, 1974.

4. Fischer-Dzoga, K., Jones, R.M., Vesselinovitch, D. and Wissler, R.W.: Increased mitotic activity in primary cultures of aortic medial smooth muscle cells after exposure to hyperlipemic serum. In: Atherosclerosis III, Proceedings of the Third International Symposium, p. 193. Schettler, G. and Weizel, A., eds. Springer-Verlag, Berlin, 1974.

5. Dzoga, K., Wissler, R.W. and Vesselinovitch, D.: The effect of normal and hyperlipemic low density lipoprotein fractions on aortic tissue culture cells. Circ. 44 (Suppl. II):6, 1971.

6. Ledet, T., Fischer-Dzoga, K. and Wissler, R.W.: Diabetic macroangiopathy: In vitro study of the proliferation of the aortic smooth muscle cells. Am. J. Path. 74:50a, 1974.

(4)

THE ARTERIAL SMOOTH MUSCLE CELL: STIMULATION OF CHOLESTEROL ESTERIFICATION BY PLASMA LIPOPROTEINS

Richard W. St. Clair, Ph.D.

Department of Pathology and The Arteriosclerosis Research Center
Bowman Gray School of Medicine
Winston-Salem, North Carolina, U.S.A.

A major feature of atherosclerosis is the accumulation of lipid within the arterial wall. Most pronounced is the increase in the cholesterol concentration with the greatest increment occurring in the concentration of cholesteryl esters, first recognized by Windaus in 1910 (1).

In early fatty streak lesions most of the cholesteryl esters are found within fat-filled cells ("foam cells"). The cholesteryl esters within these "foam cells" are different in composition, however, from those of the plasma cholesteryl esters, in that there is a considerable enrichment in oleic acid at the expense of linoleic acid (2). This observation is consistent with results from several studies indicating a stimulation in cholesterol esterification in "foam cells", with cholesteryl oleate being the major cholesteryl ester synthesized (3).

A stimulation of cholesterol esterification occurs quite early in the development of atherosclerosis. Such a stimulation has been demonstrated in pigeons after only 14 days of cholesterol feeding (4) and in rabbits after three days of cholesterol feeding (5). In both cases this metabolic change occurred prior to the appearance of grossly visible atherosclerotic lesions. A stimulation of cholesterol esterification can also be demonstrated *in vitro* after one day of exposure of normal segments of pigeon aorta to hypercholesterolemic serum in organ culture (6). These studies suggested that cholesterol esterification in smooth muscle cells of the arterial wall was capable of being stimulated by some component or components of the serum. In order to study this more fully we conducted the following studies using arterial smooth muscle cells grown in culture.

For these studies smooth muscle cells from explants of the aortic media from rhesus monkeys were grown in culture using essentially the procedure of Bierman, et al. The culture medium consisted of Eagles' Minimum Essential Medium supplemented with twice the normal concentration of vitamins, 2 mM L-glutamine, 100 units penicillin/ml, 100 µg streptomycin/ml and 10% fetal calf serum. For experiments cells were grown to approximately 90% confluency in 100 mm tissue culture dishes and culture medium containing 5 mg/ml of lipid deficient serum (LDS) (8) was added. After 24 hours, 5 ml of culture medium containing LDS, the lipoprotein to be tested, and cholesterol-1,2-^{3}H or oleic acid-1-^{14}C as substrate, was added for periods up to 48 hours. Following incubation cells were washed with balanced salt solution, removed from the dishes by trypsinization, and lipids extracted, separated, and quantified, as described previously (6).

As shown in Figure 1, incubation of smooth muscle cells for up to 48 hours with hypercholesterolemic rhesus monkey serum results in only a slight increase in the concentration of unesterified cholesterol within the cells but greater than a 5-fold increase in the cellular cholesteryl ester content. Associated with the increased

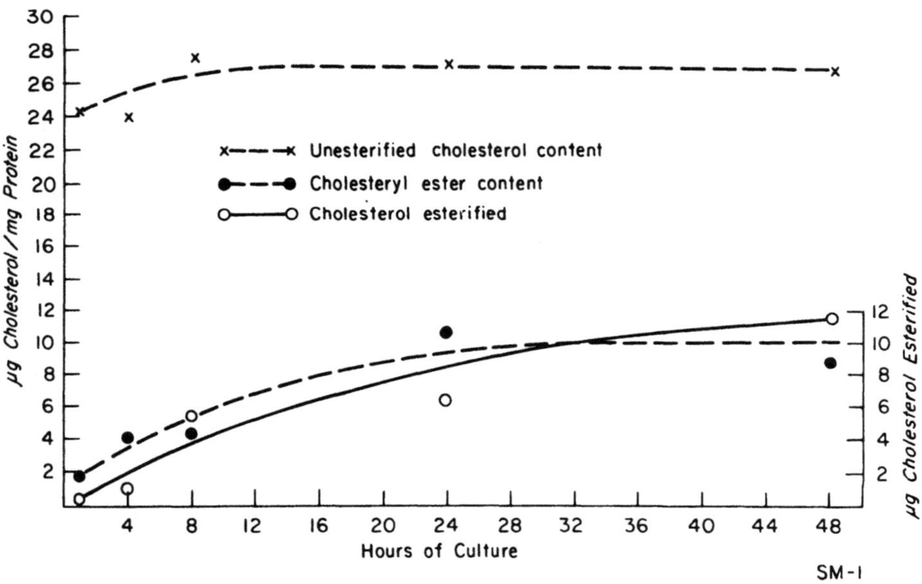

Fig. 1. Influence of hypercholesterolemic rhesus monkey serum on cholesterol esterification in rhesus monkey aortic smooth muscle cells. Smooth muscle cells from the 6th cell generation were cultured for up to 48 hours in culture medium containing cholesterol-1,2-^{3}H and 10% hypercholesterolemic rhesus monkey serum (9.4 mg cholesterol/ml). Results are the mean of duplicate cultures.

content of cholesteryl esters was a greater than 20-fold stimulation in cholesterol esterification. The time course of the stimulation in cholesteryl ester accumulation and cholesterol esterification were similar, reaching a maximum after about 24 hours of culture. For these studies cholesterol-1,2-^{3}H was added as substrate complexed to LDS. Cholesterol esterification was calculated using the specific activity of the unesterified cholesterol actually isolated from the cells.

In order to determine whether this effect was due to lipoproteins in the serum we isolated low (LDL) and high (HDL) density lipoproteins (9) from cholesterol-fed rhesus monkeys having plasma cholesterol concentrations ranging from 500 to 900 mg/dl. The isolated lipoproteins were dialyzed against several changes of culture medium prior to addition to cells in culture.

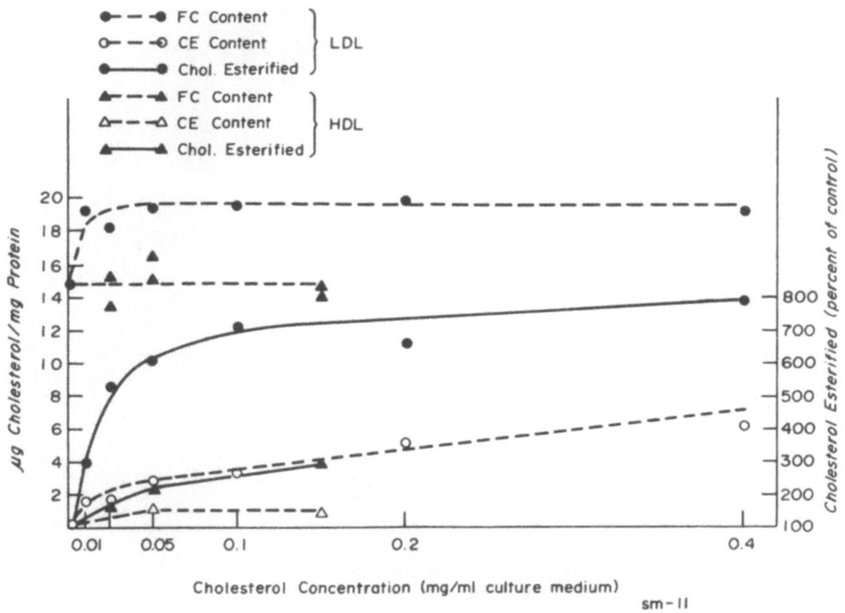

Fig. 2. Influence of rhesus monkey LDL and HDL on the accumulation and esterification of cholesterol in rhesus monkey aortic smooth muscle cells. Smooth muscle cells from the 18th cell generation were cultured for 24 hours with medium containing LDS then for an additional 24 hours with medium containing LDS + HDL or LDL. Cholesterol-1,2-^{3}H was added complexed to LDS and controls represent cells cultured without added lipoprotein.

Results of the influence of LDL and HDL on cholesterol content and cholesterol esterification are shown in Figure 2. Low density lipoprotein stimulated cholesterol esterification at even the lowest concentration used and reached a maximum stimulation at approximately 0.1 mg LDL cholesterol per ml culture medium. There was an associated small but consistent increase in the free cholesterol concentration of the cells that did not change with addition of increasing amounts of LDL. The cholesteryl ester content of the cells increased progressively as the amount of LDL was increased, at least to 0.4 mg LDL cholesterol per ml culture medium.

Similar concentrations of HDL cholesterol had little if any influence on the concentration of free and esterified cholesterol within the smooth muscle cells. Likewise, there was only a slight stimulation of cholesterol esterification with HDL. These results are similar to those recently published by Goldstein and Brown (10) using aortic smooth muscle cells obtained from a six-month-old human fetus.

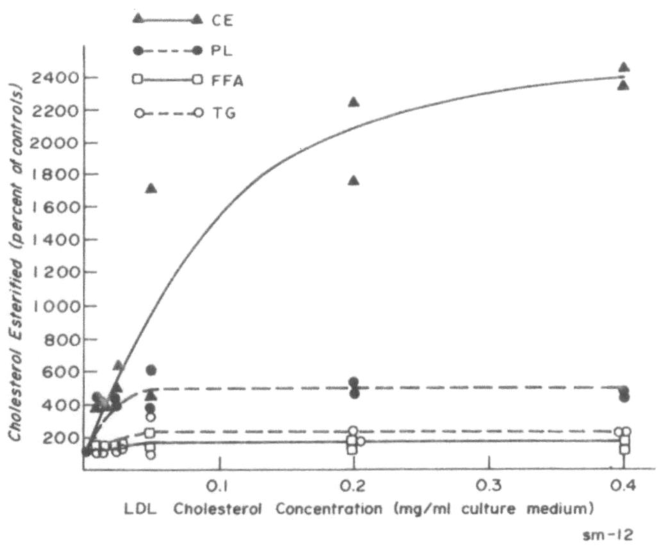

Fig. 3. Influence of rhesus monkey LDL on esterification of oleic acid-1-^{14}C in rhesus monkey aortic smooth muscle cells. Smooth muscle cells from the 18th cell generation were cultured for 24 hours with medium containing LDS, then for an additional 24 hours with medium containing LDS + LDL and oleic acid-1-^{14}C complexed to albumin.

It is also possible to show a stimulation of cholesterol esterification using oleic acid-1-^{14}C as substrate (Figure 3). In smooth muscle cells in culture, as was true for hypercholesterolemic whole serum in organ cultures of arterial tissue (6), LDL promotes a preferential stimulation of esterification of fatty acids to cholesterol compared with incorporation into other complex lipids.

Consequently, the stimulation of cholesterol esterification in arterial smooth muscle cells is similar to that which occurs in organ cultures of pigeon aorta exposed to whole serum (6) or isolated lipoprotein (Figure 4). Thus, the response of smooth muscle cells in culture to lipoproteins does not appear to be an abnormal reaction of the cultured cells but rather a reaction that occurs even in the smooth muscle cells contained within the arterial wall.

The stimulation of cholesterol esterification in arterial smooth muscle cells from rhesus monkey aorta by LDL appears to be similar to that described by Goldstein, et al. (11) for skin fibroblasts from human beings. This, coupled with the observation that LDL inhibits cholesterol synthesis in arterial smooth muscle cells (12),

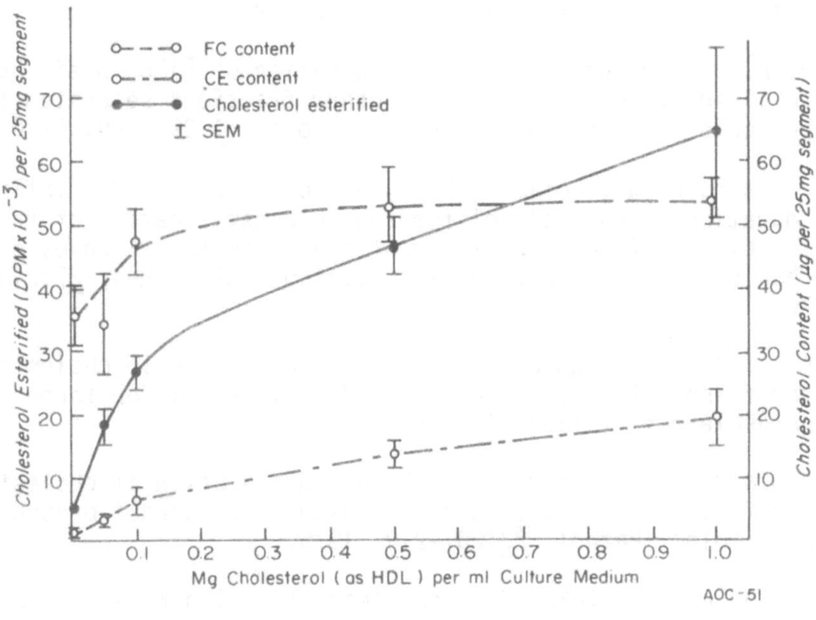

Fig. 4. Influence of pigeon HDL on the accumulation and esterification of cholesterol in organ cultures of White Carneau pigeon aorta. Arterial segments were maintained in organ culture for 96 hours with medium containing cholesterol-1,2-^{3}H complexed to LDS + pigeon HDL. Each point represents the mean and SEM of four cultures.

much as it does in skin fibroblasts, suggests that regulation of cholesterol synthesis and esterification in arterial smooth muscle cells may be controlled by LDL concentrations within the arterial wall. Thus, the reaction of the arterial smooth muscle cells to lipoproteins traversing the vascular endothelium may be critical to the initiation of atherosclerosis. Genetic and environmental factors may act to modify this response either at the level of the arterial smooth muscle cell or by subtle alterations in the composition of structure of the circulating lipoproteins.

References

1. Windaus, A. Über den gehalt normaler und atheromatoser aorten an cholesterin und cholesterinestern. Ztschr. F. Physiol. Chem. 67:174-176, 1910.

2. Smith, E. B., Evans, P. H., Downham, M. D. Lipid in the aortic intima. The correlation of morphological and chemical characteristics. J. Athero. Res. 7:171-186, 1967.

3. Day, A. J. and Tume, R. K. Incorporation of [^{14}C] oleic acid into lipid by foam cells and by other fractions separated from atherosclerotic lesions. Atherosclerosis 11:291-299, 1970.

4. St. Clair, R. W., Lofland, H. B, and Clarkson, T. B. Influence of duration of cholesterol feeding on esterification of fatty acids by cell-free preparation of pigeon aorta. Studies on the mechanism of cholesterol esterification. Circ. Res. 27:213-225, 1970.

5. Day, A. J. and Proudlock, J. W. Changes in aortic cholesterol-esterifying activity in rabbits fed cholesterol for three days. Atherosclerosis 19:253-258, 1974.

6. St. Clair, R. W. and Harpold, G. J. Stimulation of cholesterol esterification *in vitro* in organ cultures of normal pigeon aorta. Exptl. Molec. Pathol. 22:207-219, 1975.

7. Bierman, E. L., Stein, O., and Stein, Y. Lipoprotein uptake and metabolism by rat aortic smooth muscle cells in tissue culture. Circ. Res. 35:136-150, 1974.

8. Brown, M. S., Dana, S. E., and Goldstein, J. L. Regulation of 3-hydroxy-3-methylglutaryl Coenzyme A reductase activity in cultured human fibroblasts. J. Biol. Chem. 249:789-796, 1974.

9. Rudel, L. L., Lee, J. A., Morris, M. D., and Felts, J. M. Characterization of plasma lipoproteins separated and purified by agarose-column chromatography. Biochem. J. 139:89-95, 1974.

10. Goldstein, J. L. and Brown, M. S. Lipoprotein receptors, cholesterol metabolism, and atherosclerosis. Arch. Pathol. 99:181-184, 1975.

11. Goldstein, J. L., Dana, S. E., and Brown, M. S. Esterification of low density lipoprotein cholesterol in human fibroblasts and its absence in homozygous familial hypercholesterolemia. Proc. Natl. Acad. Sci. 71:4288-4292, 1974.

12. Mahley, R. W., Assmann, G., Brown, G., Brewer, H. B., and Weisgraber, K. H. Swine plasma lipoproteins and their effects on cholesterol synthesis in aortic smooth muscle cells in tissue culture. Circulation 49&50:III-70, 1974.

(5)

PRODUCTION OF GLYCOSAMINOGLYCANS, COLLAGEN AND ELASTIC TISSUE BY AORTIC MEDIAL EXPLANTS

A.S. Daoud, K.E. Fritz, J. Jarmolych, J. Augustyn and T.P. Mawhinney
V.A. Hospital and Albany Medical Center Hospital

Albany, New York, U.S.A.

Collagen, glycosaminoglycans and elastic tissue are the principle extracellular substances of the early atherosclerotic plaque. It is well established by *in vivo*[1-7] and *in vitro*[8-10] studies that these elements can be synthesized and secreted by arterial smooth muscle cells (SMC). In this laboratory we have devised and characterized an *in vitro* system which, under our standard culture conditions, develops a peripheral growth having many features resembling those found in the early atherosclerotic plaque.[11] Both cell proliferation and cell death, which are two important components of atherosclerotic lesions, are observed early in the culture period and continue throughout the life of the explants. The cells in the peripheral growth are SMC and are indistinguishable from those described in early atherosclerotic lesions. The cells secrete collagen, elastic tissue and glycosaminoglycans.

Explants cultured in chemically defined medium (M199) alone show less necrosis, and are less actively synthesizing DNA and protein than those grown in the presence of any whole or dialyzed serum. Such M199 only cultures never develop a peripheral growth although they remain viable and lose none of their potential for synthetic activity.[12] However, the presence of 20% whole serum in the medium results in the initiation, at about 4 days, of a peripheral growth which increases until the termination of cultures maintained up to 21 days. The amount of peripheral growth occurring in explants from the same aorta varies from serum to serum. The same serum used on explants from different aortas also results in different amounts of peripheral growth which suggests an interaction between some tissue component and the serum in the medium.

Histochemical staining for glycosaminoglycans, collagen and elastic tissue shows that glycosaminoglycans are present in the peripheral growth at the end of the first week, while collagen and elastic tissue are demonstrated only after 14 days and in some instances become abundant by 21 days. Electron microscopic studies of the peripheral growth show the typical electron opaque granules and thin fibrils characteristic of mucopolysaccharides as early as 7 days and continuing thereafter. From this early stage on, the extra-cellular space also contains amorphous osmiophilic material and microfilaments varying in size from 5 to 10 mμ. The amorphous material, similar in appearance to basement membrane, sometimes is mixed with a few microfilaments. The microfibrils resemble those described by Ross[9] and by Haust[1] as elastic microfibrils and by Goldberg and Green[13] as collagen fibrils. In addition to the microfibrils, fibers showing the periodicity typical of collagen fibers, singly or in groups, are demonstrable at 14 days and both are abundant at 21 days. Electron microscopy at 14 and 21 days also shows a roughly circular structure composed of a homogeneous clear or slightly electron dense center surrounded by an electron dense border, the structures referred by Haust et al as elastic units. The homogeneous centers, according to Haust, are composed of elastic matrix and the periphery consists of elastic filaments. The size of the unit varies from 40 to 300 mμ and the filaments average 10 mμ in thickness. The elastic units are sometimes found singly but generally form aggregates and sometimes fuse with adjacent elastic fibers. When the units are cut longitudinally, they are found to consist of a clear center and an electron opaque periphery composed of thin fibrils.

Quantitative studies of collagen and glycosaminoglycan synthesis as related to total protein and DNA synthesis were carried out in explants grown for 9 days in the presence of human sera. The sera were derived from patients admitted to the hospital for cardiac catheterization and/or coronary angiography. For collagen synthesis 4 experiments using a total of 58 different sera and tissue from 4 aortas were performed. For synthesis of glycosaminoglycans, one single experiment using 18 different sera was carried out.

In the collagen studies ^{3}H-thymidine was added to the cultures 2 hours before termination and ^{14}C-proline added 48, 24 or 2 hours before termination. The longer periods of ^{14}C-proline inclusion in the medium resulted in higher levels of incorporation, but all experiments gave essentially the same results. At termination the cultures were exposed to ice-cold non-radioactive medium, washed in 0.9% NaCl and 5% trichloroacetic acid (TCA), lyophilized, homogenized in TCA and lipid-extracted. Aliquots of the delipidized tissue were used for determination of specific activity of DNA and for determination of the radioactivity of both proline and hydroxyproline.[14]

As a measure of collagen synthesis we use the dpm hydroxyproline/µg DNA, while the dpm proline/µg DNA indicate total protein synthesis.

For glycosaminoglycan studies $^{35}S-SO_4$, 5 µc/ml, was added 24 hours before termination of culture with ^{3}H-thymidine for the last 2 hours. Following exposure to non-radioactive substrate and 0.9% NaCl washes, the tissue was lyophilized, papain-digested 24 hours and precipitated with TCA. The precipitate was used for determination of DNA specific activity while the supernatant was used for determination of uronic acid[15] and hexosamine[16] and of ^{35}S radioactivity incorporated into glycosaminoglycans. The dpm $^{35}S-SO_4$ incorporated, expressed per µg DNA, is considered the measure of glycosaminoglycan synthesis.

Within experiments the human sera varied as much as three fold in their capacity to stimulate not only DNA synthesis but also collagen and total protein synthesis. Figures 1 and 2 are plots of the data of a representative experiment in which 18 sera were each tested in triplicate. Figure 1 is a plot of the ^{3}H-thymidine incorporation against the ^{14}C-hydroxyproline incorporation for each culture while Figure 2 is a plot of the ^{14}C-hydroxyproline against the ^{14}C-proline incorporation. Regression analysis shows a high degree of positive correlation between collagen synthesis and synthesis of both DNA ($r=0.77$) and total protein ($r=0.94$), each significant at $p < 0.0005$.

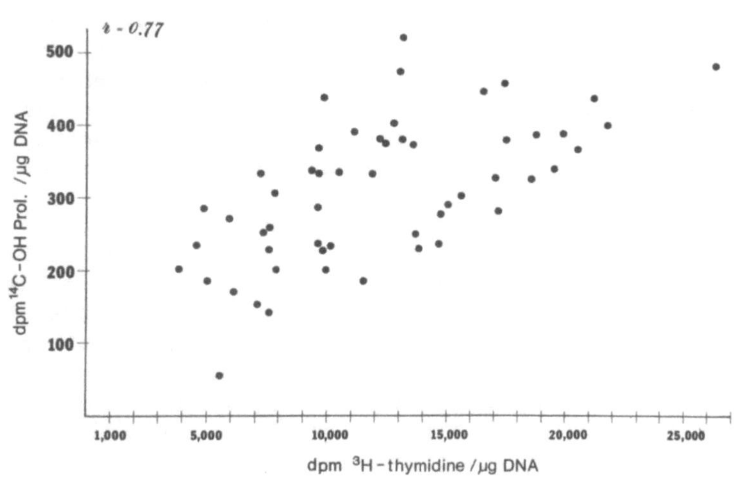

Figure 1

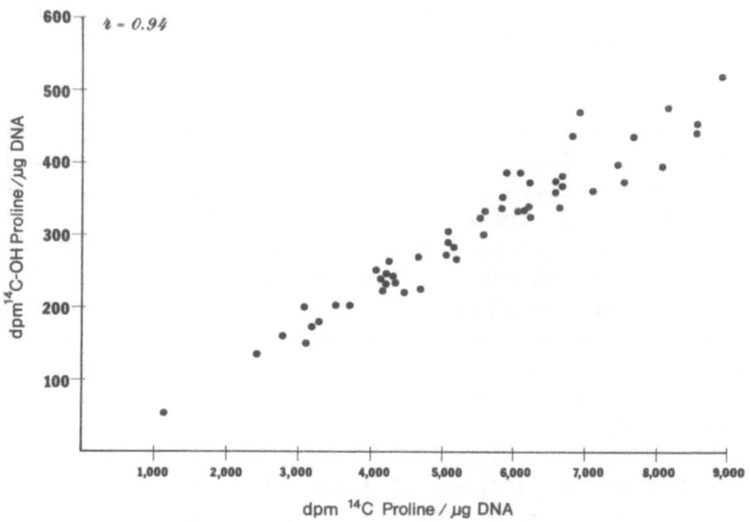

Figure 2

The synthesis of glycosaminoglycans, as illustrated in Figure 3, which is a plot of $^{35}S-SO_4$ incorporation against ^3H-thymidine incorporation, is significantly and positively correlated with DNA synthesis (r=0.79) ($p < 0.005$). There is no significant correlation, however, between either total DNA or DNA synthesis and uronic acid

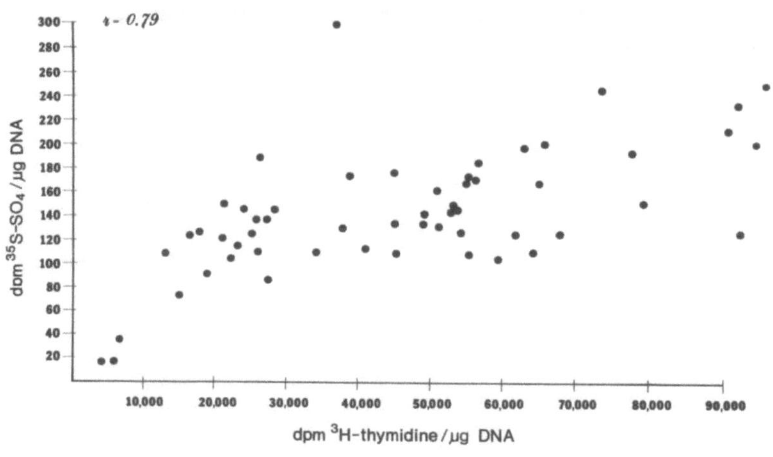

Figure 3

content, hexosamine content or total glycosaminoglycan content, as represented by the sum of uronic acid and hexosamine, except for a negative correlation between total DNA and hexosamine content ($p < 0.025$).

In summary, an explant system consisting of segments of swine aortic medial tissue cultured in semi-synthetic medium containing human or swine sera develops a new peripheral growth having many of the characteristics of the early atherosclerotic plaques. The cells in the peripheral growth are capable of secreting glycosaminoglycans, collagen and elastic tissue. Quantitative studies of collagen and glycosaminoglycan synthesis on the ninth day of culture in the presence of the human sera showed a positive correlation between the synthesis of these substances and of DNA. A positive correlation between collagen and total protein synthesis was also demonstrated.

These results are suggestive of either a coupling of synthetic processes, DNA, total protein, collagen and glycosaminoglycan, all of which react to a single stimulant, or, alternatively, that several synthesis-stimulators are present in relatively constant proportions. Support for the concept of correlation of DNA, total protein and collagen synthesis has been presented by Davies _et al_[17] who found that in synchronized diploid rat cells both collagen and total protein synthesis continued through S phase with their peak slightly after the peak DNA synthesis and, further, that collagen synthesis fluctuates with total protein synthesis. Similarly, parallel glycosaminoglycan and DNA synthesis has been demonstrated.[18] Also, a factor derived from rat liver cells has both DNA synthesis and sulfate incorporation stimulating capacity (Dulak).[19] The explant system is proving useful both in discriminating among human sera and in bringing out relationships among fundamentally important synthetic processes.

REFERENCES

1. Haust, M. D., More, R. H., Bencosme, S. A., and Balis, J. U. (1965). Exp. Mol. Pathol. 4, 508.

2. Haust, M. D., More, R. H., and Movat, H. Z. (1960). Amer. J. Pathol. 37, 377.

3. Parker, F., and Odland, G. F. (1966). Amer. J. Pathol. 48, 451.

4. Imai, H., Lee, K. T., Pastori, S., Panlilio, E., Florentin, R., and Thomas, W. A. (1966). Exp. Mol. Pathol. 5, 273.

5. Wissler, R. W. (1968). J. Atheroscler. Res. 8, 201.

6. Karrer, H. E. (1960). J. Ultrastruct. Res. 4, 420.

7. Paule, W. J. (1963). J. Ultrastruct. Res. 8, 219.

8. Daoud, A. S., Fritz, K. E., Singh, J., Augustyn, J. M. and Jarmolych, J. (1974). Arter. Mesenchyme Arterioscler. 43, 281.

9. Ross, R. (1971). J. Cell Biol. 50, 1972.

10. Wissler, R. W. (1973). Hospit. Pract. 8, 61.

11. Jarmolych, J., Daoud, A. S., Landau, J., Fritz, K. E., and McElvene, E. (1968). Exp. Mol. Pathol. 9, 171.

12. Daoud, A. S., Fritz, K. E., and Jarmolych, J. (1970). Exp. Mol. Pathol. 12, 354.

13. Goldberg, B., and Green, H. (1964). J. Cell Biol. 22, 227.

14. Rojkind, M., and Gonzales, E. (1974). Anal. Biochem. 57, 1.

15. Wardi, A. H., Allen, W. S., and Varma, R. A. (1974). Anal. Biochem. 57, 268.

16. Antonopoulos, C. A., Gardell, S., Szirmai, J. A., and DeTyssonsk, E. R. (1964). Biochim. Biophys. Acta. 83, 1.

17. Davies, L. M., Priest, J. H., and Priest, R. E. (1968). Science. 159, 91.

18. Delaunay, A., and Bazin, S. (1964). Int. Rev. Connect. Tissue Res. 2, 301.

19. Dulak, N. D., and Temin, H. M. (1973). J. Cell Phys. 81, 153.

(6)

SUMMARY (TISSUE CULTURE II)

Abel Lazzarini Robertson, Jr., M.D., Ph.D.

Case Western Reserve University
School of Medicine
Cleveland, Ohio, U.S.A.

For those of us who have been interested for some time in applying arterial cell, tissue and organ culture technique to the study of atherogenesis (1), it has been most rewarding to note recently a significant increase in the number of investigators using these methods and in the amount of data being generated under a variety of experimental conditions.

While direct extrapolation of such information to the behavior of vascular cells in the living animal cannot be made without carefully considering some of the obvious limitations of an in vitro system, the latter allows an almost infinite number of laboratory models - difficult or impossible to carry out in vivo - for the study of specific metabolic and functional characteristics of the vessel wall.

It is only fitting that in this International Workshop, organized by our Canadian colleagues, well deserved emphasis has been placed on the behavior of vascular smooth muscle cells since Haust and More (2) and Haust, et al. (3) were one of the first groups of investigators in recent times to stress the key role of this cell type in atherogenesis.

This session on Tissue Culture studies has provided further evidence of the interaction of specific lipoproteins or their apoproteins and lipid constituents with smooth muscle cells from several animal species.

Dr. Olga Stein described studies on the mechanisms of uptake, esterification and hydrolysis of lipoproteins by rat aortic medial cells. They emphasized, by trypsin treatment, the differences between cell surface binding of the lipoproteins and their intracellular uptake. The results obtained resembled those previously reported with human arterial cells showing differences in uptake rates between lipid and apoprotein moieties (4) and underscore the regulatory role of cell surface coats on the intracellular incorporation of lipoproteins. Dr. Stein also stressed the role of cell number and density in such cultures since they showed a reverse relationship with lipoprotein uptake. While her interesting results emphasized species differences in total lipoprotein uptake between rat and human cells, the highest rates were obtained in both instances with low density lipoprotein fractions.

The studies reported by Dr. Robert W. Mahley relate to the effects of lipoproteins on cultured smooth muscle cells and fibroblasts using cholesterol-fed miniature swine as laboratory models. This investigator had previously reported the appearance of an unusual lipoprotein fraction (HDL_c) in cholesterol-fed dogs and has now identified it in pigs. While this fraction has a particle size and cholesterol content similar to that of homologous LDL, it lacks the B apoprotein. Using cultures of swine thoracic aorta, Dr. Mahley noted that this HDL_c fraction had little influence on smooth muscle cell proliferation in contrast to the characteristic growth promoting effects of LDL. This finding suggests that this action of LDL in hypercholesterolemic pigs is related to its apoprotein composition and is in agreement with the mitogenic properties found for human LDL from Type II homozygous donors (5). He also showed competitive binding and uptake of HDL_c and LDL at cell level with both fractions exerting similar regulatory effects on HMG-CoA reductase activity in vascular smooth muscle cells and in skin fibroblasts. As in Dr. Stein's studies, in the presence of dietary hyperlipemia, apoprotein composition and lipoprotein particle size seem to be major factors in regulating intracellular uptake and rate of cholesterol synthesis.

Dr. K. Fisher-Dzoga provided new information on the influence of hyperlipemic sera on the growth rates of primary explants of isolated aortic media. The results reported emphasized proliferative stimulation and striking variations in morphology and size of cultures after incubation in media containing hyperlipemic serum not observed in control preparations. Qualitative reduction in the synthesis of extracellular material by smooth muscle cells and accelerated cell degeneration were also noted, particularly with a lipoprotein fraction identified as LDL_2. It corresponds to a density gradient of 1.019-1.063 and is only found in hyperlipemic sera.

The studies reported by Dr. R. W. St. Clair summarized interesting observations on the incorporation of free and esterified cholesterol by aortic smooth muscle cells obtained from rhesus monkeys.

The data showed that while a limited increase in free-cholesterol was found, a five fold rise in intracellular cholesterol ester would occur in the presence of hyperlipemic serum simultaneously with significant stimulation in cholesterol esterification. Again, the LDL fraction from cholesterol-fed animals was by far the most effective agent to induce these metabolic changes while HDL had little or no effect. The findings are in agreement with previous studies by the same investigator utilizing organ cultures of pigeon aorta exposed to either hyperlipemic sera or its isolated lipoproteins. They are also similar to results obtained by others with human aortic and skin cells and strongly suggest that the intracellular regulation of cholesterol esterification and synthesis by LDL may be rather general phenomena to be found in various cell types of several animal species.

Finally, Dr. A. S. Daoud reviewed studies on the synthesis and secretion of collagen, glycosaminoglycans and elastin by swine aorta in culture. They noted that the growth response of such explants varied from donor to donor and with the type of sera used. The investigators observed stimulation of glycosaminoglycan synthesis within one week after implantation, followed by that of collagen and elastin in two-three weeks. While most of the extracellular material appears amorphous at first, microfibrils may be identified as the culture becomes older. Utilizing sera obtained from patients undergoing cardiac studies, they noted significant differences between individual donors in their ability to stimulate swine aortic cells to increase DNA synthesis as well as collagen and protein production.

These reports are encouraging for they show that in spite of the limitations of methodology currently available, common denominators of specific cell functions may be found that transcend species, tissue and cell individualities. It is our hope that more extensive application of recent advances in tissue and cell culture techniques, such as the routine use of clonal selection and karyotyping to identify homogeneous populations of diploid cells after short-term cultivation, may significantly broaden the use of tissue and cell culture methods in atherosclerosis research. It seems reasonable to expect that they should provide timely and productive data to further our understanding of the complex cellular changes accompanying the multifaceted pathological process we call atherogenesis.

BIBLIOGRAPHY

1) Robertson, A.L., Jr.: Functional characterization of arterial cells involved in spontaneous atheroma. In: Schettler, G. and Weizel, A. (eds.), Atherosclerosis III, pp. 175-184. Berlin, Heidelberg, New York: Springer-Verlag, 1974.

2) Haust, M.D. and More, R.H.: Significance of the smooth muscle cell in atherogenesis. In: Jones, R.J. (ed.), Evolution of the Atherosclerotic Plaque, pp. 51-63. Chicago, London: The University of Chicago Press, 1963.

3) Haust, M.D., More, R.H., Bencosme, S.A. and Balis, J.U.: Electron microscopic studies in human atherosclerosis. Extracellular elements in aortic dots and streaks. Exp. Mol. Pathol. 6: 300-313, 1967.

4) Robertson, A.L., Jr.: Transport of plasma lipoproteins and ultrastructure of human arterial intimacytes in culture. In: Rothblat, G.H. and Kritchevsky, D. (eds.), Lipid Metabolism in Tissue Culture Cells: Wistar Inst. Symp. Monogr. 6: 115-128. The Wistar Inst. Press, 1967.

5) Robertson, A.L., Jr.: The artery and process of arteriosclerosis. Pathogenesis. In: Wolf, S. (ed.), Advances in Experimental Medicine and Biology, Vol. 16A, pp. 24-25, 104-107, and 229-239. New York, London: Plenum Press, 1971.

(7)

DISCUSSION (TISSUE CULTURE II)

DISCUSSION AFTER DR. STEIN'S PAPER

Dr. Wissler (U.S.A.) asked if Dr. Stein had information regarding possible cell export or egression of partially degraded lipoproteins. He referred to previous studies by Drs. Bierman, Stein and Stein that had suggested mobilization of altered lipoproteins out of cells. Dr. Stein answered that further information on this subject is not available.

Dr. Rothblat (U.S.A.) then asked if crossover studies have been carried out to investigate whether specificity for intracellular uptake rests with the cell types or lipoprotein fractions used. Dr. Stein answered that specificity relates to both. Human LDL for example is not incorporated by either human or rat cells. Rat HDL interaction with human cells has not been tested due to technical problems involved in obtaining them in adequate volumes.

Dr. Trowell (U.S.A.) requested information regarding the effects of cell size on lipoprotein uptake. Dr. Stein answered that a confluent culture has higher density and thus more surface area than a nonconfluent one and that lipoprotein uptake was found to be proportional to total cell surface.

DISCUSSION AFTER DR. MAHLEY'S PAPER

Since inhibition of HMG-CoA-reductase turns on cholesterol esterification, Dr. Mahley was asked if the same holds true for HDL_c. He answered that cholesterol esterification measured by incorporation of ^{14}C oleate is different for HDL_c than for LDL. In the former, a lag of 5-7 hours occurs.

He was then asked what concentrations of LDL and HDL fractions were used to stimulate growth. Dr. Mahley answered that the studies were done using concentrations in culture media corresponding to 10 micrograms of lipoprotein cholesterol. He emphasized the fact that serum factors other than lipoproteins may stimulate cell growth. This has been demonstrated by other investigators.

Dr. Paoletti (Italy) asked if any phospholipid differences were identified between HDL_2 and HDL_c to which Dr. Mahley replied that such studies have not yet been carried out.

DISCUSSION AFTER DR. FISHER-DZOGA'S PAPER

Dr. Kramsch (U.S.A.) briefly reviewed his studies on the formation of elastin by arterial cells in culture with appearance of sheets of elastin on monolayer cultures.

Dr. Björkerud (Sweden) then asked if cell heterogeneity was found in cultured cells that would suggest a nonhomogeneous smooth muscle population in the arterial wall or species differences that could be interpreted as genotypic variations of such cells. Dr. Fisher-Dzoga answered that, in their studies, clear-cut evidence of heterogeneity in smooth muscle cell cultures had yet to be found.

DISCUSSION AFTER DR. ST. CLAIR'S PAPER

Dr. Wissler (U.S.A.) asked if the pigeon HDL fractions used in the study were obtained from hyperlipemic animals. Dr. St. Clair answered that this was indeed the case.

Dr. Robert (France) then commented on differences between smooth muscle cells in culture and aortic cells *in vivo* which may be considered age-dependent using glycosaminoglycan synthesis as an example. Dr. St. Clair agreed with the need to carry out systematic studies to identify this important question.

Dr. Y. Stein (Israel) mentioned that in their studies, the rate of cholesterol esterification does not continue to be exponential after incubation. Similar results were also obtained by Dr. Chang (U.S.A.) working in Dr. Wissler's laboratory. Questions were then raised regarding the meaning of these phenomena and the suggestion was made that they could be an expression of temporary saturation of cell esterification sites. Dr. Björkerud then mentioned that he had found considerable esterification capacity in non-reendothelialized arterial lesions which also - in contrast to normal aortic tissue - showed a high rate of glucose uptake into sphyngomyelin.

Enhancement in the rate of cholesterol esterification relative to glyceride and phosphatide synthesis as well as sites of intracellular localization of cholesterol esters were also discussed. Dr. St. Clair mentioned that a weak relationship seems to exist between rates of glyceride synthesis and cholesterol esterification. In their studies there was approximately a 1:5 ratio. He revealed also that their studies have failed to provide good morphological evidence of the location of cholesterol ester accumulation in cells, but some of it seems to be present in membrane-bound vesicles.

DISCUSSION FOLLOWING DR. DAOUD'S PAPER

Comments were made regarding initiation of synthesis of glycosaminoglycans before collagen and other extracellular constituents. Dr. Daoud said that their morphological studies suggested early production of mucopolysaccharides preceding formation of recognizable collagen or elastin microfibrils. Histochemically, glycosaminoglycans appear around the seventh day in culture while collagen and elastin take longer.

Dr. Wissler (U.S.A.) questioned the nature of the increase in DNA synthesis observed by the authors. Dr. Daoud's answer indicated that tissue explants from the same artery responded with varied growth rates to different sera.

Dr. St. Clair (U.S.A.) then asked if the reported results on collagen synthesis expressed either by per/mg cell protein, as total cell number or as cell DNA varied with serum cholesterol concentrations in the sera used. Dr. Daoud responded that such comparisons had not been carried out in studies with human sera but that in previous experiments with hyperlipemic swine sera there was some correlation between severity of hyperlipemia and growth rate response of arterial cells in culture.

Dr. Robert (France) emphasized the importance of the donor's age in the expected arterial response to synthetic rates *in vitro*. Dr. Daoud concurred and added that in their studies with swine aortic cell cultures, all animals weighed about 150 lbs. and were approximately 6 months old at the time of slaughter.

GENERAL DISCUSSION

Dr. Wissler (U.S.A.) emphasized the importance of recognizing that variations in results obtained by different investigators may be related to the cell culture techniques employed, ranging from the behavior of cells after enzymatic cell isolation and subculture to attached or floating arterial explants. He stressed further that such methodological differences must be kept in mind when evaluating the morphology and function of arterial cells *in vitro*.

Dr. Robertson (U.S.A.) concurred with these comments and pointed out physical differences, depending on culture methods used, for the availability of lipoprotein receptor sites on the arterial cell surface. As an example, he cited the advantages of monolayer cell preparations over multilayered cultures and primary explants for quantitative studies on lipoprotein uptake.

Comments were requested from the audience regarding comparative rates of uptake of free and esterified cholesterol by arterial cells. Dr. St. Clair (U.S.A.) pointed out that his laboratory has not yet been able to answer that important question by use of either organ or cell culture systems. Free and ester cholesterol specific activities in cells were found to be different due to dilution of the ester fractions; the metabolic significance of cholesterol esterification vs. accumulation has not been determined.

Dr. Rothblat (U.S.A.) mentioned that in their studies with hepatoma cell lines - which are known to accumulate large amounts of cholesterol ester compared with arterial cells - 40% of endogenous or extracellular cholesterol accumulates as ester in lipid inclusions whereas the remaining 60% derives from esterified cholesterol outside the cell. He also emphasized variations in the response of different cell strains to severity of hyperlipemia.

As one mechanism for accumulating cholesterol, Dr. St. Clair referred to increased free cholesterol uptake in skin fibroblasts followed by their incorporation in secondary lysosomes as recently demonstrated by Goldstein and Brown. Another pathway is the direct enrichment of cellular membranes as it occurs in red blood cells in the presence of severe hyperlipemia.

Dr. Mahley (U.S.A.) then stressed variations in uptake between similar cells from different laboratory animals. Dog arterial smooth muscle cells, for instance, incorporate considerably more free and ester cholesterol from the tissue culture medium than identical cells from pigs.

Dr. Daoud referred to studies with heterologous culture systems, i.e., swine and dog arterial cells incubated in media containing human serum compared with human cells incubated in media with swine or dog sera. By far, the slowest growing cells of all these various combinations proved to be dog arterial explants.

Dr. Y. Stein (Israel) commented on the complexities of tissue culture systems. He believes that part of the cholesterol is taken by cells in culture as particle cholesterol; the free cholesterol may then be redistributed in the cell membrane or returned to the extracellular compartment.

Dr. Rothblat (U.S.A.) referred to the complexities of growing cells in chemically defined medium and to the fact than a protein free medium is not available that can consistently support cell growth for long periods.

Referring to the studies reported by Dr. Daoud, Dr. Wissler raised the question of the role of platelet growth factors that may be present in sera obtained in a clinical setting. The studies done at Albany, however, failed to find stimulation of cell growth in cultures incubated in media containing sera from normal donors. Dr. Robertson indicated that in his studies with short-term monolayer cultures of diploid human arterial cells, serum or platelet-rich plasma was needed as part of the culture medium and that plasma from the same patients did not sustain adequate cell growth.

Dr. Björkerud suggested that efforts should be made to differentiate growth factors as nonspecific cell nutrients from those that may act as essential trigger mechanisms for cell proliferation. He also referred to Dr. Daoud's finding that serum factors stimulate cell migration as a counterpart to changes found in early stages of experimental atherosclerosis. Dr. Daoud pointed out that, in their studies, such substances could be isolated by dialysis from growth stimulating agents.

Finally, Dr. Fedoroff (Canada) commented on the variability of human sera and warned investigators about the use of heterologous systems because most mammals, with the exception of Old World monkeys, have cell surface antigens that may interact with human serum antibodies and significantly alter growth cell characteristics. He further emphasized the role of dietary conditions in experimental animals preceding collection of tissues in preparation of primary cultures since this too may induce severe alterations in cell membrane composition and function.

CHAPTER 16
ENDOTHELIUM AND PERMEABILITY

(1)

THEORETICAL MODELS FOR TRANSPORT OF LOW-DENSITY LIPOPROTEINS IN THE ARTERIAL WALL

R.L. Bratzler*, C.K. Colton†, and K.A. Smith†

M.I.T. Arteriosclerosis Center and the
Departments of Chemical Engineering, †Massachusetts
Institute of Technology, Cambridge, Mass. and
*Princeton University, Princeton, N. J., U.S.A.

The accumulation of blood-borne plasma constituents, such as low-density lipoproteins (LDL), in the arterial wall is a complicated process dependent not only on the plasma LDL concentration but also on the transport properties of the arterial wall. In an attempt to learn more about this accumulation process, theoretical transport models have been developed which account for the movement of labelled plasma proteins into and through the arterial wall and for the interactions between the plasma proteins and constituents of the arterial wall. The labelled protein concentration profiles predicted by these models are compared with experimentally measured profiles of radioiodinated LDL in normal conscious rabbits *in vivo* in order to assess the suitability of the models and to estimate the magnitude of the various parameters which characterize intramural LDL transport.

The physical basis for the theoretical models is presented schematically in Figure 1. The description is applicable to the transport of LDL in rabbit aorta: it may also apply to other plasma proteins and other large blood vessels as well. Recent studies have demonstrated the presence of immunologically reactive LDL apoprotein in pathologically normal regions of human aortic intima (1). Thus, it is likely that plasma LDL is able to penetrate intact endothelium by transendothelial vesicular transport (2, 3). Diffusion and/or convection of LDL through the junctions between endothelial cells is possible but not likely. Both mechanisms are included in the model for the sake of generality.

Another possible route of LDL entry into the aortic media is by transport across capillary endothelium present in aortic adventitia. Regardless of the point of entry, LDL which has gained access to the subendothelial intima or media will diffuse radially in a direction consistent with the local concentration gradient. Since there exists a pressure difference across the rabbit aortic wall, a filtration flow may also affect LDL movement by convecting entrained solutes radially toward the adventitia. There are the numerous possible interactions which may also influence the movements of LDL across the wall. For example, LDL may bind to acid mucopolysaccharides (AMPS) (4), elastin (5) and/or collagen (6). The situation is further complicated by the fact that aortic smooth muscle cells are capable of interiorizing and degrading LDL (7). Thus, depending on the relative kinetics of cellular uptake and the catabolic process, smooth muscle cell metabolism may be an important determinant in LDL removal rates. Another mechanism for clearance is the lymphatic system. Presumably the interstitial space surrounding the adventitial capillaries is drained, as in all capillary beds, by lymphatic terminals. A compromised rate of lymphatic clearance could affect the rate of intramural LDL accumulation. In short, the concentration of LDL in the arterial wall is likely to be affected in a complicated fashion by the plasma LDL concentration, the permeability of both capillary and intimal endothelium, and the rates of diffusion, convection, cellular uptake and reaction,and/or binding within the arterial wall, and the lymphatic clearance rate.

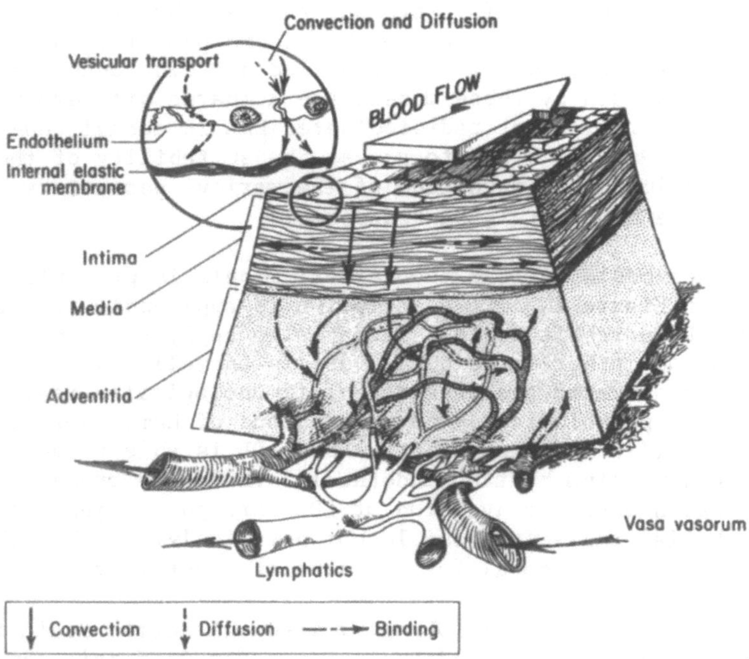

Figure 1 - LDL Transport in Rabbit Thoracic Aorta

While the foregoing qualitative description of LDL transport is somewhat speculative, it does provide a reasonable physical basis for modelling the accumulation process. In order to develop a mathematical model, we have assumed that the arterial wall may be treated as a continuum. A material balance over a differential element in the media yields the following conservation relation for freely diffusable labelled protein:

$$\underbrace{\frac{\partial}{\partial x}\left(D\frac{\partial C_f}{\partial x}\right)}_{\text{diffusion}} - \underbrace{\frac{V}{\varepsilon}\frac{\partial C_f}{\partial x}}_{\text{convection}} - \underbrace{\mathcal{P}(C_f - C_i)}_{\text{cell permeation}} - \underbrace{r_1}_{\text{binding}} = \underbrace{\frac{\partial C_f}{\partial t}}_{\text{accumulation}} \qquad (1)$$

where D = effective diffusion coefficient; V = superficial filtration flow velocity; ε = tissue porosity; r_1 = rate of LDL binding to wall constituents; $\mathcal{P}$ = smooth muscle cell wall permeability coefficient; C_f = concentration of freely diffusable LDL; C_i = intracellular concentration of labelled LDL; x = distance from intimal endothelium; and t = time.

Equation (1) shows that at any position within the arterial wall the rates of diffusion and convection must equal the rate at which LDL accumulates, binds to wall constituents, and permeates into smooth muscle cells. Cartesian rather than cylindrical coordinates are used since the thickness of the aortic wall is less than 10% of the internal radius.

Expressions for the rate of accumulation of bound and intracellular protein are given by

$$\frac{\partial C_b}{\partial t} = r_1 \qquad (2)$$

$$\frac{\partial C_i}{\partial t} = r_2 + \mathcal{P}(C_f - C_i) \qquad (3)$$

where the rate of permeation into the cells is assumed to be linearly proportional to the concentration difference. The kinetic expressions for the rate of LDL binding (r_1) and the rate of LDL intracellular catabolism (r_2) are presently unknown. For uptake of labelled solute they may be expressed as linear functions of concentration, whence

$$r_1 = k_1 C_f - k_2 C_b \qquad (4)$$

$$r_2 = - k_3 C_i \tag{5}$$

where k_1, k_2, and k_3 are kinetic rate constants. Equations (1) - (5) are the governing partial differential equations which apply throughout the media and subendothelial intima. Boundary conditions are used to describe transport across the intimal endothelium (x=0) and across the media-adventitia interface (x=L):

at x = 0:

$$\underset{\text{transport in junctions}}{VC_p(1-R_E)} + \underset{\text{vesicular transport}}{K_E\left(C_p - \frac{C_f}{\varepsilon}\right)} = \underset{\text{convection in media}}{VC_f} - \underset{\text{diffusion in media}}{D\frac{\partial C_f}{\partial x}} \tag{6}$$

at x = L:

$$\underset{\text{transport to lymphatics}}{VC_f(1-R_L)} + \underset{\text{vesicular transport from capillaries}}{K_c\left(\frac{C_f}{\varepsilon} - C_p\right)} + \underset{\text{vesicular transport to lymphatics}}{K_L\frac{C_f}{\varepsilon}} = \underset{\text{convection in media}}{VC_f} - \underset{\text{diffusion in media}}{D\frac{\partial C_f}{\partial x}} \tag{7}$$

where C_p is the plasma labelled LDL concentration; R_E and R_L are phenomenological rejection coefficients for the intimal endothelium and lymphatic terminals, respectively; and K_E, K_c, and K_L are vesicular mass transfer coefficients for intimal, capillary, and lymphatic endothelium, respectively. It is assumed in equation (7) that the labelled solute concentration in the lymphatic terminals is zero and that macrosolutes cross the intimal endothelium only by vesicular transport or by convection and/or diffusion through the endothelial junctions. At the media-adventitia interface, the same transport modes are assumed across the capillary endothelium with one important difference, however. Since there is convection of fluid out of the arterial end of the capillary but back in at the venous end, the net rate of convection may be relatively small and is neglected in the analysis. The lymphatic vessels are taken to clear solute by both convective and diffusive means.

Equations (1) - (7) have been solved using Laplace transforms to yield $C_f(x,t)$ for the case where the initial concentrations of bound, mobile, and intracellular LDL are everywhere zero. This condition applies to the experimental situation wherein protein-labelled ^{125}I-LDL is administered to a rabbit at t = 0 and intramural distribution of labelled protein is monitored at various time intervals thereafter (8, 9). Thus, the validity of the model can be tested by comparing experimental results with theoretical predictions.

As posed to this point, the model [equations (1) - (7)] requires quantitative estimates of not only a diffusion coefficient, D, and a filtration velocity, V, but also estimates of kinetic rate constants k_1, k_2, and k_3 ; vesicular mass transfer coefficients, K_E, K_c, and K_L; and the cell permeability coefficient, P. To test the necessity of including reaction and cell permeation effects in the model, a simplified version is examined in this initial analysis wherein k_1, k_2, and k_3 are set equal to zero and the models are compared with labelled LDL distribution data from relatively short time experiments (t = 10 and 30 minutes). This model corresponds to the case where the third and fourth terms on the left hand side of equation (1) are neglected. It is also assumed that solute crosses the intimal endothelium only by vesicular transport (R_E=1), but that LDL freely permeates lymphatic endothelium (R_L=0).

A wide range of parameter estimates have been investigated in order to find combinations which yield reasonable agreement between theoretical predictions and experimental data. Representative theoretical concentration profiles are plotted on Figures 2a and 2b for different estimates of V, D, and K_E (as tabulated in Table I). Also shown are experimentally determined labelled LDL concentrations 10 and 30 minutes after injection (8, 9). The tissue label concentrations are expressed as the fraction of the maximum attainable concentration, which is taken to be εC_p. ε is taken to be 0.42 (10). The distance from the intimal surface, x, is normalized with respect to the distance to the media-adventitia interface, L, where L has been experimentally determined to average 96µ for rabbit

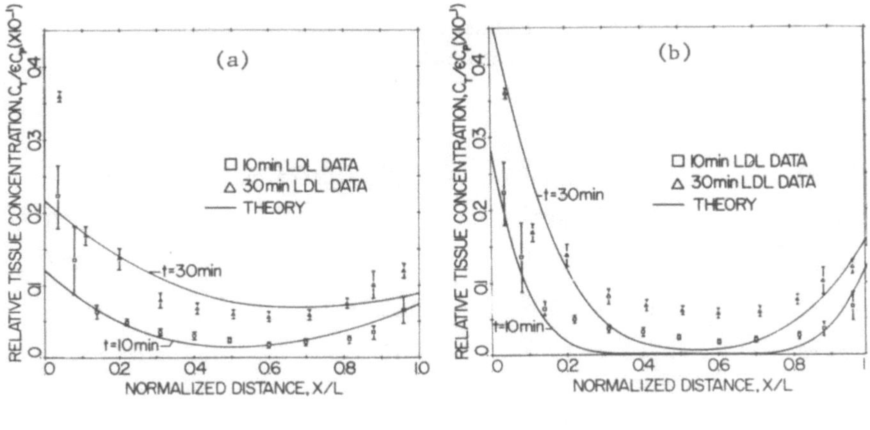

Figure 2 - Theoretical and Experimental Labelled LDL Distributions

thoracic aorta. In one case (Figure 2a) theory and experiment compare favorably in the center and outer media but not near the intima where the experimental concentration gradient is much steeper than that predicted by theory. In the second figure (Figure 2b) the predicted profile near the intima approximates the experimental data nicely, but agreement is less satisfactory in the center media.

Numerous variable combinations have been tried to improve the correspondence of the theory with experiment. However, it was not possible to fit the data over the entire thickness of the aorta with a single set of parameters. The two values of the LDL diffusion coefficient (Table I), which differ by a factor of about 6 and may bound the true value(s), are approximately a factor of 100 lower than the diffusion coefficient in aqueous solutions. Such a large reduction may not be surprising in view of the microporous and heterogeneous nature of the aortic wall. The vesicular mass transfer coefficient (K_E) employed in the prediction is a factor of 10 lower than that deduced from experiments performed with capillary endothelium. The fact that aortic endothelium is being considered in this work may explain the difference. A range of values for hydraulic flux were used in the calculations. While they are somewhat smaller in magnitude than those measured experimentally, one must not attach too much significance to this fact since the theoretical concentration profiles are relatively insensitive to variation in V at the short times investigated here. It should also be noted that the extracellular volume fraction (ε) for LDL is not known, and departures from the value employed here would lead to commensurate changes in the estimates of the transport parameters.

The curves presented on Figures 2a and 2b were based on a Peclet number (VL/εD) of 0.1 so that the relative rate of convection was small compared to that of diffusion in the media. It is interesting

Table I - Parameter Estimates Used in Theoretical Predictions

	Fig. 2a	Fig. 2b	Literature
$D(cm^2/sec)$	7.5×10^{-9}	1.2×10^{-9}	2.3×10^{-7}[a]
$V(ml/cm^2 hr)$	$\leq 3 \times 10^{-3}$	$\leq 10^{-3}$	$3 \times 10^{-3} - 10^{-2}$[b]
$K_E(cm/sec)$	1.6×10^{-8}	1.6×10^{-8}	10^{-7}[c]
$K_C(cm/sec)$	3.3×10^{-8}	1.1×10^{-8}	—
$K_L(cm/sec)$	3.3×10^{-6}	4.1×10^{-7}	—

a. diffusion coefficient of LDL in aqueous solution (11);
b. *in vitro* data (8, 12); c. capillary transport (13, 14).

to examine the consequences of a significantly increased filtration velocity while keeping all other transport parameters the same as in Fig. 2. As shown in Figures 3a and 3b, a 100-fold increase in Peclet number results in considerably lower relative tissue concentations and much flatter profiles. The effect is even more pronounced in Figures 4a and 4b where theoretical predictions at longer times are presented. Thus, a higher hydraulic flux, with all other parameters held constant, tends to depress tissue concentrations, especially at long times. This makes sense if one envisions the hydraulic flow as clearing solute to the lymphatics and if one assumes that all solute crossing the intimal endothelium does so only by vesicular transport and not by convection through gaps between

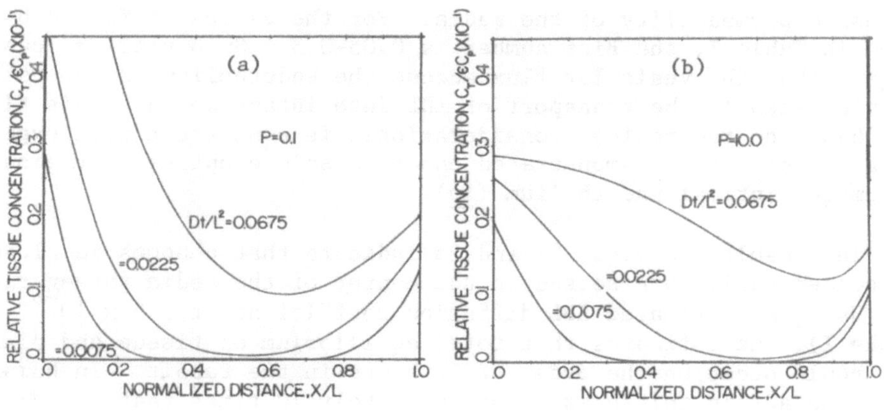

Figure 3 - Changes in Theoretical Profiles with a 100-Fold Increase in Peclet Number(P)-parameters same as in Fig. 2b

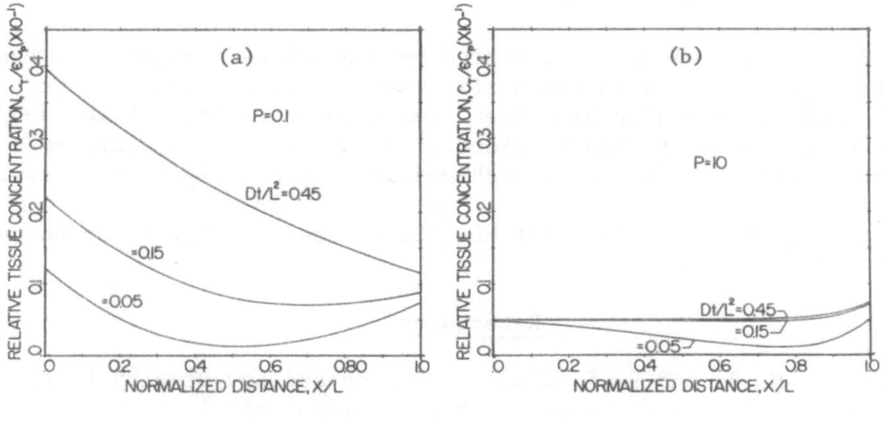

Figure 4 - Changes in Theoretical Profiles with a 100-Fold Increase in Peclet Number(P)-parameters same as in Fig. 2a

adjoining cells. Preliminary comparisons between predicted and experimental data 4, 24, and 67 hours following injection suggest that Peclet numbers of order unity are required to prevent theory from overpredicting tissue label concentrations. This implies that diffusion and convection play equally important roles in LDL transport through the media.

An interesting observation from the results in Table I is that the endothelium is the limiting resistance to LDL transport in the arterial wall. Given the small magnitude for the LDL diffusion coefficient, one might have suspected that diffusion was the rate-limiting step. However, when equations (1) - (7) are cast in dimensionless form, there arises a dimensionless Biot number ($K_E L/\varepsilon D$), which is a measure of the permeability of the endothelium relative to the diffusive permeability of the media. For the values of K_E and D given in Table I, the Biot number is 0.05-0.3. Such small values suggest that the vesicular flux across the endothelium is the rate-limiting step in the transport of LDL into intact aorta. This finding, based on theoretical considerations, is consistent with experimental studies that demonstrated enhanced solute uptake in regions of damaged intimal endothelium (15).

The results in Figs. 2a and 2b indicate that changes in plasma LDL concentration are sensed in the center of the media rather rapidly. Using an estimated LDL diffusion coefficient of 7.5×10^{-9} (Table I), one estimates that total equilibrium of tissue and plasma LDL should occur on the order of 10 hours in the rabbit. In humans, where the aortic thickenss is approximately 10 times that of the rabbit, equilibration times on the order of 1000 hours, or 40 days, are to be expected. Although clearly speculative, this might explain, in part, why atherosclerotic lesions can be induced in rabbits in only a few months whereas human lesions may develop over much longer periods of time.

The simplified model presented here provides insight into the LDL transport process in the aortic wall. More complete models, which include metabolic processes (reaction, cellular uptake) and/or position-dependent transport properties, are likely to yield even better agreement. Work with such models is currently is progress.

Supported in part by NIH Grant HL 14209-01 and the Princeton University Computer Center

References

1. Smith, E. B. and R. S. Slater, "Lipids and Low-Density Lipoproteins in Intima in Relation to its Morphological Characteristics," in "Atherosclerosis: Initiating Factors," A Ciba Symposium Series, 12, pp. 39-62, Elsevier, Amsterdam(1973).

2. Watts, H.F., "Basic Aspects of the Pathogenesis of Human Atherosclerosis, "Human Path.", 2, 31-55 (1971).
3. Stein, O., Y. Stein, and S. Eisenberg, "A Radioautographic Study of the Transport of ^{125}I-Labelled Serum Lipoproteins in Rat Aorta", Z Zellforsch, 138, 223-237 (1973).
4. Iverius, P.-H., "Possible Role of Glycosaminoglycans in the Genesis of Atherosclerosis", in "Atherosclerosis: Initiating Factors", a Ciba Symposium Series, 12, pp. 185-193, Elsevier, Amsterdam (1973).
5. Kramsch, D.M. and W. Hollander, "The Interaction of Serum and Arterial Lipoproteins with Elastin of the Arterial Intima and its Role in the Lipid Accumulation in Atherosclerotic Plaques." J. Clin. Invest., 52, 236 (1973).
6. Bratzler, R.L., unpublished result.
7. Bierman, E.L., O. Stein, and Y. Stein, "Lipoprotein Uptake and Metabolism by Rat Aortic Smooth Muscle Cells in Tissue Culture", Circ. Res., 35, 136-150 (1974).
8. Bratzler, R.L., "The Transport Properties of Arterial Tissue", Ph.D. Thesis, Massachusetts Institute of Technology, Cambridge, Massachusetts (1974).
9. Bratzler, R.L., G.M. Chisolm, C.K. Colton, K.A. Smith, and R.S. Lees, "The Distribution of Labeled Low-Density Lipoprotein Across the Rabbit Thoracic Aorta in Vivo", submitted to Circulation Research (1975).
10. Torok, J., O.A. Negergaard, and J.A. Bean, "The Distribution of Inulin Space inthe Rabbit Thoracic Aorta, "Experientia", 27, 55 (1971).
11. Shumaker, V.N., "Hydrodynamic Analysis of Human Low Density Lipoproteins", Accts. Chem. Res., 6, 398 (1973).
12. Yamartino, E.J., Jr., "Determination of the Arterial Filtration Coefficient of the Rabbit Aorta", M.S. Thesis, Massachusetts Institute of Technology, Cambridge, Massachusetts (1974).
13. Karnovsky, M.J. and S.M. Shea, "Transcapillary Transport by Pinocytosis", Microvas. Res., 2, 333-360 (1970).
14. Bruns, R.R., and G.E. Palade, "Studies on Blood Capillaries: 1. General Organization of Blood Capillaries in Muscle." J. Cell. Biol., 37, 244-275 (1968).
15. Somer, J.B., and C.J. Schwartz, "Focal (^{3}H) Cholesterol Uptake in the Pig Aorta, Part 2. Distribution of (^{3}H) Cholesterol Across the Aortic Wall in Areas of High and Low Uptake In Vivo", Atherosclerosis, 16, 377-388 (1975).

(2)

THE MORPHOLOGIC BASIS OF ARTERIAL ENDOTHELIAL PERMEABILITY: SOME ULTRASTRUCTURAL ASPECTS OF THE EVANS BLUE MODEL

Ross G. Gerrity, Mary Richardson, and Colin J. Schwartz

Department of Pathology, Faculty of Health Sciences, McMaster University and the Southam Laboratories, Chedoke Hospitals, Hamilton, Ontario, Canada.

Much of the available information on vascular endothelial permeability has been derived from studies on either small arteries or capillaries, from which the pore theory of capillary permeability has evolved.(1-3) Using a variety of molecular probes, a number of studies have concluded that the structural equivalents of such pores are located within the intercellular junctions of endothelial cells.(4-6) With myoglobin as a probe others have shown that in muscle capillaries the plasmalemmal vesicles represent the morphologic equivalents of both large and small endothelial pores.(7) Recently Simionescu, Simionescu and Palade,(8) using two small heme-peptides, each of some 20Å diameter, haveshown that these probes cross the endothelium primarily by vesicular transport, with no early or preferential accumulation of reaction product in the intercellular junctions.

To what extent the many observations on capillary endothelium may be extrapolated to the endothelium of large arteries has yet to be clarified. However, studies on large arteries using horseradish peroxidase (HRP) as a probe(9-11) have demonstrated reaction product not only in intercellular junctions but also in plasmalemmal vesicles, suggesting either that endothelial transport in large arteries differs from that of capillaries, or alternatively, that the endothelial transport of HRP differs from that of other probes.

Over a number of years we have developed and explored the Evans Blue model in some detail, in the hope that it might not only clarify some of the problems associated with transendothelial transport in large arteries, but also contribute to a better understanding of the early biological processes involved in atherogenesis. The protein-binding azo dye Evans Blue, after intravenous administration, exhibits a characteristic and relatively consistent focal uptake pattern in the aortas of the dog,[12] rabbit,[13] and pig.[14-16] The dye-uptake pattern is significantly modified in experimental aortic coarctation,[16] and cannot be reproduced by simple in vitro incubations in media containing Evans Blue.[17] These findings are consistent with the view that the focal uptake pattern reflects focal differences or disturbances in aortic hemodynamics. Areas of dye uptake (blue areas) show significantly greater aortic endothelial permeability to both ^{131}I-albumin and ^{131}I-fibrinogen in vivo[14,18,19] relative to adjacent areas showing no dye accumulation (white areas). Such areas of spontaneously-occurring greater permeability to proteins also exhibit an increased endothelial cell turnover, as measured by ^{3}H-thymidine autoradiography,[20] together with a number of differences in en face morphology.[21]

Areas showing a greater aortic endothelial permeability to proteins (blue areas) have been examined by both transmission and scanning electron microscopy, and compared with adjoining areas of lesser permeability characterized by the absence of dye accumulation.[22] Details of the procedures employed in fixation and processing are described in detail elsewhere.[22]

A consistent and striking feature is the markedly thickened and edematous subendothelial space (SES) observed in blue (Figure 1) but not in white (Figure 2) areas. This thickened SES was found to contain both collagen and elastin elements, together with a variable number of undifferentiated cells, dispersed in a floccular matrix of relatively low electron density (Figure 1).

Endothelial cells in blue areas were generally cuboidal in shape (Figure 1), in contrast to those in white areas, which appeared much flatter and elongated (Figure 2). Intercellular junctions also exhibited a number of morphologic differences. In blue areas, the junctions were relatively short, end-to-end, and frequently showed a segmental vacuolation or dilatation (Figure 1a). In white areas, by contrast, the junctions were elongate, tortuous, with many complex interdigitations (Figure 2a). Tight junctions appeared with a similar frequency in both areas.

A glycocalyx layer, visualization of which was facilitated by Ruthenium Red-staining, was observed over the surface of endothelial cells in both blue and white areas (Figures 3a, 3b). In the latter, (Figure 3b) the surface layer measured up to five times the thickness of that in blue areas. The glycocalyx in both areas consisted of a dense lamina closely applied to the plasmalemmal membrane, and superficially, a finely fibrillar mesh of lesser density (Figures 3a, 3b). Nodular densities, having no discernible periodicity, were more prominent in white areas. Material of a density and appearance similar to that of the glycocalyx was present in some, but not all plasmalemmal vesicles in both blue and white areas, and was also observed within the luminal aspect of intercellular junctions.

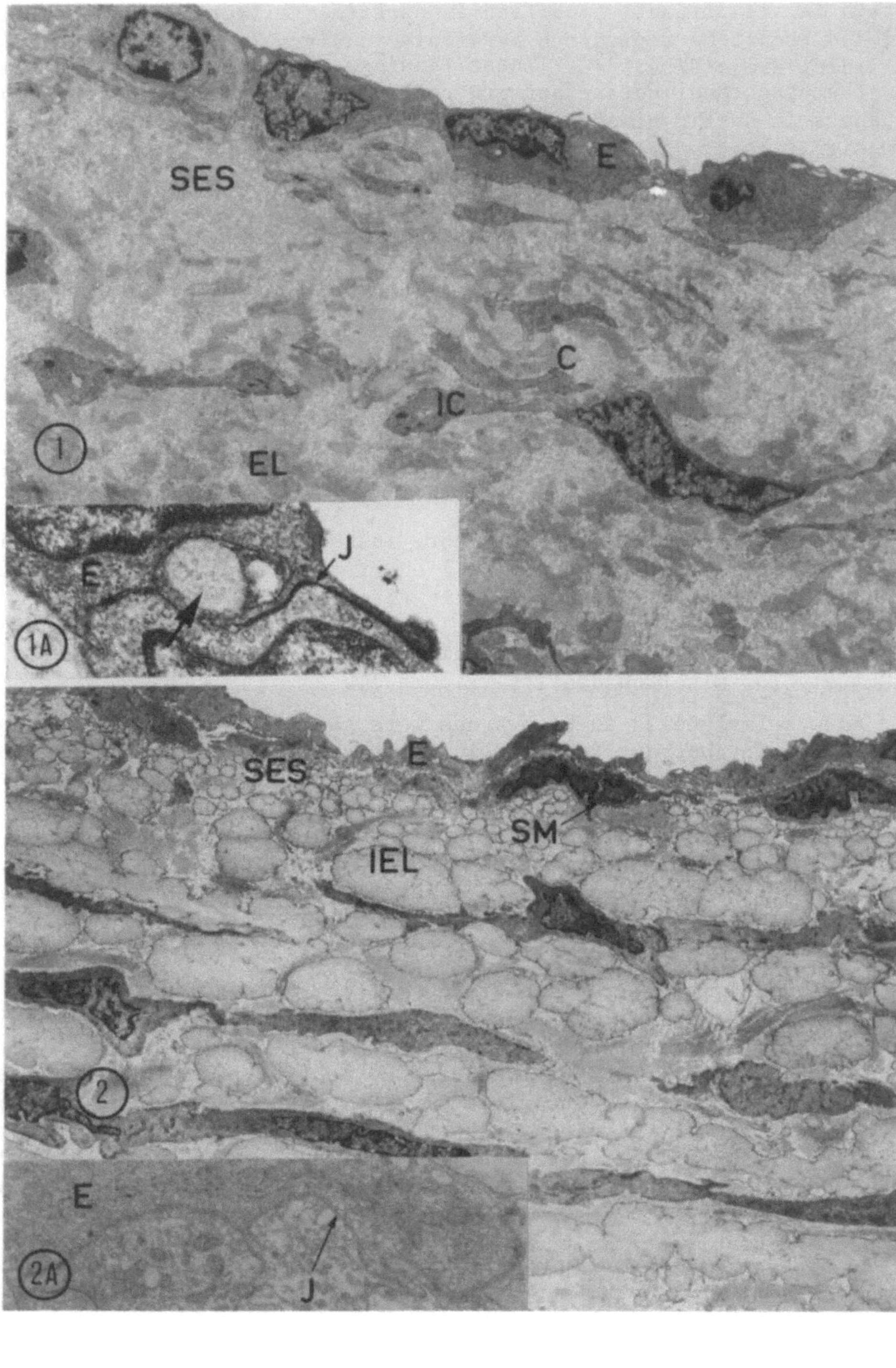
SES
E
C
IC
EL
1
E
J
1A
SES
E
SM
IEL
2
E
J
2A

Severely injured or dead endothelial cells showing loss of cytoplasmic density and organelles, peripheral condensation of nuclear chromatin, and cytoplasmic vacuolation were not infrequently seen in blue (Figure 4) but rarely in white areas. Some such cells appeared partially lifted, while in other foci within blue areas, defects in the endothelium, presumably reflecting denudation of dead cells were present, covered by attenuated and degranulated platelets.[22] Although the frequency of such foci of endothelial cell death could not be determined electron microscopically, with en face silver-stained Häutchen preparations, dead cells, appearing as areas of intense silver-staining, sharply delineated by the cell boundaries, were observed with a four-fold greater frequency in blue than in white areas.[22] This demonstration of a greater frequency of endothelial cell death in blue areas is consistent with the significantly greater endothelial cell turnover described for these areas. (20)

Studies with ferritin as an electron probe have shown that this tracer appears earlier and in greater quantities in the SES of blue (Figure 5) relative to white areas, and that it appears to cross the endothelium primarily by vesicular transport. Thus far, the contribution of defects or "ultra large pores" resulting from endothelial cell death or loss in blue areas, to the transendothelial transport of macromolecules has yet to be assessed.

Some aspects of endothelial ultrastructure associated with spontaneously-occurring areas of differing permeability to proteins in the aorta of the healthy young pig have been described. That the normal aortic endothelium is not an homogeneous entity, either functionally or ultrastructurally, is emphasized. Areas of greater endothelial permeability within the aortic arch have been shown to exhibit a thickened and edematous SES, and a significantly greater frequency of endothelial cell death, which may contribute to the greater transendothelial transport in blue areas.

←

Figure 1. Cross-section, aortic intima, blue area. Endothelial cells (E) are cuboidal, subendothelial space (SES) is edematous, and contains collagen (C), elastin (EL) and intimal cells (IC). x 3,600. Figure 1a. Blue area, end-to-end junction (J) between endothelial cells (E) showing saccular dilatation (arrow). x 19,200. Figure 2. As in Figure 1, from a white area. Endothelial cells (E) are flat and elongate with modified smooth muscle cells (SM) lying parallel to the endothelium in narrow subendothelial space (SES). Internal elastic lamina (IEL) is forming directly below. x 3,600. Figure 2a. White area, complex interdigitating junction (J) between endothelial cells (E). x 15,200.

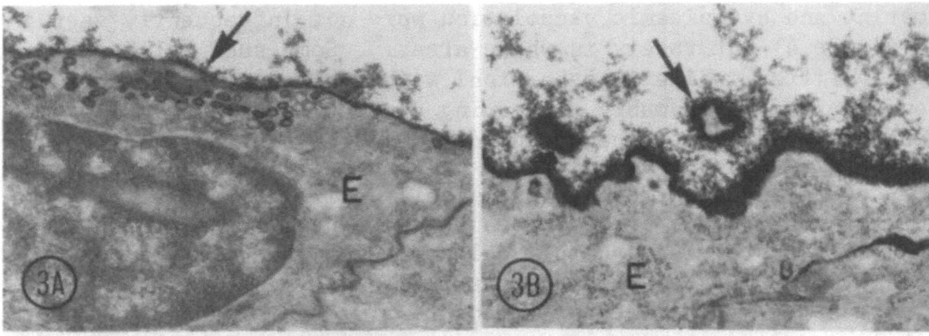

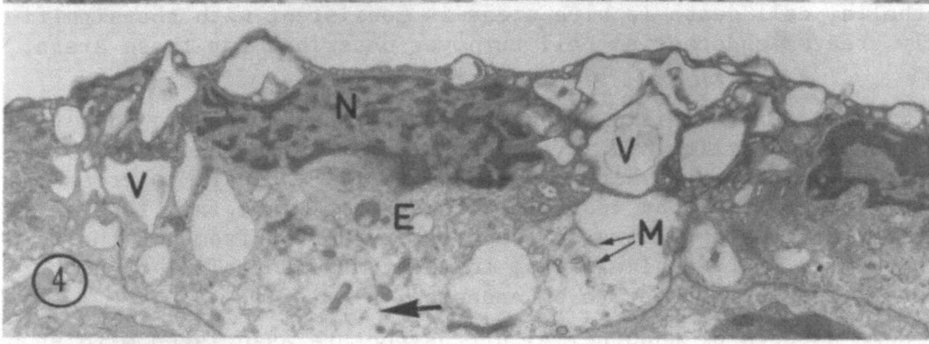

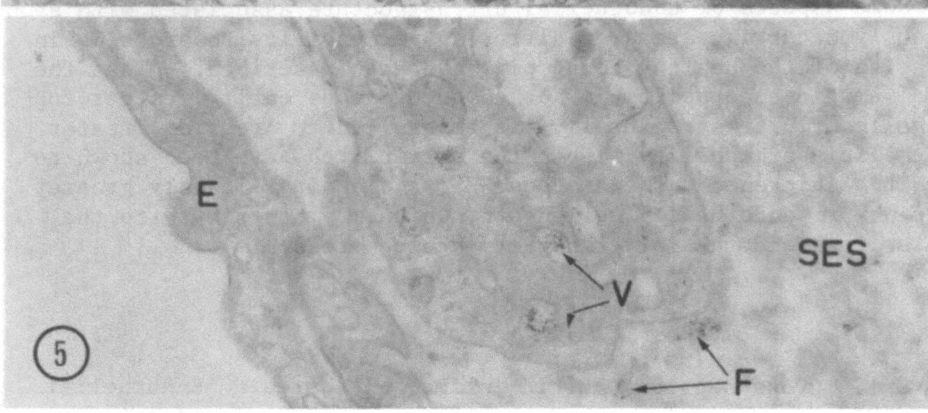

Figure 3a. Blue area endothelium (E) showing thin Ruthenium Red-stained glycocalyx (arrow). x 22,000. Figure 3b. White are endothelium (E) with thick Ruthenium Red-stained glycocalyx (arrow). x 22,000. Figure 4. Injured endothelial cell (E) in blue area, showing loss of cytoplasm (arrow), vacuolation (V), membrane disruption (M), and condensation of chromatin in the nucleus (N). x 11,000. Figure 5. Blue area, 5 min after ferritin injection. Ferritin (F) has passed through endothelium (E) and is located in subendothelial space (SES) and in vacuoles (V) of intimal cells. x 35,000.

While the biological role of the endothelial glycocalyx remains uncertain, it is tempting to suggest that the thicker glycocalyx observed in white areas might partially account for the lesser permeability of these areas, either by limiting access of molecules to plasmalemmal vesicles or binding sites on the plasma membrane. This surface layer might also modify or limit contact between circulating lipoproteins and plasmalemmal membrane, thus influencing unesterified cholesterol exchange, a mechanism which might explain the differing uptakes of ^{3}H-unesterified cholesterol in blue and white areas.[15,23] In terms of endothelial permeability, however, it is of some interest that in experimental hypercholesterolemia, which results in an increased permeability to albumin,[24] a thinning of the glycocalyx has been observed.[25,26]

ACKNOWLEDGEMENTS

The work on which this report is based is supported by the Medical Research Council of Canada (MT.3067), and the Ontario Heart Foundation.

REFERENCES

1. PAPPENHEIMER JR, RENKIN EM, BORRERO LM: Amer J Physiol 167:13, 1951
2. PAPPENHEIMER JR: Physiol Rev 33:387, 1953
3. LANDIS EM, PAPPENHEIMER JR: Handbook of Physiol, Washington, D.C. 2:961, 1963
4. KARNOVSKY MJ: J Cell Biol 35:213, 1967
5. KARNOVSKY MJ, RICE DF: J Histochem Cytochem 17:751, 1969
6. KARNOVSKY MJ: Academic Press Inc., New York, 341, 1970
7. SIMIONESCU N, SIMIONESCU M, PALADE GE: J Cell Biol 57:424, 1973
8. SIMIONESCU N, SIMIONESCU M, PALADE GE: J Cell Biol 64:586, 1975
9. FLOREY HW, SHEPPARD BL: Proc Roy Soc Lond (B) 174:435, 1970
10. HÜTTNER I, MORE RH, RONA G: Amer J Pathol 61:395, 1970
11. SCHWARTZ SM, BENDITT EP: Amer J Pathol 66:241, 1972
12. McGILL HC, GEER JC, HOLMAN RL: Arch Pathol 64:303, 1957
13. FRIEDMAN M, BYERS SO: Arch Pathol 76:99, 1963
14. PACKHAM MA, ROWSELL HC, JØRGENSEN L, MUSTARD JF: Exp Molec Pathol 7:214, 1967
15. SOMER JB, SCHWARTZ CJ: Atherosclerosis 13:293, 1971
16. SOMER JB, EVANS G, SCHWARTZ CJ: Atherosclerosis 16:127, 1972
17. BELL FP, SOMER JB, CRAIG IH, SCHWARTZ CJ: Atherosclerosis 16:369, 1972
18. BELL FP, ADAMSON IL, SCHWARTZ CJ: Exp Molec Pathol 20:57, 1974
19. BELL FP, GALLUS AS, SCHWARTZ CJ: Exp Molec Pathol 20:281, 1974

20. CAPLAN BA, SCHWARTZ CJ: Atherosclerosis 17:401, 1973
21. CAPLAN BA, GERRITY RG, SCHWARTZ CJ: Exp Molec Pathol 21:102, 1974
22. GERRITY RG, RICHARDSON M, SOMER JB, BELL FP, SCHWARTZ CJ: 1975 Submitted
23. SOMER JB, SCHWARTZ CJ: Atherosclerosis 16:377, 1972
24. STEFANOVICH V, GORE I: Exp Molec Pathol 14:20, 1971
25. WEBER G, FABBRINI P, RESI L: Virchows Arch Abt A Path Anat 359:299, 1973
26. BALINT A, VERESS B, JELLINEK H: Path Europ 9:105, 1974

(3)

LIGHT MICROSCOPIC LOCALIZATION OF ACTOMYOSIN AND TROPOMYOSIN IN TISSUES BY IMMUNOPEROXIDASE TECHNIQUE FOLLOWING FIXATION IN DIMETHYLSUBERIMIDATE AND EMBEDDING IN POLYETHYLENE GLYCOL

Carl G. Becker and Arlene Hardy

The New York Hospital-Cornell Medical Center,

New York, N.Y., U. S. A.

In experiments previously reported from this laboratory, it was observed that actomyosin extracted from human uterine smooth muscle and actomyosin (thrombosthenins) extracted from human platelets were functionally, structurally and immunologically similar (1). Antisera prepared in rabbits to either of these proteins were, by direct or indirect immunofluorescent technique, observed to stain specifically endothelial cells and smooth muscle cells of systemic arteries and veins, endothelial cells of liver sinusoids and certain capillaries, mesangial cells of renal glomeruli (2), endothelial cells cultured from umbilical veins, blood platelets and mature megakaryocytes (1,3). These antisera also stained specifically, myoepithelial cells, perineurial cells of peripheral nerves (4) and "fibroblastic" cells of granulation tissue. In corollary experiments, essentially similar observations were made using rabbit antisera to human uterine tropomyosin (5). All of these experiments employed acetone "fixed" frozen sections of human tissues or acetone "fixed" smears of human peripheral blood and direct or indirect immunofluorescence microscopy. Frozen sections and acetone "fixation" were used because the antigenicity of actomyosin and of tropomyosin were destroyed by other fixatives such as formaldehyde, paraformaldehyde, and glutaraldehyde. The purpose of this communication is to report the results of experiments in which human tissues were fixed in dimethylsuberimidate, a diimidoester, and embedded in polyethylene glycol prior to sectioning and treatment with rabbit antisera to uterine actomyosin or tropomyosin and peroxidase labeled antibodies to rabbit IgG.

Materials and Methods:

Preparation of Antisera: The details of extraction and purification of uterine actomyosin and tropomyosin, the production of rabbit antisera thereto, and the measures of specificity of these antisera were described previously (1, 5) as were the details of preparation of goat antisera to rabbit IgG.

Preparation of Peroxidase Labeled Antibodies to Rabbit IgG: Horseradish peroxidase (HRP, Sigma, grade) was conjugated to goat antirabbit IgG antibodies using 1% fluorodinitrobenzene, sodium periodate and ethyleneglycol as described by Nakane (6). Excess peroxidase was removed by chromatography on G-200 Sephadex.

Preparation of Tissues: Samples of human papillary muscle obtained at surgery and of left ventricular wall and of kidney obtained at necropsy were cut into cubes measuring 1-2 mm in greatest dimension and fixed with agitation for $2\frac{1}{2}$ hrs in dimethylsuberimidate as described by Hassell and Hand (7). The tissue blocks were then dehydrated in a graded series of alcohols and embedded in polyethylene glycol (PEG) as described by Mazurkiewicz and Nakane (8). Sections 3μ in thickness were cut from these blocks at room temperature on a conventional paraffin section microtome and floated on a water bath with 0.1% glycerol for one hour. They were then transferred to glass microscopic slides, subbed with gelatine, and dried at 40°C.

Treatment of Tissue Sections for the Detection of Actomyosin and Tropomyosin: After washing in phosphate buffered physiological saline (PBS) to remove PEG the sections were overlayed with either rabbit antisera to human uterine actomyosin, uterine tropomyosin, or cardiac actomyosin, or with pooled normal rabbit serum and incubated at 37°C for 30 minutes. All antisera were diluted 1:10 with PBS. The sections were then washed in three changes of PBS for twenty minutes and treated with HRP conjugated goat anti rabbit IgG antibodies. The sections were incubated for 30 minutes at 37°C, again washed in PBS, incubated with 3-3-diaminobenzedine and fixed in osmic acid as described by Graham and Karnovsky (9). The sections were dehydrated in alcohol and xylene and mounted. Absorption controls were essentially similar to those described previously (1, 3, 5). Companion sections not stained with antibody were stained with hematoxylin and eosin and mounted.

Results:

Fixation of tissues in dimethylsuberimidate followed by dehydration in alcohol and embedding in polyethylene glycol did not destroy antigenicity of either uterine actomyosin or tropomyosin or of cardiac actomyosin.

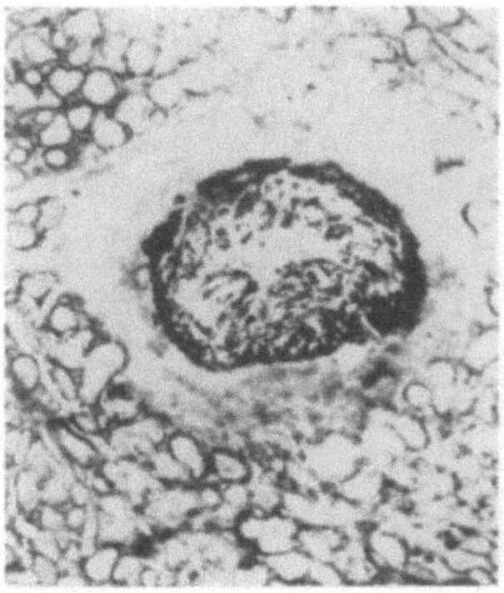

Fig. 1.

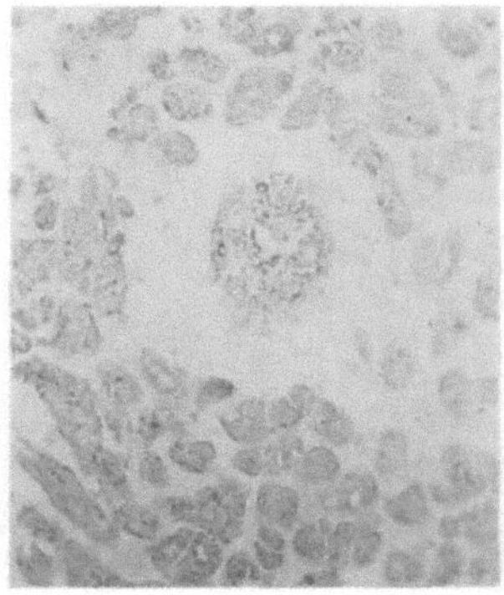

Fig. 2.

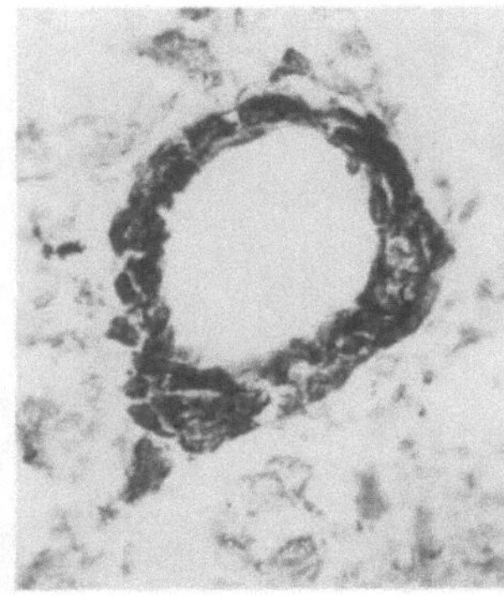

Fig. 3.

Figure 1. Section of human papillary muscle, fixed in dimethylsuberimidate (DMS), embedded in polyethylene glycol (PEG), and treated with rabbit anti human uterine actomyosin serum (R-AUAM) followed by horseradish peroxidase conjugated goat anti rabbit IgG antibody (GARG-P*). Arterial endothelial cells, intimal cells, and medial cells as well as the walls of myocardial capillaries are stained. Striated heart muscle cells are not stained. (X 156)

Figure 2. Section of human papillary muscle fixed and embedded as above. R-AUAM was previously absorbed with human uterine actomyosin before treating section. This was followed by GARG-P*. Staining of arterial endothelial, intimal and smooth muscle cells and walls of capillaries is inhibited. (X 156)

Figure 3. Artery in human kidney fixed and embedded as above. Section was treated with rabbit anti human uterine tropomyosin serum followed by GARG-P*. Arterial endothelial cells and medial cells are stained indicating that they contain tropomyosin similar to that of uterus. (X 500)

When sections of human heart and kidney were treated with rabbit antibodies to uterine actomyosin (AUA) followed by HRP labeled goat antibodies to rabbit IgG, and immersed in 3-3 diaminobenzidine solution, endothelial cells and smooth muscle cells of arteries and veins, and the walls of myocardial capillaries were stained (Fig. 1). Renal glomerular endothelium was not stained, but glomerular mesangial cells were. The same structures were stained

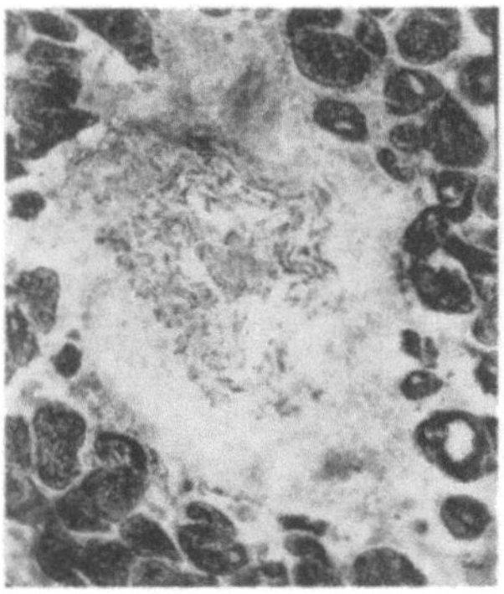

Fig. 4.

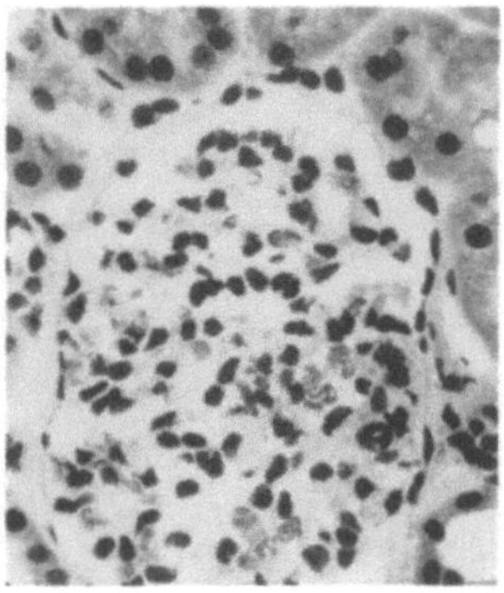

Fig. 5.

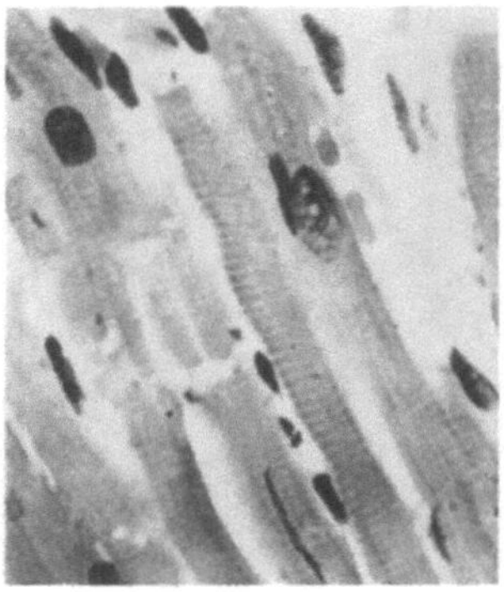

Fig. 6.

Figure 4. Human papillary muscle fixed and embedded as above. Section was treated with rabbit anti cardiac serum followed by GARG-P*. Cardiac muscle fibers, but neither endothelial cells, arterial smooth muscle cells, nor capillaries, are stained. (X 312)

Figure 5. Human renal glomerulus and adjacent tubules in autopsy specimen of kidney fixed and embedded as above. (H & E, X 312)

Figure 6. Human heart muscle in autopsy specimen fixed and embedded as above. Striations of muscle and nuclear detail are well preserved. (H & E, X 500)

when anti-uterine tropomyosin serum (AUT) was substituted for anti-uterine actomyosin serum (Fig. 2). Previous absorption of AUA with uterine actomyosin or of AUT with uterine tropomyosin completely inhibited staining (Fig. 3). When sections of heart were treated with anti cardiac actomyosin (ACA) as the primary antibody and then processed similarly, striated cardiac muscle, but neither endothelial cells nor smooth muscle was stained; staining of cardiac muscle was inhibited by absorption of ACA with cardiac actomyosin (Fig. 4). When sections of heart or kidney were treated with normal rabbit sera followed by HRP conjugated anti-rabbit IgG there was no staining of any structures.

Hematoxylin and eosin stained sections of these PEG embedded blocks were comparable in quality to sections of tissues fixed in formalin or other conventional fixatives and embedded in paraffin (Fig. 5, 6).

Discussion:

Diimidoesters have the general formula:

$$\begin{array}{ccc} {}^{-}Cl + H_2N & & NH_2\ Cl^{-} \\ \| & & \| \\ H_3CO - C - & (CH_2)_n & - C - OCH_3 \end{array}$$

Dimethylsuberimidate (DMS, n = 6)

These are a class of bifunctional reagents which cross-link proteins by binding to α and ε-amino groups. At higher pH values (9.5 - 10.0) the preferential reaction is with ε-amino groups (7, 10, 11). At this pH, cross linking of proteins involves largely lysine residues, unlike glutaraldehyde or other aldehydes which react with phenolic and imidazole rings of tyrosine and histidine, sulfhydryl groups of cysteine, and α and ε-amino groups of proteins as well.

It is probably the relative specificity of DMS for the ε - amino group of lysine that results in retention of antigenicity of actomyosin and tropomyosin in tissue fixed in DMS. In our experience, antigenicity of these proteins in tissues is destroyed by fixation in aldehydes.

The results of experiments described here indicate that fixation of tissue in DMS and embedding in polyethylene glycol permits study of the distribution of contractile and regulatory proteins by immunoperoxidase techniques as well as good quality sections which can be stained with conventional histologic stains. This obviates the need for frozen sections and dark field immunofluorescence microscopy previously necessary to localize these proteins by immunohistochemical technique.

These observations also are in accord with previous observations from this laboratory indicating that endothelial cells of many blood vessels contain actomyosin and tropomyosin similar to that of smooth muscle.

Bibliography

1. Becker CG and Nachman RL: Contractile proteins of endothelial cells, platelets and smooth muscle. Am J Path 73:1, 1973.
2. Becker CG: Demonstration of actomyosin in mesangial cells of the renal glomerulus. Am J Path 66:97, 1972.
3. Becker CG and Murphy GE: Demonstration of contractile protein in endothelium and cells of heart valves, endocardium, intima, arteriosclerotic plaques and Aschoff bodies of rheumatic heart disease. Am J Path 55:1, 1969.

4. Becker CG and Murphy FL: Demonstration of contractile protein in perineurial cells of peripheral nerves. Am J Path 66:67a, 1972.
5. Becker CG, Hardy AM and Dubin T: Contractile and relaxing proteins of smooth muscle, endothelial cells, and platelets, in Platelets, Thrombosis and Inhibitors, ed by P Didisheim, et al. FK Schattauer Verlag, 1974, pp 25-34.
6. Nakane P: Personal communication, April 1973.
7. Hassel J and Hand AR: Tissue fixation with diimidoesters as an alternative to aldehydes. J Histochem and Cytochem 22:223, 1974.
8. Mazurkiewicz J and Nakane PK: Light and electron microscopic localization of antigens in tissues embedded in polyethylene glycol with a peroxidase labeled antibody method. J Histochem and Cytochem 20:969, 1972.
9. Graham RCJ and Karnovsky MJ: The early stages of absorption of injected horseradish peroxidase in the proximal tubules of the mouse kidney. Ultrastructural cytochemistry by a new technique. J Histochem and Cytochem 14:291, 1966.
10. Hartman FC and Wold F: Cross linking of bovine pancreatic ribonuclease A with dimethyladipimate. Biochem 8:2439, 1967.
11. Hunter MJ and Ludwig ML: Amidination. Method Enzymol 25:585, 1972.

(4)

THE MORPHOLOGIC BASIS FOR NORMAL ENDOTHELIAL PERMEABILITY; Intercellular pathways*

Maia Simionescu

Yale University School of Medicine

333 Cedar Street, New Haven, CT., U.S.A.

The vascular endothelium represents a porous, semipermeable barrier at the level of which exchange of substances may occur either across the endothelial cells (through their special features), or along the intercellular spaces. Among the still controverted aspects of endothelial permeability is the pathway taken by lipid-insoluble molecules which by their nature cannot penetrate directly the endothelial cell membrane. In the most common type of endothelium, designated "continuous" endothelium (encountered in large vessels and in capillaries of somatic tissues), the only possible continuous water-filled structures are the intercellular spaces. The patency of these spaces depends on the general geometry and the degree of tightness of the junctions linking together the apposed endothelial cells.

Better knowledge than currently available on the organization and the extent of permeation of the endothelial junctions in different segments of the vasculature, is needed in physiology as well as in vascular pathology. Evidence has been accumulated that under stress conditions focal separations of the endothelial cells at the level of their junctions occur preferentially in certain vascular segments. Such separations are involved in inflammatory reactions, hemorrhage and thrombosis. Moreover, at present it is assumed that alterations in endothelial permeability play a substantial role in atherosclerosis. Hence, it is important to obtain more

*This work has been done together with Drs. N. Simionescu and G.E. Palade; part of it was published in The Journal of Cell Biology, 1973,57,2, and 1975,64,3, and part of the results have been submitted for publication to the same journal.

information about the intimate organization of the endothelial junctions and about the degree of their tightness/patency. This information may help to clarify the role of the junctions in the normal and abnormal permeability of the endothelium.

For the reasons mentioned above, we focused our attention on the continuous endothelium of muscular capillaries. Because of its similarity with that of the large vessels, the results obtained may be of interest for those working on vascular pathology.

The structural organization of the endothelial junctions in the blood capillaries has been investigated on thin sectioned specimens (which give information on the organization at the level of cell to cell contact), and on replicas of freeze-fractured vessels (which show intramembranous differentiations of the junctional membranes).

In thin sections, the endothelial junctions of true capillaries appear either as lines (bands) of close contact (or fusion) of the two outer leaflets of the joined membranes, the width of the two fused leaflets being equal to that of one membrane leaflet (densitometric studies); or as lines (bands) of fusion with complete elimination of the dense outer leaflets, resulting in a bridge between the corresponding intermediate hydrophobic layers. Such appearances indicate that along the lines of membrane fusion, the tight junction obliterates the intercellular spaces and functions as a gasket or sealing device. From the examination of sectioned specimens only, it cannot be ascertained whether such sealing devices take the form of continuous belts or that of discontinuous bands.

The freeze-fracture preparations have the advantage of exposing large areas of junctional membranes with their intramembranous differentiations, but they also have the limitation that the true cell surface cannot be visualized directly. Our investigations were carried out on muscle capillaries (mostly diaphragm and heart), and on capillaries dissected from well identified microvascular units isolated from the omentum and mesentery, and made up by an arteriole, its capillaries and the emerging venule (ACV units). The pattern of endothelial junctions of capillaries was compared with that observed in the preceeding arteriole and in the emerging venule.

Systematic examination of such isolated vessels showed that the organization of the endothelial junctions varies characteristically from one microvascular segment to another.

In arterioles, the junctional membranes display a continuous and elaborate meshwork of tight junctions with large intercalated gap junctions (communicating junctions).

The capillary endothelium is provided with 2-6 ridges or grooves generally similar to those found in arterioles, except for the absence of gap (communicating) junctions. The ridges/grooves are either continuous or quasi-continuous. In the latter case, they form a staggered arrangement along the junctions.

The venules (pericytic and muscular venules) exhibit loosely organized, discontinuous junctional elements of occluding type. Small and rare gap (communicating) junctions are present in muscular venules only.

There are reasons to assume that at least part of the ridges and grooves seen in freeze fracture correspond to the lines of cell to cell adhesion or membrane fusion seen on sectioned specimens, but this correlation is not yet firmly established.

The intramembranous differentiations found at the level of the junctions differ consistently and characteristically from one segment of the microvasculature to another. The findings suggest that the junctions are mechanically strong and functionally "tight" in arterioles, and weak and possibly "leaky" in postcapillary venules. In the capillaries they appear to be nearly as tight but less strong than in arterioles. These differentiations probably represent adaptations of the vascular endothelium to local conditions of physical stress along the microvasculature.

The arterial endothelium (aorta, large arteries) has junctions comparable to those found in arterioles, while the venous endothelium (cava inferior, large veins) has a mixture of continuous occluding junctions (predominant component) and discontinuous, "venular" junctions (minority component).

To explore directly the permeability of the endothelial junctions, we have carried out tracer experiments using probe molecules of small dimensions: myoglobin (Mb) (mol. wt. 17800; mol. dimensions 25x34x42 Å), hemeundecapeptide (H11P) (mol. wt. 1900; mol. diam. $\leq$ 20 Å) and hemeoctapeptide (H8P) (mol. wt. 1550). These probe molecules have been put in contact with the two faces of the continuous endothelium of muscular capillaries in two ways: a. intraluminal injection; b. interstitial injection in the cremaster muscle. These probes have peroxidatic activity and are located in the tissues by a cytochemical reaction which gives an electron dense reaction product. The behavior of the probes in the endothelium of other segments of the vasculature has not yet been studied; the findings apply exclusively to the continuous endothelium of muscular capillaries.

After intravenous injection, these probe molecules (which were found to circulate in predominantly monomeric form in the plasma) cross the endothelium via plasmalemmal vesicles which can function either as isolated units shuttling from one cell front to the other, or can fuse to form patent transendothelial channels. The latter feature may represent the structural equivalent of the small pore system. Under well controlled experimental conditions, no detectable amounts of reaction product were found in the endothelial junctions.

When the same tracers were injected interstitially, it was found that they reach the capillary lumina again via plasmalemmal vesicles which are marked by the reaction product sequentially from the tissue front to the blood front of the endothelium. Transendothelial channels were also encountered in these experiments. The endothelial junctions proper, do not appear to be permeated by the probes.

With the evidence in hand and within the sensitivity of the techniques used, we conclude that in the continuous endothelium of blood capillaries and under normal conditions, the intercellular pathways (junctions) are not premeable to molecules larger than 20 Å. This does not rule out the possible diffusion of smaller molecules along the intercellular junctions, but the size limit for permeant molecules remains to be established. Molecules larger than ≃20 Å permeate the capillary endothelium through transendothelial channels formed by plasmalemmal vesicles, or are transported across it by vesicles functioning as independent units.

Since each microvascular segment has its own characteristic endothelial junctions, it would be interesting to investigate in the future by a corellated structural and functional approach, the permeability characteristics of sequential segments (arterioles, capillaries and venules) along the microvasculature.

(5)

THE MORPHOLOGICAL BASIS FOR ALTERED ENDOTHELIAL PERMEABILITY IN ATHEROSCLEROSIS

Dr. P. Constantinides

Department of Pathology, University of B.C.

Vancouver, Canada

There is little doubt that the permeability of the endothelium that lies over atherosclerotic plaques is greatly increased for all kinds of marked molecules (including lipids), as compared to the endothelium over the normal wall. At least, this is the conclusion from experiments with animal models of the human disease - we have not experimented with human lesions yet. The question now is: does the increased permeability promote atherosclerosis or does atherosclerosis promote increased permeability? Current research provides strong support for the first possibility, and this is what I will talk about today, although the second possibility may also be true to some extent, i.e. once an atheroma is established in any way, it may become leakier than the rest of the wall for some time. Let's look at the present data. There is growing experimental evidence that the normal arterial endothelium is <u>not</u> constantly traversed by a stream of lipoproteins, but rather that it acts like a barrier and allows only a trickle of them through. When, however, it is injured in any way, it becomes much more permeable than normally and allows lipids to pour into the arterial wall "by the bucketful", where they accumulate because they become trapped, they cannot get out, and they are coming in faster than they can be locally metabolized.

Thus, e.g., if we take a species such as the rat, we find that even after 2 months of cholesterol feeding and a terminal blood cholesterol level of about 500 mg% these animals do <u>not</u> develop any grossly visible plaques, but if we <u>first</u> injure their arteries in any of a dozen ways and <u>then</u> expose them to hyperlipemia, we get plaques at the sites of injury in only 7 days and with only 150 mg% cholesterol. We observed that such quantitative relationships apply to rodents and Bruce Taylor found that they apply in exactly the same manner to primates[1]. In fact, if we use the electron microscope (E/M), we see that atherosclerosis can be promoted by injury in much less than 7 days. Several years ago, when we injected intravenously massive amounts of egg yolk lipoproteins into rats 3 times a day for 3 days, not a single lipoprotein particle penetrated through the arterial endothelium of normal animals but when we injured the arteries with calciferol we discovered that lipoprotein particles entered into the arterial wall through gaps in the damaged endothelium within only 5 minutes of a single injection, and that mini-atheromata were produced within only 3 hours[2].

What are the specific mechanisms through which injury can produce gaps or otherwise increase the permeability of the arterial endothelium and promote massive entry of lipids?

Experimental E/M studies in recent years indicate that injury can "open doors" in the endothelial barrier through at least 7 different mechanisms, depending on the nature of the insult, its intensity, the chemical environment and the animal species in which it acts: when it is severe, it can produce real physical gaps (1) by killing individual endothelial cells and causing them to slough off, before regeneration of the lining seals the holes again, (2) by causing the endothelial cells to contract away from one another, and (3) by destroying the glue that binds them together. When it is mild, it can increase the permeability of the arterial lining without producing any physical gaps, namely (1) by increasing the number or size of pinocytic vesicles that bubble through the endothelium, (2) by causing confluence of pinocytic vesicles leading to giant transport vesicles or trans-endothelial canals, (3) by increasing the chemical capture of some lipids by the endothelial plasma membrane (PM), and (4) by increasing the direct passage across the PM itself of certain lipids. The first 5 of these mechanisms represent morphologically documented phenomena while the last 2 represent at the moment,theoretical possibilities.

What agents can injure the arterial lining?

With the help of the E/M it has recently been recognized that, when in excess, a great variety of agents we never even suspected before can punch little holes in the endothelium of arteries within an incredibly short time. Some of these are exotic factors that hit only a few people under rare circumstances (e.g. choleratoxin, cadmium, snake venoms), but many represent very common insults that hit millions of people during their everyday life and are therefore clinically important. The growing list of the latter now includes (1) hemodynamic stresses such as hypertension and blood turbulence, (2) vaso-active peptides and amines such as angiotensine, catecholamines, serotonine and tyramine, (3) carbon monoxide, (4) antigen-antibody complexes, (5) certain lipids such as fatty acids and cholesterol, and (6) certain lipid derivatives such as keto-acids, bile acids and lysolecithine. With the exception of hypertension, all of these insults have been studied, so far, in animals only. We shall now summarize the ultrastructural endothelial effects of each of these common agents.

(1) Hypertension has 3 documented effects: (a) it accelerates pinocytic traffic across the endothelial cytoplasm, as found by Hüttner et al.[3], in confirmation of our theoretical prediction of several years ago[1], (b) when prolonged, it stimulates marked proliferation of apparently contractile actin microfilaments in endothelial cells, practically transforming the latter into smooth muscle cells, as shown by Gabbiani et al.[4], and (c) it opens endothelial junctions in muscular arteries of animals and man as found by Wiener et al.[5], Suzuki et al.[6], and Jones[7], a finding which may explain the arterial wall edema and the greatly increased atherogenesis in hypertension.

(2) Vaso-active peptides and amines. We do not yet know what agency opens the junctions in hypertensive arteries, but there is an excellent chance that the culprits may be angiotensine and epinephrine. Several years ago we perfused angiotensine through rat arteries and found that at 1 μg/ml. this substance opened the endothelial junctions within 20 seconds, because the endothelial cells contracted away from one another [8,9]. Robertson in Cleveland repeated and confirmed our results [10] and found that they could be obtained even with 5 ng/ml., i.e. with an angiotensine concentration close to that which actually arises in some human patients with malignant hypertension. Thus, angiotensine may be the agent responsible for the opened junctions in hypertensives with high blood levels of this peptide. I think we must also explore the fascinating possibility that the essential factor here is not so much the increased angiotensine stimulus in the blood, as an increased responsiveness of the hypertensive endothelium to that stimulus, in view of the recent finding that endothelial cells become much more myoid and presumably much more contractile in hypertension. Finally, it is possible that catecholamines may also be involved in this. When we perfused epinephrine through rabbit arteries for 20 seconds, we found that at 1 μg/ml this catecholamine opens endothelial junctions and at 100 ng/ml it causes microcontractions of the endothelial cell surfaces, just like angiotensine, but at 20 ng/ml (which is the highest concentration observed in man) it has no visible effects[11]. Future studies will tell us whether epinephrine can produce gaps in the arterial lining at concentrations encountered during stress in man when it acts on the much more contractile endothelium of hypertensives, when it is synergized by other factors, or when it acts for longer than 20 seconds.

(3) Blood turbulence. It has been noticed repeatedly more than half a century ago that the earliest lipid deposits of human atherosclerosis, as well as those of cholesterol-fed animals, tend to develop at sites of the arterial tree that are exposed to special hemodynamic stresses (turbulence, shear) such as branchings, curves, etc., but it is only recently that we began to explore precisely how these stresses promote lipid deposition. It now emerges that at least one mechanism through which they work is that they increase the local permeability of the endothelial regions they affect; Mustard and Schwartz[12] e.g. have certainly shown that this is the

case in regard to permeability for certain blood proteins and cholesterol. It further emerges that they increase permeability at branchings because they alter the endothelium in at least 3 ways: (a) by injuring individual endothelial cells, as shown by Fry[13] and by Björkerud[14] with the light microscope, (b) by loosening and opening endothelial junctions, as shown by Gutstein et al[15] with the E/M for the iliac bifurcation, and (c) by increasing pinocytic entry, as can be postulated in certain cases. Thus, it begins to appear that the endothelium at certain bifurcations, etc. is "permanently injured" by turbulence and that this is the reason lipids first penetrate and deposit in such areas when a hyperlipemia is produced in any mammal or bird. As to the causes of such injury we have to consider mechanical cell deformation, endogenous histamine release or release of platelet serotonine at such sites, as suggested by the work of Fry, Hollis and Mustard, respectively.

(4) Carbon Monoxide (CO). This respiratory poison may well play an important role in the promotion of atherosclerosis by heavy smoking that is reported by epidemiologists[16]. Recent work by Danish workers[17,18] has shown that a blood concentration of CO that can materialise in heavy smokers (about 20% saturation) will increase atherosclerosis in lipemic animals, apparently because it loosens or opens endothelial junctions. This, together with our previous finding that cyanide perfusion of arteries opens all junctions in seconds[19], indicates that junctional integrity somehow requires continuous oxidative energy expenditure, among other things.

(5) Antigen-Antibody Complexes. When we sensitised rats to hemocyanine, a foreign antigen, and later infused this substance into their arteries, we found that it severely damaged many endothelial cells within less than 2 minutes, apparently as a result of the activation of cytotoxic complement factors by antigen-antibody complexes that formed on the arterial lining[9]. This effect probably explains the great intensification of experimental atherosclerosis by serum sickness as shown by Minick et al.[20] and others, and it suggests that every time an antigen to which we have become sensitized enters our circulation, it may silently punch holes in our arterial lining and promote atherosclerosis.

(6) Finally, there is increasing evidence that prolonged and excessive elevation of blood cholesterol levels will in itself act on the arterial lining and greatly increase its permeability for intravenously injected albumin, cholesterol and other substances, as shown by studies of Gore[21], Adams[22] and others. We explored this phenomenon morphologically with E/M autoradiography by giving labeled cholesterol to normal and chronically hyperlipemic animals orally, so that it would enter their blood in a physiological manner as a radioactive lipoprotein, and so that we could visualize directly its movements across vascular walls. We found that the normal arterial endothelium has a very low permeability for cholesterol - much lower than that of capillaries - but that prolonged hypercholesterolemia changes it, opens some of its junctions and

makes it extremely permeable to this lipid[23]. Cholesterol molecules apparently penetrated through this changed arterial endothelium in 3 ways: (a) straight through the cytoplasm of the altered endothelial cells (the majority mechanism), (b) as free lipoprotein particles through the gaps in the lining, and (c) as passengers in the cytoplasm of blood monocytes that also crawled through opened endothelial junctions[23].

Apart from the effects of high cholesterol there is evidence that elevation of blood fatty acid levels will also injure the arterial lining. We found that a single large load of fatty acids given to rats by mouth will cause within only a few hours marked swelling of endothelial cells leading to their rupture and to endothelial gaps[24], and similar results were obtained more chronically with high fatty acid diets in chicken by Yu *et al.*[25]. There are indications that fatty acids may act by building into the endothelial plasma membrane and disrupting its cation pumps. Furthermore, we observed that similar endothelial edema and disintegration was also produced in arteries by lipid derivatives such as keto-acids[24], bile acids[26] and lysolecithine[26]; the bile acid effect has been recently confirmed by Gutstein and Park[27], who found that even the endogenous high blood cholate levels of experimental icterus will exert such effects. Thus, ketosis and liver disease could promote atherosclerosis through endothelial injury.

The broader implication of the above effects is that when present in prolonged excess, lipids may become "aggressive", they may injure the arterial lining and greatly increase their own entry and that of other molecules into the arterial wall. We must also explore the possibility that once an advanced atheroma is established, local lipid breakdown products may act on the overlying endothelium from the gruel side and keep it abnormally permeable for a long time.

In closing, I should say that I consider the following objectives as the most important future research goals in this area: (a) we must continue to study endothelium-injuring agents in animals in order to identify their whole spectrum, to analyse their mechanism of action, and to develop effective pharmacological treatments, such as e.g. the complete prevention of serotonine injury by its specific antagonist, lysergic acid[24]. (b) We must start the systematic study of human arterial endothelium with the electron microscope in order to check out in man some of our experimental animal findings; this is a laborious task that has to be done with great care and painstaking special procedures in order to avoid artifacts. (c) We must find ways of diagnosing the presence of endothelium-injuring agents in individual patients, i.e. we must set up "endotheliotoxin profiles", the way we now do it for "lipoprotein profiles"; because if we identify them we can neutralise them.

Addendum: Marked development of actomyosin by human arterial endothelium in hypertension was shown with immunofluorescent technique by Becker and Hardy [28], in agreement with subsequent E/M findings.

REFERENCES

1. Constantinides,P.: Experimental Atherosclerosis,Elsevier Publ., Amsterdam 1965.
2. Constantinides,P.: AMA Arch.Path. 85:280-297, 1968.
3. Hüttner,I.,Boutet,M., Rona,G. and More,R.H.: Lab.Invest.29:536-546, 1973
4. Gabbiani,G., Badonnel,M. and Rona,G.: Lab.Invest.32:227-234,1975
5. Wiener,J. and Giacomelli,F.: Am.J.Path.72:221-240,1973
6. Suzuki,K.,Ookawara,S. and Ooneda,G.: Exp.Mol.Path.15:198-208,1971
7. Jones,D.: Lab.Invest.31:303-313,1974.
8. Constantinides,P. and Robinson,M.: AMA Arch.Path.88:106-112,1969
9. Constantinides,P.: Proc.Lindau Sympos.1970 in Adv.Exp.Med.Biol. 16A:185-212,Plenum Press Publ.,New York, 1971
10. Robertson,A. and Khairallah,P.: Science 172:1138, 1971
11. Constantinides,P.: Fed.Proc. 32:855, 1973
12. Bell,F.P.,Day,A.J., Gent,M. and Schwartz,C.J.: Exp.Mol.Path. 22: 366-375, 1975
13. Fry,D.L.: in "Atherogenesis: Initiating Factors", R.Porter and J.Knight (Editors), Ciba Foundation Symposium,pp.93-126, Elsevier Publ., Amsterdam 1973.
14. Björkerud,S. and Bondjers,G.: Atherosclerosis 15:285-300,1972
15. Gutstein,W., Farrell,G. and Armellini,C.: Lab.Invest. 29:134-149 1973
16. National Heart & Lung Institute, U.S.A. "Risk factors and prevention in "Report of Task Force on Arteriosclerosis", p.30, N.I.H. Publ., Washington,D.C., 1971
17. Astrup,P., Kjeldsen,K. and Wamstrup,J.: J.Atheroscler.Res. 7:343-349, 1967
18. Thomsen,H.K.: Atheroscler. 20:233-240, 1974
19. Constantinides,P. and Robinson,M.: AMA Arch.Path.88:99-105,1969
20. Minick,C.,Murphy,G. and Campbell,W.: J.Exp.Med. 124:635-644,1966
21. Gore,I.,Miyaski,T.,Kurozumi,T. and Hirst,A.: Am.J.Path.66:47a, 1972
22. Adams,C.W.,Morgan,R.S. and Bayliss,O.: J.Atheroscler.Res.11:119-124, 1970
23. Constantinides,P. and Wiggers,K.D.: Virch.Arch.A, Path.Anat.362: 291-310, 1974
24. Constantinides,P.: Internat.Congress Series No.269:51-56, Excerpta Med.Publ., Amsterdam, 1973.
25. Yu,W., Yu,M. and Young,P.: Exp.Mol.Path. 21:289-299, 1974
26. Constantinides,P. and Robinson,M.: AMA Arch.Path.88:113-117, 1969
27. Gutstein,W. and Park,F.: Am.J.Path. 71:49-60, 1973.
28. Becker,C.G. and Hardy, A.M.: Circul. 48(Suppl.IV):44, 1973.

(6)

THE INFLUENCE OF HYPERCHOLESTEROLEMIA UPON ENDOTHELIAL GLYCOCALIX

Dr. G. Weber

Institute of Pathological Anatomy

University of Siena, Italy

The influence of hypercholesterolemia upon endothelial "glycocalyx" has been studied in rats by A. Balint et al. (1974) who made use of the Ruthenium red technique and in rabbits by G. Weber et al. (1972; 1973) who made use of the Concanavalin A reaction after Bernhard and Avrameas.

G. Weber et al. (1973; 1974) observed an increase of the Concanavalin A reactivity at the surface of aortic endothelial cells in rabbits on a short-term hypercholesterolemic diet and in endothelial aortic cells of rabbits subjected to immunological injury.

E. Konyar et al. (1974) observed a thickness increase of the Ruthenium red positive external coat of the vascular endothelium in the muscular arteries of rats with experimental renal hypertension. The surface coat was instead thinner in the aorta.

The amount of Ruthenium red-OsO_4 complex bound by the endothelial cell surface was decreased in the observations of A. Balint et al. (1974) in hyperlipemic rats.

G. Weber et al. (1972; 1973) observed, in rabbits during cholesterol atherogenesis near the aortic areas which showed an increased reaction, other aortic areas which instead showed a decreased Concanavalin A reactivity or even a loss of any surface reactivity.

While studying the effects of hypercholesterolemia upon glycocalyx, we have observed that high levels of hypercholesterolemia did exert no influence at the fifteenth day of treatment on

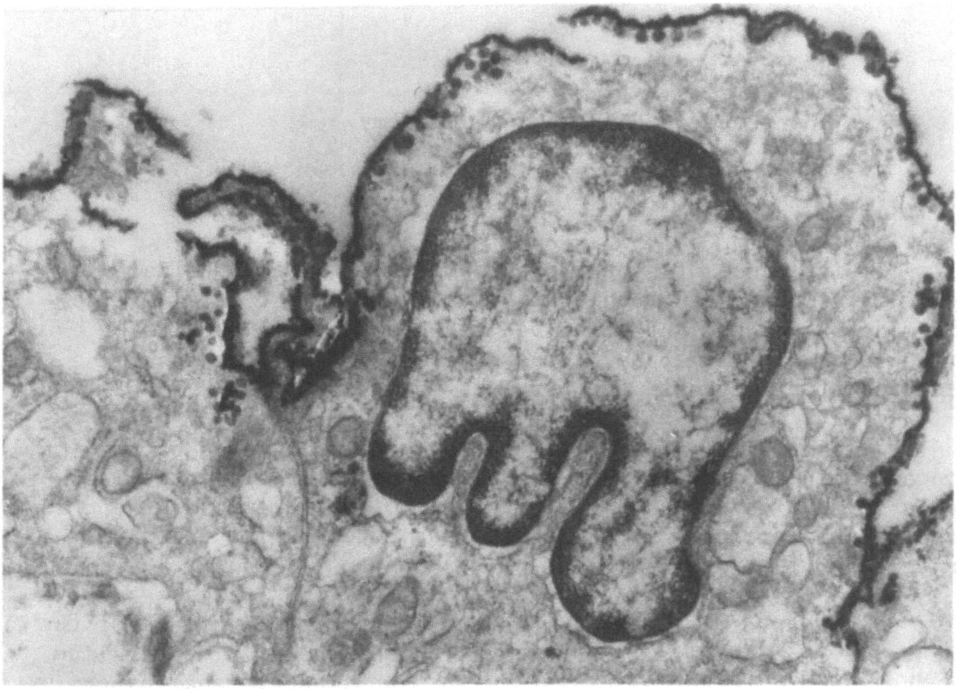

Figure 1. Rabbit (n° 209) on a very short-term hypercholesterolemic diet (7 days). Vacuoles are present in the endothelial cells. No evident modification of the Concanavalin A reactive surface coat. (Transmission electron microscopy Philips EM 300 at 60 kv). X 27,000.

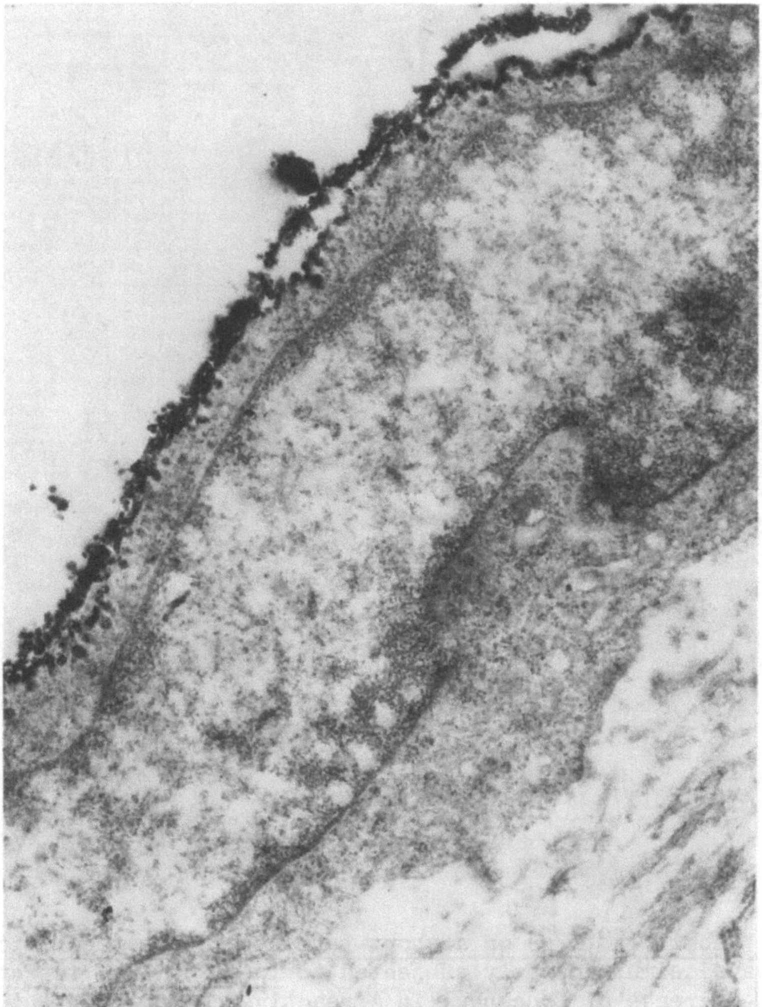

Figure 2. Rabbit (n° 365) on a short-term hypercholesterolemic diet (15 days). The Concanavalin A reactive surface coat is strongly increased. (TEM Siemens Elmiskop 1A at 75 kv) X 25,000.

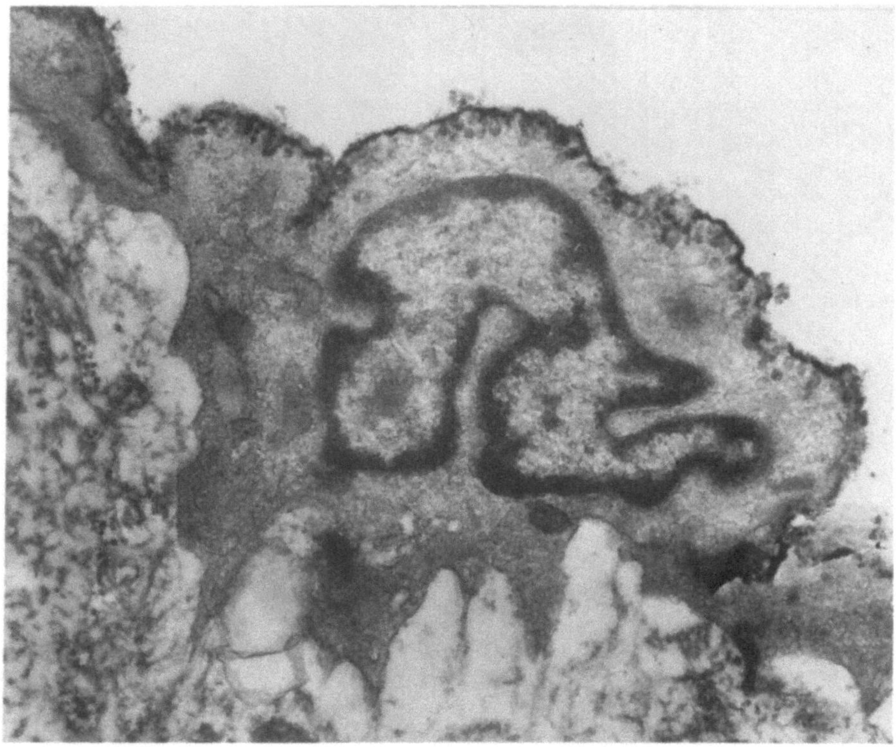

Figure 3. Rabbit (n° 174) on a short-term hypercholesterolemic diet (15 days) simultaneously subjected to Tween 80 i.v. injections. No evident increase of Concanavalin A reactive coat. (TEM Philips EM 300 at 60 Kv). X 18,000.

the endothelial surface reactivity to Concanavalin A if the rabbits on a hypercholesterolic diet were simultaneously subjected to i.v. injections of Tween 80 (G. Weber et al. , 1973). The hyperlipemia thus obtained is not atherogenic (T.P.B. Payne and G.L. Duff, 1951; G. Weber and G. Zampi, 1955; 1957; G. Weber et al., 1973).

Also in rabbits on a short-term hypercholesterolemic diet, simultaneously injected with methylprednisolone, no thickness increase of the Concanavalin A reactive coat at the endothelial surface was observed (G. Weber et al., 1973; 1974).

We are now studying the effect of alloxan diabetes (not atherogenic) hypercholesterolemia on the endothelial surface coat in rats. The work is still in progress but preliminary results suggest a decrease of the Concanavalin A reactivity on the aortic endothelial surface of diabetic rats.

E. Konyar et al. (1974) proposed that the changes of the surface coat thickness could probably play a part in increasing transcellular permeability.

One of the earliest modifications described during experimental cholesterol atherogenesis was the development of vacuoles in endothelial cells together with subendothelial oedema, at the 15th day of treatment. In rabbits, even at the seventh day of a hypercholesterolemic diet, we have observed large endothelial vacuoles and subendothelial oedema before any modification of the Concanavalin A reactive surface coat could be discovered.

We are studying also the surface coat of endothelial cells of Guinea pigs on scorbutigen diet. In this experimental condition, important changes of permeability have been observed. Also in this experimental condition we have observed early formation of vacuoles in the aortic endothelial cells and subendothelial oedema without appreciable modifications of the Concanavalin A reactive coat.

It is yet difficult, therefore, to assess a clear relationship among hypercholesterolemia, permeability changes of the endothelial cells and modifications of the surface coat.

In our opinion permeability variations of the arterial wall, at least during experimental atherogenesis, are greatly influenced also by other factors as endothelial cell "contraction" and endothelial cell detachment.

Detachment of endothelial cells, observed even in normal, is increased in different experimental conditions (H. Payling Wright et al., 1975; F. Parl et al., 1975).

Our scanning and transmission electron microscope observations on experimental plaques in rabbits and in monkeys disclosed that practically all the plaques, chiefly in their central portions, were largely devoid of any endothelial lining.

J. French (1971) postulated the possible importance of modifications of the surface coat of the endothelial cells in order to explain their changes from being normally "unwettable" to being "wettable" during pathological processes.

By scanning electron microscope observations we have observed the early appearance of a veil-like substance on aortic intimal surface of Guinea pigs and rabbits on a hypercholesterolic diet (G. Weber and P. Tosi, 1971; G. Weber et al., 1970; 1973). Many blood cells (chiefly erythrocytes and platelets) were adherent, sometimes together with cholesterol crystals (G. Weber et al. , 1973), to the surface covered by this amorphous material.

Such material appeared in areas where the abluminal cell membrane looked very thin and the surface Con A reactivity was not evident. It may be speculated that this material deposition had occurred in areas where the Concanavalin A reactive coat of the luminal endothelial surface was decreased.

REFERENCES

Balint A., Veress B. and Jellinck H., Modifications of surface coat of aortic endothelial cells in hyperlipemic rats. Path. Europ., 9, 105-108, 1974.

French J., The structure of arteries, growth adaptation and repair:the dilemma of the normal. In "The artery and the process of arteriosclerosis. Pathogenesis" ed. by S. Wolf, Plenum Press New York-London, 1-51, 1971.

Konyar E., Kerenyi T., Veress B., Balint A., Kolonics I. and Jellineck H., Study of experimental hypertensive vascular lesions by Ruthenium red staining technique. Path. Europ., 9, 167-175, 1974.

Parl F., Gustein W.H., D'Aguillo A.F. and Baez A., Endothelial injury. Association with elevation of serum bile acid and cholesterol concentration in biliary-obstructed rats. Atherosclerosis, 21, 135-146, 1975.

Payling W.H., Evans M. and Green R.P., Aortic endothelial mitosis and Evans blue uptake in cholesterol-fed subscorbutic Guinea pigs. Atherosclerosis, 21, 105-113, 1975.

Payne T.P.B. and Duff G.L., Effect of Tween 80 on serum lipids and tissues of cholesterol-fed rabbit. Arch Path., 51, 379-386, 1951.

Weber G. and Zampi G., La malltia ateromasica "endogena" del coniglio conseguente alla reversiona della xantomatosi sperimentale splancno-tesaurotica non aterogena. Arch. De Vecchi, 24, 1063-1102, 1956.

Weber G. and Zampi G., L'influsso del Tween 80 sulla reversione della xantomatosi splancno-tesaurotica non aterogena sperimentale del coniglio. Arch. De Vecchi, 25, 563-582, 1957.

Weber G., Fabbrini P., Figura N. and Resi L., Prevention by methylprednisolone of the endothelial lesions in rabbits on a hypercholesterolic diet or submitted to immunologic injury. Path. Europ., 9, 303-306, 1974. (Key references)

(F)

RESUME OF WORKSHOP-CONFERENCE

Henry C. McGill, Jr., M.D.

The University of Texas Health Science Center

San Antonio, Texas 78284

Summarizing a meeting requires the subjective selection of impressions, reactions, and interpretations. Unfortunately, to convey these impressions, I cannot write poetry like Hugh Sinclair, I cannot play the piano and sing like David Kritchevsky, and I do not have a collection of comic strip cartoons as used by Sheila Mitchell. In fact, I have no slides at all, and you must understand how greatly being without slides handicaps a pathologist.

With so many experts in atherosclerosis present, a comprehensive analysis of the current status of our knowledge and a prediction of future progress should be possible. However, atherosclerosis still defies attempts to synthesize relevant knowledge into a coherent, systematic description of etiology, pathogenesis, natural history, treatment, and prevention. Our knowledge of the subject contains many contradictions and incongruities, and these were manifested abundantly at this conference. Perhaps emphasizing the contradictions is the best way to summarize both current status and future needs, because in resolving such contradictions we make our greatest progress.

The conference program was heavy in its emphasis on lipoproteins. The material presented suggests that this special area of knowledge is progressing rapidly. The physical and chemical characterization of lipoprotein structure is well advanced, and we can anticipate that, in the near future, we will have a description of the binding of lipids to apoproteins in molecular terms. Together with this knowledge of the internal structure of the lipoproteins, we are learning where lipoproteins are synthesized, where they are degraded, and how they function. Changes in lipoproteins after feeding animals cholesterol and fat enriched diets now appear more complex than simply elevation of LDL, and investigators are finding several varieties of lipoproteins generated in response to dietary challenge. One or more of these varieties of LDL may be associated more closely with atherogenesis than total serum cholesterol or total LDL. Furthermore, specific lipoprotein fractions may help explain more of the individual variability among both animals and humans in the response to dietary cholesterol and fat. The announcement of Dr. Gotto that one of the apoproteins had been synthesized suggests the possibility of using a synthetic lipoprotein to control hyperlipidemia and, possibly, to induce regression of atherosclerosis.

In contrast to the enormous body of information about lipoprotein metabolism and structure, we know relatively little about how lipoproteins contribute to the pathogenesis of lesions. Studying the process by which lipoproteins participate in atherogenesis obviously is difficult. Isolated organ perfusion or tissue culture provide models for study, but the models are remote from the *in vivo* situation. We need better and more relevant information about the interaction of lipoproteins with the arterial wall in the intact organism. One participant suggested that chylomicrons, not lipoproteins, were the culprits in atherogenesis. One of the submitted papers reported that the ability of hyperlipemic serum to stimulate proliferation of smooth muscle in tissue culture resided not in the lipoproteins but in other serum proteins.

Thrombosis and its role in atherogenesis also received much attention at this workshop. Dr. Fraser Mustard described, in his usual enthusiastic style, many mechanisms by which platelets participate in thrombosis and by which they may participate in atherogenesis. Despite the enormous volume of knowledge about the biochemical and cellular processes involved in coagulation and thrombosis, the roles of these processes in the development of atherosclerosis remain uncertain. We formerly thought that thrombosis had a key role in the terminal occlusive event in which a thrombus on the surface of an atherosclerotic plaque obstructed the artery. As illustrated in Dr. Robert Wissler's comprehensive review of the topic, this concept has been challenged, but not disproven. I remain skeptical that thrombosis is important in the early stages of atherogenesis; it seems possible, and even likely, that it participates in the development of advanced plaques, such as the stenosing fibrous plaque; and it seems certain that it contributes to many, if not all, of the terminal occlusive episodes. Future investigators should find better ways to study this difficult problem.

A complete session was devoted to the topic of regression. As recently as five years ago, a group of papers devoted to regression of lesions in experimental animals or in humans would have been unlikely, and certainly could not have been filled with substantive data. The papers presented at this session demonstrated a healthy beginning in investigating regression, both in experimental animals and in humans. Several groups have established that lesions induced in rhesus monkeys by cholesterol feeding, as well as similar lesions induced in rabbits, undergo regression when serum cholesterol is lowered by removal of the dietary challenge. Experiments to test regression are difficult to design because individual variability among animals is great and atherosclerotic lesions cannot be measured in vivo. Despite the criticisms, one feels that it is better to perform imperfect experiments with the best design available than not to attack the problem at all.

The difficulties of studying regression are even greater in humans than in animal models. Dr. David Blankenhorn described a heroic assault on this problem. This attempt is to be admired, even though the initial results are still inconclusive. Methods of reducing hypertension, hyperlipidemia, and cigarette smoking in humans may create conditions in which regression is very likely to occur. Concomitantly, developing technology may make available better tools with which to measure the anticipated regression of lesions in both experimental animals and in humans.

A commentary on changing times was provided in the discussion of Dr. Jack Geer's electron micrograph of a lesion thought to be regressing. The discussion centered around whether a lipid filled macrophage, half in and half out of the intimal lesion, was entering or leaving. Ten years ago, this observation would have been discussed as a mechanism of lipid deposition in the progression of lesions. This time, the picture was discussed as illustrating a mechanism of removing lipid in the context of regression.

A session on the role of connective tissue in atherogenesis also illustrated a new emphasis. Techniques of examining the chemistry of connective tissue are being applied to arteries. The statement was made that approximately 50% by weight of the material in human lesions is connective tissue. This observation indicates limitations on the effectiveness of lowering of serum lipids to induce regression of lesions in both animals and humans. The high connective tissue content of advanced lesions may explain in part why the lipid lowering regimens tested in the Coronary Drug Project showed no effect on survival. The cases in that clinical trial had advanced stenosing lesions which, undoubtedly, were rich in connective tissue as well as in other relatively immobile constituents such as calcium and necrotic debris. We will await with interest future information on the dynamics of connective tissue generation and removal in the progression and regression of atherosclerosis.

Endothelium has been mentioned in connection with atherosclerosis for a long time. Increasing emphasis on the role of endothelium was illustrated by the attention given to it in a plenary session and two workshops. Another interesting contrast with the past was the presentation by Dr. Daria Haust on the multipotential capacities of endothelial cells. Ten years ago, Dr. Haust was proposing an expanded role of smooth muscle cells as enthusiastically as she was proposing the role of endothelial cells day-before-yesterday.

Unusual sessions for a conference on atherosclerosis were those devoted to myocardial perfusion, regional blood flow, and minimizing infarct size. Efforts directed toward increasing blood flow in the presence of advanced coronary artery stenosis, or maintaining the viability of myocardium damaged by ischemia, are beneficial only to the persons who survive the first few hours after suffering actual myocardial infarction. The results of the Coronary Drug Project reported by Dr. Jeremiah Stamler give a new significance to these efforts. If the best single predictor for long term survival is ECG evidence of damage remaining after the acute episode, minimizing infarct size may be expected to influence the long term life expectancy of persons who survive an infarct. Since myocardial infarction as a leading cause of death undoubtedly will be with us for some time to come, it appears that these efforts are well justified. We wish those in this field success for the benefit of all of us who may be victims as well as investigators.

The results of the Coronary Drug Project have confirmed the pessimism of those who felt that secondary prevention was too late. However, that study has generated important and useful information regarding the natural history of myocardial infarction and its sequelae. It definitely has answered the question regarding efficacy of lipid lowering agents in secondary prevention. It is satisfying to have a definite answer, even though the answer is, "No".

Along with the hope of improving chances for survival by minimizing myocardial damage, our long range hopes remain based on primary prevention of atherosclerosis and coronary heart disease, even if success means our joining the unemployed. Therefore, I went to the session this morning on "Recommendations to the public" with high anticipation. Here, I thought, would be distilled the essence of knowledge in specific prescriptions for prevention. However, nowhere else were the incongruities and contradictions more apparent in a single session of the workshop than in this one, where the purpose was to reach conclusions and plan practical applications. There was the tension resulting from wanting to do something yet not wanting to do harm. There was the contrast between the persistent hope that it will be possible to prevent coronary heart disease by modification of the diet, and the inability to demonstrate the effectiveness of such intervention in humans. There was the contrast between measures that can be applied only by the medical care system -- identification, diagnosis, and individualized prescription, and the measures that can be applied only by environmental engineering -- manipulation of the environment for an entire population. Procedures to be carried out in the course of delivering medical care, usually specific, but expensive and still questionably effective, were contrasted with procedures to be carried out by public health agencies, governmental bodies, and industry.

Environmental engineering is risky and is extremely difficult to evaluate. Nothing as specific and as simple is yet available, or even in sight, for the prevention of atherosclerosis as fluoride is for dental caries. At the same time, the difficulties that have been encountered in instituting such a simple and effective procedure as fluoridation of drinking water temper any optimism regarding feasibility of prevention by any type of intervention.

Another contrast in this session was the unanimity in recommending to the public physical exercise and control of obesity for prevention of coronary heart disease, despite weakness of the evidence that obesity or lack of exercise are causative agents for coronary heart disease, or that exercise and leanness will prevent coronary heart disease.

Those concerned with recommendations to the public appeared to agree that the primary determinants of coronary heart disease are life style, environmental exposure, and other habits or conditions rather than deficiencies in the medical care system. This emphasis contrasts with the prevalent discussions in the U.S. regarding the failure of the medical care system to prolong life and to prevent disease. The blame for failure to achieve a better health record in regard to coronary heart disease should be assigned more clearly to the individual than to his physician.

The recommendations regarding smoking were consistent with the behavior of the participants as evidenced by the low prevalence of cigarette smoking at this meeting. On the other hand, the recommendations for diet were not very consistent with the choices in the breakfast line at the residence hall.

There also was a contrast between the atmosphere of self-sufficiency in the various workshop sessions devoted to experimental work, and the atmosphere of skepticism, debate, and frustration in the sessions on prevention. Experimentalists should share the responsibility for answering some of the simple but difficult questions regarding prevention. A variety of animal models is available and selection from among these models should make it possible to obtain answers to some of the questions involving prevention. Such experiments will require larger numbers of animals and longer experimental periods than are currently popular. On the other hand, skeptics of the dietary lipid hypothesis should be more willing to accept evidence from well designed experiments, particularly those involving nonhuman primates.

The sessions on atherosclerosis in childhood were not novel, but do represent a relatively new emphasis in the investigation of atherosclerosis. They did not penetrate deeply into the problem but they were symbolic of an awakening interest in this aspect of atherosclerosis. This is another problem that should be noted by experimentalists. It is almost impossible to conduct experiments with human children, yet relatively few experiments have been concerned with animals of known parentage and very few have involved investigations of atherosclerosis beginning in infancy. These questions should provide the basis for performing some difficult but important experiments.

I do not wish to risk the folly of making predictions for the future, which was part of my assigned task. What is the perfect experiment? If I knew, I would not be telling you this afternoon -- I would be at home writing it in a grant application. It is not possible to predict scientific insight, creativity, or new syntheses. However, to insure that new insights will occur, we need to develop new methods, involve new disciplines, and recruit new skeptics in the investigation of atherosclerosis.

Finally, like all good meetings, we learned more in corridor consultations, coffee break conversations, and dining room discussions than in formal meeting sessions. Thanks to the international representation, the free and independent spirit of the country in which we met, and the hospitality of our hosts, the meeting was highly successful in achieving its objective of promoting scientific communication, scientist to scientist, whether in or out of the meeting hall.

(G)

CLOSING REMARKS

Colin J. Schwartz

Professor, Department of Pathology,
Faculty of Health Sciences, McMaster University.

It is a pleasure to have this opportunity to address the Conference on behalf of the Programme and Planning Committee. Of one thing I can be certain, that you would wish my comments to be brief. My closing remarks will therefore be conspicuous by their omissions rather than their detail.

First, it is my sincere belief that this has been a most successful conference, a comment that the Chairman of the Conference, Dr. Daria Haust, would not feel appropriate for her to make. We all owe Daria a great debt of gratitude for her tireless, selfless and devoted efforts, not only in the conception of the conference, but in her meticulous attention to the details, and her great concern that the guests would enjoy their visit to Canada, not only scientifically but socially and culturally; - Our most sincere thanks to Daria.

It has been a great pleasure to host, for the first time in Canada, the European Atherosclerosis Group. Most of us benefit from not infrequent visits to meetings sponsored by our good friends in the United States, and this conference has given us a much-overdue opportunity to return their continuing hospitality.

If I were to commence on a list of people and organizations to whom we owe thanks for their efforts or support, the list would be enormous. However, a special word of thanks to Dr. Bruce Squires, who has so ably and unobstrusively looked after the local arrangements. Also, of course, we are most grateful to the University of Western Ontario, The Ontario and Canadian Heart Foundations, and the many donors whose names appeared with the programmes.

Last, but by no means least, we are grateful to our colleagues from many parts of the world, who kindly and willingly agreed to present papers, or chair sessions. Without such support the workshop-conference could not have succeeded.

Dr. Henry McGill, with characteristic insight and a delightful touch of humour, has most succinctly presented us with a resume of the conference. I hope you will agree that we have dotted some of the i's and crossed some t's in the perplexing riddle of occlusive arterial disease. However, to me at least, major problems remain, with many more unanswered than answered. Only by encouraging new ideas, supporting creative research, and by an effective and challenging exchange of ideas will we make further progress. Such a challenging exchange of ideas has indeed occurred. To all our friends who are departing for their homes, we wish you bon voyage, and for those of you who are staying a short while in Canada may your travels be most enjoyable. Come back again soon.

WORKSHOP-CONFERENCE ON ATHEROSCLEROSIS -- SEPTEMBER, 1975

INVITED CONTRIBUTORS AND CHAIRMEN

Dr. Colin W. Adams
Dept. of Pathology
Guy's Hospital Medical School
London, U.K.

Dr. S. P. Ahuja
Dept. of Medicine
University Hospital
London, Ontario, Canada

Dr. A. Angel
Clinical Investigation Unit
Toronto General Hospital
Toronto, Ontario, Canada

Dr. John B. Armstrong
Community Health Division
15 Overlea Blvd.
Toronto, Ontario, Canada

Dr. Mark L. Armstrong
Cardiovascular Laboratories
University Hospital
Iowa City, Iowa, U.S.A.

Dr. Joel Avigan
National Heart & Lung Institute
National Institutes of Health
Bethesda, Maryland, U.S.A.

Dr. H. J. M. Barnett
Dept. of Clinical Neurological Sciences
University Hospital
London, Ontario, Canada

Dr. J. L. Beaumont
Institute National de la Sante et de la Recherche Medicale
Hopital Henri Mondor
51, Av. du Mal de lattre de Tassigny
Creteil, France

Dr. C. G. Becker
Dept. of Pathology
Cornell University Medical School
New York, New York, U.S.A.

Dr. Earl P. Benditt
Dept. of Pathology
University of Washington
Seattle, Washington, U.S.A.

Dr. James M. Beveridge
President
Acadia University
Wolfville, Nova Scotia, Canada

Dr. Sören Björkerud
Astra Lakemedel AB
151 85 Sodertalje
Sweden

Dr. David Blankenhorn
2025 Zonal Avenue
Los Angeles, California, U.S.A.

Dr. Colin M. Bloor
Dept. of Pathology
University of California
San Diego School of Medicine
La Jolla, California, U.S.A.

Dr. D. Bocking
Dean, Faculty of Medicine
University of Western Ontario
London, Ontario, Canada

Dr. George S. Boyd
Dept. of Biochemistry
University of Edinburgh Medical School
Teviot Place
Edinburgh, Scotland

Dr. Helen Brown
Cleveland Clinic
Cleveland, Ohio, U.S.A.

Dr. Lucien Campeau
Institut de Cardiologie de Montreal
5000, est rue Belanger
Montreal, P.Q., Canada

Dr. Paul Cannon
Dept. of Medicine
College of Physicians & Surgeons of Columbia University
630 West 168th Street
New York, New York, U.S.A.

Dr. L. A. Carlson
King Gustav V Research Institute
Stockholm, Sweden

Dr. K. K. Carroll
Dept. of Biochemistry
University of Western Ontario
London, Ontario, Canada

Dr. Joe C. Christian
Dept. of Medical Genetics
Indiana University Medical School
Riley Residence, 129
100100 W. Michigan Street
Indianapolis, Indiana, U.S.A.

Dr. Thomas B. Clarkson
Bowman Gray School of Medicine
Winston-Salem, North Carolina
U.S.A.

Mr. J. L. A. Colhoun
President, Ontario Heart Foundation
310 Davenport Road
Toronto, Ontario, Canada

Prof. C. Colton
Arteriosclerosis Center
Massachusetts Institute of Technology
Cambridge, Massachusetts
U.S.A.

Dr. F. Connell
Dept. of Medicine
Queen's University
Kingston, Ontario, Canada

Dr. W. E. Connor
Dept. of Internal Medicine
Iowa College of Medicine
Iowa City, Iowa, U.S.A.

Dr. Paris Constantinides
Dept. of Pathology
University of British Columbia
Vancouver, British Columbia
Canada

Dr. Gerald R. Cooper
Medical Laboratory Section
Communicable Disease Center
Atlanta, Georgia, U.S.A.

Dr. Eva Csonka
2nd Dept. of Pathology of Medical University
Budapest, Hungary

Dr. A. S. Daoud
Laboratory Services
Veterans Administration Hospital
Albany, New York, U.S.A.

Dr. Jean Davignon
Clinical Research Institute
110 Pine Avenue
Montreal, P.Q., Canada

Dr. Ralph DePalma
2065 Adelbert Road
Cleveland, Ohio, U.S.A.

Dr. C. G. Drake
Dept. of Surgery
University Hospital
London, Ontario, Canada

Dr. S. Fedoroff
Dept. of Anatomy
University of Saskatchewan
Saskatoon, Saskatchewan
Canada

Dr. Katti Fischer-Dzoga
Dept. of Pathology
University of Chicago
950 East 59th Street
Chicago, Illinois, U.S.A.

Dr. Ivan Franz
University of Minnesota Medical School
Minneapolis, Minnesota
U.S.A.

Dr. Jack Geer
Dept. of Pathology
Ohio State University
370 West 9th Street
Columbus, Ohio, U.S.A.

Dr. Seymour Glagov
Dept. of Pathology
University of Chicago
Chicago, Illinois, U.S.A.

Dr. Charles Glueck
General Clinic Research Center
Cincinnati General Hospital
Cincinnati, Ohio, U.S.A.

Dr. A. M. Gotto, Jr.
Dept. of Medicine
Methodist Hospital & Baylor College of Medicine
6516 Bertner Blvd.
Houston, Texas, U.S.A.

Dr. R. A. Goyer
Dept. of Pathology
University of Western Ontario
London, Ontario, Canada

Dr. Ramsay W. Gunton
Dept. of Medicine
University Hospital
London, Ontario, Canada

Dr. Donald B. Hackel
Dept. of Pathology
Duke University Medical Center
Durham, North Carolina, U.S.A.

Dr. J. R. Hampton
Dept. of Medicine
General Hospital
University of Nottingham
Nottingham, England

Dr. H. Hauss
Medizinische Klinik und Poliklinik der Universität Münster
Westring,
44 Münster, Germany

Dr. M. Daria Haust
Dept. of Pathology
University of Western Ontario
London, Ontario, Canada

Dr. Richard J. Havel
Dept. of Medicine
University of California Medical Center
San Francisco, California
U.S.A.

Dr. R. Heimbecker
Dept. of Surgery
University Hospital
London, Ontario, Canada

Dr. David Hewitt
School of Hygiene
Dept. of Biometrics & Epidemiology
University of Toronto
Toronto, Ontario, Canada

Dr. William Hollander
Dept. of Medicine
Boston University Medical School
Boston, Massachusetts, U.S.A.

Dr. W. L. Holmes
Division of Research
Lankenau Hospital
Philadelphia, Pennsylvania
U.S.A.

Dr. Louis Horlick
Dept. of Medicine
University of Saskatchewan
Saskatoon, Saskatchewan
Canada

Dr. G. Hornstra
Unilever Research
Vlaardingen, The Netherlands

Dr. A. N. Howard
Dept. of Medicine
Addenbrooke's Hospital
Hills Road
Cambridge, England

Dr. William B. Insull, Jr.
Center for Prevention of Premature Arteriosclerosis
Rockefeller University
New York, New York, U.S.A.

Dr. Björn Isaksson
Dept. of Clinical Nutrition
Sahlgren's Hospital
Gothenburg, Sweden

Dr. H. Jellinek
2nd Dept. of Pathology
Semmelweis Medical University
Budapest, Hungary

Dr. Richard J. Jones
Dept. of Medicine
University of Chicago Medical School
950 East 59th Street
Chicago, Illinois, U.S.A.

Dr. W. J. Keon
Division of Cardiothoracic Surgery
Ottawa Civic Hospital
1053 Carling Avenue
Ottawa, Ontario, Canada

Dr. B. S. Langford Kidd
Division of Cardiology
Dept. of Paediatrics
Johns Hopkins Hospital
Baltimore, Maryland, U.S.A.

Dr. Gerald A. Klassen
Cardiovascular Division
Royal Victoria Hospital
687 Pine Avenue West
Montreal, P.Q., Canada

Dr. Anatoli Klimov
Laboratory of Lipid Metabolism
Institute of Experimental Medicine
Kirovski Prospekt 69/71
Leningrad, U.S.S.R.

Dr. Dieter Kramsch
Dept. of Medicine
Boston University Medical Center
Boston, Massachusetts, U.S.A.

Dr. R. M. Krause
Rockefeller University
66th Street & York Avenue
New York, New York, U.S.A.

Dr. David Kritchevsky
Wistar Institute
Philadelphia, Pennsylvania
U.S.A.

Dr. A. Kuksis
Banting & Best Dept. of Medical Research
University of Toronto
112 College Street
Toronto, Ontario, Canada

Dr. Peter O. Kwiterovich
Lipid Research Clinic
Dept. of Paediatrics
Johns Hopkins University School of Medicine
Baltimore, Maryland, U.S.A.

Dr. K. T. Lee
Dept. of Pathology
Albany Medical College of Union University
Albany, New York, U.S.A.

Dr. Lena Lewis
Cleveland Clinic
Cleveland, Ohio, U.S.A.

Dr. L. J. Lewis
Cell Culture Laboratory
Dept. of Medicine
University of Iowa College of Medicine
Iowa City, Iowa, U.S.A.

Dr. J. Lindner
Universitäts-Krankenhaus Eppendorf
Pathologisches Institut
Martinistrasse
2 Hamburg 20, Germany

Dr. J. A. Little
Lipid Research Clinic Project
University of Toronto
1 Spadina Crescent
Toronto, Ontario, Canada

*Dr. Hugh B. Lofland
Dept. of Pathology (Biochemistry)
Bowman Gray School of Medicine
Wake Forest University
Winston-Salem, North Carolina
U.S.A.

Dr. P. J. Lupien
Centre Hopitalier de l'Universite Laval
2705 Laurier Blvd.
Quebec City, P.Q., Canada

Dr. Robert H. Mahley
National Institutes of Health
Section on Experimental Atherosclerosis
National Heart & Lung Institute
Bethesda, Maryland, U.S.A.

* Deceased

Dr. Attilio Maseri
Fisiologia Clinica
Laboratoria del Consiglio Nazionale delle Ricerche
Via Savi, 8
Pisa, Italy

Dr. Neville Marsh
Queen Elizabeth College
University of London
Dept. of Physiology
Campden Hill Road
London, England

Dr. H. C. McGill, Jr.
Dept. of Pathology
University of Texas Medical School
7703 Floyd Curl Drive
San Antonio, Texas, U.S.A.

Dr. G. W. Manning
Dept. of Medicine
University Hospital
London, Ontario, Canada

Dr. Maurice McGregor
Royal Victoria Hospital
687 Pine Avenue West
Montreal, P.Q., Canada

Miss Valerie McGuire
Nutrition Coordinator
St. Michael's Hospital
30 Bond Street
Toronto, Ontario, Canada

Dr. W. W. Meyer
Institute of Pathology
University of Mainz
Mainz, Germany

Dr. T. Miettinen
Second Dept. of Medicine
University Central Hospital
Helsinki, Finland

Dr. C. Richard Minick
Dept. of Pathology
Cornell University Medical School
New York, New York, U.S.A.

Dr. C. J. Miras
Dept. of Biological Chemistry
University of Athens School of Medicine
Goudi, Athens, Greece

Dr. Maurice Mishkel
Lipid Research Laboratory and Clinic
Hamilton General Hospital
Hamilton, Ontario, Canada

Dr. J. R. A. Mitchell
Dept. of Medicine
General Hospital
Nottingham, England

Dr. S. C. Mitchell
Atherogenesis Branch
Division of Heart & Vascular Disease
National Institutes of Health
Bethesda, Maryland, U.S.A.

Dr. S. Moore
Health Sciences Centre
McMaster University
Hamilton, Ontario, Canada

Dr. Robert H. More
Dept. of Pathology
Pathology Institute
McGill University
Montreal, P.Q., Canada

Dr. Ethel Morrison
Dept. of Pathology
Albany Medical College
Union University
Albany, New York, U.S.A.

Dr. J. Fraser Mustard
Dean of Medicine
McMaster University
Hamilton, Ontario, Canada

Dr. E. A. Nikkilä
3rd Dept. of Medicine
University of Helsinki
Helsinki, Finland

Dr. Kaare R. Norum
Institute for Nutrition Research
University of Oslo School of Medicine
Blindern
P.O. Box 1046
Oslo, Norway

Dr. R. M. O'Neal
Dept. of Pathology
University of Oklahoma
Oklahoma City, Oklahoma, U.S.A.

Dr. Marian A. Packham
Dept. of Biochemistry
University of Toronto
Toronto, Ontario, Canada

Dr. Rodolfo Paoletti
Universita degli Studi
Instituto di Farmacologia e di Terapia
via Andrea del Sarto 21
Milan, Italy

Dr. J O. Parker
Dept. of Medicine
Queen's University
Kingston, Ontario, Canada

Dr. J. Patelski
Medical Academy
Dept. of Biochemistry
ul. Świecickiego 6
Poznań, Poland

Dr. H. Peeters
Simon Stevin Institute
Jeruzalemstraat 34
Brugge, Belgium

Dr. R. Pick
Experimental Atherosclerosis Section
Cardiovascular Institute
Michael Reese Hospital & Medical Center
Chicago, Illinois, U.S.A.

Dr. O. J. Pollak
Dover Medical Research Center
Dover, Delaware, U.S.A.

Dr. J. C. F. Poole
Sir William Dunn School of Pathology
University of Oxford
South Parks Road
Oxford, England

Dr. Jürgen Rauterberg
Medical Clinic and Policlinic
West. Wilhelms University
Münster, Germany

Dr. David Redwood
Cardiology Branch
National Heart & Lung Institute
National Institutes of Health
Bethesda, Maryland, U.S.A.

Dr. S. Renaud
Inserm
Unite 63
Lyon, France

Dr. J. Renais
Hopital Boucicaut
78, rue de la Convention
Paris, France

Dr. Leslie Robert
Laboratoire de Biochimie du Tussu Conjonctif
Universite Paris-Val de Marne
Faculte de Medecine
6, rue de General Sarrail
Creteil, France

Dr. Robert Roberts
Cardiovascular Division
Washington University School of Medicine
St. Louis, Missouri, U.S.A.

Dr. Abel L. Robertson, Jr.
Case Western University
Cleveland, Ohio, U.S.A.

Dr. Paul S. Roheim
Dept. of Medicine
Albert Einstein College of Medicine
Yeshiva University
1300 Morris Park Avenue
Bronx, New York, U.S.A.

Dr. J. Roland
Laboratoire d'Anatomie-Pathologique
Hopital Tenon
4, rue de la Chine
Paris, France

Dr. George H. Rothblat
Wistar Institute
Philadelphia, Pennsylvania
U.S.A.

Dr. G. Schettler
Medizinische Universitäts-klinik
Bergheimerstrasse
6900 Heidelberg, Germany

Dr. G. Schlierf
Medizinische Universitats-klinik
6900 Heidelberg
Bergheimer Strasse, Germany

Dr. C. J. Schwartz
Dept. of Pathology
McMaster University
Hamilton, Ontario, Canada

Dr. R. Foster Scott
Dept. of Pathology
Albany Medical College of Union University
Albany, New York, U.S.A.

Dr. A. G. Shaper
MRC Social Medicine Unit
London School of Hygiene and Tropical Medicine
Keppel Street, (Gower Street)
London, England

Dr. Takio Shimamoto
Japan Atherosclerosis Research Institute
1-12 Kanda-Awaji-Cho, Chiyoda-Ku
Tokyo, Japan

Dr. F. Brian Shorland
Dept. of Food Science & Human Nutrition
Michigan State University
East Lansing, Michigan, U.S.A.

Dr. Maia Simionescu
Section on Cell Biology
Yale University School of Medicine
333 Cedar Street
New Haven, Connecticut, U.S.A.

Dr. Elspeth Smith
Dept. of Chemical Pathology
University of Aberdeen Medical Buildings
Foresthill
Aberdeen, Scotland

Dr. Jeremiah Stamler
Dept. of Community Health & Preventive Medicine
Northwestern University Medical School
Ward Building, 9th Floor
303 East Chicago Avenue
Chicago, Illinois, U.S.A.

Dr. Frank Rees Smith
Dept. of Medicine
College of Physicians and Surgeons of Columbia University
New York, New York, U.S.A.

Dr. Richard W. St. Clair
Bowman Gray School of Medicine
Wake Forest University
Winston-Salem, North Carolina
U.S.A.

Dr. Olga Stein
Lipid Research Laboratory
The Hebrew University
Hadassah Medical School
Jerusalem, Israel

Dr. Y. Stein
Lipid Research Laboratory
The Hebrew University
Hadassah Medical School
Jerusalem, Israel

Dr. George Steiner
Room 7302, Medical Science Building
Dept. of Medicine
University of Toronto
Toronto, Ontario, Canada

Dr. Jack P. Strong
Dept. of Pathology
Louisiana State University School of Medicine
1542 Tulane Avenue
New Orleans, Louisiana, U.S.A.

Dr. A. Studer
Dept. of Experimental Medicine
F. Hoffman-LaRoche & Co. AG.
Grenzacherstrasse 124
Basle, Switzerland

Dr. H. J. C. Swan
Cedars Sinai Medical Center
Box 54265
Medical Advisory Board
Los Angeles, California
U.S.A.

Dr. C. B. Taylor
Veterans Administration Hospital
Albany, New York, U.S.A.

Dr. Wilbur Thomas
Dept. of Pathology
Union University
Albany, New York, U.S.A.

Dr. S. D. Vesselinovitch
Dept. of Pathology
University of Chicago
Chicago, Illinois, U.S.A.

Dr. A. C. Wallace
Dept. of Pathology
University of Western Ontario
London, Ontario, Canada

Dr. K. W. Walton
Dept. of Experimental Pathology
Rheumatism Research Wing
Medical School
University of Birmingham
Birmingham, England

Dr. G. Weber
Instituto Anatomia e Istologia Patologica
Universita di Siena
Siena, Italy

Dr. Bernard Weigensberg
McGill University Pathology Institute
3775 University Street
Montreal, P.Q., Canada

Dr. A. B. Chandler
Eugene Talmadge Memorial Hospital
Medical College of Georgia
Augusta, Georgia, U.S.A.

Dr. H. M. Whyte
Dept. of Clinical Science
Australian National University
Box 4, P.O.
Canberra, A.C.T. Australia

Dr. D. R. Wilson
Dept. of Surgery
Toronto Western Hospital
Toronto, Ontario, Canada

Dr. Robert W. Wissler
Dept. of Pathology
University of Chicago
950 East 59th Street
Chicago, Illinois, U.S.A.

Dr. R. Witty
Canada Packers Limited
2211 St. Clair Avenue West
Toronto, Ontario, Canada

Dr. Stewart Wolf
Marine Biomedical Institute
200 University Blvd.
Galveston, Texas, U.S.A.

Dr. Bernard M. Wolfe
Dept. of Medicine
University Hospital
London, Ontario, Canada

Dr. Neville Woolf
Dept. of Pathology
St. George's Hospital Medical School
Hyde Park Corner
London, England

Dr. Donald B. Zilversmit
Cornell University Graduate School of Medicine
Ithaca, New York, U.S.A.

CONTRIBUTORS

ADAMS, C.W.M.
AGETA, M.
ALEXANDER, K.M.
ALEXANDER, N.
ALLCOCK, J.M.
ALLEN, D.M.
ANTONUCCI, M.
ARAVANIS, C.
AUGUSTYN, J.M.
AVIGAN, J.
BAHLER, R.C.
BARNETT, H.J.M.
BARNICOAT, K.T.N.
BEAR, R.A.
BEAUMONT, J.L.
BEAUMONT, V.
BECKER, C.G.
BELL, F.P.
BELLON, E.M.
BERARD, M.
BERENSON, G.S.
BJÖRKERUD, S.
BLACKET, R.B.
BLANKENHORN, D.H.
BLOOR, C.M.
BONDJERS, G.
BOWIE, E.J.W.
BOYD, G.S.
BRADBY, H.
BRATTSAND, R.
BRATZLER, R.L.
BRECKENRIDGE, W.C.
BROWN, A.L.
BROWN, H.B.
BUCKLEY, G.
CAMPEAU, L.
CANNON, P.J.
CARLO, I.A.
CARROLL, K.K.

INDEX

MIX
Papier aus verantwortungsvollen Quellen
Paper from responsible sources
FSC® C105338

If you have any concerns about our products,
you can contact us on
ProductSafety@springernature.com

In case Publisher is established outside the EU,
the EU authorized representative is:
Springer Nature Customer Service Center GmbH
Europaplatz 3, 69115 Heidelberg, Germany

Printed by Libri Plureos GmbH
in Hamburg, Germany